THY DAUGHTER'S NAKEDNESS

novels by Myron S. Kaufmann

Remember Me To God

Thy Daughter's Nakedness

THY DAUGHTER'S NAKEDNESS

Myron S. Kaufmann

J. B. LIPPINCOTT COMPANY
Philadelphia and New York

First edition
Printed in the United States of America
Library of Congress Catalog Card Number 68–24134

to Paula

THY DAUGHTER'S NAKEDNESS

1

When the commencement exercises were finished, the family stopped in again briefly at the apartment of the Chicago grandaunt that Millicent had stayed with while at the University. Then they got into the old car and headed east.

Millicent was the eldest child, but in the back seat of the sagging Plymouth she felt squashed. The tremendous roll of Patty's hip pressed against her on the left, and Roland fidgeted and squirmed on her right. The day was bright and humid and the car had old gasoline smells. In the front seat Charles was at the wheel, arguing with both his parents about why they ought to let him quit school.

"What's the matter with you?" their mother said, her voice rising. "Don't you want to get into college? Don't you want to wear a cap and gown like Millicent? Didn't she look adorable up there? All kinds of honors—"

"This cram school isn't gonna get me in anywhere," Charles said. "It's just money thrown out. It bothers me. You can't afford it."

"You can't afford to drop out," their father said. "That's what bothers me."

"Look," said Charles. "I can go back to high school in the fall and take a p.g., and make a fresh start. And over the summer I can start to amass some capital. I've got two jobs offered me. I can work in Moon's Garage and I can drive a cab."

"That's too dangerous," said his mother.

"You and your capital," said his father. "You're getting ahead of yourself. Millicent's got capital. A degree. An education. That's capital."

"You can't take a p.g. if you don't even graduate, dopey," said Patty.

Their voices both ignored the desolate stuff on the radio and competed with it.

Patty sang with it.

"—In the winter of our love, dear,
While the winds of sorrow wail—
I'll weave together snowflakes
To make a wedding veil—"

"How pukey can you get," said Roland.

The song went into a refrain. "Woo, woo, waa, waa—" Patty sang. She was slumping and leaning with her head cocked in such a way that she mourned almost into Millicent's ear, and Millicent felt Patty's red tresses on her cheek.

Out here their Boston accents had struck her for the first time as quite strong. She had noticed it whenever she introduced any of them to anybody. It was provincial-sounding, narrow-sounding. And she recognized in it also the accents of her own childhood—she had not realized how much her own speech had changed during the university years. And being fetched home now was like being carted off back into her childhood.

She wished she had had the foresight to sit by a window. She closed her eyes, thinking it might help ward off car sickness, but the darkness only brought the vibration and endless engine noise up into her head.

And she wished she could say something effective to Charles. Because he did have brilliance, that he was in danger of wasting. And she knew her parents would not have let him and the younger kids miss school for this Chicago trip if there were any chance of his graduating. Nor would they have moved to a new town in the closing months of his senior year.

"So, what are you going to do, Millicent Audrey?" her father asked her.

For a moment everyone seemed to await her answer. She had given various answers to that question in the past, always vague, but lately her thoughts had crystallized.

"Politics," she said. Her voice quavered weakly.

"Not teaching?" said her father.

"What do you mean, politics?" said her mother.

"You mean you're gonna run for something?" said Patty.

"Well, not right away," she said. "I'll have to start at the bottom." Her voice continued to quaver.

"What's at the bottom?'" asked Patty.

"Well, in the wards. Political clubs. I'll have to work in other people's campaigns, and just work hard, I guess. Try to get noticed."

"What party?" asked her father.

"Well, one or the other of the major parties. I haven't decided."

"It can be a slow process," said her father.

"I know it. Well, I might learn typing and shorthand first, so I can support myself, and go to law school nights, in Boston somewhere."

"You can do better than typing and shorthand, with your brains," her mother said. "Your education."

"Well, it's only temporary."

"I've never pictured you practicing law," said her father.

"Well, not practicing, necessarily."

"You ought to get married," Patty said.

"For that you need a man," her mother said.

"You mean not one of those guys would marry her?" said Patty. "All those guys she was in college with?"

"I'm sure a lot of them would," said her mother. "But she has to find the right one."

The problem of beginning a career now that would give her adult status threatened her with the difficulty of it. She wanted to begin—otherwise a girl whose four college years were behind her was like an overage child. A superannuated child. If you meant to meet the real world, and have an effect upon it, the time was now, before you sank into the silly condition of a graduated girl doing nothing serious.

But she was out of touch with Massachusetts. And the town where the family lived now was completely strange to her—they had moved only a couple of months ago, making the three younger kids change schools in midterm, because her father had been called to a new pulpit. But even apart from that, she felt totally without know-how, unsure that she could even persuade the professionals to let her begin. It made her feel small.

It was easier for a boy to make the transition. Her friend Eugene had run against the Cook County Democratic machine in the primary though only a student in law school, and despite having only a few hundred dollars, and despite his professors' advising him against it. And though he was defeated badly he had begun to have the feel of things and to be known a little.

And he had done it without making a fool of himself. She did not feel that she could.

It would be much easier to make a start if she could continue to collaborate with Eugene, or at least be able to go to him now and then for advice. She had nominally been his campaign manager, though actually it had only meant mimeographing and mailing and handing out flyers, and giving him a few ideas to use in speeches. He had had no staff.

But having graduated, there was no practical way for her to stay on further in Chicago. Her parents expected her home, and Eugene had not suggested that she remain. If he had, she might have considered looking for a job there. And for a while she had expected he might, because they worked well together.

They had kept it human being to human being, without the corruption of romance. But apparently he was too ambitious even to have time for friendship. So it was just as well they had had the maturity not to cheapen it.

The family spent the night at a motel, and Millicent had to share a double bed with Patty, who snored a little in a bubbly way. The next morning they were all out on the asphalt early, repacking the car. The day already promised to be another scorcher. Her father told Patty to quit bitching. Roland seemed to Millicent an eleven-year-old savage. He had a way of making disgusting sucking noises by pressing a hand to his armpit or behind his knee. He could also slack his jaw and emit an inhuman foghorn noise that seemed to rise from the hollow of his stomach.

Her mother told her father he had better shave, but her father kept trying to wedge the suitcase among the valises.

"If a cop ever stopped you for any reason he'd never believe you're a clergyman," her mother told him. "You look like a bum."

"I am a bum," he said.

Millicent wished her parents would act their age. Her mother was in shorts, and though at forty-two she still looked athletic and slim her thighs had tiny broken blue-red veins that seemed to Millicent to make shorts inappropriate.

"What's the matter, Cockeyes?" Charles asked quietly. He was looking down at Millicent with solemn blue eyes, his face young and thin under a blondish crew cut.

"I'm not cockeyed," she said in her tremulous voice, turning from him.

In the car she got a window seat this time, but Patty's bulk was next to her again, and the singing and the radio began almost immediately. She has a fair-enough voice, if only she had some taste, Millicent felt like telling her.

"Rock-a-bye, rock-a-bye,
 Just us two-oo—
Rock-a-bye, rock-a-bye,
 Me and you—
Hold me tight, till the night
 Turns to blue-oo—"

Charles was not driving this morning, and the back of his close-cropped head was directly before Millicent. He had a nerve, she thought, the way he took this grown-up manner with her, ever since he had grown taller than she. In the first place, he was more than three years her junior. And his calling her a nickname based on a supposed physical idiosyncrasy just showed how immature he was.

Anyway she was not cross-eyed. The convergence was slight and perfectly symmetrical, and the doctor had told the family it was more apparent than real. Her vision was normal, she wore no glasses, and everyone agreed that she shared in the family's good looks.

She watched her father driving. From this angle she could almost see through his sunglasses toward the sun. He seemed to sit carelessly. He needed a shave, and the stubble already showed some white among the black, the same as at his temples. A cigarette hung from his lips, and the hot wind from the window kept stirring his hair. He turned the radio away from Patty's songs, as though searching for news, but the first he found was about Senator McCarthy. Just right for this weather, Millicent thought.

There was a downpour, that made them close the windows and slow the car, and turned the brilliance to dim gray. Water running on the glass enclosed them, and the wipers wagged and rubbed. Then it was sunny, and hot once more. A radio voice that whistled on the sibilants talked about potato bugs. Storms continued, off and on.

Roland was explaining a plan he had to get several kittens from a kid named Bobby O'Shaughnessy, who had a pregnant cat, and rent them out to other kids. As the cats grew big he would call them in and give out new kittens of the next generation, so that his rental customers would always have a kitten, never a cat. It was a new idea that would make a fortune.

"Where would you breed all these cats?" said Patty. "In the cellar? Or the barn?"

"No," their mother said. "You're not breeding cats."

"The A.S.P.C.A. will get after you," said his father.

"Why?" said Roland. "What's cruel about that?"

"It would frighten the birds from the birdhouse," said his mother.

"No it wouldn't. I'll put a fence around the birdhouse pole, out of chicken wire or something."

"The birds would still smell the cats," said his mother.

"Birds don't smell," he told her.

"It's too commercial anyway," Patty said. "It's too mercenary. People would get the wrong impression."

"Yes," said their mother.

"Where do you learn those big words?" Charles said to Patty.

"Oh, poo," she said to him.

"The nesting season's over anyway," said Roland.

"They only sound big to you," Patty added to Charles.

"I don't know about every kind," said their mother. "And they'd get the little birds in the porch eaves."

"Buy him a fishing rod and let him open up a fish market," said Charles.

Millicent wished they wouldn't argue. She let herself doze off. But when she awoke her head had lain on the vibrating metal, and it seemed to ache down into her brain.

She talked little most of the trip home, but kept to her thoughts, recalling the recent past and feeling anxious about the future. "Why are you so quiet, Millicent Audrey?" her father asked her once. She explained that long rides disagreed with her.

But toward the end of the third day, as they came into Massachusetts, she asked what the house was like that the family had taken in Wilmerding Crosswalk.

"George Washington died in it," said Patty. "A lingering death."

"No he didn't. It's very nice," her mother said.

Patty said it was an outpost, but her mother said there were some neighbors.

It was dark when they drove into the town, and for the last hour Millicent had been feeling nauseated, but she could see an oblong common, with a smallish pointed monument in an old style. There were large trees, and store fronts closed for the night, and a white church opposite one end of the common. Patty said this was Corporal Kevin Aloysius Murphy Square. They went to the left of a fork and over a stone bridge amid venerable trees and Victorian houses. She hoped they would in the next instant be there, because she felt ill and stiff, but they continued for what seemed a long time, as though leaving the town. She was aware of arching trees, and of each rise and depression in the road.

At last she felt the turns and bumps of a dirt driveway. The headlights shone on an old brown barn door. She dragged herself forward and almost fell out onto the grass.

"You missed the apple blossoms," Patty said. "They were about two weeks ago."

Millicent went with the family over the porch, hardly looking at the house. Patty led her up the worn carpet of the staircase, and showed her the bathroom with wood floor and overhead tank and pull chain, and the bedroom they would share.

Working together Patty and Millicent folded their bedspreads, their hands meeting, and then Millicent went to bed at once, taking the iron cot as the big bed was now Patty's.

There was a constant sound of young frogs, broken every now and then by the vibrant throaty bung of an older frog.

She was still awake in the darkness when Patty went to bed. Her eyes felt gritty. But Patty talked a while, mostly about not liking the kids out here nearly as well as in Brighton.

"Well, you'll meet other kids," Millicent told her.

But Patty said she had had only one date since moving to Wilmerding Crosswalk, and he was an ick.

"What would you say," she asked in the dark, "if a boy said your bosom made him think of the full-blown sails of a Spanish galleon?"

"I wouldn't dignify it with a reply," Millicent said.

2

*I*t was still night, though she knew she had slept for some hours, when the yowling bawl of a train awakened her. It fell in pitch as it passed. She heard the pandemonium of wheels. The windows of her bedroom hummed.

The clatter receded, diminishing. She lay in darkness on the metal cot and heard Patty's deep, throaty breathing in the bigger bed. Then she could hear also the sound of her own pulse, inside her head, where it pressed the pillow. Its throb was disconcerting—it made life itself seem uncertain and tenuous.

Far off in the night a dog barked. The family's old dog did not answer. But the bark came again, and this time an even more distant one answered, quite faint. The two called back and forth to one another. She tried to sleep again. There was a genteel bong, single and lonesome, as though from some steeple. She wondered what time it was. The carved wall clock in the downstairs hall gave a chime. In the air was a mild scent of skunk, not unpleasant.

She lay curled in the sheets a long time, but her dozings did not sink far. At daybreak she heard a rooster. She tried to sleep longer, but then there were bird twitterings and considerable quacking of ducks. She heard a squirrel's noisy scrambling on the roof. It was a sound she had not heard since the family lived in Abbottsford, in the Berkshires, many years before.

She went to one of the two windows and stood watching for the sunrise. The tree outside had a branch near enough to touch. In one field, diagonally across from her own yard, a couple of old horses lumbered freely about. Patty lay with eyes closed and lips parted, her breathing not audible now, and the reddish tresses flung about her on the pillow as wildly as if they had floated under the sea.

Though the cross ventilation gave the room a pleasantness it was not very big, and rather crowded. Besides the beds there was a big brown dresser with a mirror, and Patty's dressing table, with Millicent's own little alarm clock ticking on it, and a curvy white highboy with chipped paint. A big teddy bear with a gray wound in the seam sat before the mirror, beside Patty's little white phonograph, and toilet articles and clothing of Patty's were strewn here and there. From the other window Millicent looked down on the slate roof of the kitchen. The back yard was not deep, and beyond some live stumps that sprouted a mess of branches a scrub forest bound it.

It occurred to her that to discover what lay through that forest, and explore the new surroundings, would be an agreeable way to pass the morning. She did not want to waste time. But now that the day for walking cold into a real party ward club was actually here, she felt timid about it.

She did her calisthenics, in an open pajama top, and then went downstairs, in shirt and jeans. The staircase had a carpet worn out and frayed by earlier residents who were unknown to her. It was molded to the stair and imbedded with the odor of dust. But there was a fine carved banister, its varnish dark and smooth, that encouraged her to slide her fingers on it. Roland had the downstairs bedroom, and from the stairs she saw him still sleeping, the room half darkened by a green window shade that leaked pinpoints of light, and his collections of butterflies and moths on the wall above him.

She crossed the big porch and went down its steps to the big yard. She saw that the house was set far back. The grass was uncut, except near the house, and a winding dirt drive led down to the tumbly stone wall and open gate. The clapboard of the house was dusty green, and she saw some blistering in the paint.

She looked for Roger, the aged collie, and found him lying at the door of the barn. A gray squirrel passed quite near him. She watched the arc of its back as it made its way across the grass in little jumps. She knelt and stroked the long fur, speaking to the dog. A couple of insects circled near him. Only his moist eyes moved. But she knew he recognized her. They had gotten him as a pup, in Abbottsford, and he had been with them all the years in the apartment in Brighton. In the dimness of the barn rafters swallows circled. Deep inside, behind the rusting Plymouth and Charles's high squarish Model T, she saw a damaged station wagon suspended in mid-air. It was a striking sight, tilted upward as though it might fly and pass just over her head. Ropes and pulleys held it from the high rafters. That must be some piece of junk Charles is working on, she thought. The barn swallows kept swooping.

She knew that the household had begun to waken. Her father was in the habit of rousing Charles, to make him join him in morning prayers, and she heard her father urging him to come on.

She had breakfast with the family, and then went adventuring out back. She passed a rusted old harrow in the high grass by the barn and found an overgrown path in the forest. She pushed through underbrush. A rabbit dashed out of her way, giving her a start. Twigs broke under her sneakers on the mat of last year's leaves and pine needles. But the woods did not last very long, and soon she came upon the railroad track. Beyond it was a marsh, a maze of still waterways among tangled shrubs, flowers and weeds. The reflection of clouds was broken by floating lily leaves.

She hiked along the track, toward the west. You come out of college and you're faced with a blank wall, she thought.

When the track cut out into the marshland, with open ties above water, she left it and looked for firm ground to walk on. Alongside the ooze the growth was impenetrable. But she retraced somewhat, and came out of the woods again where the waters narrowed for a small dam. There was a duck farm above it, and a bit further upstream a covered bridge, beyond which the water was only a noisy brook in woods. The road from the covered bridge turned and climbed steeply in forest. She could hear the brook in a steep gully, though foliage hid it. Then near the top of the hill the road curved again, and she saw it was her own street. At a distance she saw the barn again and the house, and the handful of other houses beyond, and the two horses pasturing. Her house had an old television aerial, though they had no television.

When she got to her gate she found that it leaned and the hinge was rusted, and the gate could not be shut. There was a new galvanized mailbox on a post, with the name Gordon.

Still she put off going to Boston. She helped her mother hang out the wash. There was everyone's underwear—her father's, her mother's, Charles's, Roland's, Patty's, her own.

In the afternoon she wheeled Roland's red bicycle from the barn and followed the road in the other direction, not toward the duck farm and covered bridge but toward Wilmerding Crosswalk.

Near Corporal Kevin Aloysius Murphy Square she dismounted, walking the bike over heaves that the roots of big trees made in the shady sidewalk. For a while she watched men with ladders, who sawed at a rotten branch. Then on Muckanaug Street she found her father's temple, past an intersection and a weedy corner lot. It was of orangey stucco, low like a basement intended to be built upon later. She got off the bike and tried the door, but it was locked. There was a tablet with movable letters displaying her father's full name, Edward Bernard Gordon, and his phone number, and the hours of services.

It seemed strange to her that her parents should have ended up in this town, of which she had scarcely ever heard.

She did not get home until the family was already starting supper, and she joined them at the long heavy unpainted table in the kitchen, taking a chair opposite Charles. She noticed for the first time that the kitchen had its own fireplace.

"I'm not half as much of a pig as Rollo is," Patty was saying.

"Pig or not, you'll turn into a horse," her mother said. "You're growing tall, and if you let yourself spread out you'll be enormous."

"It isn't my fault," she said. She was eating half a large roll spread with butter.

"Whose fault is it then?" said her mother.

"I'm big-boned. I can't help it."

"The biggest bone must be in your behind then," said Roland.

"Some people have a certain kind of glands," Patty insisted, ignoring Roland. "I could go on a diet of two crackers a day, and I could even die of starvation, and I'd still keep on gaining weight until I actually died. It's a certain kind of glands."

"That's not true," her father said, without any particular emotion and not looking up.

"See?" said Roland.

Her father passed Millicent the salad and she took some.

"Where have you been all day?" her mother asked her.

"Oh, exploring. Exploring the town." Even now her voice quavered. There didn't seem to be anything she could do about it.

"Did you find the Indian reservation?" Roland asked her.

"No."

"There aren't any Indians on it," said Patty.

They ate silently for a moment and the conversation changed, but Millicent took no part in it. Apparently the station wagon hanging in the barn was a wreck that her father and Charles had bought for nearly nothing, to rebuild for the congregation to use in transporting children to the temple. Her father was remarking that Charles was a mechanical genius—for a kid not even eighteen years old to have such a touch with motors was fantastic.

"You wouldn't let me put in the supercharger though," Charles said.

"No, no," said his father.

"I'm a genius until I get an idea."

"You don't soup up a Sunday-school bus," his father said. "It just isn't appropriate."

"Listen, trust me. If I tell ya it's safe it's safe."

Millicent decided to find the Boston Globe directly after supper and study the Female Help Wanted ads. She offered first to walk the dog, but she was told the dog didn't walk any more. She found the newspaper in the living room and sat with it in the tall rocking chair, which was placed at an angle in the bay window. She turned to the classifieds, folding and refolding. But before she got settled her mother handed her another paper, taking it down from the top of the upright piano. It was a local weekly with a story in it of her father's arrival in town. His picture was there, high on the front page, which had some blackish group picture elsewhere on it but was otherwise a mass of type, with very small headlines. It was called the Wilmerdingian. She considered the awkwardness of it, wondering if it were pronounced Wilmerdingyan or Wilmerdinjan. But she didn't ask—there might be two opinions and the whole family could get involved. She handed it back to her mother, saying it was nice, and tried again to read the ads.

Her mother settled at the sewing machine, just inside the wide arch to the dining room, and told her they wanted to plan a housewarming. They had been putting it off until Millicent came home from college. Patty began playing at the upright piano.

Most of the jobs were offered through agencies.

counter girls, exp $25 tips
elevator opr, exp $25
stuffers, $28
folders & gummers, $30

She heard her father running a hand drill somewhere in the back of the house—putting up shelves or hooks, or fixing something. Patty's hands waved and beat and tickled the piano keys as though she heard only her own playing. Neither the drill nor the occasional whirr of the sewing machine seemed to bother her. And she played exceedingly well, Millicent thought. She marveled that Patty could go in for such classical stuff in her piano-playing and for such tripe in popular recordings.

Her mother was saying that the furniture ought to be rearranged before the housewarming party. She was not satisfied with where she had put the big chair or the lamp table. Millicent could see that it was a difficult room in which to place things—there was very little wall space. The piano covered the only expanse that would fit it, on the same side as the bay window, and the opposite wall was broken up by the French doors and a fireplace. The sofa was backed against the windows to the porch, and most of the fourth wall was the open arch to the dining room.

"Why don't you let Roland practice the trumpet with you," her mother said to Patty, "and you could play a duet at the housewarming. I think it would be very nice."

"He plays lousy," Patty said, without interrupting her playing.

"Just one or two numbers," said her mother.

"No. He makes mistakes on purpose," said Patty.

The classified ads made Millicent's task seem harder than ever. She listened to Patty's playing over the noise. Her gaze wandered to the photograph atop the piano, of herself and the other three children when they were small. She had been the biggest then. Now she was smaller than all but the littlest. She went outdoors, nervously. The sun still hung in the sky, though it was already enlarged in anticipation of sunset. There were bird calls, especially from the woods in back. One kept saying bobwhite so clearly that it might as well have spoken.

She suspected uneasily that walking into a political club and volunteering her services was not really the way to begin. The hard-bitten men she would find there probably didn't welcome ambitious college-educated youngsters. She would be laughed right out of the place, and her attempt would only show her ignorance.

The next day she still could not find the courage and went walking again, even though the weather was chilly and overcast. She was not even certain yet whether her services should be offered to the Democrats or to the Republicans. The Republicans she considered backward. But in Massachusetts the most unprincipled thieves were reputedly Democrats, whereas there were Republicans who tried to maintain the old New England values. She had heard that the more sophisticated people around Boston and Cambridge were accustomed to splitting their tickets. Besides she had a distrust of the President, because of his dropping the bomb, even though Eugene admired him.

She had asked her father what kind of government the Town of Wilmerding had, and he had said it was an open town meeting that wouldn't be held again for nearly a year.

She walked slowly in the direction of the town. The sun was an ill-defined blotch of warmth behind a veil. She knew now that the street that passed her house was called Massapeequit Road, and that the stream under the covered bridge in the other direction was Massapeequit Brook, and that the train that woke her each night was the Montreal-to-Boston express. She took a turnoff where a sign pointed to Sachem Hill, and followed a road that wound higher and higher in a forest of pine and oak and scattered white birch.

A moist film of drizzling rain now chilled her face, and she cut in among the trees. She thought she could see bits of white sky through the woods almost at ground level, as though there must be a drop-off and a view. Presently she did in fact come out to the rim of a cliff. There was a panorama of tiny houses, thickly settled in a straggling and elongated shape—not the town she had explored yesterday—but its colors were already muted in mist. On the hills that stretched away there was bank after bank of foggy trees, each further bank grayer than the one before it, until they were lost. The sky rolled in and out upon itself in a dozen shades of smoke gray and blue-gray, coming down quite near her in ghostly spreading structures. When the downpour began she backed in among the trees. She could not see the panorama now—beyond the cliff it was blind gray-whiteness. The noise of rain in foliage was all about.

She wondered if she should send Eugene a book or something, for his birthday. Then he would write, and they would correspond.

The trouble was that he would be practically bound to misunderstand, in some part of his mind, in spite of knowing better. Any move a woman made toward a man was taken to mean that she wanted to fall in love, and the result was the degrading situation known as pursuit.

Why did people make such a universal thing of sex? Because of it, she could not seek the friendship of any male, married or single, without the risk of being misunderstood. Half the minds of the human race were forbidden to her. For practical purposes she was restricted to the friendship of women. It was an absurd and crippling restriction. Really intelligent, congenial people were so rare and so hard to find. If someone had a stimulating brain, and was also stimulated by hers, why could they not meet to discuss, to debate, to think, to grow by the intercourse of ideas? Why do they insist that a person's identity lies not in his brain but in his pants?

Mating so dominated people's minds that it was impossible simply to make friends. She resented it bitterly.

It would be a stupid thing for her and Eugene to fall in love, when neither of them was anywhere near ready to get married. Yet if she made any efforts to continue the friendship, she would appear to be a hunting female. But if she did nothing and merely waited for him to write first, that was passive and hence female too. Whatever she did, it would be interpreted as having to do with being a woman.

Certainly someday you married, to reproduce yourself, but it should be to some close friend, without silliness, without letting it get out of proportion, as part of the plan of your life. Meanwhile, if people could transcend sex, she thought, they could truly know one another. They could give their attention to one another's skills and abilities. She wanted to have friends, not just classify people according to their sex organs.

The chill damp made her give a sudden little shiver, even as the sound of rain softened.

If she had her way, she thought, not even matrimony should cut off a man or a woman from wide-ranging decent friendships, regardless of the sex of the friends. Maleness or femaleness was a small part of the totality of a person.

3

The rain became less severe but it did not stop, so after a long time she went home. Her shirt clung to her shoulders and she kept sneezing. Her mother bawled her out for the stupidity of hiking in such weather, but Millicent insisted that it was not a cold but her allergies. In late afternoon, when the sun came out, she went to a Dr. Yarrish in Wilmerding Crosswalk, that her mother recommended, and got some allergy pills.

The following morning she felt guilt and urgency at having delayed so long, and set out for Boston to find whatever employment she could.

There was a little brown bus that she had seen pass the house, and after breakfast she hailed it, neat in her tailored suit. It took her down through the covered bridge and after about twenty minutes left her at the depot in Sparkstown, where she awaited the Boston train.

She bought all four of the Boston papers there. The train had two cars, pulled by steam. While she rode she tore out the help-wanted columns. But only one listing sounded as though the work might be rewarding in itself—a girl of all work was needed by the Society for the Prevention of Cruelty to Children.

The city street was sunshiny when she came out of the terminal, but blowy and dusty, and she raised an arm to her eyes a moment to avoid cinders. A ragged old man with a white stubble began to speak to her and she gave him a quarter from the leather bag that was slung at her hip.

"That's for something to eat, not for alcohol," she told him.

"God bless you, kid," he said.

"I mean you're very foolish if you don't spend it the way I said."

"God bless you," he said again with a little salute, turning away.

She misjudged the direction somewhat from North Station to Beacon Hill, and after several uphill blocks she decided it had been a mistake to have walked, but she had gone too far to proceed in any other way. She did not like suits and had only this blue woolen one, and as it had grown exceedingly hot she began to feel sticky and disheveled. The shoulder strap of her bag felt heavy. The address she carried on the torn slip of newsprint she found in a brick building with a narrow front. The office was small, and there was a fortyish man with a dark, sour face seated at a desk. He was in shirt sleeves. No one else was there. He didn't rise. He asked if she took shorthand.

"No, but I expect to. I'll be learning it, I mean." She had entered panting from the heat and felt she didn't look her best.

"You're not of working age, are you?"

"I'm twenty-one," she said, reddening. "I have a master's degree."

There were dead pauses between all his questions but his expression never changed. "Why do you want to work for the Society?"

"Well, I saw the ad. I want to prevent cruelty to children." She wished the tremolo wasn't always in her voice. It made her sound frightened.

"I don't think we can use you."

She came out from the stone stairs. In college she had been on the verge of adulthood. In college it had seemed that the time after college would be a great unfolding of a wider battlefield. It probably was, for people like Eugene, who knew what to do.

She walked slowly down the shady street, sneezing a few times, to the wide thoroughfare at the bottom of the hill, where her Aunt Gwendolyn had a little apartment. She phoned her aunt from a booth and went there to use the bathroom and wash.

The slim, pretty, blondish aunt greeted her at the door with smiles and a warm hug, saying she had heard she was back. She ushered Millicent into the little kitchen and made her sit. The baby was standing in the high chair and shouting, a mess of beets over her face and bib and coveralls. There were bits of other vegetables on the floor. Gwendolyn forced the baby to sit again, wrestling with her legs. Then she sat down herself, with legs crossed, and tried to feed the baby while conversing with Millicent. She wore tight trousers and her hair was in a ponytail. The baby took the spoon and fed herself, and then began to mash the beets. Millicent noticed the complexity and intelligence of her bright-eyed expressions.

"She's certainly bigger," Millicent said.

"Of course. When did you see her last? September? She's eighteen months."

She asked how Millicent liked the new house. Gwendolyn hadn't seen it yet. Then she asked what Millicent would do now, and Millicent said gloomily that she had made up her mind to get a job this afternoon, whatever she could get, whatever it was, and enroll immediately in evening classes for typing and shorthand.

"First I want to feel that I'm not a child, and can pay my way," she said. "That's the first thing."

"I keep forgetting what you majored in," Aunt Gwendolyn said.

"Classical archaeology."

"Oh, that's right. What is that exactly?"

"Greeks and Romans. Pottery and stuff, ruins."

"Oh. Well, I'm sure you'll get something." The baby flung the spoon to the floor. "I guess she's had all she wants," Gwendolyn said, and lifted the baby out. She carried her to the sink.

Millicent said she really wanted to get into politics, and was counting on the idea that shorthand was supposed to be an entree into almost anything. "There was even somebody that got to be president of Cuba by knowing shorthand," she said. "He was secretary to the previous president, and learned the job."

"Well, you'll get something. I don't know about President, or president of Cuba." Her aunt set the baby standing on the floor. "I've got to start looking for something too. As soon as I find someone I can trust with the kid." She put a pot on the stove and began opening a can. "It's tough, you know. The alimony's only twenty-five a week and sometimes he skips. And it's hard to find what you want. I did some selling at Christmastime."

"How do you get along?" Millicent asked.

"Well, my mother helps out—Grandma. Grandma Annie. And I don't pay much rent, knock on wood."

She asked Millicent to share lunch with her—she was only having some soup and bread and tea. Millicent was uncertain about accepting, but she did. The baby meanwhile had toddled to her and showed her the flat pages of a picture-book, naming objects.

"Look," Millicent remarked to her aunt, "the way a child learns things. You couldn't tell if she's a boy or girl. I mean, to listen to her, and watch her. I mean, don't you think too much distinction is made over sex?"

"I think she's very girlish," Aunt Gwendolyn said, stirring the pot.

Millicent knew that her aunt hadn't understood her. She let her baby cousin show her pictures, and cuddled her a little. "What I mean is," she told her aunt, "if nature or a God had intended the sexes for the roles they play in society, females would have been made with lower intelligence than males. But the fact is they're not."

Aunt Gwendolyn set the table and poured the soup.

Directly after lunch Millicent set out for the employment bureaus. She went to two, down in the gray heart of the city, and the most convenient way to get there seemed to walk. She filled out cards. The second place sent her to an insurance company, still deeper down in the city, on a high floor of an office building, to be a file clerk. She was interviewed there, at the back end of a big floor that had many desks and cabinets, by an ancient lady, thin and quite tall, with white hair in a bun on top, named Miss Bancroft. Millicent sneezed during the interview but said she didn't have a cold. Miss Bancroft seemed frail and stiff. She was very pale, and on her cheek were a couple of brown spots, as if she were beginning to rot. She asked Millicent's age.

"Twenty-one," said Millicent.

"You look younger than that," she said.

"I know it."

"Tell me, child, do you use tobacco, or alcohol?"

"No, I don't."

"Well, I don't know but what you look as though you might be a serious type—it's the very young ones I don't like," Miss Bancroft said at last. "There's nothing hard or difficult about filing, but that's all the more reason to be exacting. You have to keep your mind on it. You'll have thirty-five dollars a week. It's flagrant the way salaries have gone up since the war, but you get the benefit of it. Now I notice you're not wearing stockings. I must insist on stockings. And when I say nine I mean a quarter to. I don't like last-minute people."

Millicent agreed to begin the next morning at nine, punctually, and left. At a phone booth she studied the ads for business and secretarial schools in the Yellow Pages, and called a few. There was one that had begun classes only a week before and that promised to give her special attention so she could catch up. So Millicent said she'd be there tomorrow night.

She thought that perhaps she ought to begin right away, tonight, but she was tired. Besides she didn't have money for supper and didn't want to impose on Aunt Gwendolyn again.

She used her last two nickels to call old friends. The first one turned out to be married and living in New Jersey. She conversed with the girl's mother until the nickel ran out.

The next one she called, Ruthie Meyers, she knew was married and living in the Back Bay. Ruthie sounded delighted to hear from her—she had left work early because she had a cold, and that was why Millicent had found her at home. Besides she wanted to pack—she and her husband were sailing in two days for Europe. Millicent said she was coming down with a cold too. Ruthie invited her for dinner. Millicent declined, but they talked a long time.

"Oh, the job situation's awful," Ruthie said. "Boston's a dead town. It's a depressed area or something. All the boys get out. The men and the jobs are in New York."

Millicent agreed finally to come to Ruthie's the next evening—not for dinner, as she would have to rush directly from work to her classes. But on her train back to Sparkstown she felt as though she had been begging for companionship.

In the morning Miss Bancroft complimented her on not wearing lipstick and said there was nothing prettier than natural color. In the afternoon the venetian blinds did not shield her from the baking sun. There were many men and women busy at desks. She made a mistake once, and Miss Bancroft asked if she knew the alphabet, but giggled throatily as though to soften the insult.

An extraordinary proportion of whatever she needed seemed to be filed in the drawers nearest the floor, and the constant squatting in the narrow skirt made the backs of her knees and thighs ache. It became hard to balance. Moreover there was a man who gazed at her behind whenever she stooped. There was also a garter that rubbed and scraped her whenever she bent, no matter how she readjusted it. In addition she felt the onset of a menstrual period that she had not expected quite yet.

It seemed the longest day of her life. She wondered if the daily replacement of stockings would be a substantial budget item on which she hadn't counted.

The secretarial school she had chosen was far uptown, past Copley Square, so she had time only for a doughnut and a cup of milk before taking the underground trolley.

The class had both men and women, mostly older than herself. The teacher was tiny, mild-mannered and very pregnant. She set Millicent to doing a pair of typewriter exercises and left her repeating them for the hour. The shorthand hour followed, and no matter how slowly the pregnant girl dictated it was slightly too fast, in a tantalizing way, so that she felt herself slipping hopelessly behind, and the maddening effort made her edgy until she wanted to scream, but the torment went on. She wondered why dull-looking housewives about her could do it and she could not.

It was past nine when she arrived at Ruthie's. The furniture was low and oblong and modern. She had met Ruthie's husband only at the wedding and didn't care for him. He was pudgy and soft and though tall he did not look a finished adult.

"Just ginger ale for me," she said, on a corner of the couch. "Don't put anything in mine, Sheldon."

"Justin," his wife corrected her.

"I'm sorry," Millicent apologized.

She kept feeling that Justin spoke to her in a patronizing way—so she wanted to get into the rough and tumble of politics, hey?

"You weren't in government though, were you?" Ruthie asked her.

"No. But I went pretty deeply into the Athenian republic."

When Justin had gone to the kitchen for more drinks Ruthie asked Millicent how she was fixed for guys. Millicent said she was pretty much out of touch with just about everyone. Ruthie said she had a second cousin who had just come up from Connecticut to intern in surgery at the Mass General. "I know he hasn't met anybody."

"Is he bright?"

"Well, I suppose, within limits. He made a brilliant record and all that. You know how doctors are."

Justin spent the evening slung in the principal chair, talking knowledgeably and making little witticisms. Ruthie chuckled at them but Millicent was unable to.

She did not have a good time. She felt she was being a bore. But Ruthie smiled.

On the train she kept thinking of Ruthie laughing at all Justin's embarrassingly poor jokes.

It was terribly hard for a bright girl to find the right mate. Ruthie had been her best friend during the years of growing up in Brighton, and at Girls' Latin.

Her train stopped everywhere. She would get to Sparkstown past one, and have to take a cab from the depot.

Above all, she thought, the person you married had to be someone whose efforts at humor didn't cause you to gag inwardly. You had to find someone whose affectations and unawarenesses did not make you retch in your heart, or wince for shame.

4

Ruthie's second cousin telephoned Millicent at the insurance company. His name was Leslie Hollander. Miss Bancroft warned afterward about receiving phone calls.

The company closed Saturdays at one, and Millicent arranged to meet him at three-thirty in the Public Garden. She had hoped to buy a dress immediately after work, and she still meant to squeeze it in. She told him by what statue she would sit, and that she was five-three, with black hair cut short, fair skin, blue eyes, and would have a small leather bag with shoulder strap.

"Are you fat or skinny?" he asked.

It was clearly a kind of banter, but she didn't know how to answer except seriously. "Well, neither one—I suppose I'm more or less decently proportioned," she said, her voice shaky, at once embarrassed by the unintended import of her phrase. "I weigh a hundred and seven. I'm sure we'll find each other."

She did find a summer dress suitable for office wear, a pale summery cord, and sat waiting, neat and trim, near a green bronze statue of a long-haired man in a greatcoat. It was a polished little park in the center of the city. Much of it was taken by a shallow curvy pond. A box containing her old suit was on the bench slats beside her—it occurred to her belatedly now that she ought to have had it sent.

Leslie Hollander had said he would smoke a pipe, and she kept scanning the walk in both directions for anyone who could be he. He was apparently a good half a head taller than she, and had said he had brown hair and wore glasses.

It was odd, she reflected, that custom provided for men and women meeting sight unseen, locating each other stumblingly, half by guesswork in a park, on the basis of descriptions they had given one another.

But you had to have men among your friends. To have only women for companions was in its way as hopelessly female as boy-chasing. Only by having friends of both sexes could you transcend sex.

On a bench diagonally opposite an elderly lady tossed peanuts among the pigeons.

When at last he did appear he stared so questioningly that there was no doubt it was he.

"Hi," she said, rising.

"Hi." He removed the pipe, which did not seem to be lit. He was quite slim, and looked tired. He was perhaps twenty-five. The line of his jawbone stood out all the way to the ear. He dropped his pipe into a rumpled seersucker jacket. "I'm sorry I'm late."

"Oh, that's all right."

"I took a nap, and I overslept."

He motioned to the bench, and they sat. He leaned back in a leisurely way and rested an ankle upon a knee. The hairy leg showed above the sock, and the flannel trousers were unpressed.

She searched for a way to begin conversation, but he started easily enough, about his work at the hospital, and about Ruthie. Then they talked a little about their homes and schooling, and again about his work at the hospital. At some distance before them a swan boat in the pond was making a turn, slow as a raft, its pontoons rising in front like the points of two Persian slippers. Leslie had worked round the clock, and had been praised for a diagnosis. An emergency case had been suffering from a coronary and a diabetic coma at once. He described how later the resident had asked him questions, not to quiz or instruct, but rather by way of testing his own thoughts.

"Will he live?" Millicent asked. "The man in the coma?"

"He might. I looked in on him again before I came over here."

Millicent was impressed. "You'll probably save lots of lives," she said.

"Well, this time I was right—I happened to see it, or I thought I did. But now I'm still where I can consult people. One of these days I'll be in a spot where there's nobody to consult."

They watched the swan boat creep like a barge, bench after bench of quiet children and their elders, and when the turn was made they saw the pedalman in his bird.

"Do you believe medicine is a science or an art?" she asked.

"How do you mean?"

"Well, I mean, not bedside manner exactly. But it includes that. The rapport. The human side."

"You're always dealing with a human." He had put the unlit pipe in his teeth but took it out again. "And you try to grasp the whole patient in all his aspects—all the personality and all the chemistry. But suppose he's in a coma. Where's your bedside manner then?"

He's very bright, she thought.

"Even take a little girl with a lye burn," he said. "A five-year-old. What she cares about is that you know how to fix her burn. She's smart enough to sense it. And that's what comforts her. Not a lot of guff like 'What's your dolly's name.' "

"In other words you think medicine is a science and not an art."

He tightened his expression and ran a hand through his hair, as if she were beginning to irritate him. "Look, science itself is an art. What I'm saying is that if you give everything to your work, you're too busy to be anything but honest and man-to-man with people."

She hadn't meant to be exasperating. However, he rose, and the pigeons fluttered noisily from his feet.

"Want to walk?" he asked her.

They followed a path. He carried her parcel with her old suit inside. It was the week for roses, and in the oblong beds were regiments of them, each in its own color.

"Being involved in medicine must give you a scary perspective on things," she began again.

"Scary?"

"Do you know what I mean?"

"In a way, sort of." She was glad that he didn't sound irritated any more.

"I mean it's always right in front of you. The heartbeat. The adrenal cortex oozing chemicals."

"So?"

"You're always reminded. Forced to think about it."

"Of what?"

"Of our dependence on our bodies. It's frightening."

"Would you rather be a disembodied spirit?"

She didn't answer. She walked pensively.

"That would have its limitations too, I think," he added.

He bought peanuts at the stand and offered her the bag. She reached in absently. With her thumb and forefinger she cracked the dusty pod.

"Some people think the human body is just sort of a lovely Greek statue," she said, "but it must be awful to be a surgeon. Aren't people awful horrible colors inside when you cut them open?"

"Eat that peanut."

Then he offered the bag again and she took a small handful.

"Let's try the boat ride," he said.

They went through the ticket pavilion, eating peanuts. Talk grew easier and easier. The boat's motion could not be felt. It pushed aside the silent ripples. The bridge moved darkly over their heads. Her parcel lay on his lap.

They came into the sun again, and peanut shells glided past on the black water. There were brown ducks. His voice was soft, and sometimes hesitant. He told her of the year he had spent in Baltimore. After four years in New Haven he had not wanted to go on to medical school in the same town, and entered Johns Hopkins instead. But his mother had kept writing and nagging, so after a year away he had transferred back to Yale, so his mother could come down from New Britain once in a while to do his mending and bring a hunk of chicken, leaving his kid brother in charge of the store. He said his mother was a nut.

On the slope of the city's red skyline the great low golden dome dazzled so with sunlight it could not be looked at.

"What's that?" he said.

"The State House."

When they had left the boat she asked if he would like to see the historic buildings. They set out walking, but bought more peanuts first near the garden's sculptured gate. He explained he had had no lunch.

"That's terrible," she said. "I'm surprised at you, living on a diet like that. A doctor should know better."

They waited for a signal, and he tried to take her arm at the crossing, but she withdrew it. She talked for some time of her political ambitions, but finally he asked whether she was a Democrat or Republican and found it amusing when she couldn't tell him.

"I have to look things over first and see where I can do the most good," she explained, hurt by his laughter. "Local politics are very complicated here."

They walked through the shopping district, and eventually toward the produce market, and the city changed again from gray to reddish.

Millicent pointed out a building that rose with high Georgian windows over fruit and vegetable stalls which it sheltered all around it on the cobbles. She told him it was the cradle of American liberty. Men in soiled smocks were helping unload a truck.

"It's got flies on it," he said.

"It's quite graceful," she contradicted him.

"You'd think they'd clear away the barrels, and put a park around it or something."

"Then it wouldn't be alive," said Millicent. "It's always been a market."

They continued walking, and the streets grew narrower and the people more foreign. Sometimes there were pushcarts.

At last they entered a tall brick church, and she said she would show him the steeple where Paul Revere's lantern was hung. He signed a register in the vestibule. There was no one else there except a broad, elderly white-haired gentleman, who showed them the main part of the church, pointing out some curios. He said he belonged to the congregation and that he was retired.

At last Leslie and Millicent went up the narrow staircase to the steeple alone. It was a tight defile, and Millicent climbed behind. The wooden steps were worn into cradles.

"Quite a Boston accent on that guy," Leslie said.

"It's a lovely accent," said Millicent. "You hardly ever hear that kind any more."

The stairs led only into an empty room, with walls of unadorned brick, and another ladder of wood stairs going still higher.

"Kind of rickety," he said.

"And don't say it's got flies on it. It's just a poor church, and the members keep it up so people like you can make fun of it."

"I haven't made fun of it."

"You were getting ready to."

The tower was built of a series of rooms, one over another. The next one up was dark altogether, and Leslie bumped his head on a timber before he steadied himself on the next ladder of stairs, but he said nothing. The air was dense and moist. They climbed higher, into a room that was filled almost entirely by a carillon, and stopped for breath. A stingy bit of daylight filtered dustily through a panel of louver boards onto the huge black bells and timbers, as though the whole room were a sound box. They crept around the still bells to the stair, stepping carefully, and touching the timbers or the bricks.

"Are you afraid of bats?"

"Bats are utterly harmless," she told him.

"Spooky," he said.

The rooms became smaller, and of boards instead of brick. Leslie reached from the stair and poked into the unprotected works of a great clock. The only light came from the open floor hatch overhead.

"Don't," said Millicent.

" 'The clock struck one and down he run,' " he said.

The little lookout room was bright and refreshingly breezy, with its windows open on all four sides. It came as a relief. They stood there together, as though in the air. He wiped his glasses and put them on again. They had clear frames of colorless plastic. Down in the confusion of roofs some window was a gleaming speck of mirror. Arms of the harbor wound amid tanks and hoists, small and far off. A ferry was slowing for a passing vessel.

She glanced at Leslie and he was gazing out, smiling. She felt a sway in the tower—it would seem to inch sideways in a series of barely perceptible starts, and then quietly right itself. But they didn't comment on it. One of his hands came to rest on hers at the window sill, so she found a new spot for hers.

"So Paul Revere belonged to this church?" he asked her.

"Oh no, he didn't belong to it—it was Anglican, and Paul Revere was Congregational. But they used it for espionage because it was high."

"High Episcopal?"

"Tall—this was the tallest building in the city then." But he looked down at her smiling and she realized he had been joking.

"Is that a Phi Beta Kappa key?" he asked.

"Yes." She wore it as a centerpiece in the row of tiny white beads at her neck.

He looked into her eyes, but just as she became uneasy he began to study the moldings of the woodwork instead, and the lipstick smearings on the panes.

"Why don't they turn the place over to the Government?" he said. "Instead of the members trying to run it."

"Oh, they'd never do that."

"Why?"

"Well, they just wouldn't. Things aren't done like that here. If you were a New Englander you'd understand."

"I am a New Englander."

"Oh, that's right. I sort of never think of Connecticut as part of New England, actually. Somehow."

They were looking down toward the nearest row of shuttered windows, which was quite far below. On a tar-covered roof she could almost make out their own shadow, and the needle of the spire over them. She wanted to explain why it was not given to the Government.

"Tradition is a responsibility—" she said.

"Isn't it about time for you to get something in your eye?"

"What?"

He was staring down at her brightly through his eyeglasses. He grabbed her in a violent embrace, pressing down a kiss, and she felt a panic of anger and embarrassment. She tried to dodge his lips and twist free, but he held and his lips followed hers. She told herself in an instant not to compound the confusion by creating a scene. Their lips met stiffly.

He let go and she turned her back, staring out the rear window. She felt her whole body shaking. She thought of telling him that perhaps his long hours of overwork had confused his mind as to what is expected when a man and a woman find themselves alone in a steeple. But she knew she could not yet say anything effectively. He moved to her and put a hand gently on her shoulder, but without turning to him she gave a stiffening shudder that cast it off. Do you think being male gives you the exclusive privilege of deciding that there's to be an encounter of that kind, and in such and such a time and circumstance, of your own private contriving?, she imagined herself asking him. Would you care to be suddenly manipulated and manhandled in that fashion?

"You seem bothered," he said.

"I'm disappointed. I thought you were more sensible."

The shake was there in her voice. He didn't answer. She turned and looked up.

"And I thought your remark about 'time to get something in my eye' was quite insulting. And if it wasn't I'd like to know what you meant by it."

"Well, you know, a cinder in the eye. It's kind of breezy up here." But his smile was already losing its easy certainty and she saw she had succeeded in puncturing him somewhat.

"Oh, I see," she said contemptuously.

"Sometimes it brings two faces together."

"That's what I thought you meant. And it's both insulting and conceited. You think women are just awed admirers of men, don't you. Like dogs and children. You throw a stick and we fetch."

"Aw, no—" He was smiling again, almost laughing at her, and it infuriated her.

"And I think we better go down."

"Well, the sign down there did say we come up at our own risk." He tried to smile at her but her expression did not permit it and it faded.

She stepped carefully into the hatchway, steadying herself when she was far enough down to reach the crude rail. "You're a conceited bore."

"You don't sound bored."

"Well, conceited. You, I mean." She descended with caution in the darkness.

"Actually," he said behind her, "you don't have anything to fear from me, because I'm too damn tired." She heard the tone of sullenness and knew that he too was somewhat angry.

She circled in the dimness to the next set of narrow stairs. They seemed more hazardous descending, and steeper. Here there was no rail and she kept some fingertips to the wall.

"I suppose," she said, "if I turned my ankle on these stairs you'd assume it was a ruse, to have you pick me up and carry me."

"Well, I have to admit you passed up an opportunity to fall off the swan boat and be rescued."

"Oh yes indeed." Her agitation was increasing.

"We could have had some fun with artificial respiration."

"Are interns always so—" She choked on her own breath.

"So what? Cynical?"

"I'll never go anywhere with a doctor again as long as I live."

"I'll spread the word around the hospital."

Between staircases she hurried, but he kept a leisurely distance. Descending past the carillon she again slowed, picking her footing and using both hands.

"I always thought politicians were the cynical ones," he said.

"I don't intend to go into politics out of cynicism. There are still some idealistic people left in the world. Even if you don't think so."

She lowered herself a step at a time, half sideways.

"Want me to help you down the stairs?"

"Don't touch me!" She stumbled as she said it, because she thought she was already at the floor when actually there was another step. But she recovered her balance.

Suddenly the white beads slid from her neck and she heard them popping and bouncing in the darkness. She stooped and went feeling about for them, hot in the prisonlike mugginess, and keeping her skirts tucked. The biggest bells hung nearly to the floor and her hands felt about rapidly under them on the splintery dust, reaching over the bottom timber. The boards had wide crevasses stuffed with soft dirt. Leslie was also on his knees, searching about. She kept her back to him as though he were not there.

"Have you got the key at least?" he asked her.

"Yes, I've got the key." She heard her tremolo.

This is ridiculous, she thought. She would never find them in this light, even if she crawled among the timbers, and anyway they were inexpensive to the point of worthlessness. But she kept searching out of nervous tension. His manhandling upstairs had probably been the real cause of the string's breaking, she thought. She found a run in her stocking.

"I'm surprised you're not afraid to bend down with me in the room."

She sprang erect. She feared she might weep. She wanted to ask him if he were going to be vulgar in addition to everything else. She saw that he had collected a few of the beads, but she hurried on down, through the remaining rooms, as rapidly as the light would permit. In the vestibule the old gentleman of the congregation was potbellied in his chair. He gave her a look of alarm.

Out in the sunshine she continued to hurry, dodging people, without looking behind. Leslie came beside her with long strides.

"Good-bye," she said, not looking at him.

"I'm sorry about the beads."

"You wanted some disaster."

"Can I take you somewhere?"

"No. I'm going to the subway."

"Okay. I'll walk you to the subway."

"You don't have to. I can get there myself."

But he continued beside her.

"I can't just leave you here."

"I wish you would."

"It isn't done."

His gallantry irritated her. "You don't—you just won't understand at all," she said.

"What?"

"Your whole attitude isn't flattering, it's humiliating."

She went as fast as she could, beginning to pant, and pausing only at curbs when the traffic forced her. He continued beside her in silence.

When she got to a large open square, where she could see a subway entrance far off, Leslie suddenly opened the door of a cab. "Come on," he said. "Get in. Where do you want to go?"

She slipped in, sliding to the far corner of the leather. He sat beside her, slamming the door.

"North Station," she told the driver directly.

They rode a block in silence, quite slowly. Her face was hot, as if she had been running.

"Cat got your tongue?" Leslie's voice was quite low.

"No, the cat hasn't got my tongue."

"Look, I made a simple little pass, that's all. It's not so unheard of."

"Just routine, I suppose." But her eyes fixed on the back of the driver's head and the roll of thick neck. She hoped Leslie would not press the conversation further. However, he seemed to feel the driver's presence also, and nothing more was said. She realized all at once that they no longer had the parcel containing her old suit. It must have been left somewhere in the church, among those display cases. But her inclination now was to abandon it.

When at last she got out he did also, and reckoned at the driver's window.

"Aren't you going to keep the cab to go home?" she said.

"I can't afford it."

He restored the wallet to his pocket and stepped toward her. She was standing there among the passersby before the doors of the railroad terminal.

"Well," he said, "it's too bad we couldn't part on speaking terms."

"I think it's time you—" She put a hand to her face briefly, with a nervous brush of her eye and hair, and tried to regain control of her emotions.

"Time I what? Grew up?"

"I think you spoiled a lovely afternoon."

"Don't you think your reaction is a little exaggerated?"

"No I don't." She knew there were tears in her eyes. "I just don't see why a man and a woman can't be dignified together."

They remained looking at each other a moment. Then she turned and hurried toward the trains.

5

That Sunday her parents gave their housewarming. Her mother's sisters, Aunt Celeste and Aunt Gwendolyn, had come early with cakes they had baked. There were scalloped paper napkins and coasters everywhere with ***Lucinda & Ed*** on them.

Her father, as it happened, was called to officiate at a funeral almost at the last moment, and did not get back to the house until the guests were arriving. When he did he brought a young man with him—one of the undertaker's assistants. Millicent wondered if it had been with the idea of steering boys to her. She hoped her father hadn't done anything as embarrassing as that. The boy's name was Chester something, and when introduced he was unsmiling and visibly self-conscious. His uneasiness increased her own uneasiness, so that she took a dislike to him. He still wore the black suit of the funeral, with white boutonniere, and was only slightly taller than herself, thin and dark, already balding at the temples though he could scarcely be more than twenty-four. But the house was becoming crowded, with relatives, with lots of members of her father's new congregation, a few of the other clergymen of Wilmerding Crosswalk, and even a sprinkling of old friends of her parents from Brighton, so that she was able to get away from the young undertaker by going to the kitchen to replenish a tray of hors d'oeuvres.

Her mind had also been on Leslie Hollander a lot since yesterday. She was dissatisfied with the way she had handled that. After all, it should be possible to laugh off those foolish gambits. It was not easy for boys these days to know how to behave.

But she didn't know how to make light of it. It seemed to her that a certain coyness was required of women in such situations, a coyness that was essentially false, and therefore degrading.

As she brought the tray down the center hall beside the staircase she sneezed, turning her face sharply to her shoulder to avoid the food. She tilted the tray away from the sneeze, righting it barely in time to avert spillage—the hors d'oeuvres had already slid and bunched. It hurt sharply up in the softness of her palate. Those sudden, convulsive sneezes often did that to her, unless she could lift a hand in time to pinch her nostrils. She saw that the double front doors with their tall glass panels had opened again, and against the light she made out the stout little figure of her grandmother, entering into the crowd with her second husband, Mr. Krupchick, and being greeted by her mother and others. There was a purple mole on her cheek. A long fox was flung about her neck.

"We got lost—who can find this place?" her grandmother was saying. Her voice was husky. She squinted through metal-rimmed glasses and a tiny veil at Millicent, who was trying to work past toward the French doors of the living room. The grandmother threw out her arms, so that Millicent drew back lest the tray be bumped. "Ah, there's the prodigal! Did you take good care of my sister out there?"

"She's fine," Millicent said.

"Your mother gave us bum directions," Mr. Krupchick said glumly to Millicent.

Her grandmother clasped her by the arms, smiling, and the tray pressed both their stomachs. "I bet she told you she's younger than me, didn't she. She's a liar. She was born on the other side, not me. I was born in Boston. You can look it up in City Hall. Ha ha!" Her laughter had the same huskiness as her voice, not loud, and harsh and flat-sounding in the back of her throat, yet hearty. "I bet they didn't teach yiz to cook a square meal out there. Tell me, you got yourself a boy friend yet? Ah, here's the other one! Mm, a boolky." She released Millicent and reached up joyously to Patty's cheek, giving it a hard pinch and tug. Her darting eyes caught everyone present, and with a quick motion of her head she indicated to Lucinda her approval of Patty.

Her husband took an hors d'oeuvre from the tray. He was a small man, dressed in grays, with a thinly knitted sweater under his jacket. Millicent sensed that the young undertaker Chester had come very close to her, a little behind and to the side, but she did not look at him.

"Look at ya, the two of yiz!" her grandmother exclaimed, a sweep of her white gloves encompassing Patty and Millicent. "Ooh, what's that?" Her smile faded a moment and she squinted up through the veil at Patty. "Mascara?" She swayed her head. "I thought somebody gave her a black eye. Imagine, a party this size. She's out of her head, your mother. She should have traded in the two of yiz for a nigger maid. You know it? That's what she should have done. Look, he's looking at me," she said with a smirk, having noticed Chester's stare. "Don't mind me," she said to him. "They been looking to put me in the bughouse for years—I'm too smart for them. They're fixed, anyways, the bughouses. He thinks I'm crazy."

"Hi, Grandma Annie!" two young boys shouted, one after the other, running from the staircase and sliding across the floor.

"Look out!" she said. "You'll split your head open. Oop!" They caught her hands in the white gloves.

"Want some champagne, Grandma Annie?" Patty asked her.

"Trying to get your grandmother drunk?" she answered. The boys were pulling her. They looked about nine and seven.

Mr. Krupchick asked Patty for whisky in a shot glass. He indicated the size with a thumb and forefinger.

"Champagne, getting extravagant," the grandmother said.

Lucinda began to shepherd them through the French doors. Millicent tried to follow her mother, carrying the tray.

"Gary, Evan! Let Grandma alone," Aunt Celeste said. "Behave! Or you'll have to play outside."

"There's the darling!" Grandma Annie said to Gwendolyn's baby. "Come to Gammah. Oof, she isn't so light any more, you know it?"

"Are those your grandparents?" Chester asked Millicent.

The two boys suddenly dashed around behind Lucinda and in front of Millicent, grasping an edge of one of the doors as if to use it for a pivot, so that she had to draw back. "Let's try the banistairs," she heard one of them say.

"My grandmother's remarried—he's not my grandfather," she answered Chester. "Unless you want to call him a step-grandfather. Excuse me, I've got to pass these."

"Can I help you?"

It seemed an awkward remark. She didn't see how he could help her pass a tray of refreshments.

However her mother relieved her of it, and when she moved out of her mother's way she found herself standing between Chester and the fireplace irons. She fingered a button of her dress nervously.

"What's that they call your grandmother—Grandma Annie or something?" he asked.

"Well, it's sort of a compromise. She wanted us to call her by her first name."

The room was a hubbub of voices, but she heard Chester draw a breath. She wished he would go away, but he seemed to cling as though insisting that they make conversation. She saw Aunt Celeste shepherding her grandmother and

Krupchick now, and someone moving to a folding chair to make room on the sofa.

"It's disgusting, a woman that age thinking she needs a man," Millicent began.

"Maybe she's lonely."

"Even so," Millicent said. "I don't see what a woman with false teeth needs a husband for. The answer for lonesomeness is to get busy."

Through the dining-room arch she saw her brother Charles trying hard to open a bottle of champagne. His face was strained and earnest, and her father's half-brother Franklin, big and florid with a gray mustache, was trying to help him. She saw Charles blink as the cork popped. Her Aunt Gwendolyn's child was crawling out from under the table, behind some lady's legs, and she had an impulse to rush over before the baby could be stepped on. But then her little cousin Nan gathered the child up in her arms, and kissed it and smiled, showing the brace on her teeth, and sat down with the baby on the square leather hassock. The people she didn't know outnumbered those she did. Her father's dark-eyed twin sister Rosalind was sitting with a Nordic-looking thirty-ish man whose head was braced stiff in some kind of great surgical collar. At one end of the sofa her grandmother was laughing up at a man who stood with his back to Millicent, and at the other end Patty sat on the arm of it, her crinoline showing under a bouffant skirt, and giggled at something her cousin Stephen said. Patty gave a little screech and almost fell off.

"I've just never had that gift of laughing," Millicent said.

"What?" said Chester.

"That social giggling. I don't know, I suppose it's a knack of laughing at pleasantries, but I've just never been able to make myself laugh if I'm not amused—I just physically can't. And when somebody starts telling me a joke my heart just sinks—it's awful. I worry that the punchline won't be funny and what if I can't laugh. I don't know, can you laugh at will? Any time you want to?"

"Well, I don't know—"

"I was supposed to laugh in a school play once, and they had to give the part to somebody else. I don't know, how do people do it? To me—I can't stop myself from laughing when something's funny, and I can't make myself when it isn't."

"Well, I'll remember not to tell you any jokes."

"That's good—I'd rather you didn't chance it. It just scares me to death. Knowing that something's coming that I'll be expected to laugh at."

She thought she saw her father beckon to her. He was on the other side of the room, sitting with some elderly people in the bay window. It was an opportunity to break away from Chester.

"Excuse me," she said.

She tried to work her way across the room, past knees and behind chairs. Mr. Boland, who had once been her father's partner in the used-car business, put up a hand to her and asked if she remembered him. She told him she did. The degree to which he had aged shocked her. Her spinster Aunt Rosalind, sitting between her cousin Jill and the blond man in the surgical collar, also caught her hand, but Millicent said she'd be back.

Her father had in fact beckoned. Two elderly men rose for her in a courtly way, one of them stocky and bald with glasses, and the other tall and gaunt, white-haired but balding, and offered their seats, but she declined. Her father introduced them as Newton Stillman, pastor of the Congregational church, and Caleb Folger of the Unitarian, and a plump smiling old lady with thick glasses as Mrs. Folger.

"Please sit down," Millicent said. Her voice quaked.

She made a little effort at conversation, and learned that the Unitarian church was the tall white one she had seen in Murphy Square. Its clock of black and gold was the one she heard by night.

Lucinda called to her from a little distance. When she had excused herself her mother told her to show Aunt Gwen where the pots were so she could warm a bottle for Sharlene.

Millicent began to edge her way toward the dining-room arch. That name Sharlene sounds like a chemical, she thought. Aunt Gwen has no taste.

A lady stopped her and said her son had just graduated from college, and asked if she remembered her son. But then her mother told her never mind, Aunt Gwen had found a pot.

"No stockings?" her mother asked.

"I haven't got any," said Millicent.

"Not one good pair?"

Millicent tried to make her way back to Aunt Rosalind as she had promised, but she was accosted by a whole party of stylish men and women who stood laughing and smoking and holding glasses of champagne. She had not realized they were a group until she tried to pass between and found herself in their midst. Apparently they were from her father's congregation and knew who she was.

"You better be nice to my husband, because he's chairman of your daddy's building fund," a sunny-faced young woman among them said gaily. Her summery dress was scooped out on a wobbly freckled bosom.

"Oh," said Millicent.

"Have you had any champagne?" a skinny man in a tattersall vest and sport jacket asked Millicent.

"Nah, she don't drink that cheap stuff," another man in a sport jacket said. He had a tiny cigar.

Aunt Rosalind rescued her, seizing her hand. "Let me borrow my favorite niece," Aunt Rosalind said. Her aunt looked at her brightly and dimpling. Her dark hair was pulled tight into a chignon and her dress was the color of burgundy. She took her to where she had been sitting before, next to Jill. Jill was a sour-faced teen-ager with long stringy hair, but she greeted Millicent with a moment of warmth.

"Tell me," Aunt Rosalind asked Millicent, "what will you do now? Will you do anything with your archaeology?"

"No."

"I could introduce you at the Museum."

Working in a museum, particularly with her aunt, seemed to Millicent a road to nowhere. Before she could answer, the tall blond man with the big leather surgical collar appeared before them. His handsome young head sat in it as if in a bowl. In his hands he managed three bubbling glasses of yellow champagne. Below the big collar there was a black front inside his suit, with no necktie.

"Did I take your seat?" Millicent asked, rising.

"Oh, stay where you are," he said.

Aunt Rosalind introduced him as Ralph Briggs, the rector of St. Timothy's, and he made a stiff little bow, without spilling champagne, and his head quite rigid. He offered Millicent a glass, but she refused. She was aware suddenly that the balding young undertaker Chester had crept up beside her again.

"Hi," Chester said.

"Hi," she answered. She considered for an instant omitting to introduce him, but it seemed too rude, so she began. She was unable to remember the undertaker's last name and put a hand to her face. He supplied it, and then she couldn't remember the minister's either.

"I think there's some chairs over here where we can sit," Chester said, and as he seemed to expect her to follow, and as Jill went along with him, sipping the champagne the minister had given her, Millicent followed too, still embarrassed at her ineptness.

They zigzagged among people with difficulty until they were near the French doors.

"Well, I thought there were some chairs along here, but I guess there aren't," Chester said.

If I'm going to be a politician I better start learning to remember names, she thought. She had a depressing suspicion that she was a fool who had no real aptitude for the things she sought.

In the hall behind her she heard the rattle of the double doors opening again and when she glanced that way she saw her Uncle Maxwell and Aunt Tessie. "Anybody home?" her Uncle Maxwell shouted.

"No, go 'way, nobody home!" Her mother sang cheerily from the midst of the living room.

"The guy with the thing around his neck likes your Aunt Rosalind," Jill said.

"He's probably being polite," said Millicent.

Jill alternately looked into her champagne and sipped it. There had always been something about Jill's eyes that looked a little mad, Millicent thought. Millicent saw that Chester had a glass too—apparently he had accepted the one the minister had meant for himself.

"What is that thing around his neck?" she asked.

"He said he fell off a horse," said Jill.

"It's a brace," said Chester.

"That Steve," said Jill. She was watching Steve, how he spun Patty back and forth in a dance, even though there was no music, using her raised fingers for a handle. "Poo. Not my cousin, yours."

"He's a savage," said Millicent. It struck her how agile Patty was. Her cousin Steve was big but in an athletic way—a fine chest and shoulders tapering to slimness. He had a pointed nose and curly hair and a perpetual lascivious grin. He was older than Millicent.

"He puts his arm around and pinches me," Jill said, "and he says, 'hi, junior, how's your love life.' Right with all those ministers standing around."

They watched the silent dance. Patty's hair flew back and forth. Despite her bigness and overweight she was remarkably light-footed. And she did have a very pretty face and a clear complexion, Millicent thought. But the bouffant underpinnings made her hippier than ever. It seemed to Millicent that Patty had a fascination with clothing like that of a two-year-old girl. The skirts billowed with each turn.

From nearby chairs her father's cigarette smoke rose to her face, and she heard her father tell Mr. Boland they had rented the house with an option to buy. The land would be worth something someday, but he wasn't sure yet if he would like the congregation or if the congregation would like him. Besides, the house needed seven hundred bucks' worth of a paint job. And there was other work—he wasn't sure about the well. Lucinda wanted to buy so they could paint—that's how a woman figures.

"Want to dance?" Chester asked Millicent suddenly, leaning a little to talk around Jill. "Oh, there isn't any music, is there." He seemed to become confused.

To get away from him Millicent said she had to help her mother again with serving. She excused herself. She had to push Chester gently to make him stand aside.

She found her way through toward the dining room. She overheard a lady say it was remarkable how Lucinda kept her figure, especially after four children.

In the kitchen Millicent cut a cake, carefully between walnuts, and arranged the pieces on a tray.

Patty came into the kitchen, singing softly to herself, and with a dance step in her saunter.

"I just had a kind of crazy feelin'
You were meant for me—"

She took a piece of the cake from Millicent's tray, and sang with food in her mouth.

"My head is swimmin' round the ceilin';
Can it truly be?"

"I thought you were supposed to be starting a diet," Millicent said sourly.

Patty smacked frosting sharply from her thumb, with a quick gesture between blowing a kiss and thumbing her nose.

A stocky, middle-aged lady whom Millicent didn't know appeared at the kitchen door and asked if there were another bathroom besides the one upstairs. "It's so busy up there you need a reservation," the lady said.

"There's a toilet in the cellar, but it's filthy," Patty said.

The lady looked at her uncertainly.

"You can use it," Patty assured her. "My father uses it, like when he's chopping wood or something. But there's spiders and toads and mice and everything down there."

When Millicent came out of the kitchen to serve the cake her mother told her they were having the ceremony first. She saw people going out to the porch and front yard. Chester was upon her again and asked if he could get her some champagne.

"I'm a teetotaler," she said.

"Oh. Well, do you mind if I have some?"

His awkwardness irritated her. There was no way to answer the things he said.

"I think everybody's going out now," she told him, and set her tray down on the piano bench.

Outdoors the crowd had spread about on the wide porch, on the steps, and the grass below. At a little distance, before the barn and down beside the road, many cars were parked, and the sunshine was bright on them. Steve was sitting in shadow on the porch railing. She averted her gaze quickly from his grin.

Her father was passing out black skullcaps, and she saw Caleb Folger, the lean white-haired minister, look at one whimsically and put it on. Evan and Gary came running from between the house and the barn shouting that there was a train track out back, in the woods. Jill told them to pipe down. Over by the barn the old dog watched sleepily in the sun.

"Okay, padre, let's get the show on the road," her Uncle Maxwell said to her father. Uncle Maxwell held his cigar out a little distance from his face.

Her father seemed to her the only man who could wear a skullcap rakishly, somewhat forward and down to the side. He opened his prayer book and cleared his throat, and someone told someone else to be quiet.

"What's it for," said Grandma Annie, "it's supposed to be to chase the witches out—what."

"No, no, it's just a housewarming," Millicent's father said.

"I never heard of it," said Grandma Annie. "He's strict by the letter, that one. My son-in-law."

"What do ya do, Ed, bust a champagne bottle on the door?" Uncle Maxwell asked him.

"He'll bust the door," said Uncle Franklin.

Millicent looked at them darkly and caught Maxwell's eye for an instant, but he scarcely seemed to notice. He was also a half-brother, and resembled Franklin, except not quite so old and burly, and without the mustache. Under his jacket he had a colored sport shirt with no tie.

"Is he gonna bust the door, Ma?" Evan asked, looking above and behind him.

"No, he's kidding," said Aunt Celeste. She stood with hands on shoulders of both young boys.

"Of course not," said Gary.

Ed began reading psalms, and Millicent noticed that Mr. Boland crossed himself. Chester had come near her, but she pretended not to have noticed and turned her back a little, as though trying to see the text in her father's book, and its translation on the facing page. Her father read along, not loudly, in the ancient original. The ministers were also standing fairly near her father, and she saw that they had shut their eyes tight, and except for the youngish one who wore a surgical contraption they had bowed their heads.

> *And I pleaded with my God: What use would my death be, what good would it do to put me in the grave? Will the dust praise Thee? Will the dust testify to Thy steadfastness?*

Her father kept reading. "Okay, is the house warm now?" Uncle Maxwell said.

Ed continued as though taking no notice.

"I seen the way the goyim do it," said Grandma Annie. "On the television, did you see that? The bishop, the whachamacallit. They shpritz. With a shpritzer, shpritz here, shpritz there—"

"We haven't got a television," said Patty.

"You've got an aerial," said Steve.

"This guy doesn't leave anything out," Uncle Maxwell said to somebody. "What do you say, padre," he said to Ed, "isn't it warm yet?"

"That was here before," Patty told Steve.

> *I will enjoy my house, in the integrity of my heart—*

Chester's hovering annoyed Millicent. She told herself angrily that he was a pest.

Ed finally closed the book.

"Okay, finis?" said Uncle Maxwell, looking about. "Where's Lucinda. He's got to pick her up and carry her over the doorpost."

"The threshold," said Uncle Franklin.

"The threshold. The goal post I should have said. It's a good thing she doesn't take after the Powerful Katrinka here." Maxwell pushed Patty's shoulder back and forth.

But Ed had ascended into the shady porch, and the edge of the crowd began to draw after him. Charles was with him, near the double doors which rounded up to a point, and he held a carpenter's tack hammer. Ed said a brief sentence of worship, and Charles produced from his pocket a thin brass cylinder, about two inches long, and began hammering it to the doorpost, high above the level of his eyes.

"Be careful, Charles," Lucinda cautioned him. "Watch out you don't hit your thumb."

It was a small-headed hammer, and its clap sounded against the wood.

Charles was jacketless, in a white sportshirt and chino pants, but neat, and the skullcap was round on the back of his close-cropped head. He drove a single brad at the top and another at the bottom.

"You gonna put one on the barn, Ed?" said Uncle Maxwell.

"How about the car," said Franklin. The Boston accents were very flat.

Ed moved into the house and people followed, but he stopped and the hall and entrance became quite crowded. The acknowledgment and hammering were repeated at the doorways of the living room and the study, and then they moved deeper into the house, to other doorways. Millicent saw that sometimes the little Deuteronomy passages were encased in plastic, so that some of the tiny lettering showed through, but at other rooms they were enclosed indifferently in brass or wood. Charles apparently had an assortment of them in his trousers pockets. The crowd was drawn along, ambling and bunching, inspecting the rooms. Chester said nothing and yet was with her constantly.

"And a fireplace in the kitchen, look at that," a lady said. "What have they got, two fireplaces?"

Sometimes Charles or Roland said the ancient words of worship instead of their father, Charles low and embarrassed and Roland childishly clear. Behind Millicent there was a vastness of conversing, buzzing, and occasionally here and there some convivial laughter. But she migrated along, paying attention to the ambulatory ceremony, as though to lag would invite conversation with Chester. They dragged upstairs, and she saw her mother smile as ladies admired the drapes in her parents' bedroom.

Chester managed to stay next to her. Suddenly the thought struck her, like a clear insight or revelation all at once, that women never marry the men they should. Eugene, for example, was the exceptional kind of man she could have willingly followed anywhere, but it doesn't happen like that—Eugene was like other men, self-centered. So women end up talking themselves into believing they feel love for their third-raters, their second-bests, their poor substitutes. Her eye fell upon the blondish, chunky, lined face of her Aunt Celeste, who looked older than her mother although she was really younger—Uncle Ira had not even the capability to manage his own dry-goods store, so that Celeste had not only to work in it with him but run it for him.

Or her mother standing here vacuously while the boys tacked the Lord's words upon the doorposts. Her mother was not even an atheist—religious questions, like mathematics, just didn't touch her. Her mother would never have gone along with this constant image if her father had not maneuvered her hopelessly into it, by giving her a couple of babies and then going into the clergy. His becoming a rabbi had forced her mother to go along with religious observance—she probably wouldn't have put up with it otherwise.

The hammering moved back down past the carved upstairs railing to Charles's door. Every marriage is a mismatch, she thought. Her parents had nothing to say to each other that did not pertain to the house or the children.

How had men managed it, this world of abstractions? Religion, Republicans, Democrats, nations—it was all abstraction, actually. Like the whole nomenclature of learning. Men had invented a whole imaginary world, made of principles and war aims and everything else, but they had made it the real world, until there was nothing else. Men could philosophize, lecture, worry about man's stance, our posture in the universe. And their wives cleaned up their cigarette butts. Her mother had made this party, prepared the hors d'oeuvres. With some help from herself and Patty and the aunts. The frantic scrubbing. And now here was her father's part, to occupy the center, to perform. Just as he had chucked a going business to go to the seminary, and gone off as a chaplain in the Navy—his place was to be the poet, the adventurer.

He had been old enough to have avoided the war if he wished. When he enlisted her mother had accused him in tears of wanting to be rid of her and the children, and yet how quickly her mother had forgotten all that in her joy at having him home. A woman must be rich or poor, as her husband's ego dictates.

She waved away her Uncle Maxwell's cigar smoke.

They turned to the room she shared with Patty. She somehow caught Chester's eye, though she didn't want to. The skullcap sat on the top of his head. She detested his witless face as though he had already proposed.

The crowd was tight at the doorway. She felt the guests all about her examining the room, and she also saw a pair of her white underpants, lying wrinkled and soft, with a touch of soil, in the middle of the floor. A white bra hung nearby from a chair. She had meant to tidy up, and realized now she had forgotten it in the rush. She shrunk within herself, her face hot. Chester, her cousin Steve, those ministers, including the Episcopalian with his head braced—the kids Evan and Gary, old Krupchick—she could almost feel them appraising and contemplating. They could know it had to be hers. Those various circles were too small to be Patty's.

6

On her lunch hour Monday Millicent telephoned the Democratic State Committee and asked the location of the ward club nearest where she worked.

Whatever work she did for the club during the week would have to be limited to lunch hours and late at night, after her classes, she thought. But she could do a lot on weekends.

At noon the following day she walked there at once, without stopping to eat anything. It was about five blocks. She found the address in a shabby two-story building of brick, over a dingy shoe-outlet store. The doorbell in the entry was broken, and when she pushed the door open the stairs were unswept. At another door at the top she knocked again, and a bald little man opened it in such a way as to bar entry. He had sleeve garters, and looked up at her without a trace of a smile. His cheeks were fleshless and hung loose. "Who you looking for?" he said brusquely.

She asked if this was in fact the club she sought. He made no reply. He did not even change the expression of his face. One of his hands held the doorknob and the other a chrome loving cup and a polishing cloth. Behind him the room was long and darkish, with little furniture. There was shelving with stacks of paper, not very neat, and some crates of empty soda bottles.

Her voice grew shaky. "Can you tell me when your club meets, please?" she swallowed, embarrassed by his silence. "I'd like to find out about dues, and joining."

"Who sent you?" he said.

"The Democratic National Committee—I mean the State Committee," she said, correcting herself and reddening. "I mean I asked them to send me."

Behind him a big important-looking man emerged in the shadows from one of the interior rooms and came toward them. He looked at Millicent with a fixed smile, as if he thought she was someone he ought to know. He had a cream-colored vest and a walking stick. But his eyes and his whole broad face had a kind of glaze.

The little man widened the door to make way for him. "This is a college kid, some professor sent her over from Radcliffe," the little man said. "The Plan E crowd."

"That's not true—I have nothing to do with Radcliffe or Plan E!" Millicent protested.

The big man was venerable-looking. The vest had brass buttons on his rounded front, under a dark coat. His smile remained, but Millicent saw that his face had almost a bloated sleekness. "Ah," he said.

"Can you help me, sir?" Millicent appealed to him. "Will you put me on the mailing list?"

"Why of course. Fitz, put this pretty maid on the mailing list." He put on his hat and went slowly down the stairs with his walking stick.

The little man began to shut the door.

"Please!" Millicent said sharply, and the door paused.

She cleared her throat and looked down the stairs to appeal to the big man. But he had gotten to the bottom and gone out.

"Excuse me, Mr. Fitz," she said. "Can you tell me that man's name, that just went out?" She felt she might need to contact him.

"What you checking up on him for?" the little man asked.

She looked at him angrily. "Will you put my name on the mailing list, please?"

"Sure, I'll put it on." The door shut in her face, with a groan of wood and a click of metal.

She knocked, sharply, and it opened.

"Do you have a pencil?" she asked him. He had not taken her name.

"Sure, I got a pencil." The door shut again.

Her blush renewed itself. But she gave up and went downstairs.

In the sunshine she felt too outraged to decide at once what to do. She walked aimlessly.

But at last she went to the phone booth in the luncheonette across from her office building and called the Democratic State Committee again. She tried to tell the lady what had happened, but she could not find the right phrases and she felt she sounded emotional. Finally the lady said she ought to join a club in her own district, and asked where she voted.

"Well, I live in Wilmerding Crosswalk—I suppose I'll be voting there."

She remained in the booth for some minutes while the lady went to search. Then the lady's voice came to her ear again and told her there was no organization in the Town of Wilmerding.

"Nothing?" said Millicent. "You mean nothing at all? The Democratic Party doesn't exist?"

"Well, I wouldn't say it doesn't exist," the lady answered her.

For some days Millicent could not decide on her next approach. Work in the office continued drearily. Once, when Miss Bancroft was out of sight for a moment, and the large office happened to be fairly empty, she reprimanded the fortyish claims adjuster who always stared at her from his desk. She told him it was rude and that she didn't like it.

He said that with a face like hers he couldn't help himself.

She refused to accept the compliment. "The fact that I have normal attractiveness doesn't excuse it," she told him. "I don't gawk at nice-looking men or women. Or even at attractive children. It's discomforting."

The next morning he asked her to have lunch with him, and she refused curtly. But her conscience bothered her during the forenoon. Perhaps he had only wished to make amends for yesterday, she thought as she worked among the filing cabinets. And now it was she who had been rude. She knew she had a tendency to be snobbish. Yet she wanted a career in politics, which meant a love of humankind—she told herself she was inconsistent.

Toward lunchtime she told him she would eat with him, if he still wanted company. But she insisted on the busy, unpretentious counter where she always went, and on paying for her own milk and sandwich. Nor was the conversation agreeable. He talked about people in the firm and referred to Miss Bancroft as an old biddy. Millicent at once cut him off, saying he mustn't use that expression. "I don't have any great love for Miss Bancroft," she told him, "but I object to the use of any of these contemptuous words for women. It's just like saying 'wop' or 'guinea,' and I won't have it. I'm sorry, Mr. Durfee."

Miss Bancroft meanwhile had begun a monumental project of revising the entire filing system—she said she had been waiting until she had a reliable girl before starting this—and then in the midst of it she had discovered that Millicent wrote with an exquisite hand, so they began anew, with folder designations written by Millicent instead of typed. Millicent wrote with appealing clarity, the consistency of the slant and the grace of the loops making a pattern as delicate as lace, set off now and then with angry downstrokes. But she had the regular filing and fetching and locating to do at the same time, and with a small part of the system changed over and the rest not she made mistakes.

Later in the week the young undertaker Chester Walberg phoned her at the office, explaining that her mother had given him the number. Miss Bancroft's mouth and cheeks had tightened as she handed Millicent the phone.

"I can't talk to you," Millicent said hurriedly, half losing her breath. "I can't take calls at the office." She hung up immediately, a little flushed.

"Well, don't resent it, child," Miss Bancroft said. "You know we can't have your patootie calling the office." Millicent turned and busied herself arranging folders in a file drawer. She was shaking a little. "I suppose you think an old maid doesn't understand such things," Miss Bancroft added.

Millicent thought of confiding that she did not resent it. But she feared it would only lengthen the protestations.

" 'Old maids are honorable, frisky flirts are abominable,' " Miss Bancroft said, resuming her work.

When Millicent got home in late evening her mother asked if Chester had reached her. There was also a tiny package that had come for her, with no return address. It turned out to be from Leslie Hollander, the intern—a white necklace, perhaps a bit nicer than the one that had come apart in the tower. Her mother asked what it was, and Millicent said it was nothing.

Sometimes she thought of her old blue suit, lying tied in its box in the Old North Church. She had meant to go there after work and retrieve it, but with her typing and shorthand she never had time. And she did not feel like facing that old gentleman—he must have known from the way she ran out of the tower that some upsetting quarrel had taken place. Maybe she had better write them a letter before they gave her suit away to the poor.

She couldn't afford to lose that suit. She didn't have much else suitable for the office, except her new cord dress. She had worn a blouse one day, but the fit of it gave some prominence to her breasts and made Mr. Durfee keep looking.

There was no money for more. Since Charles had started summer school at the Sweetser Hall preparatory academy Millicent had been riding to Boston with him every morning in his high, squarish Model T coupe, which was a saving in fares, but she still had to return by train and bus at night, after her typing and shorthand. She had had to let her parents pay for the cord dress, and she had not even been able to give any board money yet because of the typing manuals and shorthand books.

Tuition for the classes cost her by the week, but by Thursday she was very discouraged. She had reviewed and reviewed the symbols, and had known them on the train. But before she could sort them and bring the right one to mind the instructress would be on to the next word, until Millicent's brain never knew which way to jump, whether to chase the word just past or meet the new one oncoming. It was heartbreaking. The men and women around her did not look especially clever, but they wrote pages and pages. The pregnant little instructress only glanced toward Millicent's nearly blank sheet and passed silently, pausing to bend over the next pupil.

Saturday Leslie Hollander surprised her in the lobby of her building when she came down at one o'clock.

"Oh dear!" she said, startled.

"Hi." He looked more tired and drawn than the other time, and he still needed a haircut. "I hope you don't mind my stopping by unannounced—it was just on impulse."

"Oh," she said. "No. No, I don't mind. As a matter of fact I'm glad you did, because the lady I work for doesn't like personal calls."

He said he was just out walking, and had Saturday afternoon off again. He normally had only every other Saturday but someone had asked him to swap.

"Oh," she said. "Have you had lunch?"

When they stood watching at the curb she let him take her hand, as traffic was quite heavy. He switched his folded newspaper to the other arm. When they were at last on stools at the counter it occurred to her that she perhaps should pay for his lunch. She had heard in Chicago that interns earned very little and she presumed it could not be much different here in Boston.

She thanked him for the necklace. "I thought that was really quite kind, and beyond the call of duty," she said. He replied that it was nothing.

But she said that he must basically be a very considerate person. He smiled as though he thought her silly.

"No, really," she said. "You probably wouldn't have become a doctor otherwise."

He ordered a sandwich and she ordered soup and salad. He took off his glasses and massaged his closed eyes, near the bridge of his nose. He stifled a yawn. When he opened his eyes she saw they were quite bloodshot.

"Were you up all night again?" she asked.

"Well, a good part of it. I was on call. Emergency seems to get busy on the weekends."

"You should be home in bed instead of out walking."

"When would I ever get out then? All I get's a day and a half every other week."

The luncheonette was not crowded Saturdays and they sat a long time. She told him how she had tried to join a political club, and of its dreadful backwardness. She didn't see how it could thrive if they discouraged ambitious young people. She had even been thinking of joining a Republican club if the Democrats wouldn't have her. She really would, she said, provided she could have their assurance that they didn't condone McCarthy. She had heard anyway that in Massachusetts some of the Democrats supported McCarthy more than the Republicans did.

She said she was sorry that the Town of Wilmerding had an open town meeting. If it had a representative town meeting, she could run for town-meeting member. And as there might be several members from every street, that would be a small enough office to run for. She obviously couldn't start off running for selectman or town clerk, against all the entrenched people.

"Why don't you run for school committee?" said Leslie.

"Well," she said, "that's a thought."

She watched him dangle his tea bag. It twisted in the steam. But she knew nothing of the realities of school committees either, she thought unhappily. She wondered if there were lots of angry parents fighting for those jobs.

She told him that there were two small parties in Massachusetts, the Socialist-Labor and the Prohibition, and it might even be good to work in one of those a while for the experience. The Prohibition Party appealed to her a little. But on second thought, she added, there was no future with a small party.

He gathered both their checks and took money from his wallet.

"No," she said. "Let's make it dutch."

"Don't be silly."

"No, I mean it. Really."

"Come on. It's not done."

She followed him to the cashier and he paid. The folded newspaper had soiled his jacket.

"Well," she told him, "it's my treat next time."

On the sidewalk he asked if she'd like to see a movie. There was one about Irish fisherfolk on an island off Donegal, which was said to be sensitively photographed and to have captured moods.

They walked to it, though it was far uptown. They walked all through downtown, and across the Common and the Public Garden, and up an avenue that had a dirt walk and grass under big trees in its center, with truck and auto traffic on either side. She kept trying to think of a way to prevent him from paying for the tickets. But when he got to the box office she said nothing. It was silly to fight custom all the time, she thought, and apparently his pride demanded that she be escorted in the usual fashion.

In the theater he quickly fell into a deep sleep. She would have let him rest upon her shoulder under the circumstances, but he had fallen asleep in a different position, with his head leaning the other way. His snoring was throaty and not at all bothersome. However she knew the lady behind was growing annoyed. "Please don't wake him," she asked the lady softly. "He's a doctor and he worked all night."

She had seen the film one and a half times when he wakened. But she wanted to stay so that he might see it. "No, that's all right," he said. He was blinking, and stretching the kinks out of his face and body.

That poor boy, she thought on the train ride home. He works so hard, and when his day off comes he's worn out.

It occurred to her that he might not have telephoned her in order to save the nickel.

It was good to have supper at home again. But during the meal Roland asked her father how they used to get sleighs through the covered bridge. "Did the horse pull it on bare wood or what?" She too looked to her father for the answer. He nodded, with a thoughtful shrugging motion of his lip. "I don't know," he said finally. "It seems like quite a problem, doesn't it. I'll have to work on that. Maybe I can ask some old-timer around town."

It bothered Millicent even after supper. It could wreck your whole concept of what life was like in the nineteenth century, she thought.

She changed into her jeans, and went down to her father's study for some postcards. She found them in a drawer of the desk. Then she settled on the living-room sofa. She wanted to write to Americans for Democratic Action to ask to be put on their mailing list, to the Republican State Committee to ask if there was an organization in her town, and to the Weekly Wilmerdingian to ask what organizations there were.

But Patty came and sat on the square hassock, setting her little white phonograph and some records below her on the old reddish oriental rug. Millicent tried to compose her postcards, but the recording had a choking, whining female voice that grated on her.

"Do you have to play that trash right here?" she asked after a while.

Patty poked her tongue out at her. "You don't own the place," said Patty.

The little phonograph went on.

"Why don't you write your cards upstairs if you don't like it?" said Patty.

"Because it's not comfortable up there. It's filthy up there, thanks to you. Why don't you play your records up there?"

"Because Charles is studying, ha ha," said Patty sourly.

"—He'll pick up the pie-e-eces,
He'll dust off my hea-a-art.
He'll love me warmed o-o-over—"

Millicent took her cards to the kitchen. She needed the phone books that were there for the addresses anyhow. She worked at the heavy plank table. She wondered whether it might be reasonable to write to every member of the legislature, inquiring of each if he needed an assistant, or whether they only hired bums that they knew, or whether she should wait until her typing and shorthand improved. On a brown grocery bag she tried to draft a circular letter, just to see how it might sound.

The wall phone rang. A girl asked for Patty, and Millicent called her. Then she returned to the table, working in pencil on the brown paper. She did not even know if they had assistants.

"Oh, great, copacetic," Patty said into the phone.

Millicent scratched out and began again.

"Hold on a minute, okay?" Patty said into the phone. "I can't talk here."

"I'm not listening," Millicent told her without looking up.

Patty left, and the phone dangled from the wall. In a moment Millicent heard her through the rooms as she asked her father to vacate the study and let her use the phone there. Charles's friend Sudquist came into the yard with his motorcycle, shouting for Charles in a kind of yodel. Millicent hung up the dangling phone. She heard Charles's rapid heavy descent on the stairs. It was twilight, and dusky indoors. She pulled the cord of the ceiling light. Her letter seemed to her to have a childish ring, and she beat her forehead, looking for a way to fix it. The motorcycle made a sudden racket and she heard her mother screeching from an upstairs window.

"Charles! Charles! Do you want to get killed? I said you're not to ride that motorcycle!"

"Am I riding it?" Charles shouted back indignantly. "Am I riding it?"

Millicent ran and leaned to the windows over the sinks. The motorcycle was roaring, its exhaust fiery in the dusk, and Charles was straddling it, but it was stationary.

Presently Charles returned to the house and Sudquist left. She heard him engage in old arguments with her parents in the living room.

"You want to be more than a mechanic," her father was telling him. "You want to be an engineer, and that means math, boy."

Outside she heard a bird saying whippoorwill. She crumpled the brown paper and went out the side door of the kitchen. She heard the call again at intervals, from the woods in back. She walked across the grass in the darkness, toward the point from which it seemed to come, but it stopped. She could hear the rustling of the trees, and the distant gurgling of Massapeequit Brook.

She felt a breeze, and turned and strolled in the yard, toward the big elm. Out front Patty and Roland were on the steps, and Millicent turned that way. They were arguing about whose fault it was that the old dog hadn't been fed. She climbed the steps past them, noticing as she did that Roland chewed a stem of grass.

Millicent rocked herself on the porch glider. She could see the nest of birds up in a corner of eaves.

"It's your turn," Patty said to Roland.

"I don't care—Mama told you to."

Millicent slapped at a mosquito. She watched Patty. Her sister often irritated her, yet she thought now that Patty had striking looks. She was tall and had a big frame, with green eyes, reddish chestnut hair, and clear skin.

Patty told Roland he was cruel to animals, and they argued about a jarful of grasshoppers that Patty had allowed to escape.

"It wasn't cruel," said Roland. "I had air holes in the cover. And they weren't all plain grasshoppers, either. There were some pretty rare species there."

"Oh, yeah, I bet," said Patty.

"There were. And if you do it again I'll make trouble." He appealed to Millicent. "You know what else she did?" he told her. "She took all my unmounted butterflies and dumped them in my trumpet. Busted wings and everything."

"We're not running a bughouse," said Patty.

"Yeah? Do you know I had one there that was good enough to be in a museum? And you wrecked it."

"Fish bait, probably," Patty said.

"It wasn't fish bait. It was a kind they don't even have around here. It came from South America or some place."

"Yeah," Patty said sceptically.

"Yeah. I'll show you right in a book."

"Yeah, you and your rare species. How'd it get up here then?"

"Ever hear of air currents, stupid?"

"Yes, stupid. And I don't believe it, stupid."

"All right, stupid. We're gonna find out who's stupid. This is the end."

"You're stupid. Why don't you learn something besides bugs?"

"Insects are important. There are more different species of insects than everything else put together."

"There are not."

"There are too. You ask any scientist. This is called the Age of Insects."

"You should have been one. And I'm gonna tell Mama you set a snare for a rabbit, too."

"So what. I didn't catch anything."

"If nobody else is going to feed Roger I will," Millicent said. She rose and went through the house to the kitchen.

She brought the dog his dinner. She found him on his old quilt, just inside the open door of the barn. She rubbed his head, and he worked his ears a little. She returned by way of the porch.

"I hope you didn't give him those bones," Patty said. "His teeth are no good."

"He can do what he wants with them," said Millicent. "He's got other things."

"Somebody ought to wash that dog, too," Roland said. "They won't let me give him a bath because he's too old, and he stinks."

"He doesn't stink half as bad as you do, with your onion grass," Patty said.

Her mother pushed open the screen door and looked about. The brownish light was behind her. "Is Charles out here?"

"No," said Millicent.

"He disappears, I don't know," her mother said. "I thought he went up again to study."

7

In the morning Millicent tried to write to Eugene. She sat on her bed with a little box of blue stationery, a leg tucked beneath her.

Dear Gene,

She wanted to ask his advice. She thought of telling him he didn't realize how much easier things were for a boy. A boy wouldn't take a filing job, or bother with typing and shorthand.

She put it in a drawer, with only the salutation written, when she went down to help her mother hang the wash. But when she came up again Patty held the little blue page and the drawer was open.

"Who's Gene?" Patty asked.

"Give me that!" Millicent said breathlessly, and rushed to snatch it. She crumpled it. "And get your things out of my bureau!" The tremolo in her voice was violent. "Get 'em in your own bureau!"

"I haven't got room!" Patty protested, sitting back on the iron cot.

But Millicent took a bulky sweater of Patty's from the white bureau and flung it sideways against Patty. "Here!"

"Hey!" said Patty, springing up as Millicent snatched up a fistful of another one. She tried to snatch Millicent's arm and the sweater with both hands, but Millicent elbowed her sharply. "Ooh you—!" Patty squealed, bringing down her fist in an axlike blow that missed, and as Millicent turned Patty fell upon her with her weight and her fists, eyes wild and moist, and Millicent tumbled to the floor between the iron cot and the carved bench of the dressing table. She fought back, and got at least one good punch in, to Patty's lip, but Patty came down upon her, straddling her, and brought down her beefy right fist as if pounding a table, pinning her shoulder meanwhile with the other hand. The blow glanced on Millicent's cheek and mouth, and the next one came like a mallet on the forearm that Millicent raised to fend it.

Millicent sobbed, and Patty relented, but with a self-satisfied expression. Patty rose and restored her sweaters to the third drawer of Millicent's bureau, folding, dusting, and smoothing with brisk motions. Millicent picked herself up, sobbing involuntarily. She sat cross-legged on the cot, not looking at Patty, and feeling the humiliation of impotent fury. It seemed utterly degrading to be beaten up by a sister who was six years her junior, even though taller and heavier and stronger. She touched the sore places in the briefest way, anxious that Patty not see her do so. She couldn't stop crying, even when she lay back and pretended to rest, looking at the ceiling. She wished she hadn't lost her temper. But Patty had no right to use Millicent's bureau, just because Patty was such a clotheshorse and had so much stuff. It meant that Patty at least had a bureau to herself, while Millicent's could always be rummaged in.

She would have gone down and appealed to her parents, except that continuing sobs kept disgracing her. She couldn't bear having the family know that Patty had drubbed her like a child.

This is the end, she told herself. She would have to get out of here, perhaps to a room at the Y. Living with these children was keeping her a child.

But she knew she couldn't get out.

She locked herself in the bathroom to wash her face and calm her nerves. She found no bruises.

At lunch she scarcely spoke to anyone. Then she went to the sofa with part of the Sunday paper.

But in time Patty came by. "Want to make up?" Patty offered. She said Polly Cook was supposed to go with her to Squonkamesset Pond, but now

Polly had to visit her grandmother instead. So she wondered if Millicent would like to go.

Millicent sighed, and did not answer immediately. Then she said she'd go on condition that Patty didn't bring her record player.

They rode together on the little brown bus, carrying a rolled blanket their father had had in the Navy, and their suits and towels in a shopping bag. They had to change buses in Sparkstown but it was a pleasant ride, and they saw cows grazing. She was grateful that Patty did not ask again who Gene was. Giving herself away like that had been the most childish thing of all, she thought.

She was a fair swimmer, taught by her mother, but she kept her nose out so as not to sneeze. She bobbed with a leisurely breast stroke, feeling the ripples about her face. Distances seemed great when seen from water level. If she could swim down under water like Patty, she thought, it would make for a peace and isolation.

She saw Patty's tall frame, high on the diving board. Patty leaped high, and made a big splash. The blinking head reappeared, the red hair dark and stringy now. She swam speedily, with a technique that kept her body relatively unsubmerged. Then the big thighs flexed up as though waving to the sky, and she slid from view like a whale.

They lay side by side on the Navy blanket, presenting their bodies to the sun with closed eyes. Some people sprawled nearby had a radio and after a time Patty sang softly with it.

> "—I'll play today and I'll sorrow tomorrow,
> Be gay while I may and I'll cry by and by."

Two boys sat down hard on either side of them and they started up. Millicent looked at a grinning face of perhaps seventeen years. His chest was all droplets and his sopping trunks oozed into the blanket. His friend was beside Patty.

"Go away!" Millicent ordered them. "At once! Or I'll call the guard."

The boys rose sheepishly. They walked down the beach without looking back.

"Aw, they were cute," Patty said.

"I thought we came to swim."

Millicent began to daub herself with lotion. Patty sat gazing after the boys, who were kicking sand now in a game of ball at some distance.

"Heck, I can't meet anybody with you around," said Patty.

"I'm not stopping you."

"They're all in pairs. What do you think I am?"

When they got home Aunt Celeste was there with Nan, and Millicent was told that the young undertaker had phoned and had said he'd call again.

When Millicent had changed she went down to the dining room where her mother sat doing the mending and talking with Aunt Celeste. Aunt Celeste was blond and squat. She looked tired and puffy-faced. Millicent sat, to be sociable, and Aunt Celeste said she knew of a nice boy, a neighbor of hers, that she could ask to call. He hadn't gone to college but he was very intelligent, and took courses, and was in business with his father in a hardware store. The whole family were lovely people. Not rich, but comfortable.

"I'd rather you didn't," Millicent said uneasily.

"Why?" her mother said, looking up. "Don't turn up your nose because he's a businessman. A businessman can read books and go to concerts too, you know." She returned to her sewing. "Some girl will appreciate him and grab him, and he'll probably make her very happy. Shower her with everything."

"I suppose you won't look at a man unless he's a college man," said Aunt Celeste.

"And what if Chester calls again tonight, when you're sitting at Aunt Gwen's," her mother asked her. "Shall I give him the number there?"

"No."

"Maybe it's just as well," said her aunt. "Let him think she's out."

"No," said her mother. "I'll say she's baby-sitting and I'll give him the number. It's the second time he's called today. He doesn't know if she's really out."

"Please—the grand strategy just embarrasses me," said Millicent. "We're not congenial and if he had any sense he'd know it."

"Boys know other boys, you know," said her mother. "Just because you don't like a boy, that's no reason. Through one boy you meet other boys. Young people go in groups. I may not have gone to college but I do know some things."

"Please—I'm not in the marriage market."

"Oh, don't be so independent! You can't just sit home!"

"I didn't know there was a law against it," she told her mother. Her voice was weak and shaky and she was blushing at the ears.

It bothered her too to have her little cousin Nan standing there silently, watching and listening. Poor Nan's already learning what it is to be female, she thought.

"And there's a Winkler boy," her mother said, "Mrs. Herzlinger's nephew. A professor at M.I.T. Studying for his Ph.D. Is that good enough for you at least? Or are you gonna turn him down too when he calls?"

"We'll see when he calls," she said shakily.

"It's too bad you went to college so far away," said Aunt Celeste. "That makes it hard. You have to get acquainted all over again."

"Well, you know my daughter," Lucinda told her. "She couldn't stay home and go to Wellesley or Radcliffe like other girls. No, she always has to be different. She had to go where nobody goes."

"Why don't you take evening courses at the Harvard Summer School," said Aunt Celeste. "Harvard should be a good place to meet people."

"Harvard doesn't have evening courses."

"Or a receptionist job—that's good for meeting people," her aunt said. "You know, I bet Steve could introduce you to boys. But I suppose a pharmacy college isn't a real college by you. According to you."

Later, when Aunt Celeste and Nan went home, they gave Millicent a lift, dropping her off in Boston at Aunt Gwendolyn's, as Millicent had promised to baby-sit.

The child was already in pajamas. She practiced her few words on Millicent, and then Millicent entered into her baby games, sitting on the rug and helping to fill a truck with blocks.

How identical with a little boy a girl of that age is, she reflected. Watching a boy or a girl play with blocks, you would not know one from the other. Their interests, their dexterity, they're all the same. The sexual difference is purely departmental, like their clothing and haircuts, and of little significance.

Up until a couple of years short of adolescence, a girl can still climb trees, climb the jungle gym, ride on rafts. But then her body and her clothing and society combine more and more to nag her, to convince her that the prime purpose of each generation is only to produce the next. As in the vegetable kingdom—no more sensible purpose than to scatter your seedlings and dry up.

Men were allowed to let the reproductive function be only a part-time one, she thought, as it ought to be. And that's why men were more stimulating—because they were more often doing things. The world of women was full of people not doing much. As the subjugated sex they become concerned with their roles as sexed creatures, whereas men could still be people part of the time.

The difficulty with men was to keep them acting like people when a woman is around, she said to herself. When a woman is around they often stop being people and start thinking of themselves as males, which is just as bad.

The baby fell asleep quickly, and Millicent looked for something to read. But her aunt's books were few and trashy. She wished she had brought a book of her own. She played the radio a while and listened to the news, but it was all bad. Two children had smothered in a refrigerator in Roxbury and North Korea had invaded South Korea. Next thing you know East Germany will invade West Germany, she said to herself. She had never thought that freezing those occupation zones into separate governments was a good idea. It had been bound to lead to this.

She slept the night at Aunt Gwendolyn's and walked to work from there in the morning.

When she got home, after the typing and shorthand, Chester had not telephoned again but he had sent flowers. Gladioli in pink, shading to yellow, rose tall and spreading from a slim wicker basket under an arching handle. They were stuffed around with ferns and tiny white and lavender auxiliary flowers she could not name. Her mother had stood the basket in the center of the dining-room table.

"He's certainly persistent," her mother said.

Millicent looked at it in silence.

"Do you think he had them left over from a funeral?" Roland asked the next morning, breakfasting in pajamas.

"Yeah," said Patty.

"No, I don't think so," said Lucinda. "The funeral parlor may have a cut-rate arrangement with a florist, or something. But I think it's very sweet. A lovely gesture. And I hope you appreciate it," she said to Millicent. "Nobody ever sent me any flowers."

Millicent ate a little of the breakfast without answering. Then she asked whether the North Korean invasion would be the start of World War Three.

"No," both her parents answered quickly.

"We ought to drop a few atom bombs," said Roland. Millicent saw her father glance at him.

"They ought to drop one on you," Patty said to Roland.

"All right, let's drop the subject," said her mother. "Everybody. Including Millicent."

The Model T did not start easily on wet mornings and by the time Charles tooted for her the drizzling rain was like a dewy sweat on his sad face, on the close-cropped blondish head, and on the shaker sweater full of holes. She got in beside him with her shoulder-strap bag.

"You're all filthy greasy," she said. "Do you go to school like that?"

"I'll wash when I get there," he said. "We're late."

He seemed more depressed than usual, and talked to her all the way into Boston, calling her Sis and occasionally Cockeyes. He said Mother was against Sudquist because Sudquist had quit school. Just like in Brighton she had wanted him to go around with a kid called Norbert because Norbert got A's. Sudquist could have gotten him a job in Moon's Garage.

And what he needed, he said, was to get his hands on that first hunk of capital. He had another chance for a job now. A friend of Sudquist's by the name of MacFarland worked for a Boston newspaper as a copy boy, but he was getting drafted.

"They won't let you," said Millicent.

"Why not?" he said. "It won't interfere with school. It's the night shift. I could study on the job—it's mostly sitting around. And two days off in the middle of the week—you work weekends." He said he had no interest in the newspaper business itself, because newspapers had no future—he only wanted to save enough dough to buy an old truck. "Once you own that first piece of capital equipment," he said, " like if I could get my hands on a truck, you've got something to start expanding with. You're not just peddling your time by the hour. And a loan on the first truck buys the second. Guys have ended as millionaire road builders starting like that. Or they clear land, and lease it for industry."

"Why don't you think newspapers have a future?"

"They're not expanding, Sis. No newspaper stock is rated as a growth stock any more."

She was impressed by the way his mind worked. She barely knew about growth stocks, let alone thought of them as a guide to where one ought to seek employment. And Charles was only seventeen.

He let her out in downtown Boston and she walked the few blocks to her building thinking of him. She felt he was a boy who turned loose in the world would grow rich. Perhaps he was right, and her parents were wrong to think success stemmed from formal schooling. She remembered a time when her father asked him what he would do if he suddenly needed calculus, and Charles had replied that he would hire someone who knew calculus.

It occurred to her for the first time that perhaps Charles saw things much as she did—the activity of the nation was like a working system, and when you were young, a beginner, a child, the nation's activity was a closed economy that you were outside of. You had to find a way to break into it, and that beginning, that claiming of a share, was not easy. It had all its own connections already, functioning without you, and no loose ends.

Even so, she thought, her parents were right in not letting him do anything that would interfere with summer school. They had spent a lot of money on it, that they could scarcely afford. He had better try to get into college while he could. She still felt the Korean fighting could expand into a World War, because it seemed to her the United States would have to intervene. She was surprised that the radio stations and newspapers did not yet foresee this.

There were no phone calls for her that night. Chester's bouquet was still in the living room, and she looked forward to its withering, so that her mother would let her throw it into the garbage.

The next night her mother said a lady from the Young Women's Republican Club had phoned and had asked if Millicent baked. But both her parents seemed agitated, and upstairs Patty told her they had had a terrible fight with Charles. He had gone and applied for the newspaper job after school and actually worked a couple of hours, phoning home to explain where he was. "Were they ever furious!" Patty said. "Mama even spoke to the city editor, and they made him quit and come home witout any supper. Boy, they were so mad they'd have taken his car away. Except that he needs it to go to school."

Millicent went down in her pajamas for a glass of milk. Her mother was in the kitchen in a bathrobe, but Millicent did not ask about Charles.

Charles was bitter next morning when he told her the story on the way to Boston.

For some miles he grew silent. Then he told her that even in the country there were ways of making a living. "Take that guy Featherstone, that pumped the cesspool. He's got the whole cesspool business, all over town, with no competition, and he does plowing for the town, and his whole investment's only a few thousand. And besides he's Tree Warden. He makes a decent living without killing himself and he doesn't punch a time clock. And he grows his own food. Waits for jobs, that's all. And he's got time to go in the woods in the middle of the week and shoot himself a pheasant."

"Does he have a family?"

"Sure he has a family."

Somehow the thought of applying herself for the newspaper job crossed her mind. She dismissed it, but it came back while she worked with Miss Bancroft, and more and more strongly in the afternoon. The weather was sweltering and

Mr. Durfee sat red-faced in shirt sleeves, his eyes closed, fanning himself with a paper booklet.

Directly after work she looked for the newspaper Charles had spoken of. She felt a little frightened. She didn't know if they took girls in such jobs, and besides she would never catch up in shorthand after skipping like this. Yet it seemed that they must have needed someone urgently to have put Charles to work immediately, and her best chance was to apply at once and hope they had not had time to find someone new.

The streets were still hot, though the sunlight was turning orange. She paused only to open her shoulder-strap purse and comb her hair, bending at a gum-slot mirror.

The newspaper turned out to be in brick buildings of an old type—five stories with roof slanting back at the top—and curved along a bend in a narrow main street where the traffic moved one way only. At street level there were blackboards, where news flashes had been chalked for public viewing, and middle-aged newsboys hawked all four of the Boston papers. Directly across was one of the rival papers.

The elevator was old-fashioned, encaged all around, and a pudgy old man slammed the gate open and shut again. There was a steady, rhythmic rumble overhead that she thought must be the presses. The sound excited her.

She stepped into what seemed a maze of angular corridors, made by partitions of wood and stippled glass that did not go quite to the ceiling. The gate of the elevator shut behind her. She stumbled down three little steps, and when she looked about she realized that old buildings of different levels had been joined. Two boys of her own age or younger were fooling at a drinking fountain, spitting mouthfuls of water upon one another. She asked again for the city editor and one of them pointed down a corridor that had a bend in it, belching water upon his friend and laughing. She passed disdainfully, close to the wall.

The room she came into was large and long, with many desks, not all facing the same way, and none of them neat. Lights hung from the ceiling by black cords, some with conical shades of green glass and some plain bulbs, all of them on though it was still day. Down the middle a row of columns made of painted pipe supported the ceiling, and at one of them a big dictionary rested open on a stand. At the far end some chest-high machines stood in a row and chattered with an incessant clicking. Only a few of the desks were occupied, and near her a great pear-shaped man with a drooping mustache sat frowning into a typewriter.

She cleared her throat. "Excuse me," she asked him. "Can you tell me where I can find the city editor?"

He glared up at her, hunched, with eyes close together. The mustache was fairly big and hung around his mouth. He tossed a finger and returned to his typing.

"Oh." She turned. "Thank you."

The man he had pointed to sat behind a catercorner desk across the room, and leaned far back in a swivel chair holding a phone to his ear. "Yeah—yeah—" he was saying peevishly.

She cleared her throat, turning again to the man with the mustache. "Excuse me, may I bother you again, please? Can you tell me his name, please?"

"Killian," he said without looking up. She noticed that he typed with only two fingers.

She moved to wait near Mr. Killian. She allowed herself to lean a little on a vacant desk behind her, but then decided it was more proper to stand erect. His free hand was reaching down into his shirt behind his neck and scratched his back. A great shock of brown hair was swept sideways across his head, but stuck up slightly as though magnetized.

"You want to see me?" he asked, catching Millicent's eye and taking the phone an inch from his ear.

"Yes—"

But he plunged back into the phone conversation. A foot was on an open bottom drawer of the desk, and he used it to rock the swivel chair. He seemed to be arguing with someone. He kept running a hand through the shock of hair.

She saw his eyes glance for an instant at her chest, and it irritated her. Always even the most respectable and courteous of men would manage to flick their eyes that way even as though unaware of it, elderly men and young boys—her father and her brothers even—she had been accustomed to it since before she was twelve. She felt it was a meaningless thing and yet a nasty thing, as though a man must always remember that you're of the so-called weaker sex, not simply a person. Even if he meant nothing lascivious, his eye must check your breasts as if they were a yellow badge.

He played with a spindle that had been stabbed through some papers—his fingers held the point and its iron base rolled like a wheel on his desk, behind a row of reference books. At last he put down the phone and met her eyes.

"What," he said.

She stepped nearer, feeling her heartbeat. Her mouth was dry. "Mr. Killian, I'm Millicent Audrey Gordon. I'm the sister of Charles Gordon—you know—that couldn't take the job yesterday? The copy-boy job?" Her voice sounded faint in her ears. She swallowed. "I'd like to apply. If you haven't got anybody yet."

He creaked back in his swivel chair, a foot on the drawer and his hands behind his head. She could hear the steady clicking down the room and the rhythmic rumbling, still above her. "You're his kid sister?" he said.

"His older sister."

"You got working papers?"

"I'm twenty-one years old." She felt the blush beginning.

"Twenty-one?" The way he stared humiliated her. "You got a driver's license?"

"No."

"You look about fourteen."

"I'm not. I'm twenty-one. I'm a graduate of the University of Chicago."

He kept leaning back and staring.

"Will you give me a chance?" she said. She felt hot.

He rocked forward, put his arms on the desk and no longer stared. "Well, we don't hire women."

"I see at least one woman," she said. There was a skinny little lady, visibly rouged, at a typewriter far back.

"Oh, well, Maud. Maud's been here for years."

"Why don't you hire people by their ability," Millicent said, her voice quaking. "And their willingness to work, and learn. It's not fair."

"What experience do you have?"

"I can learn. And you were willing to give my brother a chance, and he's got no experience. Just because he's a boy. I can do anything he can do. And I've got four years more education than he has."

"Well, look, I'll tell you why. Suppose for instance I was short of reporters, and I had to send the copy boy out. Now, could I send you to cover a union meeting of longshoremen?"

"Why not?" she said red-faced.

He glanced up and down tiredly. "Well, you don't see why not, but I see why not."

"What else is involved," she said. "Besides longshoremen?"

"Well, you keep up with the copy, you take it up to the printers. You go out for food, coffee. You go around the city and give the outside men their checks. You go to Police Headquarters. You go to the A.P., U.P., pick up photos. And City Hall. The State House."

"I'm sure I could do that. And I'm not afraid of longshoremen."

"All right, all right," he said with a tone of exasperated impatience. "I've got your number if I want you. The same as your brother's, right?"

"Yes."

"Okay. So long." He turned to some work on his desk.

She started out, downcast. She wondered in what way the longshoremen disqualified her—whether he meant they might molest a young woman, or be obscene, or were simply prejudiced against giving news to female newspaper employees, or what.

"Hey!" Mr. Killian said.

She turned at the door.

"When can you start?" he asked her.

It occurred to her to say right now. But it would be unfair to give Miss Bancroft no notice at all. "Monday?" she asked, quavering.

"All right. Be here Monday."

There was still time for the shorthand class, if she rushed, though not for the typing. But she felt like giving herself a holiday. The sticky heat had given way to a lovely evening breeze. She ate, spending a whole dollar carelessly.

Her family was not as excited as she had expected them to be. But she lay happily in the darkness a long time. She heard the whippoorwill again. The frogs were not making the high-pitched chirping of spring any more but now and then she heard a frog sound a solitary bung, like the tuning of an instrument.

"Do you wear your garter belt over your panties or under your panties?" Patty asked from the larger bed.

There was some distant thunder.

What her parents had not grasped, Millicent thought, was how this journalistic opportunity was in fact an opening into politics. She saw herself a few years hence, sternly asking questions, reducing a shifty-eyed mayor from arrogance to humility, and then exposing venality in black headlines. She cast the glassy-eyed man from the political club in the role.

"Denise wears them under," said Patty. "Denise Saint-Onge. Pretty stupid, *I* think."

Millicent saw herself telling the humbled politician never again to turn away a young person who wanted to serve. A political party is an opportunity for service, she was explaining to him, not a private preserve. And if your career doesn't consist in service, then you're consuming and giving nothing in return. Which means, sir, that you're not part of the world's work, and hence not part of the world, but only a bystander.

"Polly and I have got a deal that we tell each other everything we do with a boy," said Patty.

Millicent tried not hear her.

"Did you ever have a deal like that?" Patty asked.

"No."

"There hasn't been anything yet because we just started," Patty said.

Millicent tried to follow her own train of thought.

"Do you think I can trust her not to hold back anything?" Patty asked.

Millicent settled deeper in the sheets. She was undecided whether, having cleaned up the corruption, she would move on to Washington as a correspondent, or leave journalism at that point to run for Congress. Her fame would be at a crest just then, and make either course possible. Perhaps she could do both at once, each career giving insights into the other. She wondered if anyone had ever thought of that. What had happened to her today could be the most important event of her life.

"Hey," Patty said. "Millicent."

"What."

"Aren't you gonna answer?"

"What."

"Should I trust Polly? I mean would you if you were in my place?"

"Oh, really, Patty, I'm not interested in things like that."

"Aw."

There had been more thunder, and now it began to rain. For a long time she listened to it. She could hear a symphony of drippings from different corners of eaves. She might even be sent to Korea as a correspondent if the fighting continued. A mosquito sang now and then in her ear, but she could not catch it. Patty snored in a soft bubbly way. What a tub of lard Patty is, she thought.

She awoke earlier than usual. She heard the neighbor's rooster. Then she heard ducks. She believed she could distinguish now which were the wild ones in the marsh and which were the farm ones. She clicked off the little alarm clock she kept on Patty's dressing table, though it hadn't yet rung. In a while she heard her father go downstairs to say his prayers and check the mousetraps. Journalism was not just the glamour of exposing corruption, she told herself. There were humdrum things to be brought to light day by day. The condition of people in the slums. The whole labor of human destiny begged for her contribution.

She mentioned it to Charles on the way to Boston.

"I know it," he said. "I've always believed in you, Sis. I think you're gonna go far."

When she got to the office she approached Miss Bancroft's desk guiltily. "Miss Bancroft, I've come to a decision," she began.

She saw that Miss Bancroft at once grasped the ominous nature of this phrase. The old lady tightened her mouth and became nearly rigid but for a slight fluttery shaking. Her color flushed as Millicent explained, but she looked only at the desk and her hands, refusing to meet Millicent's face. At last there was a silence.

"I know it's not very fair to you," Millicent added uncomfortably.

"Why do you do it then?" the old lady said nervously, her hands fidgeting about, but she still kept her eyes down.

"I mean I feel terrible especially about leaving before the change-over's finished."

"You won't get anywhere being a rolling stone," said Miss Bancroft. "I know what they used to say when I was young. 'If a task is once begun, do not leave it till it's done. Be the labor great or small, do it well or not at all.' "

"Well, I just can't afford not to take this opportunity, Miss Bancroft," Millicent said, her voice shaking. "I'd feel lots better if you'd try to understand my position."

"Terrible people work on newspapers. Especially at night."

"But I might not ever be so lucky another time. You know how hard it is for women."

"And what'll you do—walk through the streets to North Station after midnight?" Miss Bancroft's hands moved nervously and her head quivered but she still would not look at Millicent.

"Well, I don't know. If the subway isn't running I suppose I'll take a taxi if I have to."

"I don't know if it's even legal to quit before the agency's got its fee."

"Isn't it? Well, I don't know, I'll have to look into that. Isn't it legal, Miss Bancroft? Really?"

"Well, I don't know." Miss Bancroft's fingers moved about as though looking for something she couldn't find. "I should think it mightn't be."

"Well, I'll find out," Millicent said. "I think my father would know."

Miss Bancroft remained agitated, her lips parted, panting quietly. But the silence was so long that it seemed possible to leave her desk without being rude.

Millicent moved to her filing, opening a drawer nearby. She felt the burden of disappointment she had brought to the poor woman.

"It's just not possible to get good help these days," she heard her say. "Not these days. It's too bad too, because you're still young enough to learn good habits. I didn't think you were one of these flighty ones." Miss Bancroft touched a crumpled pink handkerchief to each eye and each nostril. "Ding bust it."

8

Okay," Ed Gordon said to his sons, "let's say grace." He began the Grace After Meals from memory, seated at the end of the long unpainted kitchen table. Charles and Roland gave the opening responses. Charles started muttering the wrong one but heard Roland's clear voice and corrected himself. Ed proceeded, watching the boys and at first pronouncing carefully, as if to encourage them to follow. But he had not the energy to push them tonight, and in a moment he continued more quietly and rapidly. Meanwhile his hands listlessly and absent-mindedly helped to clean his end of the table. With a butter knife he scraped some crumbs from the wood into a saucer, still saying the grace, and stacked his dishes and handed them to Millicent, who was clearing the table.

"Here, stupid, it's your turn to wipe," Patty said, tossing a towel that landed on Roland's front.

"I haven't finished grace yet," Roland told her without moving.

"Well say it faster," she said.

When Ed finished he rose. Roland asked him if he could have a fishing rod.

"Have you got a place to fish?" Ed asked.

"Massapeequit Brook."

"What do you catch there? Catfish?"

"Oh, there's minnows and stuff."

"Well, I'll shop around," Ed said. "Why don't you see if you can make one meanwhile."

"Come on, Roland," Lucinda said. "Boys have to know how to do dishes too."

Ed stepped out into the yard, and the screen door sprang shut behind him. The sun was not yet down. He was expected to sit in at a meeting of the executive board at the temple, and intended to walk there for the exercise. But it was not time to go yet. He contemplated his log pile, stacked by the barn, and the ax with which he had been working in the afternoon. But he did not want to exercise again directly after supper. Down where his dirt driveway met the road there was a wide gate of wood set into the little wall of boulders on stone pillars, but the hinges were rusted and the bottom one broken, so that the gate hung permanently open, its end wedged in the earth. He had not decided whether to repair it or remove it altogether. He walked down there and smoked a cigarette, looking at the cracked hinge, rough with rust, and listening to the whippoorwill. Without looking at the sun he saw its color on the granite change and disappear. At last he turned, and walked toward town on the black of the road, where it merged with the dirt.

There's something about a house, he mused. It's not like an apartment. His grandfather had had a house.

He had been glad of the opening in Wilmerding Crosswalk. The town itself was old and pleasing, though the congregation there was new, made up mostly of families that had gone there since the war. An accountant named Conrad Bernstein and some of his friends had started a community center and Sunday school, which grew, meeting first in the homes of members and then renting the dance hall next to the Masonic rooms over the supermarket. They acquired some land, where a street running out from the Square began to fade into fields, and began to build. This spring at last they had opened their temple, and hired Ed as their first rabbi. It was a bottom story only, of stucco, half sunk in the ground, and like his previous temples it had no organ, which disappointed Patty, since she wanted to play on one, but they hoped to raise a handsome main structure above it in ten or twenty years. Ed admired their initiative, and they seemed pleased to have found a mature man at their price, rather than a raw kid out of the seminary.

It was Lucinda who had insisted on a big house with land, rather than a smaller and newer place in the town itself. It was further from the temple than he would have liked it, but she said he could pursue his studies there. And he did have a scholarly project in mind. He had wanted for a long time to compile a huge master index, so that you could find out at a glance whatever light the various ancient and modern commentaries shed on any given subject.

He felt that in the past twenty years of his life he had accomplished little. Before coming here he had had an assistantship in a huge congregation in urban Brighton, only a few miles from downtown Boston. He was passed over when the man above him retired, but he stayed on there nevertheless as assistant several more years, until a few months ago when Bernstein's group interviewed him. And before Brighton, right after the Navy, he had gone for a year to a congregation out in Abbotsford, Mass., where there were mountains. The house had been smaller than here, with the upstairs all dormers, but Lucinda had learned to drive there, and though a city girl she loved the openness. She had hated to give up the garden when they left. Ed had become friendly with the widowed old Methodist minister down the road, who was caring for a thirty-year-old son just released from a mental hospital. But the pretty little clapboard temple there was full only on the High Holy Days—the rest of the time it was a phantom congregation. He had hoped briefly at first for some gesture toward daily prayer, and settled a week later for Sabbaths only, but only six men came, and finally one Sabbath morning only himself. Except on the anniversary of the death of some member's parent, it was impossible to scrape together a service. He was hardly more than a children's teacher. And it bothered him to teach little children about communal religious practices as though they were real and extant, when in fact they were never performed. Meanwhile, all these years, he studied and began to putter on his index project. But all that he had done that was worth doing seemed like six years' worth, or eight—it was impossible to account satisfactorily for twenty.

And already Charles, with all his years ahead of him, was headed wrong, flunking the subjects he needed. How could he make Charles know that in twenty years he will not regret having done nothing—he will regret that what he accomplished in twenty years could have been done in ten.

If the boy doesn't get into college, so you tell him it's no disgrace. But how do you give him that male unrest that makes for ambition, and at the same time not let him think his laziness or his failures disappoint you?

At thirteen Charles had rigged a transformer from a toy electric train to charge the battery of an automobile—that was how smart, how precocious the kid was.

Ed wanted to see Charles acknowledged and efficient in the career to which his talent pointed—in some branch of engineering. And at the same time, of course, as a man who knew and practiced his religion quite thoroughly. It had always seemed to Ed more pious somehow to be an amateur religionist than a professional one. His grandfather's synagogue had had no rabbi—one member or another took a turn leading the service, and if he loused it up the others interrupted him.

Ed walked the length of Massapeequit Road, under a high-roofed tunnel of arching trees, to where new houses came closer together, and then big square Victorian ones, and sidewalks began. It merged in a fork with Washington Street and took him over a small stone bridge and alongside Caleb Folger's church. The black-and-gold clock high on the white spire still caught the daylight, and he saw he was still on time. He crossed the long rectangular green of Murphy Square diagonally, past the Civil War obelisk with its old-style base and its lists of names.

The towering elms and the ancient cemetery sloping uphill beside Folger's church made for a quietness.

There was scarcely anyone around, except the teen-agers in Yerxa's Pharmacy and Bingle's Cookery. There was a light in the Hand Laundry, but the shops alongside it were dark, as were the supermarket and the doors of the fire station beyond. Far down the green he saw that a stand had already been raised for reviewing the Fourth of July parade, but now it was empty and dim.

He had thought of joining the volunteer firemen. He still had his tools and he could tune their motors. A few weeks before, as the result of a chance encounter, he had repaired Father Donahue's bicycle. The priest was an aging physical-culture enthusiast, and as the Most Precious Blood Parish covered the entire town and part of another the old priest pedaled a lot. Ed's fixing the bike seemed to have made a tremendous impression on everybody, and especially on his own congregation.

He had the feeling that the rest of his life would unfold here. He would like over the years to make this congregation a rich community, culturally and spiritually, that would link the past to the future. It was like being responsible for everyone in town. And he was sure that people who worked so hard for a brand new building did not mean to leave it empty—the one at Abbottsford had after all been built by the deceased parents of the present people. It had been Conrad Bernstein's inspiration to purchase traditional prayer books and reform ones also, using the reform ones on Friday evenings only, and avoiding affiliation, so as to please everybody. But above all, the congregation was larger than at Abbottsford. So even if lack of interest set in the hard core should still amount to a quorum for a prayer service.

Of course things hadn't really gotten going yet. He had come when summer was approaching and everything slacked off.

The wooden houses along Muckanaug Street and along the side streets that ran from it were narrow, close together, and out of date, but just past Sumner Street they petered out, and after a weedy corner lot he came upon the broad flat-roofed stucco temple, seemingly half sunk in a gentle slope of ground. In the plot of new grass before it a high flagpole arose. There were some cars parked. Ed followed the walk to the side door, and went down the corridor, not to the main hall where services were held but to one of the smaller rooms at the back. A light was on, and some of the executive board were already at the varnished table.

"Hello, Ed," said Conrad Bernstein.

"Hi, Ed," said Phil Walker, and they all greeted him. Ed took a chair. Phil's wife Sandy was there, her hair held loosely back by a ribbon, and Amethyst Gilbert, the Sisterhood president, neat and tailored, wearing purple-framed glasses that rose to points at their outer edges. Roy Herzlinger was there, a large, graying, executive-looking distributor of drugs and chemicals, whose Boston office was wholesaler to all New England, and Murray Spingarn, bald, owlish, flat-nosed and black-jowled, of the Peggy Jane Style Shop in Sparkstown.

They sat talking and waiting for others to arrive. Phil offered Ed a cigarette and someone slid an ashtray down the table to him. Conrad said Burt Seligman couldn't make it.

It crossed Ed's mind that he should make this room into a library. He could also have some of the adult education classes here, and even the older children's classes. This table would be good for seminars.

There was an architect's drawing, framed on the wall, showing how the temple would look years hence when the top was built, and the conversation turned to it. Phil Walker twisted about to look at it, leaning with an arm over the back of his chair. He was curly-haired, with wide brows curving over eyes far apart and a turned-up nose. As chairman of the building fund and vice-president he was familiar with the drawing, and explained that the idea was that it shouldn't be show-offy. They chatted a while about what inscription would be nice on the stone lintel, and Phil Walker and Murray Spingarn had an argument as to where *Love Thy Neighbor As Thyself* came from.

" 'Thou shalt love thy neighbor as thyself'—that's Leviticus," Ed told them. "Chapter nineteen."

"See what did I tell ya?" Walker said to Spingarn. "It's perfectly kosher."

Mr. Dembitz arrived, an elderly man with a large head, who ran the Superette grocery with his son down in Wilmerding Mills. His clothes hung on him. They talked about landscaping, and whether trees should be planted in the fall or the spring.

Mr. Herzlinger suggested to Conrad that they get started. Conrad looked at his watch and said he didn't think anyone else was coming. "Madam secretary, will you read the minutes of the last meeting?" he asked Sandy Walker.

Sandy opened her notebook and began to read from the last membership meeting instead of the executive meeting. She caught herself, running her tongue out in a girlish way, and began afresh. Her voice was faint and raspy, and she tried to clear her throat garglingly, with comic expressions, touching her fingers to her neck. Ed watched her. Her summer dress was scooped wide and low, and her bosom was full of freckles, but soft-looking and nice. Mrs. Walker was prettier than Mrs. Gilbert, Ed thought. Amethyst had a sculptured face, and her brown hair was pulled up and convoluted tastefully, but her mouth was her only really attractive feature. When she smiled her teeth rested on a delicate lower lip that turned down at the corners. She had pancake make-up that seemed to Ed to have a tinge of lavender.

"Can we do anything about that constant drip?" Amethyst said. The adjoining room was a kitchen.

Mr. Spingarn rose and tried to tighten the faucet, but couldn't.

"I've got some washers at the house," said Ed. "I'll take care of it during the week."

"Naw, you don't have to do that," Conrad told him. He had a narrow face and high forehead, with metal-rimmed glasses.

"Let Conrad do it," Amethyst said. "The building's his baby." Her voice was quite deep.

Sandy hadn't finished reading, so she made another of her joking little throat clearings and continued. Conrad leaned back watching her, his long skinny fingers together over the tattersall vest. There were lines in his face, and Ed guessed his age as forty. Phil Walker seemed scarcely thirty-five.

The business of the meeting was to authorize Conrad to hire a cantor without calling a membership meeting of the whole congregation. They had hoped to try out a few cantors at the spring membership meeting, but they could not get any to try out. But now, Conrad explained, there was a guy down in New York, well recommended, that they could get for six thousand, provided they grabbed him before anybody else did.

When it was settled they sat talking of other things. Conrad noted that the

Sparkstown radio station had invited Ed to give some one-minute prayer spots. Also, the ladies' auxiliaries and ladies' guilds of some of the local churches had for some years been combining in a midsummer rummage sale and carnival, down on the field known as the old Pigs Gusset Indian Reservation, and this year they had invited the temple Sisterhood to join them. Phil Walker offered to donate a freezer that could be raffled.

"New, or out of your stock?" Mr. Dembitz asked idly.

"New! What do ya mean, what do ya think. It's not a floor sample. Sure it's out of stock."

"This year's model?" Spingarn asked.

"Last year's model."

Roy Herzlinger suggested to Conrad that the meeting be adjourned.

As the group separated under the street lamp Amethyst Gilbert offered Ed a ride part way home. Her car was large and black and polished. It would have seemed unsociable to say no.

They rode a little without conversation, her gloved hand turning the steering wheel at the Square. At last she asked him how he liked living here, and how his family liked it.

She remarked on the beauty of his four children. "The plump girl has an extremely pretty face," she said, "—Patty, I think you call her."

"Yeah, Patty's a good kid," he answered her. "Outgoing. She makes friends."

At the fork Amethyst took Massapeequit Road, saying she might as well take him all the way. Ed remarked that it was out of her way, but she said it was all right.

She drove slowly, and trees passed overhead.

"'It's wonderful the way they're all spaced three years apart," Amethyst said.

"Well, just about."

"Twenty-one, eighteen, fifteen, and twelve, aren't they?"

"Well, Charles'll be eighteen. And Rollo's twelve in August."

"Beautifully planned. You must have been able to have a baby any time you wanted."

"Ya, I guess we did."

"Just like that. Some people have it, I guess. I wish you'd give Marvin a few lessons."

Ed said nothing, and her wistful pleasantry hung on the air, in bad taste.

"We've tried everything," she explained. "And they tell us there's nothing physically wrong."

"Well, keep trying."

"I'm thirty-five," she said. "I don't have too many more years."

The conversation lapsed a few moments. They rocked easily over the bumps. The car was lush and smooth-riding.

"I'm terribly unfulfilled," she said.

He searched for an answer. But before he found it she began.

"You have such good-looking children. Well, it's no wonder, I guess." Her voice became low and murmuring. "Everybody says you're really too good-looking to be a rabbi."

She drove watching the road. He did not look at her either.

"Except you ought to wear a more ivy-league style of ties," she purred. "Would you like me to pick out some ties?"

"No—"

"Marvin has a charge at Brooks."

"No, don't pick out any ties."

"How did you get into it?"

"What?"

"Into being a rabbi."

"Well—"

"Was your father a rabbi?"

"No. No, I'm the first in the family, as far as I know. My father was in the musical-instrument business."

"Oh, Gordon's—of course," she said. "In Boston. Was that your father's?"

"Yeah. My brothers have it now."

"But you must have been raised very strictly."

"No, not especially. I was brought up like any kid, more or less."

"Was Lucinda's family religious?"

"No, except residually a little."

"Then what changed you? Something had to make you religious."

"Well, I came to it by degrees, I guess. You begin to study, you know, a bit of Talmud, or a little bit of Midrash, out of loyalty, and at first you expect a hodgepodge. You think it's gonna be hard to justify intellectually. And then you find it's not. It's extremely subtle, and put together by very sophisticated men, and when you discover that, it's a shock."

"This is your place, isn't it?" she said. They had arrived at Ed's dirt driveway, and the closed white gate stopped them. The headlights shone on it.

"There's no sense in taking me up the driveway," he said. "I'd have to get out to open the gate here anyway. So thank you." The door handle clicked under his hand.

"Tell me more," Amethyst said, and shut off the motor.

"Tell you what?"

"Well, everything," she said. "What religion means to you."

"It means everything to me." He paused, sitting in the car.

Her question was thin and vague, but nevertheless it was not one that he wished to slight.

"This might sound crazy to you," he began slowly, "but the last few years I've come around more and more to the feeling that a minyan is the one situation that hasn't got lonesomeness in it."

He saw her nod a little, gravely, in the scant light that the gate and the grasses reflected back from the headlights.

"The people you love most, they don't know what's in your heart," he said. "Or you strike up an acquaintance with a guy and you swap stories—and you still know his world isn't yours. But ten, eleven, twelve guys that got together for a few minutes to pray—maybe you don't know their names, or they're not your background, not your generation, not your type. But the fact remains, ten strangers looked for each other to face the Almighty with. To ask: what is this—what are You doing—let us live. For that moment we're in the same boat—it's acknowledged. Those guys, without talking to them, and without trying to reach them, you reach. In that moment there's no loneliness."

He saw Amethyst wet her lips. "I would have thought you and Lucinda are perfectly suited," she said.

Her use of his remark irritated him.

"Well, that's not the point," he said. "You can be the ideal couple, and still one of you has to die before the other."

"How old are you, Ed?"

"Forty-four."

"That's young."

"No it's not. Girls I necked with in high school have been grandmothers already."

They sat thoughtfully a moment.

He cleared his throat. He thought perhaps he could depart now without seeming rude. But Amethyst began to talk, as if to prolong the conversation. "Were you religious when you necked?" she asked.

"I suppose I was. I always was."

"And why does one boy, out of so many boys, get a religious calling, or whatever it is? That's what I was asking. Why you and not your brothers."

"I don't know," he said. "You're somewhat religious yourself, aren't you?"

"Somewhat."

"There are actually two questions," he said, "—why was I religious, and why did I go into the pulpit. And if you ask the first I can't tell you. It seemed natural to me. I remember once when I was a kid, I had to do an errand for my grandmother in Roxbury—and I found the umbrella fixer leading a dozen men in their afternoon prayer in the back of the butcher shop, and I had to wait for them to finish before I could buy anything. No clergy, no temple, no treasurer's report, no rummage sale, no trust fund—just these men working along the block there who used to take a few minutes for daily worship. That was a living culture, you know. And it would have hurt me to see it evaporate, especially by my own remissness. And as for being a rabbi—well, there were reasons against it. I was in the used-car business when I got married, studying nights, hoping to teach history or something, but in time the reasons against it seemed less important."

"What reasons against it?"

"Well, I wasn't sure whether it would bring me closer to people, and closer to my children, or set me further apart. You know, a lot of people seem to find it hard to appreciate that a minister, or a rabbi, or a priest is a human being. Or it used to seem so. But the reasons develop as you get into it, I guess. It wasn't an overnight thing."

"You seem very human to me, Ed," she said. The low voice was huskily warm.

He saw her eyes on him through the pointed glasses.

"Well, I guess I better be going," she said. "Marvin might be jealous."

Her mouth made the pretty smile.

"But I guess I'm safe with you," she added.

He let himself out, not sure whether her words deserved an answer. "You're safe," he said.

They bid each other good night and he thanked her again. The glowing tail lights circled and departed.

He walked up the dirt road. He was annoyed with her for turning to these absurd flirtings. What kind of play-acting did she want from him? There was something sad about her having to do that.

It was true that some of the conversation he had enjoyed. He had given expression to a thought or two more successfully than he could at home. But he was old enough to realize, he said to himself, that the reason a woman you're not married to is so agreeable to talk to is that you're not forced to take her seriously. He felt sure that Amethyst's husband was not to be envied. Lucinda had her dissatisfactions and her marital disappointments, but she had too much natural dignity to twitter about them abroad.

From the lighted windows above the porch roof he guessed that Lucinda was already preparing for bed. He went to the cellar and set the mousetraps.

Upstairs he found Lucinda in bed with a magazine. She wore her reading glasses.

"Whose car were you sitting in so long?" she asked.

"Amethyst Gilbert. She felt like talking."

He began preparing for bed.

"Ed—" she said.

"What."

"We've just got to get a decent living-room rug. I mean it. That old oriental is a sight. We can put it in your study if you want, but I want a nice high pile for the living room in case the children want to sit on the floor. And if we can't afford it I'm gonna make one. I saw an ad. They send you materials and directions and everything."

"When do they ever sit on the floor?" he asked.

"Well, the girls will be entertaining boys, you know. Having parties."

"They have to entertain them on the floor? What kind of a party is that? What are they gonna do on the rug that they can't do on chairs?"

Lucinda talked more about the rug, but he said nothing further.

When he was ready he got under the covers. She was still reading and the tilted lampshade cast its yellow light. On the wall was the watercolor portrait his twin sister Rosalind had done of him.

He ran a foot playfully along Lucinda's leg.

"Ouch!" she said. "Damn it. Cut your toenails for God sakes. That's why I'm darning socks all the time."

He rolled away from her and let her read. He shut his eyes. He heard the footsteps of one of the children and the closing of the bathroom door.

Once he turned and looked at Lucinda's profile. Then he rolled back again and tried to sleep. She's still a remarkably good-looking woman, he thought. He had married Lucinda Piper when she was nineteen and he was twenty-one. He had seen himself as romantic and in love then. And perhaps as the founder of a great family. But it had not taken long to discover that husbands and wives don't really have conversations. Even if it had been possible, there was rarely the time.

Often she had seemed to feel he was a nut, and his life's work a fraud. As though the protestations of a clergyman, like those of a used-car dealer, must be taken with reservations. Yet he knew she was loyal. She was glad he was a professional man, and she did what was necessary for his success.

She can no more comprehend religion than she can comprehend science, he thought. She could learn to drive a car as a cat could learn to work a latch, without understanding. She just doesn't have a long-distance mind, that's all. To Lucinda, religion was crazy bits of orthodoxy that he tried to sneak in on her.

A woman recognizes only the present, he said to himself. Her own children, and the manners and customs of her own day. The things that mattered to a man were frequently irrelevant to a woman.

He heard her put the reading glasses on the night table. Though his eyes were closed he saw the sudden change to darkness.

He heard and felt her settle in the sheets. There was silence.

"Ed—" she said.

"What," he answered. He did not move or open his eyes.

"Do you think Amethyst is attractive?"

"Nah, she's a dog."

9

When she had said her last good-bye to Miss Bancroft, at one o'clock on Saturday, she waited a while on the sidewalk outside the building's lobby in case Leslie Hollander should happen by unannounced again, as he had the week before.

She thought he most likely did not even have the day off, and might even have chosen to stay home and sleep if he did. But in case he did come by she could not chance missing him. With her job change he would not know where to find her again.

She was even prepared with conversation. She thought him intelligent and knowledgeable, and wondered what he thought the end result would be of North Korea's invasion of the South. American ground forces had debarked yesterday in Korea, and yet it did not quite seem as though a Third World War were beginning after all. Russia had not come in. She had begun to feel that perhaps she had misjudged the situation. She thought one had to admit that Truman had done the right thing.

After some time she crossed to the luncheonette, but kept watching through the window. Finally, at two-fifteen, she left for home.

On the Sparkstown train it occurred to her that her thoughts on the Korean events and the President's response were something to write Eugene about. So was her new job—there was ample material for a chatty letter.

However, she didn't get to it. On Monday morning she was uncertain whether Mr. Killian expected her at nine, or whether she was to begin night-shift hours the very first day. But she rode to Boston early as usual, in the Model T with Charles, just in case. When she had been taken up in the slow cagelike elevator and found her way again through the partitions to the long, noisy room, Mr. Killian was not there. Someone else told her to come back at three.

So she wandered the city and meandered to a bench on the greenery near the river. In the afternoon she mailed a postcard to Dr. Leslie Hollander at the Massachusetts General Hospital, explaining her change of jobs and saying she hoped he was making progress in his internship.

She presented herself again at Mr. Killian's desk a little before three and was put at once to work. She had to rush to anyone who yanked a page from his typewriter and take it, carbon paper and all, to Mr. Hopkins, a thin, lank man of about forty who wore a green eyeshade and sat with his helpers at a long table called the copy desk. As there were many people busy at typewriters she was constantly moving about. Some even put on earphones and talked into old-fashioned upright telephones, still typing all the while. I'm coming, as fast as I can, she would think in reply when two called her at once, but she did not say it aloud. She learned that the big frowning pear-shaped man who sat near the front with a drooping mustache was called Louie Alpert. He worked very fast, though with two fingers only, and bent close over his typewriter, his deep-set staring eyes close together around a beak of a nose. Maud Dickinson, the lady whose desk was near the back, smiled in a warm, encouraging way whenever Millicent came there. Her skinny painted face was dense with wrinkles, and her legs were so spindly that her stockings hung loosely, but Millicent appreciated the friendliness of her crinkling eyes.

There was another copy boy, named Zucchino, and he was busy too, though he wore an unhurried expression, with large front teeth and uncombed hair. His shirttail hung out. He said little to her. But Zucchino had worked all day, and after an hour or two he left. She had also to tear away the stories that spewed endlessly from three clacking teletype machines that stood against the back wall and take those to Mr. Hopkins too. Her hands were stained with bluish carbon. In addition she had frequently to take bunches of stories from

Mr. Hopkins's desk and carry them upstairs to a room of huge black machines and blue fluorescent lights, where there was a smell of molten lead and a filthy floor, and hand them to a squat man named Valentino who wore a striped apron with ink smears. The stairs made her heart pound. There was no air conditioning anywhere and her face became hot. She tried to read a line or two of the stories on the run, and also the penciled headlines that Mr. Hopkins gave her on separate sheets, surrounded with cryptic directions to the printers, but there was scarcely time. She would scurry down breathlessly to find stories hanging out of the teletype machines almost to the floor.

It seemed impossible to keep up with so much, though there was an excitement in trying to. Mr. Killian was busy at his own desk, telephoning angrily, or telling men to leave their desks and go out, and talking to others that came in. Sometimes he read snatches of carbon copies, running a hand through his brown shock of hair while his chair turned and squeaked and tilted.

Mr. Hopkins told her to find out who wanted cokes or iced coffee and sandwiches and to fetch it from the spa across the street, having her own supper at the same time. As soon as she began she saw it would be complicated, as Louie Alpert was explicit about the details of his hamburger and gave her a large bill to be changed, so she jotted in pencil who wanted ketchup and who cream and sugar and so on, waving away cigarette smoke meanwhile.

The spa was deep and spacious, with dark carved wood giving an obsolescent elegance to the ceilings and walls and the separations of booths. A dark soda fountain of exquisite marble ran very long and far down a side, to where the spa, after different sections and levels, seemed to open again in the distance on yet another street. There were men who looked like businessmen, and women who might have been tired from shopping, and a subdued clanking of glasses and silver.

She was expected back in half an hour, so she did not take time to eat herself, especially as she wanted to telephone the typing-and-shorthand instructress.

From her phone booth she watched the white-capped counter boy so she would know when the orders were ready. To the instructress she explained her absence, and that she would have to drop out. The instructress mentioned in her soft voice that there were also morning classes, but Millicent said she was already hopelessly behind. At last the instructress told her agreeably that with her looks she'd never have any trouble getting a job anyway.

Millicent hurried back across the street and up the elevator with an open boxload of wrapped food and covered cups. The purse in her shoulder-strap bag was full of change. She thought of the stories that must have piled up while she was out, beside typewriters, in Mr. Hopkins's basket, or dragging from the teletypes. She wondered if some of the men had been doing her work for her. She was impressed by the fact that five deadlines had to be met every night, one for each edition.

She was no sooner back than Mr. Hopkins told her to go at once to Police Headquarters and get a copy of a certain press release. Mr. Killian had gone home and Mr. Hopkins was in charge now. He told her what subway and streets to take and how to find it. The police building had a press room, which police reporters of all the papers used in common, and there she was to ask for a reporter named Heustis Garvey.

The building was broad, of soiled granite. There was a lobby, dingy but wide, and in a corner past the elevators a very old policeman sat in an alcove behind a counter. "Can you tell me where the press room is, please?" she asked him.

Then she followed his directions, through a lonely zigzagging corridor. She tried a door that turned out to be a broom closet. But at last, in a cul-de-sac, a door with an unmarked window of frosted glass stood ajar.

"Mr. Garvey?" she said, looking in.

There were four desks, with a telephone and a typewriter on each, but only three reporters, and they all sat about one of the desks playing cards. One was much older than the others. The walls were cracked, and an absurd calendar showed an unreal young woman with nothing on, reclining long-legged against a red background. On the floor an electric fan oscillated.

"Mr. Garvey?" she asked again, and approached the older man. "I'm the new copy boy." She waved away the cigarette smoke.

The card game stopped but no one rose. He might have been fifty or sixty. He looked up and stared, squinty-eyed and florid, still perspiring from the day's heat, with tiny veins in his broad cheeks. He took his time, as though with a haughty wisdom.

"You don't look like a very good copy of a boy to me," he answered calmly, and after a split second's pause he burst into a laugh that was like a single wheeze of an asthmatic, a prolonged rasp high in his throat, his eyes shutting and his whole face wrinkling. His big hand slapped the desk. The two younger reporters smiled.

Millicent blushed.

Garvey opened his eyes for another stare and again gave a prolonged single open-mouthed rasp, shutting his eyes, his face red with hilarity. She felt a shattering embarrassment, and could find nothing to say to him or the others. But his big head and frame relaxed, as though exhausted by his laughter. She could hear his breathing above the hum of the fan and smell his perspiration. He opened a lower drawer that was stuffed to overflowing with soiled loose pages and searched in it.

"Yeah, yeah," he said. "You told Dexter Killian you could cover the dock strike."

"I told him I could try." Her voice was quaking.

"Honeybunch, it's windy down there on those docks." He handed her some mimeographed pages and shut the drawer noisily. "Your skirts might blow over your head, and then where would you be?"

His eyebrows lifted, and she thought he might burst into another of those laughs.

"Do you really think rudeness is becoming to you?" she asked quakily, trying to sound cutting, but she saw it did not affect him. What a nasty person, she thought.

Upon her return, Mr. Hopkins sent her down to the sidewalk to chalk some news flashes onto the blackboards. This part of the city was fairly empty in the evening, but some passersby did stop to watch her, as did a derelict she had seen hanging about before, and she felt both important and self-conscious, erasing the old dispatches and copying on the blackboards the words that Mr. Hopkins had printed on a little folded sheet.

At midnight, on the way home, she had a sandwich in the great hollowness of North Station. Her work had ended when all the good trains were gone, and she had to wait a long time in the concourse for one that went slowly in the small hours, with long stops every few minutes at little depots. At Sparkstown she found that the brown buses had ceased for the night and she had to waken the taxi man.

The next night also, when she was sent out for supper, she did not find time to eat, but Maud Dickinson found out and told her it was ridiculous. Maud said Dexter Killian sometimes took two hours. Millicent asked if reporters knew shorthand, and Maud said she had never heard of any.

She noticed also that no one typed properly. Few used more than two or three fingers, and Mr. Killian used only one. Maud was rapid. Her vividly polished nails flew.

Millicent's days off came, on Wednesday and Thursday. She meant to spend them reading books about journalism, since she had no training in it. She went to the town library in Wilmerding Crosswalk, on Roland's bicycle, and asked for all the books they had by Walter Lippmann.

She settled into her job. Sometimes, when stories were on deadline, they would yank them from typewriters line by line, and she would have to stand by someone's desk and dash to Mr. Hopkins and then upstairs almost a sentence at a time. Meanwhile the nervous, stuttering clack of the wire-service machines was continuous. But at four in the afternoon the low thunder of the presses shook the floor and the staccato was lost in the rolling bass. "They should have put those presses in the basement," Maud said to her. "They'll shake the whole building down someday."

Millicent changed the rolls of paper on the teletype machines when they were used up, and also brought paper stapled with carbons to the reporters' desks. She was supposed to staple more, so as to keep a supply, and to make some late at night for the daytime copy boys. Besides Zucchino there was a third copy boy, Tatro, who worked early hours and whom she rarely saw.

She knew now that the long room she worked in was called the city room. She was sent on errands to Heustis Garvey regularly, and to others who were on the staff but did all their work at certain places outside, such as Mike Gorman at the State House, who had a flattened face and nose, and who could roll a pair of loose teeth about his mouth and fit them into the bridge again, using only his tongue. She had the feeling that newspaper people knew what was happening before other people did. And it made for urgency, as though getting the facts to the public depended in part on her own promptness in climbing those stairs to Mr. Valentino.

She no longer wore a dress and stockings to work, but ankle socks and a denim skirt, since no one had seemed to mind Zucchino's tielessness. The denim took the carbon better.

In the long waits at North Station she thought about her budget. She was paid biweekly, but it came to five dollars a week more than before, and there was no school to pay and no employment agency. On the other hand her train fares had doubled, because she could not ride in with Charles any more. And there was the taxi home from the depot. She had given the derelict who hung out near the blackboards a quarter a couple of times because it seemed cruel to go by him with so much food from the spa, but she decided now she had better cut him to a dime. Especially as she had been giving some also to a blind man who sat with shoelaces.

Mr. Killian almost never spoke to her, except to grunt when she greeted him each afternoon. His foot was nearly always on a pulled-out drawer and the hair of his leg showed. He had last spoken to her during her first day at work, when he had requested that she come in as usual on the Fourth of July, and it had flattered her somewhat that she was actually needed.

On some evenings, especially after Mr. Killian had gone home, the pace of work in the city room slacked off sharply. She tried to keep busy nevertheless, because she felt she ought, and also because several of the men were in the habit of looking at her a great deal, absently, as though she were a picture on the wall, and it was easier not to notice them if she were occupied. Sometimes, at desks where no one sat, she tried the typewriters. Most had the letters uneven. One wrote only gothic capitals and jumped several spaces together. Another had no A. She knew there was no objection to personal phone calls, because she had asked Maud. Yet even if Leslie should happen to call, she thought, it would be more difficult than ever for them to get together now that she worked Saturdays and Sundays.

Mr. Hopkins invited her one evening to join the union, which he called the Guild, urging it quite seriously, and she told him she would decide in twenty-four hours. She believed in unions on principle, in the same way Eugene had, but she wanted to ask Maud first if it was an honest one. Yet increasingly she felt part of the staff. On hot nights they would send her to the spa for cold drinks several times, and she had had to learn their names in order not to confuse their orders. Some of them teased her often about how young she looked, especially a reporter named Danny McBride. He was big and about thirty, just beginning to be slightly overweight, and always had a hat on and an open-mouthed grin she couldn't stand.

"You could pass for eleven, if you'd pull your girdle up around your chest, do ya know it?" he told her one evening, standing near the teletype machines.

She kept tearing stories from the machines with a ruler, not looking at him. "I don't wear girdles."

"You don't?"

"No I don't," she said. "And I don't see that it's any business of yours."

On another occasion he told her she might look older if she grew a mustache.

"Don't let them get you," Maud said to her. Maud said a youthful appearance was something that people grew out of soon enough, and she shouldn't take them to heart. Anyway much of it was simply that she didn't wear any lipstick or anything.

"I don't regard myself as an object to be painted," Millicent replied.

The friendly smile spread again in Maud's wrinkles. Her silver-gray hair was snipped in bangs. "I don't blame you—you'd be gilding the lily," she said. "You'll be an old bag soon enough."

Later that evening, more than an hour before she was due to leave, Mr. Hopkins told her she could get an early start if she wished. "There's nothing doing," he said.

"What about the late city edition?" she asked, waving away his cigarette smoke.

"I don't see any changes."

"Well, I don't know," she said. "Do you think it's honest? I'm paid to be here until eleven-thirty."

"Scram," he said.

Mr. Killian had a way of summoning employees to his desk by beckoning with his head only, scowling, and he caught Millicent's eye in this fashion as she arrived the next afternoon. When she approached he rose, hitching up his belt.

"Millicent," he said, "I've been hearing good reports about you. And I know you aspire to be a reporter, because you told Maud." His eyes looked down sharply into hers. At last he put a foot on the bottom drawer and a hand on her shoulder. He rocked her back and forth a little. "I believe in you," he told her unsmiling. "It all takes time, but in your walks around the city I want you to try to develop a reporter's eyes."

"Thank you," she said, quite stirred, her mouth dry.

The hand on her shoulder was heavy, and gripped. "Watch for features, for human interest angles," he went on. "You don't have to witness a shooting. And read all the papers, every day—our own and all the competition, so you'll be right up on everything in case I have to send you out. Even read the Monitor. This is a great newspaper town, Millicent. Eight papers publishing every day, four on Sunday. And I'll tell you something else. The ink gets in your blood. I'd never work for a wire service. Because I love the sound of the presses. I've got to hear that edition start to roll. There's something spiritual in it. It does something to me. To go up there and watch the copper spin that endless white pulp, in and out through the steel. The news break you've sweated—to see it speeding at last over those great triangles that fold it up—it calms you. You wait. You'll see. Once I had a problem, I had a problem, Millicent, that I couldn't figure out—and it was as if voices in that rotary press told me what to do."

"Thank you, Mr. Killian," she said again, when he paused. She waved the cigarette smoke automatically with a slight gesture.

"What's this 'mister' all the time? My name's Dexter."

"Well—thank you," she said.

At last he dismissed her, with a brusque wave, still unsmiling, and sat. He seemed ill at ease.

10

Mornings she tried to sleep late. The Montreal express and the neighbor's rooster no longer waked her and the window at her head faced north, over the kitchen and toward the woods and the railroad, but the side window was so placed that the rising sun shone in her face, even past the edge of the window shade. Moreover Patty kept going in and out of the room.

"Do you have to slam drawers?" Millicent asked from the sheets.

"Sorry I woke you," said Patty. "I am. Really. Because you appeal to me more asleep than awake."

Roland was also a nuisance—his friend Bobby O'Shaughnessy was always around, and another kid called Snotsy Vaughn, and the three would swing themselves along hand-over-hand clinging from the rain gutter of the porch roof, until her mother screeched at them. "You too, Snotsy!" she would hear her mother shouting from a window on the other side of the house. Or they would sit on the peak of the barn roof, inventing outlandish shrieks. And once, while her addled head lay dozing as though half smothered, she heard them on the slate roof of the kitchen just outside her open window.

The latest train that would get her to Boston on time was earlier than it needed to be, but even so she did not have to leave the house until one. She would hang the wash, or stand folding linens with Patty. Fortunately she was away at work when the undertaker Chester telephoned in the evening.

On her day off she somehow awoke before breakfast time, though she had not gotten to bed until after two. When Mr. Hopkins released her early she could make a fast train that stopped at Sparkstown on demand only and be in bed a little past midnight, but he could not let her go so early always.

She did her calisthenics and went downstairs, her eyes smarting. In the forenoon she put on shorts and knelt in the soft blackness of the flower bed to help pull weeds. The heat penetrated and felt good. Dirt clogged her fingernails and an ant ran tickling over her hand.

Her mother was talking about Mrs. Herzlinger's brilliant nephew, the Winkler boy, who was studying for a Ph.D. at M.I.T. He had been supposed to phone for a blind date but hadn't done so. Millicent shook the soil from a mess of roots and grasses and stood to get the kinks from her knees. The shadows in the garden faded as if a cloud had crossed the sun. Her mother suggested phoning Mrs. Herzlinger again, in order to supply her nephew with Millicent's new office number.

"Mother, just don't! Don't chase him! I'd be absolutely mortified. If he happens to call I'll decide then if we're congenial or not."

"That's not chasing. Maybe he doesn't want to call away out here. It's a twenty-cent call from Boston."

"I'm not desperate to make friends with the whole world." She massaged the backs of her knees. In the tiger lilies the brightness and shadows reappeared. She knelt to work.

"He's a boy, he's not a friend," her mother continued, digging with a hand hoe. "And there's no big secret about your telephone. Boys have to know you're available—you can't advertise in the newspapers. He'll find another girl while you're sitting around."

"For goodness sakes—"

"Don't for goodness sakes me! You're just like Rosalind, and you're gonna end up the same way! This one's no good, that one's no good, an undertaker's no good, a hardware man's no good—you're your father's twin, like Rosalind, a bunch of dreamers. And so now a brilliant professor at Tech isn't good enough—not good enough for this one—what do you want, the King of England?"

"The King of England happens to be a very mediocre person, as it happens."

"Yes, to you he would be. God Himself wouldn't be right for you."

"The King of England is a married man with grown children."

"You know what I mean," her mother told her. "You turn down dates, and you won't have dates. You'll be left out of parties. Boys have to know you're not high-hat, high-falutin. They get discouraged. You're twenty-one, you're beautiful, brilliant, face, figure, educated—you don't know where a nice introduction might come from! You could have your pick now. You could be sorry some day. You don't go around saying you're not in the market, give the impression you're not interested. Now's the time to be in the market—you're young! You don't appreciate it while you have it and you'll be twenty-five, thirty, and you won't have a choice. You'll take what you can get."

The truth Millicent recognized in this gave her a chill. She worked silently, moving farther away on her knees. The crab apples were diseased and some had fallen into the garden. Her mother crouched some feet away, working with her back to her.

"And what about Chester when he calls again?" her mother asked. "Are you gonna turn him down until he's discouraged?"

Millicent didn't answer.

"At least get in circulation," her mother said. "You have to be seen. People have to know you exist."

" 'Chester,' " she muttered. "What a thing to name anybody."

"What's wrong with it?"

"I thought that name had gone out of existence."

"Well I think he's very nice. I don't say you have to marry the man. But he's been nice enough to take an interest. And he's a college man, and he'll inherit a very nice business someday. Everyone knows them. One of the biggest."

"A funeral parlor."

"All right, a funeral parlor. What difference does it make? It doesn't matter what his occupation is. As long as it's honest."

"It does matter," said Millicent. "Your occupation is what you are."

"Well if I'd gone around picking men by their occupations the last thing I would have gone out with was a rabbi."

"Dad wasn't a rabbi when you married him."

"No, he was working on a car lot, and I wasn't so keen about that either. But I fell in love with him for his character."

"Oh sure," Millicent said acidly. I'll deteriorate here, she thought.

"And you find your ideas change on a lot of things."

In the afternoon Millicent napped, but only briefly.

When she arose she started out for a walk, but apparently there had been a shower, and her mother shouted that it was still raining. "That's just off the tree," Roland said.

By supper she was exhausted again. The whole day seemed frittered. Charles teased Patty at the table, asking what she had done to her hair, and telling her she looked like a shaggy-dog story. Millicent told her father they needed new screens—there weren't enough and some didn't fit right or something.

"Are you after me too?"

"I killed three mosquitoes last night," she told him.

"Okay, okay," her father said. He said he'd patch them, and that he meant to get a few new ones.

"Roland, how about taking your bath," her mother said.

"After."

"Now."

"Please, plates aren't ashtrays," Millicent said to her father as she cleared the table.

In the evening Chester called. She had had a foreboding it was he when the phone rang, and it seemed easier to accept than to argue with her mother. He knew she was off the following evening too, so she made the date for then to get it over with. He wanted to take her to dinner.

At nine she went to bed, but the habit of nightwork had already upset her system and she could not fall asleep. After midnight she went to the kitchen in her bathrobe and had cocoa. She fell asleep toward two, but woke when the clock on the Unitarian church struck six.

"Tchk, you look so tired," her mother said to her at breakfast.

"Poor thing," said Patty.

Again Millicent could not help but waste the day. She took a book to the hayloft, hoping to avoid gardening. But though there was no hay there was a musty smell, as if wood were rotting, and it combined with her tiredness to give her fits of sneezing. She could see the dog lying in the sun down by the door, with flies around him, and he looked up at her sneezes.

In the afternoon she napped in her cot, and her mother woke her from a deep sleep at five.

She showered. As she returned to her room her mother shouted up the stairs to put on stockings. "And don't tell me you haven't got a pair, because I know you have."

Millicent opened the white bureau.

"I don't know," she heard her mother say downstairs, "Patty's the one that's supposed to be at the awkward age, but I think the older they get the awkwarder they get."

Patty came in, wearing shorts, and when she sat on the bed her thighs spread full.

The worst part about stockings, Millicent thought, was what you had to put on just to hold them up. She owned a girdle that her mother had made her get for some occasion, and she took it from the drawer. She looked at the fabricky crosshatch of its miracle fibers, the satiny paneling. The whole contraption seemed an insult. As though a woman's body was a problem for engineers. Simple pants and bras were sensible underwear, and so now and then was a slip. A bra was steadying and if you didn't wear one your breasts hurt on stairs. But once there were stockings to be held up you got into the whole mystique of the boudoir. The ridiculous pulleys and hoists and retaining walls. She dropped the girdle back in the drawer and elected to wear the garter belt instead, even though she considered it basically even more foolish.

She pulled the garter belt around her.

"Want to try my eye shadow?" Patty said.

"No."

"I knew you'd say that."

"Why'd you ask."

"I should think you'd want to be attractive. You want to be unattractive all the time."

"That's not how I look at it."

"You're tacky," Patty said.

Millicent buckled a fastening.

"Even your underwear's tacky," Patty went on. "Look, nothing the least bit pretty, nothing frilly, no color, not one single bit of lace. I don't know, I like pretty things. I like colors. I like to be as beautiful as I can."

"Do your dates see you in your underwear?"

"No."

"Well mine don't either."

"But even so."

"Well I don't like lacy underwear," Millicent said, "and all those things were designed for the cancan, if you'll think about it. The whole idea that women are objects for men to look at and be amused by." She continued dressing, with quick motions. Patty watched.

"Boy, you do hate men, don't ya."

"I don't hate anybody."

"You're maladjusted," said Patty.

"You're maladjusted too. Or you wouldn't have a weight problem."

"I'm not maladjusted. I'm just overweight physically. But I've got lots of friends and I'm very well adjusted."

"If you're well adjusted at fifteen I'm sorry for you."

"Why?"

"It's too young to be well adjusted." She went to the closet and stepped carefully into her heels. Then she took the brown dress from its hanger. It was the only one that matched the heels.

"You'll probably be an old maid," said Patty.

"Maybe I will," Millicent said, putting on the dress.

Patty rose and did the zipper.

"And heels are another thing," Millicent said to her. "Women's clothes aren't meant to be merely uncomfortable—they're meant to be disabling. High heels, tight skirts, girdles—they're immobilizing. They're supposed to handicap us. So the clumsiest male can feel like an athlete by comparison. It's part of the whole fiction of female inferiority. And that's why slips show. They're made defective on purpose, so we can excuse ourselves for repairs. And they keep changing the styles, to make us seem frivolous. Men design the styles, you know."

"Would you rather be a man?"

"I don't know. I don't think I'd be a very good one. I'm not conceited enough."

When Chester came she put on her shoulder-strap bag and went down quickly and unsmiling, almost passing him on the porch.

"Hi," he said.

He shut her into the car and went around it. It crunched slowly down the winding dirt road, past the broken gate, and headed for Boston, in the flickering shadows of the big trees, by way of Wilmerding Crosswalk center.

"I'm a little late," he said. "Your directions weren't exactly right." He pointed out where the roads did not run the way she had said.

It was going to be a long ride, and she knew the conversation would not go smoothly.

"It's pretty out here," he said.

He asked what she thought of the Korean outbreak, and turned out to agree with her about Truman and about Senator McCarthy. But he had no new ideas and the talk seemed labored. She spoke some of her new job, but not of the great hopes she had for it. He was somehow not the person to whom she wished to confide that.

"All during my teens I swore I wouldn't go into the undertaking business," he told her after a while. "But you'd be surprised. Every funeral's different. And every family's different. It's not just the logistics of traffic and routing. You're trying to be sensitive to what people want, create dignity for them. And I'm telling ya, the depth of drama I see—it's just indescribable. There's the whole tale of the life now completed, so to speak, like a world of its own, and what really opens your eyes is the survivors—people who've just lost what meant most to them."

Talk lapsed, and for a while there was only the smooth hum. The seat was wide and she did not sit near him.

"Smile," he said, glancing sideways at her, and an encouraging little smile began in his own brownish features.

"Please, I just hate anyone telling me to smile." Her solemn face hardened into irritation. "Do you remember I told you I don't like being forced to laugh at jokes?" she explained. "Well, it's the same thing. I can't smile on order. People can't just go around grinning when they don't feel like it."

"I'm sorry," he said.

"You make anyone terribly self-conscious when you tell them that. How would you like it if people kept ordering you to smile?"

"I'm sorry," he apologized again.

"It's patronizing."

He found the restaurant on a steep hill, set into a basement under brick. He hurried down the steps and held the door. The name was French, and there were checkered tablecloths on round tables and candles burning on some of them, though the electric lights made a normal brightness. Chester picked a table near a poster that showed a mountain and began to assist with her chair, but someone spoke her name quietly and she recognized the two youngest reporters from the city room smiling at her from a table diagonally across. She smiled back, only a little flustered, and stood again just as Chester knocked the chair against her. He followed her across the little room and she introduced Mr. Lyons and Mr. Tighe. But Chester's last name blacked out of her mind and she put a hand to her eyes. She thought of Walnut and of Cheeseburg. "Walberg," he said. Bob Lyons said something pleasant, and then Chester led her back to their table.

They studied their menus. It seemed as much Italian as French. A short waitress with a lined face struck a match sharply and lighted their candle.

Millicent put down the menu finally. Chester's face had a gentle mildness that made her feel sorry for him. His hair was combed neat, and she could see where he was losing it. She imagined his parents browbeating him into the family business.

"You have very strange eyes," he said in the midst of the silence.

He keeps saying these things that there's no answer to, she thought. She ordered Boston scrod. He seemed disappointed, remarking that she ought to order something French, but she said she liked fish. He ordered duckling à l'orange for himself and appetizers of pâté for them both. He asked for wine, but the unsmiling waitress said he'd have to get his own from the corner drugstore.

They sat waiting, facing each other. He drummed with one hand softly on the checkered tablecloth. She felt another embarrassed silence beginning. Then he said he ought to go out and get some wine, since it was a French restaurant. However he did not go at once, but wondered aloud whether any other city had such a system, where wine was sold in drugstores, and half the restaurants had no liquor license. She said she didn't know.

Finally he excused himself, promised to take only a minute, and left.

She studied the posters.

"Did your boy friend give you the slip?" Bob Lyons said, not loudly, from across the room. He smiled agreeably. He was personable, with freckles along his nose.

"He went out for some wine," Millicent said.

"Why don't you sit with us until he gets back?" said Lyons. "We'll keep you company."

She was hesitant. But Lyons seemed gracious, and Tighe turned and smiled also. He had a wide, compressed blond face, with prominent forehead and chin. They had both always been decent enough at work, never rude. So she took up the shoulder-strap bag she had slung from her chair and went to them. Lyons pulled a chair from an empty table.

As she sat her waitress came and asked if she were moving to this table.

"Oh no, I'm just waiting," she explained. "Visiting."

Lyons talked to her about work. Tighe was pleasant but fairly taciturn. It took her aback that they spoke with so little respect for Mr. Alpert or Mr. Garvey or even Mr. Killian. But she was encouraged to discover that Tighe had begun as a copy boy. They were eating anchovies and pimentos. Lyons offered her some on a clean fork that he took from the next table, and she protested but then tasted it. There was a delightful pungency of salt and oil.

"Waitress," Lyons said, raising his fingers with a light snap. "Another order, please."

"Oh, I couldn't," said Millicent.

It was a different waitress, a taller, washed-out one. Lyons nodded to her and she went off.

"Really, you shouldn't have," Millicent said.

"You can't just sit and watch people eat," he said.

The waitress brought her dish quickly. Millicent began to eat, and the talk continued. They speculated on what was taking Chester so long.

He appeared, carrying a bottle in a paper sack, before Millicent had quite finished all her anchovies, but she thanked Lyons and Tighe, touching a checked napkin to her mouth, and returned to her own table.

The short waitress brought two wineglasses and a corkscrew, and Chester worked at the bottle. Millicent explained the kindness of Mr. Lyons and Mr. Tighe to him, referring to them as her colleagues. Chester moved to pour the wine but she covered her glass.

"None for me, thanks."

"Why?"

"I'm a teetotaler."

He put down the bottle. "Oh, that's right. Darn it. You did tell me that. I should have remembered that."

He filled his own glass, sadly.

"Why didn't you remind me?" he said. "Before I went out?"

"I don't know. I didn't think of it. I thought you wanted some."

Their appetizers came, but the anchovies had deadened her taste and she ate only a corner, apologizing. Chester finally ate them both but did not look as though he enjoyed it. She tried to eat the fish and the peas, but they were somewhat overdone and her mouth was unbearably dry. She saw him look at the big wine bottle and it did seem a waste. They scarcely talked. At one point he poured a little wine from the bottle onto his duck. She ended by leaving most of the fish also, explaining that she ought not to have eaten the anchovies.

When the waitress offered coffee or tea Millicent asked if there was any ginger ale. Chester offered to go out for some, but Millicent begged him not to and ordered a glass of water. For dessert she suggested grapefruit, thinking it would cut the dryness, but Chester insisted that she try something French.

Lyons and Tighe had risen. They stopped by Chester and Millicent, smiling. "We're going to the fights," Lyons said. "Down the Arena. Care to join us?"

"No thanks," said Chester.

"No thanks," said Millicent.

"We can get into the press section," Lyons said.

"No, that's all right," said Chester.

"Okay," said Lyons. "Just thought I'd ask. You look sort of bored over here."

He moved away with Tighe to the cashier's desk, and Chester glumly watched them pay their bills.

"Hey," Chester said to Millicent suddenly. "Did they pay for your anchovies?" He thrust back his chair and hurried toward the cashier. "Hey, the anchovies should be on my bill," he said.

"It's taken care of," Lyons smiled at him. Tighe was already holding the door.

"Aw, come on, hey, you can't do that. How much?" Chester said. He had opened his wallet.

Lyons waved a hand coolly, still smiling. Chester reddened. "Forget it. It's our pleasure," Lyons said.

"Aw, hey, what do I owe ya?" Chester said, pressing after them, his wallet before him and open wider. But they shut the door.

Chester came back, looking humiliated. The waitress was bringing the desserts, puddings with meringue spun high.

"You should have put those anchovies on my bill," he told the waitress irritably.

"It wasn't my table," she snapped back at him. She set down the puddings huffily.

He sat down, more red-faced than ever, and dug into his dessert without looking at Millicent. She tasted it too, but her mouth had grown drier and the cooked meringue clung to her palate like glue. A sip of water only made it congeal. She put the spoon down. She saw him notice it.

"Would you have wanted to go to the fights?" he asked her.

"No."

"What did he mean by 'you look bored'? Did he mean just you, or both of us?"

"Well, I guess he meant me, mostly."

Chester looked miserable. He took a spoonful of dessert and she saw the movement of his throat as he swallowed. His fingers turned his wineglass around and around on the checkered cloth. The bottle was nearly full. Some breath from his nostrils made the candle flicker.

"Are you bored?" he said.

She was uncertain how to answer.

"Are you?" he asked again.

"I suppose so."

His fingers gave the glass stem another turn.

"Well," he said, "I'll take you home."

He pushed back his chair. He arose gloomily and she followed. When he had finished at the cashier's desk they walked down the sidewalk to the car together, not speaking.

She knew she had eaten almost nothing of the food he had provided, and it did seem impolite, although she had not intended it to work out like that.

While he drove the first several blocks they still exchanged no word, though once or twice he seemed about to.

"I tried not to be boring," he said, not looking from the road. "But it's not easy."

She made no answer.

"You're boring too," he said.

"I know it," she admitted.

"You're not even trying. I'm at least trying. Why don't you at least try to be a little gay or something?"

"I am trying," said Millicent.

"You don't seem like you're trying."

"Well, I can't."

He sighed drearily. "I must be congenitally a lousy date or something," he said after a moment. "I don't know, I just don't have it. Girls expect a guy to be gay and entertaining all the time—buoy their moods up—"

It was only beginning to be dark. Some cars burned headlights and some did not. She felt badly to be taken home so early and wondered how she would explain it to her mother and Patty.

She had realized only belatedly that it might have been best not to be truthful when he asked if she were bored. But even so, she had not meant that he was boring her, or that it was his fault, or that she wished rudely to be rid of him. She had been trying to take the blame, but it hadn't come out right.

"It's pretty damn depressing," he said.

"I know it."

"You won't even let a guy tell you jokes. I don't know. It seems to me other guys I know don't have this trouble. I must be the lousiest date in the world."

"No, I am," Millicent said. "I'm such a lousy date I'm defrauding people if I even accept."

"Do you feel as rotten as I do?" he asked.

"I guess so."

"Because I feel pretty terrible. Maybe we're just a couple of depressives. Do you think that's it? If you say you have trouble on dates too. Maybe it means we're made for each other. Or maybe it means just the opposite. I don't know."

They rode a long time in silence. It was dark when they passed the square in Wilmerding Crosswalk.

"I notice you didn't have any trouble talking to those two Irishmen," he said.

There seemed no way to explain that. She felt dissatisfied with herself.

She sneezed, explosively, before she could get the handkerchief from her shoulder-strap bag. It hurt the roof of her mouth and left her nostrils tickling and raw. The next sneeze was just in time for her to crouch forward into the handkerchief. It wrenched the bones of her neck and shoulders. Her eyes were moist and hot. The third hung fire, leaving her heaving breathlessly. Then it burst with force, shaking and exhausting her, but all the nerves of her nose were excited anew. Chester looked at her alarmed.

"Let me out," she gasped, and sneezed helplessly. She could scarcely open her eyes.

"What's the matter?" he said. "Do you need air?"

The car halted and she opened the door. They were somewhere on Massapeequit Road. There was a low retaining wall, with overhanging lilac, and she sat on it. There was another sneeze, strong and wrenching. Chester got out too, leaving the motor running and the lights on. He stood before her and she could see the concern on his face. A sneeze blasted up her throat against a tenderness of membrane. It was as if her nose was too little for such big sneezes. She tried to wave Chester away, to motion him back toward the car. She pressed the crushed handkerchief under her nose and breathed through her mouth. Air itself always seemed to irritate her nostrils when they were in this state.

"Don't you want me to take you home?" he said.

She shook no.

"I can't leave you here," he said.

She shook yes. She wanted to tell him she would be all right, but she couldn't. Every sneeze triggered new open-mouthed heaves that pulled wind down her throat. They made her whole body a bellows.

"What can I do?" he said confusedly. "What should I do? Should I get something from the drugstore?"

She shook her head. The wet of each sneeze brought a relief that vanished in an instant, the build-up recurring, and she had to give them all her attention. If she did not pinch her nostrils at the right moment, to direct all the force down through her open mouth, it would hurt stabbingly against her soft palate. She felt it subsiding, but it was far from done.

"You want me to just leave you here?"

She nodded again.

She watched with half-shut eyes, wearily. The car departed.

She kept the handkerchief to her nose and mouth. Her nostrils needed that wrapping. She heaved several times, while a sneeze teetered uncertainly. She thought the tingling diminished. Then it sharpened anew in one nostril and was ignited suddenly. She heaved again.

She breathed exhaustedly. Even when the sneezes were gone she needed the pressure and assurance of the handkerchief. The heat in her eyes made them too tired to open. The hurt remained in her mouth even when she swallowed.

At times she had even taken pills for this kind of thing, only to sneeze the pill out in a spray.

She opened her hot eyes. She looked at the stars. Her body shivered. She swung her legs a little against the wall.

It occurred to her that she could stroll down to the covered bridge, and hang around there over the gurgling water until she heard the church clock strike midnight, and then pretend to her mother that her evening out had run a normal course.

Her mother would remark on not having heard the car. But she could say that Chester had a funeral at sunrise and had bid her good night at the foot of the long dirt driveway with no time to come in.

11

She lay in the iron cot next morning, thinking of Chester. How many evenings of my unmarried life must be spent like that? Utterly dismal first dates, this compulsory exploring of all the uncongenial men in the world?

Still, if she had to do it, she wished she were better at it. She would have to learn to smile and laugh, and all that. She had not meant to be disagreeable to him. She had the unhappy feeling that she was not a very nice or friendly person.

Anyway, though, his anger had at least kept him from trying any necking business.

It was sunny, and when she had done her calisthenics and dressed she went out to the yard. She saw the mail car stop at the galvanized box down by the broken gate, and she went down there. Besides the brochures and notices for her father and the flyers announcing sales there was something for her—a mimeographed invitation to join the Independent Citizens' Committee for Theodore Victor Miecznesliwy. It must be a result of the postcard she had sent to Americans for Democratic Action, she thought. Her card to the Weekly Wilmerdingian, asking about political clubs in the town, had brought no answer, and her father had told her meanwhile that there were none. The town elections were nonpartisan.

As she strolled back to the house her mother called her and said Mr. Killian was on the telephone. Mr. Killian asked her to come to work a few hours early as the copy boy Tatro had quit to join the Army. She liked receiving calls from the office.

As routine as her job was, she seemed to learn new things daily. She was impressed by how exactly the city-room people designed their material to fit a prescribed space, even while they banged it out so fast on the typewriters. If someone wrote a line too many, or if a headline were a comma too long, Mr. Valentino would be left with a piece of lead that would not go into the form, no matter how it were squeezed.

Louie Alpert, the big, plump mustachioed man, was mad at her because twice she had forgotten to watch whether the boy in the spa put ketchup on his hamburger. But she read all the newspapers carefully, as Mr. Killian had said, and remembered to try to develop a reporter's eyes, though she hadn't seen anything to report yet. And one night when Mr. Hopkins released her early she went up to the rotary presses and stood amidst the noise, watching the great machines whirl and trying to capture the feeling Mr. Killian had described. It was in fact impressive, the way rolling blankness sped in one end and finished newspapers rode endlessly out the other, already neatly folded.

She hoped that some day she would even be allowed to try her hand at some of the editorials. One they had had about McCarthy had been quite noncommittal and mealy-mouthed.

Yet if she chanced in the city room to catch Mr. Killian's eye by accident he would look away nervously. He was a strange person, she thought. He always hung his jacket on the rounded back of his swivel chair, though it slid off several times a day in a heap, and sometimes the casters rode upon it before anyone noticed.

But she detected also that he did not laugh easily, and did not feel at home amid joking and banter, and she felt that this side of his nature she could recognize and understand.

He hired a girl named Dawn to replace the copy boy Tatro. Millicent felt that it was her own work that had broken the ice, and that Mr. Killian would now hire women more often. But when she met the new girl she was not impressed. Dawn was a skinny teen-ager who seemed to sleep most of the time, in a sitting position, but would awaken at once if anyone yelled copy. It was impossible to get any conversation out of her. After a few days she was assigned to Tatro's old hours, however, and Millicent no longer saw her.

Bob Lyons asked Millicent for a date, and so did a wire-service reporter named Aptaker, who sometimes worked with Mike Gorman in the press room at the State House, but she refused them both. She hoped they would not resent it. While she did believe in making friends, regardless of their sex, she distrusted the dating custom and its overtones; the tendency to understand such invitations as more than mere friendship, as a kind of courtship or at least a mock courtship, was far too widespread. The whole dating concept was invested with too much that was quite unnecessary. Eventually there could be embarrassment in laying these overtones to rest, and she did not feel up to it.

And even if, as her mother thought, she should date as a matter of policy, toward the eventual time of marriage, neither Lyons nor Aptaker justified that kind of effort. Aptaker at least was denominationally acceptable. But he was intellectually inferior.

It occurred to her sadly that when a girl has not managed during her four years at college to gather a group of suitable men who will be her friends afterward, all is lost; once you were out of the campus environment it was very hard to find decent men. Her mother was right that she shouldn't isolate herself, but where could you meet them? While at home for vacation last winter she had gone once to a big shloompy benefit affair, a denominational one to avoid complications, and paid a dollar admission, but it had been nightmarish—girls stinking and hardly a genuine university man in the room.

At college there had always been nice boys in your classes, and at the parties, and in your extracurricular projects. Where did you find nice men friends now? The intern Leslie Hollander hadn't answered her postcard. Anyway she needed more than just one.

Danny McBride came by while she tore stories from the wire-service tickers and gave her a buttock-grasping spank.

"Please!" she said.

"Please what?" he grinned down.

"How disgusting," said Millicent.

The Independent Citizens' Committee for Theodore Victor Mieczesliwy, as it turned out, was to be formally organized at a meeting on one of her nights off, so Millicent rode to Boston to attend it, reading the mimeographed literature on the train. Mieczesliwy apparently had attracted much attention in the State Senate, leading the reform elements in his party and trying to get the Governor's Council abolished, but after two years the regulars had knifed him in a primary. Now he sought a nomination to run for Congress, and the party regulars were out to get him again. A printed handbill with a photo of Mieczesliwy was included, and he even looked intelligent. He was educated and honest, besides which he had voter appeal, with a baby and a pregnant wife, and membership in all sorts of Catholic lay organizations, in addition to having been in a Japanese prison camp.

She found the meeting in a carpeted parlor of a seedy hotel, on the shabbiest of the avenues that fanned out past Copley Square. Mieczneslíwy was unable to be there as promised. However a tall, white-haired old man in tweedy clothing spoke humorously but effectively, in a pleasing kind of New England accent that was both urbane and archaically upper class, and as he detailed the incompetence of the party regulars, and the depravity of their associates, Millicent felt herself grow incensed. They seemed to have stolen everything but the gold off the State House dome, and she agreed in her mind that the decline would soon become irreparable unless the civic-minded fought now to reverse it. There was an audience of about fifty men and women on folding chairs, but except for a somewhat mousy-looking dark-eyed girl with curly hair, whom Millicent sat next to, they all seemed considerably older than herself. She gathered that a middle-aged busy lady who rose and spoke a lot was the wife of a Harvard professor.

The urbane tweedy gentleman wanted teams of one man and one woman each, who would tour the streets with a portable speaker's stand and take the message into the wards. Millicent's throat went dry as she thought of herself trying to speak to crowds on sidewalks—yet it seemed as though that was what she must do. There could be no career in politics if she were frightened to stand up before the people.

In the turmoil of the meeting's end Millicent and the little dark-eyed girl spelled out their names to a harried lady who sat behind a crude table.

"Address?" the lady asked.

"R.F.D. two," Millicent told her. "Wilmerding Crosswalk, Massachusetts."

She had noticed that the dark-eyed girl leaned on a cane, and had irons on a skinny leg that she swung stiffly. Her name was Ella Jane Jespersen.

They descended the carpeted stairs together, Ella Jane clinging to the banister. But they found a pelting rain. Water poured from the glass points of the marquee.

"Let's go to the coffee shop until this lets up," said Ella Jane.

They opened the glass door from the lobby and found a plastic table top lined with chrome near the window. Millicent tried to help Ella Jane with her chair, but Ella Jane seated herself competently and hung the cane on the back of it.

"My you're brave," Ella Jane said when they were both seated. "Are you really gonna go down there and harangue savages on street corners?"

"Well, I think I should try it. It's none too soon to start getting experience."

"I hope you carry brass knuckles," said Ella Jane. "Stamping envelopes is about my speed. Two coffees?" A uniformed waitress was approaching.

"I'll have cocoa," said Millicent. "Coffee's not really good for people, I think." Ella Jane's remark about brass knuckles made her anxious. Though the idea of addressing crowds on sidewalks was scary enough it had not occurred to her until now that there might be physical danger. "Maybe I'll ask them to put me in one of the better neighborhoods," she said. "At the beginning, anyway."

"Sweetie, in that district there aren't any better neighborhoods."

They gave the waitress their orders.

Millicent told Ella Jane about Eugene's campaign for the city council in

Chicago. Ella Jane said she had gotten interested in politics because of a man too, but he had stood her up tonight.

They talked a long time. They sipped at their cups, watching the rain blur the lights beyond the plate glass. They could hear its steady sound. Millicent said it was a disgrace that the Boston Yellow Pages did not have a section for political organizations. "I've noticed that too," said Ella Jane. "The categories go straight from Polishing Equipment to Pool Rooms."

They talked about the fighting in Korea, and Millicent said she had begun to feel confident that it would not be a World War after all. Especially now that the United Nations was involved.

"Are you gonna go all the way out to Wilmerding Crosswalk at this hour?" Ella Jane said after a time, when the rain had diminished. "Why don't you come and stay over with us?"

"Oh, I couldn't really."

"Why not? I'm sure my roommate wouldn't mind."

Millicent began to protest but found herself and Ella Jane talking at once. "What?" she said.

"As a matter of fact," Ella Jane began again, "we're looking for another roommate. If you think you might be interested."

"Well, gee. I don't know. I'm flattered."

"Spend the night anyway, and you can meet my roommate. And we can all decide."

There was an electric clock over the counter. Her next train was not for a while. But she did not want to spend the night without her own toothbrush or pajamas or a change of clothing. Besides she had the next day off also and nothing to do in the city.

"How long would it take just to look at the apartment?" she asked.

They found a cab.

It did not go far, and stopped on a cross street in the Back Bay. Ella Jane began to pay, but Millicent insisted on paying half. Ella Jane let herself out onto the wet street, her good leg first. Millicent tried to help her but Ella Jane pulled away. "I've learned to help myself," she said. "I'd be lost if I didn't."

The building was sturdy, with whitish stone facing on the bottom story and brick behind fire escapes above. The entry was set back in a kind of indentation; they passed first through a stone arch that seemed to have no function but decoration, and then a narrow outdoor passage with flagstone paving that led to a heavy door, made of glass set in wood and reinforced by several vertical bars of black iron. When they had pushed open the door Ella Jane pressed one of the doorbells quickly several times.

"I want to give Natalie some warning in case her date came up," she explained.

Millicent saw the two names at the doorbell, Jespersen and McCartney. The inner door buzzed. It had carving around a central panel, but the view through the glass was closed by a stretched ruffling curtain of tan. Millicent pressed the latch and opened on a lobby of white marble. The smell was musty and there was a crumpled cigarette package.

Stairs cut in at the right, and after a flat marble square they mounted forward again. Ella Jane swung herself up a step at a time, pulling on the banister and pushing the cane. It was a long flight.

"How many more?" asked Millicent at the second flight.

"One more. Third floor. There's an elevator but it's busted."

On the third floor a door was opened for them. A girl with a round healthy face stood smiling, wearing tortoise-shell glasses, a short red jacket of corduroy over pink pajamas, and slippers with pompons.

"Hi," she said.

"Hi," said Ella Jane. "You didn't let him up?"

"Not this time."

"I've brought us a roommate. Potentially."

Ella Jane introduced Millicent. It was a large room, painted white. Against the opposite wall a dull-blue studio couch ran from the window end to an open door. Then there was a small table, against the same wall, with hanging round leaves, and a lavender telephone on it, and two more doors. Behind her there was a fireplace with glazed green tile and no logs or andirons, and a mirror over the mantel. The end wall, furthest from the windows, had a delicate old cabinet with inlay, and the open door of a closet.

"You'd sleep there, on the studio couch, as the newest roommate," said Ella Jane.

"Unless one of us has a date," said Natalie, "and then whoever has the studio couch takes one of the bedrooms, so the one that has a date has the living room clear—you see what I mean?"

Millicent nodded. Her eyes went to the rather good-sized crucifix of dark wood that hung above the little folding table.

Millicent moved to the venetian blinds and looked down through their angled slats, at the fire escape and a smallish tree. The pavement still glistened moist. Natalie opened the nearer door and showed a tiny bedroom. Its window faced the same way as those in the main room.

"This is mine," she said. "The shade's busted. I undress in the dark."

One of the doors led to a very small kitchen, in which there was no room for chairs, though a table was wedged at the end. Dishes were stacked in the sink, and a decorative little garbage pail sat on the floor, its lid propped open by a corn-flakes box.

But the bathroom was of a convenient size. Stockings were piled dry in the sink. She squeezed past the tub and the hamper to a door that opened beyond. Ella Jane's bedroom was there, quite cozy, with a lamp shining yellow by the bed, and a table radio. The room was a dead end, with no access except through the bathroom. Its window faced on a building nearby.

They went back to the living room. Millicent sat on the studio couch. "Where do you eat?" she asked. Natalie put the phone on the floor and showed her how the little drop-leaf table unfolded.

The expenses, when split three ways, seemed quite reasonable. Especially when you considered the saving in train fare.

"Why don't you spend the night?" said Natalie.

"I asked her. She doesn't want to," said Ella Jane.

"I have to get back," Millicent said.

"Well, you think it over," said Ella Jane, "and meanwhile we'll talk it over."

"I don't have to talk it over," Natalie said. "It's okay with me."

"Well, thanks," said Millicent, "you're really awfully nice. But I ought to talk it over with my parents first."

"Why?" said Natalie.

"Well, I don't know. Just because, I guess. To talk it over."

She rose in time to catch her train.

"I really do like the idea," she told them at the door.

At home she lay awake a long time. She knew that her heart had decided at once to accept the girls' offer. There was no reason not to. And she felt she had better settle it quickly, before they found someone else.

She thought of the Mieczneslíwy campaign, and in the darkness her mind concocted a slogan. Here's the pitch—switch to Mitch. She wondered if it were good enough to use.

She heard the distant clock, strange and mournful and slow in the night. Once the sun rose the sound of that bell was always somehow different. The carved clock followed, chiming in the hall downstairs.

In the morning she had a fight with Patty over the housework. It made her angry with herself, because she felt she should avoid those fights. But Patty seemed determined to pick one.

Later, while she helped her mother hang the wash, she told about the apartment.

"No," her mother said. "It isn't necessary."

"Well, I feel ready for my own place."

"You have a home," her mother said sharply.

"It's your home," Millicent corrected.

"What do you mean! Your parents' home is your home! What's the matter with you! Do you want people to talk?"

"Why should they talk?"

"Because it doesn't look right. Because there's no good reason why a respectable girl needs an apartment when her parents live in commuting distance!"

"Please, Mother, you're being insulting."

"I'm not being insulting! Home is where an unmarried girl belongs."

"I'm not a girl. I'm a woman."

"That's what you think. A girl's a girl until she's married, I don't care how old she is."

Millicent dropped it for the time being, but she knew it was in fact up to herself.

In the evening she watched Patty sit at the dressing table and primp for a date.

"You'd have dates too, if you weren't so choosy," Patty said.

"Does he still think you're a Spanish galleon?" Millicent asked.

"Oh, not him. This is a different one. That bum, I wouldn't go out with him."

Patty went out to the bathroom in her robe.

"There she goes now—the toast of the icks," Millicent heard Charles say in the hall.

"Oh, you're so funny," she heard Patty retort. "You should pose for cartoons."

Millicent knew her mother was in a bitter mood, having argued with Charles about his homework and with Patty because Patty wanted an extension telephone installed in her bedroom. But after Patty had gone she brought up the apartment again anyway, in the presence of both her parents, and said the inconvenience of commuting made it a necessity. Especially at night, when sometimes she didn't get home until three.

"What do these girls do?" her father asked.

"Ella Jane's a secretary in a brokerage office and Natalie teaches second grade," Millicent told him.

"Where?"

"Winchester. And in the summer she directs children on a playground."

Her father asked how long Natalie and Ella Jane had known each other and Millicent said they had grown up together in Springfield, or Chicopee actually.

"I'll be coming home often," Millicent assured her parents. And she pointed out that the apartment was not too far from Aunt Gwendolyn's, and that it would be useful for Charles if he had to stay at school occasionally or study at the library late at night, and that her mother could drop in often when she shopped in Boston, and that her father was in Boston sometimes for meetings or lectures.

Finally it was left that her mother would look at the apartment Sunday, to see whether she approved. But Millicent knew this was only a device to save her mother's face. She phoned to ask if the offer was still open and said she thought she would move in Sunday. She told Ella Jane her Miecznesliwy slogan.

"Here's the pitch—switch to Mitch," she said.

"Marvelous," said Ella Jane. "You're a genius."

"Do you like it?"

"Terrific. You should tell them."

"I will," said Millicent.

By Sunday her mother already seemed to have forgotten the idea of approval and talked as though her only purpose was to help Millicent get settled.

Around eleven they took the rusting Plymouth, leaving Charles home to study. Ed and Patty and Roland were at Sunday school. Millicent's round valise was packed full, and there was also a square one with bedding in it.

Ella Jane answered the door for them in her nightgown, leaning on her cane, and Natalie came from the bathroom wearing a terrycloth robe. Lucinda looked approvingly at the high ceiling with its ornate moldings. The phone was on the rugless floor and the drop-leaf table was unfolded, with dirty cups and saucers and scraps of toast. Lucinda sat visiting, on the studio couch, next to Millicent, the valises on the floor before them.

"That elevator should be fixed," Lucinda told them. "You should speak to the landlord."

"Fat chance," Ella Jane said.

"But you're entitled," said Lucinda. "Especially in your condition."

"You make me sound pregnant," said Ella Jane.

Natalie brought Lucinda some coffee, to hold on the couch, and Ella Jane returned to her own at the dirty table, her deformed leg stretched out. The cane hung from the back of her chair.

Millicent unpacked. She put her little alarm clock on the mantel. Natalie cleared a large drawer and one of the little ones in her bedroom for Millicent's use, and they pressed back the hanging suits and dresses and coats to make space in the living-room closet. Lucinda went about fingering soot on the venetian blind slats and asked for a pail and a brush.

"Mother, you can't," said Millicent.

"It's filthy dirty," said Lucinda. "You'll all get sick. I can't let you live like a bunch of bohemians." She went to the kitchen and knelt to the sink cabinet.

"Mother, please!"

"We'll get to it, Mrs. Gordon. I promise," Natalie said.

"I might as well make myself useful while I'm here," said Lucinda. "It's not your fault. You girls go to business every day." She took a box of granulated soap.

Millicent left for work, but phoned during the evening to apologize for her mother. Ella Jane told her that her mother had left finally, after scrubbing the woodwork, and the bathroom floor down on her knees and the toilet and the tub, with nonstop energy, and washing the windows inside. "Your mother's a real nut," Ella Jane said. "You should have seen her. She got down in her slip and cleaned the whole cruddy little refrigerator. I couldn't stop her. Oh, and you know what else she did? She washed Natalie's laundry. All that stuff in the sink. And hung it up to dry."

"Did Natalie let her?"

"Natalie'd gone out," Ella Jane told her. And she said Lucinda had cooked supper too, mushroom soup and an omelet.

Millicent remembered the waist-high refrigerator as particularly horrid and neglected, with bulging ice and papery lettuce and patches of dried cream. The gas range that sat on it had been caked in dusty grease. Even so, she could tend to those things herself, or with her roommates' help. She felt irritated with her mother.

She got back to the apartment toward midnight, bringing the latest edition of the paper for her roommates to read at breakfast. But she found them nowhere near ready for bed. Ella Jane lounged in the tub. Natalie was ironing, on a board she had opened up in the living room, and wore the pink pajamas and short corduroy jacket in which Millicent had first seen her. She had curlers.

Millicent prepared her linens and the afghan her mother had given her upon the studio couch, moving a floppy-eared stuffed dog that belonged to Natalie to the floor. But even after she was between the sheets the girls sat about, Natalie with her knees curled beside Millicent's feet, and Ella Jane on the bare floor, talking a long time, especially Natalie, all the lights blazing. The little clock Millicent had brought from home ticked beside the pussy willows, above the fireplace, and she wondered if the girls always stayed up so late. She did not mind, but she was glad she did not have to rise as early as they did. Ella Jane toyed with the cane upon her lap.

Natalie asked if Millicent's mother had made the afghan and said Millicent's mother was very pretty and very young-looking. Millicent said her mother was forty-two and had eloped to New Hampshire at nineteen. Natalie said it must have been lovely, and Millicent said it wasn't. Natalie talked of her own childhood, and said that actually human beings just weren't fit to be parents.

Millicent philosophized that there were two worlds, the real one and the imaginary one, and that women lived in the real one and men in the imaginary one, which consisted of ideas and concepts. "I admit I'd resent the imaginary one less if they'd let us in more," she told them. "They keep it like a club." She said that war and religion and politics were big male games, built upon concepts thought up by men, not by women. Even concepts like liberal and conservative were imaginary concepts that men invented, not women, so they could fight about them. And so were order, freedom, money, value. The whole work of civilization, the whole culture, was essentially based on idea structures, and was designed to give men interesting things to do. And that was why men as individuals have always seemed to be doing such interesting things—theorizing, fighting, building. And because men could thus be more interesting women went gaga over them, and so the vicious cycle continued. She said it made her angry. Women were so gaga over men that they let them keep putting it over—it was not that men were cleverer.

"Men are bastards," Ella Jane said, almost in a drawl.

"No, I don't think that," said Millicent. "You can't blame individuals for the cultural situation they find. But it's a fact that women live under men's law. Just as much as the Indians had to live under the law of the Massachusetts Bay Colony. It was no creation of theirs. If you see the parallel. I've really been thinking lately that I feel about men the way the Indian tribes must have felt about the white settlers—they've got a highly complicated society, with all kinds of technology and high-level religion, and they raise your living standards, and they tempt you, but the price is nothing less than your total destruction. No matter how fair they pretend to be—they leave you no chance to be anything on your own. You end up living the white man's law. All because they know how to keep us divided."

"Well," said Ella Jane, "I don't know that much about the Indians, but women are the ones that end up naked, and wearing beads and feathers, I suppose. You've got a point there."

"No, I'm not kidding," Millicent said. "We're like Negroes then, if that makes it clear. We might just as well ride in the back of the bus. I know I feel it in my work, and I'm sure you do."

"Oh, I suppose," said Ella Jane.

"It's true," said Natalie. "It really is."

"I was given a chance," Millicent said, "I don't know why. Either they needed someone very badly or he just believed in me somehow. But lots of them resent me. They expect women to be menials while men seek their own self-development. I remember when my father went into the Navy—oh well. It's stupid. Whether you seek a career, or marriage, it's all set up to favor the men."

"Have you ever been in love?" Natalie asked her.

"Do you really think war and religion and politics are male games?" Ella Jane asked. Millicent opened her mouth to answer Ella Jane, but Ella Jane continued. "Do you think women would abolish them?"

Millicent closed her mouth a moment pensively.

"Generals even talk about war games," said Natalie.

"That's right, they do, don't they," said Ella Jane.

"I don't think a woman President would have dropped the bomb," Millicent answered finally.

"Yes she would," said Ella Jane. "Because we had to drop the bomb."

"No we didn't," Millicent told her. "Because we had control of the sea by then, and control of the air, and that was enough to effectively nullify Japanese control of any territory outside of their own islands. Which was all we really cared about. We could have ended the war right then, with no invasion and no bomb."

"Have you ever been in love?" Natalie asked again.

"No."

"You're twenty-one, and you've never been in love?" Ella Jane asked, staring.

"No." She was starting to color somewhat.

"Not even a schoolgirl crush?" asked Ella Jane.

"I don't think so. I've had friendships with men from time to time. I believe in friendships."

In the silence they both kept looking at her, Natalie on the afghan at her feet and Ella Jane upon the floor.

"Well," Ella Jane said, "the main difference between love and friendship is that love has more hatred in it."

"Well, I don't think sex should be a barrier," Millicent said. "People can't help what sex they are."

Toward two o'clock Ella Jane lifted herself upon her cane, yawning, and in a while the apartment was dark and quiet.

Millicent heard tires on the street. A light outside made a curious fixed pattern on the ceiling, formed of spreading shadows from the fire escape.

It had been a good conversation, she thought. It occurred to her that the problems that had overwhelmed and depressed her after graduation had already disappeared. She had a promising job, and on her own time she had found an entry into political work. And now an apartment, and friends.

You have to have a faith that your problems would be solved, she thought.

12

Bobby O'Shaughnessy stopped by with several tiny kittens in a grocery box and offered to swap them for some rabbits that Roland was hoping to catch. But Roland had no interest in cats apart from his scheme for raising them for rental, which his parents had vetoed anyway. Patty said the old dog would be jealous of a new kitten. Bobby said his father had told him any kittens he could not find takers for would have to be drowned, so Millicent, who was home again for one of her days off, asked for one to take to Boston. She picked out a completely black one, with tiny eyes like hard blue gems. It was very small, and when she held it to her its claws made scratchy noises in the cotton of her blouse. In the morning Charles let her off with it at her apartment. She also had a heavy box of sand that Charles had given her for the cat, and a potted red-leafed coleus that her mother had given her to set on the window sill of the apartment.

Her roommates were fascinated by the kitten, as she had known they would be. The first evening all three girls spent hours with it, tossing balls of paper and dangling string. On the uncovered floor his paws slid unsteadily.

Millicent had quickly come to feel at home here. The other girls arose early and breakfasted in the room where she slept, but after a few mornings the sound of doors and coffee cups scarcely wakened her, and she did not arise until long after they had gone.

She had more time than before. She took care of Sharlene during the day sometimes so Aunt Gwendolyn could be interviewed for a job, and once she brought the kitten for Sharlene to see but it kept her busy—if she set him down in order to warm lunch or rinse a diaper the baby would get to him. But if she went out pushing Sharlene in the stroller the kitten could ride in the carrier. She named him Theodore, after Theodore Victor Mieczneslíwy.

She fell into a pattern of waking about ten in the morning, on workdays and days off alike. She would close the venetian blinds and do her calisthenics in her pajama top, and then tidy the apartment. Usually she found Natalie's pajamas and red corduroy bed jacket lying about on the fat worn chair with broken springs. Her own bed had to be put into shape again as a studio couch and its linens put out of sight with her mother's afghan, and then the goggle-eyed stuffed dog with floppy ears had to be put on it. The dog wasn't much to her taste, but it had always been kept there and she didn't want to disturb her roommates' ways. She also filled some hours by doing much of the marketing, and at night the three calculated what was owed her.

She told the Independent Citizens' Committee her slogan, but they did not give her much to do yet. The street-corner speaking teams were not yet organized.

The apartment needed a careful dusting every day because of city grit, and she would have to move everything on the mantel this way and that, the little framed pictures of her roommates' relatives, the pussy willows reflecting in the mirror, and her clock. The wall fixtures on either side of the mirror were convoluted and ornate, but she had gradually gotten them clean. The wooden-and-upholstered dining chairs were rickety and needed gluing. And the inlaid cabinet that stood near the closet was also unsteady. When she moved Natalie's record player that sat on top of it there was a square in the dust, as though it hadn't been played for a while. The player was finished in tan fabric and was larger than Patty's white one.

Sometimes before going to work she would lie on the dull-blue studio couch and fondle the kitten. Her fingertips felt the soft black fur slide over the two knobs of the shoulder bones. He didn't scratch her.

Already she had learned much about her roommates, as though they were friends of long standing. She knew about Ella Jane having a romantic attachment to a broker in her office. And she knew about Natalie's parents being divorced, and that Natalie had been brought up for a time by her father's parents, who had disliked both her parents, and that her father was a renegade Catholic and that her mother had taken up Christian Science. She even knew Ella Jane's shrunken leg with a pathetic intimacy now, having helped her in and out of the tub several times. It was like skin on a frail bone.

She was impressed that Ella Jane read The New York Times on Sundays. Ella Jane said the Boston papers were awful. "With all due respect to you," she told Millicent, "you can't get any news out of them."

"Mr. Killian said Boston's a great newspaper town," Millicent answered.

Natalie was not as bright as Ella Jane. If a young man telephoned Natalie would snatch the lavender phone, which had a long cord, and settle and curl with it in the fat worn chair, the phone tucked between ear and shoulder while she lighted a cigarette. Once Millicent heard her go on and on softly with a caller who for a considerable time refused to identify himself. Another time she heard her answer detailed questions about her appearance.

Ella Jane was often taciturn. If she withdrew and shut herself for an evening with a book in her room beyond the bath Millicent was disappointed, because she enjoyed the discussions they had at other times. There was a series of stimulating arguments about whether the President was a drunkard—Ella Jane liked him as a sort of common man, but Millicent felt that the well-being of the republic demanded that a President bring dignity to the office.

On another occasion she told Ella Jane that only a male would be a Hitler or a Stalin, playing at being a god and trying to reshape the human race according to his own imagination. Playing soldier and playing divine were male sports—

women rarely went in for such stuff. Only males would have nothing better to do with their surplus energy than to invent the bomb. "Men want to be gods," she said, "and women just want to be people. That's what the whole trouble is."

Natalie listened, but it was with Ella Jane that one could exchange ideas. Once, at two in the morning, Millicent said that the phrase "women and children" was in the language as though women and children constituted a single class, and that she resented it. Another time Ella Jane asked her why she didn't look for a job in Chicago, so as to be near Eugene, and Millicent replied that she was not a puppy dog and did not believe in following people about.

At night, when she returned to the apartment bringing her roommates the late city edition, she usually took the subway, but by day it was less than a half-hour stroll to work, by the edges of the Public Garden and the Common. Sometimes Mr. Hopkins phoned her to come in early and work overtime. In the city room Maud still gave her encouraging smiles, and sometimes told her little pointers on how a news item should be put together, in case Mr. Killian should ever give her any to do. Millicent had learned meanwhile that other women worked on the paper, though not in the city room. There was Alice Dingley, who wrote an advice column in a frosted glass cubicle of her own down the corridor, and Phyllis Richmond, who edited the society page and had youthful brown hair in ringlets around a lined and powdered face. Phyllis and Alice were small and shriveled, like Maud, and once when Millicent saw the three of them cross the street to the spa together she thought they all looked much alike, especially from the rear.

She met Theodore Victor Miecznesliwy finally, at an evening reception, and was impressed by him and by his wife. She wanted to tell him about her slogan, and about naming her cat for him, but there were imposing people around him all evening long, conversing constantly, and an agitated timidity took hold of her whenever she thought about breaking in.

Ella Jane had not come with her, being in one of her withdrawn moods, and after the reception Millicent walked to the apartment alone. She found that Ella Jane had already retired, with her door shut. The kitten slept on the folded green bath mat under the bathroom sink.

Millicent found her white pajamas in Natalie's bureau. She would have to sleep in Natalie's bed tonight, because Natalie had a date and would have the living room and the studio couch.

Millicent made sure the living room was tidy, and then the kitchen and bath, so that Natalie might bring her friend up without embarrassment. Then she decided she had better go to bed early so as to be out of the way.

She lay on the painted iron bed. There was no window shade, at least none that could be drawn. The street lamp put a drab illumination on the pattern of the wallpaper, and she could see the shadow on it of some fluttering insect. The room was exceedingly small. When she had opened the bureau drawer it had bumped the bed, so that she had had to climb on the mattress.

She could not sleep. Apparently she was too unused to being in bed at this hour. She thought some ovaltine might help. She went to the kitchen and heated a tall glassful.

She lay on the bed again, with eyes shut, and tried to let herself drift into slumber. But after half an hour she gave up and simply lay on her side under the sheet, her mind wandering idly.

There was a sound of a lock turning, and she heard the voices of Natalie and a man. Natalie sounded drunk, or pretending to be drunk, although not loud. But a moment later she sounded sober, so that Millicent thought she had been mistaken. She did not like the voice of the friend. He spoke too rapidly.

She heard the door of the rickety cabinet, and in a few moments water running in the kitchen. After a while there were footsteps in the living room again, and as someone moved past her door vague shadows flickered in the orange-yellow light beneath it.

She thought she heard Natalie kick off her shoes.

She tried again to sleep. She was sorry now she had drunk that big glass of ovaltine, because she had to go to the bathroom, and there was no way to. She realized now that Ella Jane's bedroom, which she had thought the least desirable, queerly situated as it was back there, was actually the most convenient.

There was murmured conversation. She ought to be asleep, she thought. Yet she knew she was unlikely to sleep until she got to the bathroom. She hoped Natalie's company would not stay long.

The living room was silent for so long that she wondered if perhaps he had left without her hearing. The ray of light beneath the door also seemed more dim. But then there was a noise as though a glass had fallen, although it didn't break, and again a murmur of unclear conversation. "Al! You're crazy," she heard Natalie say.

"Relax," the man's voice advised softly after a moment.

"I'm trying to," said Natalie.

"Comfy?" the man's voice asked.

There was another silence.

"Do you think I have pretty legs?"

"Come on," she heard Al's voice. "There's no sense getting it wrinkled."

"Well, okay," Natalie said, in a tone of reluctance. "But that's all I'm taking off."

Millicent felt her cheeks grow warm in the dark. She felt embarrassed for Natalie's sake, to be lying here awake and hearing what she had no business to hear. There was a giggle beyond the door.

She put her head under the sheet. But it was hot. And the need for the bathroom was becoming more intense.

She was too uncomfortable to lie still. She sat up in the bedclothes, and yawned. There was no handkerchief in her pajama pocket. Her nose was not bothersome just now, but to be without a handkerchief made her uneasy.

There was more murmuring.

She saw Natalie's eyeglasses lying here on the bureau. Apparently Natalie had deliberately left them at home, and endured the movie as a blur.

"What are you *doing!*" she heard Natalie say. The voice was a squeak.

"You don't need a thing like this, with your figure," Al's voice muttered.

"I wore it for protection," she heard Natalie answer.

There was more silence, and then a little exclamation or cry, and Millicent thought they both snickered. There was a thump as if the studio couch had moved an inch and struck the wall.

I feel sorry for her, I really do, Millicent said to herself. She felt sure that Ella Jane must also realize how shallow Natalie was. But Ella Jane was the type who kept her own counsel, and would certainly not discuss the failings of a girl she had known since childhood. Ella Jane had a quiet self-sufficiency and did not talk about people.

There was silence, and then murmuring, and more silence.

She offers her lips in return for his companionship, Millicent thought, and he understands the bargain. She offers her skin to be pinched and insulted, and he offers the pleasure of his company. How conceited men are, and how degraded women are.

And in a way the most degrading thing of all was her going to the movie without her eyeglasses.

There was no sound now from beyond the door. Millicent sat rocking on the mattress. Maybe it was safe now to hazard a knock on the door, and pretend she had only this moment awakened.

But even if they got quickly presentable, she had no bathrobe and did not want that creature looking at her in her pajamas.

She looked at the window. This room was a little prison. She would never again drink anything before going to bed here.

"We've got to make you comfortable," the man's voice pleaded.

"No."

"Come on. You can't tell me it's too much trouble to get it on again. We're at your place now."

"Why don't you believe me when I say no?"

Even in these erotic sessions, Millicent thought, it's the woman whose clothes are removed, and the man who observes.

Like an adult supervising the undressing of a child. Like a clothed adult sponging a naked child—the child may have no secrets from the adult. And as in everything else, it's the man who can play the adult, while the woman must play the child.

For since women are a class of beings who are accorded no dignity in the first place, she said to herself, it follows inevitably that their privacy need not be taken seriously—that their underclothing and flesh may be smirked at.

She bent forward to get a handkerchief from one of the smaller drawers.

"Be nice, Al," she heard Natalie ask softly.

"I am nice, but I can't even cuddle. I like to hold a woman, not a bunch of two-way stretch."

The drawer gave a wooden groan and Millicent's heart gave a frightened leap.

"Sh!" she heard Natalie say almost in a whisper. "I think my roommate's awake."

Millicent stayed frigidly still. Natalie must be mortified, she thought.

She let herself silently back on the bed, abandoning the drawer. The living room became silent too. The pale light still glowed at the keyhole and beneath the door. She shut her eyes, the sheet loosely upon her head, and lay curled with her discomforts, wanting to seem asleep. Even when he goes home, I can't come out immediately, she thought.

She heard Natalie say something, quietly and unintelligible. Then there was silence again.

Her mind kept working. Children are shown naked before adults, and women before men. And slaves on the block, and concentration-camp inmates before their guards. Only the truly free citizen is spared this humiliation.

13

For several nights Millicent worked her full time, but then, on a slack evening, Mr. Hopkins released her a half hour early.

It was warm, and the theater lobbies and coffee shops were still bright, so she decided to walk at least part way. Then, as the streets seemed wide and well-lighted and peaceful, she continued on foot all the way.

She climbed to the apartment and let herself in, and for an instant it seemed that Ella Jane, sitting in her bathrobe by the drop-leaf table, looked at her with an odd expectancy. Then she saw her brother Charles in the fat worn chair.

"Charles!" she said.

"Hi." He was lounging with ankles spread out, his hands on the stuffed arms of the chair. His schoolbooks were in a pile beside his foot.

"Why aren't you home? How long have you been here?" She took a step into the room.

"Oh, twenty minutes. I had some work at the library, so I phoned the folks and said I'd be bunking here. You said I'd be able to bunk here once in a while."

"But not just like that, without any warning." From beyond the closed door of the bathroom there was a sound of a faucet. "Barging in and bothering my roommates. I don't even know if there's room."

"He didn't bother us," said Ella Jane.

"Your roommate said you'd make room."

It was true, she remembered, that she had mentioned this possibility to her mother, before she had actually moved in. But she had not thought of it since then. She crossed to the dull-blue studio couch and put down her shoulder-strap bag and her late city edition.

"Sis, I'm in the Air Force."

"What?"

"He enlisted," Ella Jane told her, "and he's afraid to go home."

Millicent sat, staring at him. He remained sprawled in the chair, not moving, and did not avoid her gaze. "You're out of your mind," she said. "You mean you quit school?"

"Well, the school doesn't know it yet. But they were gonna can me anyway."

"Charles, it's absurd. You better go straight home and tell Mother and Dad. Can the Air Force take boys just like that? It's irresponsible."

"Well, I'm not quite eighteen, technically. So I still need parental consent."

"You'll never get it. Where's your car?"

"Around the corner."

"Well you go straight home," she told him.

"Mother and Dad didn't mind my staying here."

"You didn't tell them what you were up to."

Natalie came in from the bathroom, her hair in curlers and her face aglow. She was barefoot and bare-legged, seeming to wear only the short red corduroy jacket.

"Natalie, this is my brother Charles," Millicent said.

Charles didn't rise. "I know, we met," said Natalie, and sat at an end of the studio couch, knees together. "How old are you, little soldier boy?"

"Eighteen."

"My my, think of that. And does your mother know you're out?"

"Have you got anything on under there?" he asked.

"Wouldn't you like to know," she said. The corduroy scarcely covered her hips.

"She's got panties on. Don't excite yourself," Ella Jane put in tiredly.

"Natalie! Go put something on," Millicent said.

"Why?" said Natalie. "Hasn't he ever seen legs before?"

Millicent was coloring. "That's not the point. It's elementary decency."

"I knew she had panties on," said Charles.

"Want to see them?" said Natalie.

"Natalie! Don't you dare!" Millicent said. "Natalie, really. Will you cover up please? For goodness sakes."

Natalie rose, with a sullen little twist. Then, at her bedroom door, she looked back and smiled. "He's cute," she said. She went out of sight in the bedroom, though without closing the door. There was the sound of a drawer.

Millicent felt uncomfortable, but she did not know how to resume her discussion with Charles and no one else said anything. In a moment Natalie reappeared, in slacks of a dogtooth pattern, and leaned on the doorjamb.

"You gonna let me stay, Sis?" Charles asked. "I'll sleep on the floor."

Natalie let herself fall to the studio couch.

"Give him a break," said Ella Jane. "Don't make him drive way up there at this hour."

"What's the matter, Sis? Unless you think I shouldn't be in this harem."

"I'm a perfectly adequate chaperon, as far as that goes—" she told him severely. Natalie and Ella Jane both laughed.

She reddened darker. She knew they considered her prissy. But she noticed that Charles didn't laugh.

"I'll make it up to ya," he said. "I'll fix all these chairs that are coming apart. The first thing in the morning. I'll get the glue. I've got a hammer in the car."

She leaned way back, against the studio-couch bolster and the wall, not knowing what to say to him.

"I had a test today," he said, "and I couldn't do a damn thing. And the headmaster's gonna call Dad, and what's the use of the headmaster and Dad batting me back and forth to each other and telling each other to make me study? I'll be eighteen in three weeks anyhow. I'll be drafted, with my record—I've been thinking about it a long time. But if I go in the Air Force now I can pick my service, and I'll learn to be an aircraft mechanic and I'll start my own business when I get out. So I went down there today. I was gonna enlist fraudulently and be at Otis Air Base tomorrow, but I didn't have a draft card so Dad or Mother have to give consent. I'm doing them a favor, Sis. If I wait three weeks I can go in without their consent and in the meantime the second half of the tuition's due. And it ain't cheap. That school ain't cheap. It'd be silly to stay in school another couple of weeks and waste money."

"I still think you should stay in as long as you can. They'd be heartbroken if you quit school."

"I know it. That's why I didn't want to break the news until tomorrow. Let them sleep tonight."

"I still think the three weeks might be a very useful cooling-off period. To think it over."

"Sis, I want to go in where I can learn something, in my field. I wait three weeks and the draft board's got a mortgage on me."

"You might not be drafted for a year," Ella Jane said.

"You might not even be drafted," said Natalie.

"I'd be stupid to count on that. Sis, you talk to them, will ya? So they'll give consent."

"Me?"

"Call them in the morning."

"I don't even approve. No. I will not. I refuse to be a part of it."

"He's brave enough to face the enemy, but he's not brave enough to face his parents," said Ella Jane.

"Yeah, be a man, Charles," said Natalie. "Make a clean breast of it."

"Oh sure, 'be a man,' " he answered Natalie. "It's easy for a woman to say 'be a man.' What do you know about it? Do you know what it is to be a man?"

"I still think you should do your own talking," said Millicent.

"Did you ever try to talk to Dad? It's impossible." His eyes were fixed upon her eyes, and he was spread out in the big chair. "He's too tied up in human destiny, and all that kind of crap. So he takes you for a walk, you know, his idea of getting close to you. And go on about all the joy of being alive here, the wonder. Looking at a tree or something. Boy, he thinks that's so heart-to-heart he could practically cry. All right, the universe and everything—if it's there it's still there, and so what. What I want to know is, I'm eighteen. How the hell do I get any place? How do I break into the God damn economy?"

"What could I say to him?" asked Millicent. "That you couldn't? I'm sure he won't start talking about trees."

"No. No, I know what he'll say. He'll say he's not gonna let me quit school and ruin my life."

"And what'll I say to that?" asked Millicent. "I agree with him."

"Well, tell him college should wait until I'm more mature."

"I don't know if you're right, Charles. You're the normal age now, and I don't see what you gain by putting it off and getting rusty."

"Sis, the future is in aircraft. I'll be learning all the time. My trouble is that I have to see the practicality of a problem or my mind wanders, and if my mind wanders I'm wasting time."

She tried to convey disapproval by her expression, but his blue eyes remained on her, round and sad. He looked very young, with his soft bristly crew cut and his thin face. His fingers played with the frayed upholstery.

When he spoke again there was a pleading in his voice. "You've got a way with Dad, I don't know. He listens to you."

"It's none of my business," said Ella Jane softly, "but if it was my brother I'd make the call."

Millicent was troubled.

"If a brother or a sister was in trouble," Ella Jane continued, "and asked me to phone my parents, or be a go-between, I'd phone. What do we have each other for?"

Millicent was silent. Her gaze fell away from Charles.

"Well, let's turn in," Ella Jane said finally. "How shall we arrange this?"

"Millicent can sleep with me, and he can have the studio couch," Natalie said.

"No," said Millicent. "We'll put the studio-couch cushion on the floor, and he'll sleep on the floor like he said."

"No—" Natalie protested.

"I don't mind," said Charles. "Honest."

"It'll be like a rock," said Natalie.

"No it won't," he said.

"Okay then," said Ella Jane. "I guess we better say good night. So you can turn in." She reached around for the cane that hung from the back of her chair. She rose with it, and looked at Millicent again. "Don't feel so badly," she said. "There's an old proverb—if at first you don't succeed, quit while you're still young enough to try something else."

She went out without saying anything more, but Natalie brought sheets. Natalie helped lift the long cushion from the couch and spread the sheets.

"You shouldn't have to do this," Millicent said to her.

Millicent prepared bedclothes upon the cushionless studio couch, and other bedclothes on the long cushion that lay on the floor, trying to do it quickly all herself, but Charles and Natalie both assisted. She brought her pajamas from Natalie's room.

She saw Charles stare at the flowery drapes that hung beside the venetian blinds. "Mother made those," she told him.

"I thought they looked familiar."

When Natalie was gone she asked him if he wanted some milk or cocoa.

"No thanks," he said.

"What did they say when you said you were staying overnight—who'd you talk to, Mother or Dad?"

"Mother."

"What did she say?"

"Nothing. I told her you said it was okay."

She thought of remarking that it wasn't very honest. But she let it go. She picked up her pajamas. "Well," she said, "I'll use the bathroom first and you can undress meanwhile. Have you got pajamas?"

"I'll sleep in my underwear."

She wondered briefly whether any of Natalie's pajamas would fit him, but then decided not to suggest it.

In the bathroom she found underthings and stockings hanging from the shower rod to dry. The shower light shone through a flower pattern in the half-transparent cups of a bra, and the heavy fabric of a girdle still dripped from a corner. She took them all down, that Charles might not have to see such a display, and hid them under towels on the hamper top. She saw the black kitten curled asleep on the folded green bath mat.

She returned to the living room in white pajamas. Charles was already under blankets, his head by the cold radiators and windows. She clicked out the light, and wound the little alarm clock on the mantelpiece. Then she stepped around his pallet and climbed onto the couch. She settled in her bed sheets with her face to the wall.

"You can use the bathroom now if you want," she said.

She heard him rise and walk barefoot.

The couch without its cushion was more uncomfortable than she had expected. She could feel springs. On the long cushion Charles would be more comfortable than she was, she thought.

She heard him return and settle on the floor again.

"How is it down there?" she asked. "Hard?"

"Nope."

She had spoken with her face still to the wall. She thought of asking him to trade places. But she didn't.

"If he'd accepted me today without the draft card I'd have just gone," he said.

"If who accepted you?"

"The sergeant. The recruiting sergeant. I'd be gone. Mother or Dad would have had to come in and get the car."

"That's really irresponsible."

"I'd have given you the car if you had a license. You can have it anyway if you want it."

"No."

It was depressing that her brother could go off just like that. She had not considered herself particularly close to him, and she herself had gone off to college for four years. But the family had not dissolved.

She thought of the war in Korea. But it was not just that. It was his readiness to go off and be committed in a career, with scarcely a backward glance. She seemed to realize suddenly that he would settle as a mechanic far away, and marry someday in a strange town, as though he had no kin and no sister.

"What did you do all evening?" she asked. "Did you really go to the library?" She was facing the radiating shadows on the ceiling now.

"No. I rode around. And I sat over by the river."

"Just sat there?"

"Just sat there. I talked with a girl for a while."

"What girl?"

"Just a girl that was there."

"It's a terrible time to enlist. They'll send you to Korea."

"Not necessarily. It could be Germany, Paris, Spain. Turkey, Alaska. Stateside. We've got installations everywhere."

"Will you be flying? In planes?"

"Ground crew."

"You were never interested in planes."

"Sis, I'm interested in all kinds of vehicles. When I was ten I knew every part of a steam engine, and when I was twelve I knew every part of a car. I could even name all the sails of a full-rigged sailing ship, for that matter, from pictures. Any kind of vehicles. All vehicles. Even the wind problems in the old dirigibles. Rocket ships, trolley cars, anything that moved. I used to lie awake thinking about magnetism, explosions, and momentum, and all the different ways of putting them together—the millions of tricks you could use."

"But that's just it, Charles. You have a wonderful talent with machines, and schooling will make you a success at it. Otherwise you'll just end up working for somebody else."

"Oh no. Not me."

"You have to have math."

"Now you sound like Dad. You know, Sis, part of intelligence is soul, though. You have to know when you're wasting your time. Dad used to play checkers with the minister in Abbottsford, and he never had sense enough to realize checkers is a waste of time."

"But you should finish the summer at least, and get a high-school diploma, so you'll be ready for college when you come back."

"Sis, the math in that school is trigonometry. Engineers use calculus—they don't use trigonometry. Trigonometry's for surveyors. You know what trigonometry is? It's tables. Looking up things in tables. It bores me. And in French they teach ya a tense that the French don't even use any more. Now there's guys that can put their mind on that. But I've got to cut my losses. I'd rather be a guy that flunked out of high school than a guy that flunked out of college, because people at least have a certain amount of respect for a guy that flunked out of high school. You can talk, Sis—you don't know how it feels to flunk in two schools. But the way I've been headed I'm losing. I've got to change my luck. Do you know how easy it is to be a failure? You don't have to lift a finger. It'll just roll right in. When you're little it's 'any boy can be President.' And then your ambitions go slowly down, down, till when you're eighteen it's a question of how do you get a foot in the door some place. You think I'm kidding, Sis? It's a scary thing to come of age. When you're a kid you're full of promise, and then all of a sudden you're a bum."

In the silence Millicent wet her lips.

He began again, his tone softer and slower. "There's guys I knew in high school and they're in Harvard already. I can't even talk to them. They've got it made. They've all got it made. I'm the only shmuck."

"Well," she said finally, "I'll try to tell him your point of view. But I won't recommend anything."

"You're terrific, Cockeyes." He spoke quietly, and she heard the emotion in his voice. He reached up and took her hand.

"Mother will be hysterical," she said.

"Well, that's Dad's problem. That's why I say tell Dad. Sis, you know I could have had different jobs while going to school, and amassed some capital in the meantime. Like the copy-boy deal, and I had a chance to work in Moon's Garage. But they always said no. I could have driven a cab part time in Sparkstown, and studied right there at the taxi stand. Mother said it's dangerous. And they're the ones that make me feel dumb, with all this private schools and stuff. I don't want to see them throw their money away. Especially when I can get the G.I. bill later. When I can't even put my mind on the stuff."

For what seemed a long time she felt his grasp. Then she withdrew her fingers. She turned again toward the wall, as if to sleep.

"I gave your apartment as my home address," he said.

"Why'd you do that?"

"I don't know. I just did."

"That's a crazy thing to do."

She turned and settled in the darkness. Above the radiator the coleus leaves and their pot were silhouetted on the sill.

"Does Ella Jane ever give you any stock tips?" he asked.

"No."

"I asked her about stocks," he said, "and all she knows is blue chips and mutual funds. I asked her for a growth stock, and she says Raytheon. I could tell her that myself."

He was silent a moment.

"She never let you in on a good one, did she?"

"No," said Millicent.

She stirred again, and lay looking at the ceiling.

"That Natalie's quite a dish," said Charles.

"Don't refer to a woman as a dish."

"Why?"

"Because she's not meant to be consumed. Anyway she can hear everything we say."

14

Lucinda blamed Ed, and in ways that seemed to him unreasonable and illogical. The fact was that he, not she, had been the one who had tried to interest Charles in books and in science and in scholarship generally—yet now she blamed him for interesting Charles in machinery.

It was his own influence that had inclined the children toward scholarship. Millicent actually taught herself all the twenty-six letters of the alphabet at the age of two—it was the truth, even though people sometimes didn't believe him. And at four she had known the Hebrew letters also, and so had Charles. And it was he who had kept television out, even though Lucinda would have had it. Lucinda had always been the inconstant one, who had let the children leave things undone. Patty had been sent to a summer camp as a child, but on the first Sunday, when she had cried that she wanted to go home, Lucinda had taken her home, and the child was no sooner home than she wanted to be in camp again. Millicent had shown remarkable talent in dancing school, but at the first childish boredom, at the age of nine, Lucinda had let it all go down the drain.

But when he pointed these things out now in his defense, Lucinda called him a fanatic, as though any consistency were fanaticism. He had made Charles rebel.

"Which is it?" he said. "Was I too severe or didn't I encourage him to study? You can't have it both ways."

Then she accused him of backing Charles up in using the Sabbath as an excuse to put off his homework. By now she was sobbing.

After listening to Millicent on the phone, and to Charles, and to the headmaster of Sweetser Hall at length and in detail, and considering the draft, and after some thought, and talking to Charles again, he felt he might as well consent to the enlistment. There seemed little choice. He felt in his heart that the boy was already on his own, no matter how you might plead and wrangle. He tried to clarify his thoughts, for his own benefit as well as Lucinda's, but her eyes filled up again as though he were a hostile draft board.

"I don't call that growing up," she said. "Quitting school and joining the Army Air Force."

She seemed to feel it was still possible somehow to get Charles into Northeastern in the fall and get him a deferment, because headmasters and draft boards would listen to a clergyman, and the Government didn't want boys to leave school. She also had a tearful theory now that Ed had neglected Charles as a baby by going to a seminary in New York. He pointed out that he had been willing to take the family to New York but she had opposed it, so he had come home every weekend. Her answer to that was that he had neglected the children by his time in the Navy.

There was work he had hoped to accomplish during the day at his desk, and he went back to it, feeling exhausted, and angry at Lucinda.

In the early afternoon Charles came home in the Model T, without having been to school, and bringing Millicent, since she was off. Lucinda had presented the enlistment to Patty and Roland as a disaster, and had cried on the phone to her mother and her sisters, but it struck Ed that she was much more controlled now that she confronted Charles.

"Forget about Korea," he heard Charles tell her. "Just because I enlist it doesn't mean Korea. We've got bases in England and Europe and all over the place. Including the United States. And even in Korea the mechanics are way behind the lines anyway. They have to be. Half the stuff is based in Japan."

"Maybe they'll bomb the airport," Lucinda said.

"With what?" said Charles. "What are they gonna use? Tie a junk to a balloon?"

"Well, I don't know," said his mother. "Don't they get Russian planes or something?"

"We've got mastery of the air in the Far East."

Lucinda asked what if there was a flare-up about Berlin again, or what if they began to use atom bombs, and Charles said that in that case Boston wouldn't be safe either. He said it was more likely that the Korea thing would be contained, and it might even be over by the time he finished basic. He couldn't just stay home in fear of all the possibilities that might happen.

Millicent said, in a detached way, that she had heard there were opportunities for study in the armed forces and that a high-school diploma could even be gotten, and that in any case nobody could succeed at anything he wasn't interested in.

She seemed to Ed startlingly mature, more so than he had ever seen her. He followed her out to the porch and sat on the glider, watching her loll on the steps. She sat leaning back against a column, her face and closed eyes basking. A knee was raised, and her blue jeans had gray ridges where the color had worn. She had brought her black kitten, planning to stay overnight, and it played nearby. Ed had an urge to be talking to her, yet every beginning he thought of seemed constrained.

It was as if his feeling of insufficiency toward Charles made him a little afraid of Millicent also—this one too was already out of his hands.

He saw the shabbiness of the house and the yard.

A dark, jarring feeling came upon him that perhaps his own capacities were actually far less than he had always presumed.

His gaze fell upon the cat, and upon a rent that formed two sides of a little square high in the side of Millicent's jeans. Through it he glimpsed the soft wrinkly sheen of what she wore beneath. He looked at her closed eyes. Her face leaned motionless toward the sun. He saw the slimness of her ankles, tapering from the frayed bottoms. How adult she looked. A grownup, complete. She had discussed Charles's problem, taking part in a grave family council, talking as sensibly as anyone else, and presuming to be the equal of everyone present.

Even as a child, she had always been like a little mother, an assistant mother, to the others. She was still the only girl or woman he had ever seen who squeezed a tube of toothpaste properly.

He had not exactly listened to her words this morning, but he had wondered whether to try still to guide Charles as a child if necessary—try to make him get himself into college—or whether it was perhaps time at last to give him his head, and let him maybe find himself, or even make a mistake or two. All of a child's years, from the beginning, you try to teach, but at what age exactly does he become entitled to ignore the teaching? It was like the question of daughters—do you let her go off in an automobile to wrestle with boys, or do you bind her with restrictions until she rebels?

Millicent stirred on the step, without opening her eyes.

Patty already was old enough to spend money in the beauty parlor and sit in dark cars. All right, so far so good, you teach and she's loyal. You see a daughter reach adolescence, burgeon. You think you accept it, that breath-taking sweetness, but every six months or less you're startled anew that she's grown still bigger, more beautiful. Loaded with dynamite your baby walks about, goes to school.

In the past year Millicent had mentioned to Lucinda in some connection that she never got messy with that boy she saw so much of in Chicago. Ed had said of course, but in fact he had taken comfort in it. Only now, suddenly, looking at that motionless sunning form and closed eyes, he felt he could read nothing in that face. She had reached the age of secrecy.

Ed had some appointments in the afternoon, and when he got home Millicent was in knee-length shorts. She was helping prepare supper, quickly tearing the wilted leaves from a head of lettuce. It seemed to him that her every motion and stance was grace. Every slight shift of weight, every dip of her knee or half-turn of her torso, was full of unconscious elegance. No wonder that in that childhood dancing school she had been the best in the class.

There never was a time when she wasn't beautiful, he thought. Some children have pretty ages and less pretty ones; some are gawky at one stage or another, but never Millicent. At the age of three her running laughter had been higher-pitched than the highest notes on the piano. And he remembered the beauty of a girl of nine or ten, lying on the floor with a book, the healthiness, the shape of her calves. Her serious face seemed not unhappy but sensitive. What a lovely example of a human being, he had thought. Mankind rises to a new possibility in this kid. It surprised him that Amethyst Gilbert had singled out Patty as the attractive one—Patty had a cream-puff prettiness, but Millicent had a thinking, living beauty.

She put down the bread platter, near where he sat, and their eyes met briefly. Then she was busy again.

Her eyes had always looked like that, he thought. They gave an illusion of being a tiny bit crossed, yet both eyes fixed directly and perfectly upon you, blue and large, and that illusory air of turning in seemed like the slight turning in of eyes that fix on an object at very close range. They seemed examining, fascinated, and very near. It was as if she saw nothing but you. Whether it was all only some accidental trick of her appearance that she could not help, and quite meaningless, or whether it corresponded to some truth of her nature, he could not know. And the not knowing was teasing also.

After supper Charles went out to the barn where his Model T stood, near a workbench that had cans and tools and rags, and Ed followed him. He watched Charles inspect all the car's fluids, beneath it and under the hood. Then he started the engine for him while Charles poked with a screwdriver. Charles was eager to enlist with as little loss of time as possible, in order to be shipped to a certain training school by a certain date, and he wanted to turn in his license plates and cancel the insurance. Ed had promised to raise the car on blocks in the barn, and Charles reminded him to drain the radiator, and oil the cylinders through the spark-plug holes, but Ed told him he knew how. He said he'd use logs from the log pile for blocks. Charles didn't want to sell the car. He had bought it for only thirty-five dollars, but he had heard since that such old cars brought huge sums from collectors if you could find the right party.

Watching him work, the narrow young face grease-stained and concentrating, Ed considered that at Charles's age he was already courting Lucinda. He had thought of this before, but it was like grasping it afresh. When he was only a few years older than Charles he was married. But he could not escape the gloomy feeling that Charles would of his own volition study engineering at some future time, burdened, and wishing he had done so younger. It was unpleasant to think of the middle age of one's children.

So much of a man's life is determined by what he does at the point where Charles now stands. A raw boy of eighteen makes a choice, and his whole life becomes a growth based on it. An old man becomes a judge because a kid decided to study law. In his old age the kid he once was tyrannizes over him.

Still, it was true as Charles said, that when it comes to getting rich in business, schooling is not the most important factor.

In bed he mentioned this to Lucinda, and also the aspects of Charles's nature that favored success—his intelligence, and his intensity and constancy toward the goals he set himself. Lucinda lay near him. His words seemed to comfort her somewhat. Often, when she was depressed or anxious, she had liked him to talk to her in this fashion. In her pregnancies he had assured her that the birth would be successful and the baby whole, and recounted their future joys, and night after night, as her labor drew nearer, she would ask him to tell it all again.

He felt tender and close when she sought comfort this way.

He talked a while, and then they lay quiet. In time he heard the even breathing of her sleeping.

Sometimes, when she blamed him for all misfortunes, and then denied having said what she had just said, and in mid-argument produced a new version of what the argument was about and what their positions had been, so as to frustrate his defense and put him ever further in the wrong, he had had the feeling that marriage was like being in a business partnership with an idiot.

But afterward he would tell himself that no man can be happy if he expects reasonableness from women. Lucinda had always gone along with him when the chips were down. She went where he went, and she gave in when his mind was made up. What more could you ask of her?

He could not sleep. There was a creak somewhere in the wood of the house, and then he heard a mouse in the wall. There comes a time, he thought, when your children haven't been brought up just right, and you're married over twenty years to a woman who's maybe half right for you, and your career's half shot with almost nothing accomplished, and you know then that some things won't be fixed. Then you have to learn to write off hunks of the future, the same as you write off the past.

This big house would have made more sense when the children were smaller, he thought. He had conceived of it with four kids in it, but only Patty and Roland were left.

People followed the work they had to do, as they saw it, and it was too bad a family couldn't keep together. He himself had gone off for two years as a chaplain, leaving Lucinda and four children behind. And before that even, those years of seeing them only on weekends. Those separations were to be temporary. But before he knew it Millicent took off to Lucinda's aunt in Chicago for four years, barely seventeen years old, and was scarcely back before taking her own apartment, and now Charles was gone.

He heard himself sigh, and the sheet that lay half over his face fluttered. The boy must seek his own dangers. As though he went to travel on foot in a strange land, among bandits, with all your savings entrusted to his knapsack.

Ed remembered a parishioner he had had in Abbottsford, an old man, who had lost a son decades before at the age of four. The boy had been hit by a baseball; the doctors said he was okay, after all kinds of tests, but months later he had convulsions and died. It came up somehow in some conversation about convulsions. And the man was seventy, with grown daughters and grandchildren, he had had the boy only four years and had lived on without him more than forty, yet even now he could not tell of it without his eyes filling up.

Your sons were your life. Your daughters only made it worth living. You loved your daughters as precious irreplaceable objects, like treasured furniture saved from your parents' household, like that carved clock downstairs. Girls were like brilliant gardens. Like light to the eyes. Your sons you love differently. Boys were continuity. You loved a son as you loved your grandfather, as you loved a principle, as you loved your God. Only Millicent, with her intellect, could obscure the difference sometimes. She had a mind like a boy's.

All those years in the Brighton apartment he had thought of a big house. With the yellowed photos of his parents and his grandparents in the hall, and his kids running up and down the stairs, playing in the fields and at the stream. If he could have managed it sooner, perhaps it would have imparted a majesty to all their lives.

15

When Millicent set out Friday to return to work Charles insisted on driving her to the Sparkstown depot. He would have taken her all the way to Boston if she had let him. Just before she boarded the train he bent and kissed her, with decorum, but nevertheless his emotion made itself felt. It was as if the gravity of his military enlistment all at once became real to her.

She walked to her seat down the rocking aisle, feeling suddenly the confusion her parents must feel. The remarks she had offered in support of Charles's plan seemed detached now and superficial, and she hoped her parents had in fact reached their decision without her. She had no idea whether she had done right or not.

It had been agreed that he would enlist after the weekend with his father's consent. The near relatives and a few of his friends had been invited for a Sunday-afternoon gathering, and he had asked Millicent whether she could swap days off with somebody and be at the house too, but she said it was impractical. So he said he would see her when he got a pass.

Though she had not told any of her family, she was supposed to begin street-corner campaigning for Theodore Victor Miecznesliwy on Saturday, before work. She had been supplied with a sample speech, which she found embarrassingly hackneyed and ranting. She felt it was unworthy of the candidate. But she kept it in her shoulder-strap purse with other campaign material, including a chart of his stand on various issues, which she studied on the train.

She had gotten most of it on a visit to the Independent Citizens' Committee headquarters in the shabby hotel, and had also picked up some pointers from an older lady there on street speaking. She had been told it was not difficult to collect a crowd, because once a few people had paused their presence attracted more and more.

Millicent was to be teamed with a Mr. Glidden, whom she hadn't met. On Saturday she went to the headquarters at the appointed hour. The room always seemed busy, with posters and banners on the walls, corrugated cartons on the floor and a cluttered messiness of papers on all the steel shelves. A girl turned a mimeograph on a makeshift table of thin boards. A young man in shirt sleeves was hammering nails. A bespectacled lady who seemed to be doing many things at once told Millicent to come back tomorrow, as Mr. Glidden couldn't make it.

She saw a few of the portable platforms lined up near the wall, like the one she and Mr. Glidden would share, taking turns upon it while the other passed out leaflets. Each consisted of a makeshift footstool or box for one person to stand on, and from each a three-sided railing had been erected, made of a few slim square poles that showed saw marks. The two poles forming the front of each had a cardboard placard tacked between them and a pair of stiff little dime-store American flags rising from the railing on tiny sticks.

On Sunday she returned, but apparently there had been a misunderstanding. The headquarters was closed. On Monday morning Mr. Glidden again did not appear, so Millicent asked the bespectacled lady if she could be teamed with someone else or speak alone. She lifted one of the flimsy platforms to show that she could carry it herself.

The packet of leaflets she had been given she stuffed into her shoulder-strap bag. She lugged the platform down the carpeted stair.

In the dark lobby it began to be heavier than it seemed at first. The baking street was a sudden brightness. She changed her grip to a point nearer the base, and then after half a block she set it down and switched it to the other hand. The sawed wood was rough. She tried holding the whole contraption with two hands, putting it horizontally before her. But it had to be held high enough not to bump her legs. She put it beside her again, one-handed like a valise, and at length raised one of the poles upon her shoulder. She put it all down, slung the shoulder-strap bag to the other side, and resumed. She felt quite warm in her suit. She had worn stockings too, lest informality turn people from the candidate.

In the subway she had to lift her platform over the turnstile. She pulled it up and across carefully, so as not to scrape the cardboard or snap the tiny flagpoles. Eugene never used a thing like this, she thought. He had just walked around and shaken hands. But being the candidate yourself was a different matter from speaking on behalf of someone else. Besides, Eugene's campaign had not been so professional as this one.

A man helped her lift it onto an underground trolley car, between the folded doors, while the motorman watched.

"Thank you," she said.

The car was nearly empty. But after some stations she had to switch to a real subway train, and the train didn't stop with a door near her, so that she feared the doors might slide shut on her platform's railing as she pulled it through and break it.

When she sat again she was hotter and throbbing. The dusty subway wind blowing through the car played with her skirt and petticoat, and she put a hand to her knee to hold them. On the street and on the trolley there had been few people, but here the long benches faced one another and across the car lounging men of various ages watched her idly. Her platform stood brushing her knees, and she was uncertain whether to keep the placard side toward her out of modesty or turn it about for maximum publicity.

The noise softened as the train rose to sunshine. She traveled between the upper stories of buildings. She saw clotheslines on roofs.

At last she carried and dragged her platform carefully down the long flight of suspended stairs, in shadow under the elevated station, no longer sure it had been wise to attempt this alone. A truck jounced on cobblestones in the striped sunlight beneath the elevated, its cargo clacking. She could see flies about the sunny trays that tilted before a fruit store. Near it was a shop where long white slabs of salt fish hung. All the people were Negroes. An old man with a drooping brown fedora and no shirt sat on a box. Over the stores there was clapboard. She thought the neighborhood smelled of rotten wood.

She stood her platform, with its stiff little flags, a few feet from the staircase that came down from the overhead station. Then, with some indecision, she pulled it somewhat further from the staircase. Four kinky-haired children in ragged clothing stood watching her, the eldest a girl of about ten, with two white ribbons at the base of her skull. There was a boy a bit smaller, wearing a felt beanie decorated all over with what looked like organizational pins and buttons. "You gonna give out gum samples?" the boy asked Millicent.

"She ain't giving out samples, thickhead," the girl reprimanded him in a lower voice. "She's the Salvation Army." She pronounced it Salavation.

"She ain't the Salvation Army," the boy said.

Millicent inspected her platform and its placard. She did not meet the children's eyes.

"You giving out gum?" the boy asked again.

"That's the summer uniform," the girl said.

"I'm giving out samples of political education," Millicent answered, looking at them at last, her voice unsteady. Then she moved nervously to a display window and examined the reflection of her hair superimposed on a welter of kitchen utensils. She drew a comb from her shoulder-strap purse.

In the reflecting window she could see the children still watching her. There was also a shy-looking girl of about six, and the littlest was a boy with underdrawers hanging below his pants bottoms. An old man approached her, bent and smaller than herself and dressed in rags, and muttered something she could not understand, as though his throat were full of phlegm. One eye was shut and reddened and sunken in, and he made a kind of bow, lifting a soiled stiff visored cap. There were curling white whiskers close upon his skin.

"Your slip's showing," the biggest of the children told her.

"Oh dear," she said, looking down at it.

She looked about, wondering where she might go to fix it, and whether she had better take the platform with her or leave it where it was. The man smelled sick and seemed terribly old. His remaining eye was yellow and nearly shut.

"Come on, I'll get you something to eat," she said to him, but then hesitated, looking about again. She saw two coffee-colored men, a big one and a smaller one, talking together near a massive black column where the elevated curved. "Will you watch my platform, please?" she said across the sidewalk to the bigger one.

His hands were in his pockets and he wore a cloth cap. "Sure," he smiled at her.

Past the fish store was a kind of narrow restaurant, and she hurried to it, holding the door for the old man. Inside, half a dozen men sat over coffee here and there along a counter. Everybody was colored, including a big waitress in a pink smock. The old man raised himself to the stool that Millicent indicated, and hunched over the counter.

"Give this gentleman some scrambled eggs, please," she said to the waitress timidly. "And some soup. Would you like some soup?" she asked him. She was not sure if he had teeth. "Whatever he wants," she said to the waitress. "A dollar's worth." She unfastened the purse beside her.

"Don't put your money into him," the waitress said. "He'll be dead in a week."

"Well, that's why I want him to have a square meal in the meantime," Millicent answered uneasily, putting a bill on the counter. The man's legs clutched the base of the stool, and she saw that his shoes had burst.

She asked the waitress if there was a ladies' room, and the waitress said she could go through the kitchen.

In the kitchen a burly man with a small mustache perspired at a black sizzling stove, but the bathroom was cleaner than she had expected, though cramped. She wore a half slip, and when she had shut the door and unfastened her skirt it was a simple matter to hike it up. She worried meanwhile that she should not have left her platform. She had no assurance that those men would not steal it, to use the wood. Or the children could make off with it.

She hurried. The old man had pea soup with squares of toast in it and was lifting a shaking spoon. "Good-bye," she said as she passed his stool. "And remember to vote for Theodore Miecznesliwy in the primary. For Congress."

"God bless you," said a man on another stool, putting a hand to her arm and startling her. "I seen what you done. And I'm glad there's a Christian left in the world."

"Oh. Well, thank you," Millicent said.

When she got to the sidewalk she was relieved to see the platform just as she had left it, even its fragile little stars and stripes intact. A horse and a wagon loaded with cages of live chickens were standing nearby.

"Here she comes," one of the children said.

The two men were still talking. It occurred to her suddenly that she had had no right to ask for someone's vote after buying him lunch.

"Thanks very much," she said to the bigger man when she was near enough. "For watching my platform, I mean." They nodded and smiled.

She mounted it and placed her hands on its rail, near the flags. She could smell the chicken feathers and when she glanced she saw the horse swish its tail and wriggle a knee. Perhaps the old man wasn't even registered, she thought, so she had not bought a vote after all. She hoped not. The four children had not taken their eyes from her, but the two men had turned and were wandering off. There was a scattering of people up the sidewalk, shopping or picking over fruit, and one or two sitting, but no one near, except the children. She saw a man spit into the gutter. A hefty woman came past with a nearly empty shopping bag, her short hair pulled straight, and an expression like an angry gorilla.

"Excuse me—" Millicent said from the platform.

The woman rolled eyeballs toward her but did not stop.

Millicent cleared her throat. Then she put a hand at her mouth and coughed. "I'll begin as soon as I have three grownups," she said to the children.

There were that many about the fruit display, over which an awning had been lowered, and she thought of moving her platform a little closer to them. Still, they were not terribly far as it was. She tried a couple of hand claps.

She looked again at the children. "Do your mother and father vote?" she asked the biggest one.

"My father's dead," the girl said.

"Oh," said Millicent. "Oh. I'm sorry."

The youngest child sneezed, the mucus on his lip becoming larger. Millicent went down, taking a handkerchief from her shoulder-strap bag, and wiped his nose.

When she returned to her platform she saw that a shiny police car had parked behind the chicken wagon and two policemen sat watching her. A handful of bystanders had also gathered, not close but here and there, looking at her from where they stood.

She mounted and faced them. Then she looked behind her at the two policemen. They were white men, young and ruddy.

"Am I violating any law?" she asked them, her voice shaking.

They made no answer, but continued looking at her from the car. Their faces were expressionless. Her heart was pounding, but she took their silence to mean nothing was amiss.

She turned her back to them and faced a loose audience of about seven curious men, to the right and left and back by the shops. The children were nearer. She began matter-of-factly, using the candidate's full name. Her voice quavered badly, but she believed she could be heard above the trucks that lumbered behind her. She said she wanted to analyze the incumbent's voting record and show why a younger man and a fresh viewpoint were needed.

She heard a train and looked overhead. It leaned into the curve with a prolonged shriek of metal. When it stopped she tried to get her bearings, but paused again as the train left the station. She at last resumed, but just then the sun went into shadow, the street's brightness vanishing with such abruptness that she gave a frightened start, glancing quickly toward where the sun had been. She at once caught herself, sorry for the gesture. She spoke of rent control. The quaking vibrato of her timorous voice sounded terrible in her ears. She felt herself shivering. Once she lifted a hand from the rail, but it shook so violently that she quickly restored it. She touched on labor relations and veterans' benefits and on price control. She knew the periodic shudders of her body must be quite visible. But the faces she looked at seemed gentle. She told them that while she didn't agree with the President in all particulars, the cessation of economic controls after the war had been somewhat premature. She realized almost as she said it that there was nothing about this in Mieczneslíwy's program, and wondered whether she had done wrong to inject her own views like that.

"What college are you from?" one of the policemen asked.

She looked around. "What?" she asked.

"What initiation?"

"Oh. I'm speaking on behalf of Mr. Miecznesliwy," she told him.

"Okay, like you say, we need new blood—" someone in her little audience said, and she looked front again. "But why you put up this here Mitch. Why don't you put up a colored man?"

"Show respect," a smaller man reprimanded the first one stiffly.

"No, I welcome questions—" she began. Her questioner wore a double-breasted suit, the jacket unbuttoned, and no tie. He looked at her fixedly. Behind her she heard the police car back up suddenly, shift gears and depart. She tried to answer, saying she didn't know why, but that Mr. Miecznesliwy had promised his door would be open to everyone.

"Why are they fighting over there in Korea, when we got problems right here," another one said, and an elderly man with glasses nodded his head.

She thought that was easier to answer, but before she could speak a big muscular man in shirt sleeves asked whether she knew anything about the consumer co-operative movement in Scandinavia. He was very black and stood with arms folded.

She told him she understood the principle, her voice still quavering, but that she knew nothing of it first hand, and couldn't comment on its suitability for the United States. He replied by recommending some books to her, rattling off one title after another and their authors.

"Thank you," she said.

"You can get them at the Boston Public Library," he said.

Millicent spoke a little longer and then said she was afraid that was all the material she had. She asked again that they remember to vote.

"I wish to thank each of you for your very courteous attention," she said, and let herself down with great care, as she was still shaking.

One of the smaller men clapped his hands a few times.

"Thank you, you're very kind," she said, looking at him.

She began to pick up her platform while her little audience drifted apart. The children stayed near.

"Want me to carry your stand?" the boy asked.

"No, that's all right."

But she struggled getting it into its best position, and he helped lift it by one of the outer poles. They started off with it between them, and the other children supported its end. She meant to repeat her talk to new people at each corner. It was a long way to the next intersection. She was still shivering as they walked. The sun had come out again but she felt cold, and wondered why. There was a crossing that was only an alley and then they continued.

When they reached the corner she set the platform upright, the boy helping. She mounted it, a little winded, and again the four children faced her. But there was no one else about. The store windows had a display of dusty furniture, and the buildings down the cross street looked like warehouses or garages. The sidewalks were dead.

"Well, I guess I might as well start talking to you, until somebody comes," she said, looking down at the children.

But then it seemed foolish.

"Well, I guess this isn't a very good place," she told them, stepping back down.

They all picked up the platform. As they went down from the curb Millicent stepped badly and her ankle turned painfully on the cobblestones so that she stumbled. She halted, grimacing.

"Did you sprain it?" the eldest girl asked.

"I don't know."

They held the platform and she stood on one foot, massaging her ankle. The stocking had run. She tried to walk, but the first test of weight stung fiercely and she could only limp and hobble.

"I guess I better rest a minute," she said.

The children waited, all but the littlest holding the platform. Then they set it down, crooked on the cobbles, and sat on the curb, except for the older girl, who stood with Millicent by the lamppost. Millicent thought of sitting too, perhaps on the bottom of her platform if the children would lift it to the sidewalk. But its unfinished wood had her shoe marks and would dirty her suit.

She looked down at the collection of medallions on the boy's felt cap, and it occurred to her that the Independent Citizens' Committee ought to distribute campaign buttons.

The pain in her ankle did not diminish, and she thought it was swelling. It throbbed. She wondered if something was broken. In a few hours she would have to be at the city room, scurrying up the stairs with copy for Mr. Valentino.

She told the children she had better get a cab, and the boy went off to find her one.

"You better soak it in hot water," the girl told her as they waited.

She leaned with a hand on the lamppost, wondering if she could make her way to a telephone. The leaflets stuffed in her bag came to mind. She had forgotten to pass any out.

A taxi came soon, the colored boy riding behind the driver. The door opened almost at Millicent's feet.

"What are you going to tell your mother about the primary election?" she asked the oldest girl as they helped her in.

"Vote for that man."

"Miecznesliwy," Millicent said.

They pushed her platform into the taxi beside her and the driver leaned around to help arrange it diagonally.

She rode beside it, low in the leather.

She watched the driver's thick hairy neck. She asked him whom he favored in the primary.

"Oh, they're all a bunch of crooks," he said without turning.

"Well, Miecznesliwy isn't a crook," she answered. She began to explain the reasons for supporting him. Yet even as she spoke she had the feeling she was doing so compulsively, without any chance of influencing the real world.

16

The cabdriver carried Millicent's platform up the flight to the Independent Citizens' Committee's headquarters, and she followed, pulling herself on the banister and favoring her turned ankle. The bespectacled lady had once been a nurse, and after turning Millicent's ankle this way and that she said it was not broken or seriously sprained, but that it would be good to rest it for a few days.

The cabdriver left her at her address and she climbed a step at a time, in the manner of Ella Jane. She found the kitten sharpening its claws on the fabric of the fat worn chair with broken springs. She poured it some cream in a saucer.

There was no basin, so she soaked her foot in the largest pot. She was entitled to a little sick leave under the Guild contract, but she disliked to take advantage of it. They would have to hold Zucchino overtime. Still, it seemed incautious not to, when she thought of the constant stair-climbing between the city room and the linotypes. So at last she phoned.

She lay on the studio couch. She felt badly about not having tipped the children for their help. It had crossed her mind as she entered the cab, but she had known no way to offer them money without seeming patronizing. She regretted not having thought to give them the leaflets to pass out, so she could have paid them for that.

Natalie came home at five and was surprised to find her there.

"Any phone calls for me?" Natalie asked after a while.

"No."

Her ankle felt all right the next day and she returned to the city room. But Wednesday she assisted at a major rally at which Miecznesliwy spoke holding an umbrella in the rain, and she caught cold there passing out leaflets. She spent the remainder of her days off in the apartment, nursing a sore throat and stuffed nose.

On Friday Mr. Killian beckoned with an angry toss of his head as soon as she entered the city room. He rose and seemed furious even before he began to speak. "What about this political activity?" he asked her. "I know about it. Don't think I don't know. Because somebody saw ya. In the subway there." She opened her mouth confusedly. "What are you trying to pull off?" he said before she could say anything. "Don't you know a newspaperman has to be unslanted? Impartial? Don't you know anything about this business?" He ran a hand through his wild hair and his features softened a little while he looked at her. "Millicent, in our business, we favor neither side. The public has to know the news pages are the whole truth, don't you see that? Regardless of any personal feelings. Editorial writers can do what they damn please—editorial writers aren't newspapermen. But I thought you wanted to be a newspaperman. You did, didn't ya? Isn't that what you told me? And now you've gone and compromised yourself and the whole damn paper. Maybe you're dumb, maybe you don't know the first thing about it. I hope that's it. But I have standards, and if I catch you once more in anything like that you're finished."

He brushed her away with a contemptuous wave, and she set about her work quite shaken. She sneezed once or twice, and she kept sneezing as she worked, and as she went up and down the stairs. Danny McBride took to calling her Sneezy. She felt confused and hurt.

The paper had taken no editorial stand on the Miecznesliwy campaign. And even if it had, she had thought she still had a right to be a responsible citizen, with a social conscience. At least on her own time.

But she realized that Mr. Killian had not meant that. He had meant, she told herself, that the press had unique duties in the functioning of a democracy—suppose it should be her job someday to report on facts unfavorable to Miecznesliwy? Now she understood. It seemed as though an enlightenment took place in her mind. Or suppose, more likely, she had occasion to unearth a story exonerating Miecznesliwy from some charge, or accusing his enemies—would not her known partisanship cast doubt on her disinterestedness, and on that of her paper? She saw Mr. Killian's ideal of the newspaperman now as the one whose tale could be trusted by all, because he lent himself to no faction. Even if editorialists took a stand, the reporter still covered both sides fair and square. He was not like other citizens; he must be as circumspect as a judge or juror, that a whole nation, amid all its contentions, might know of his consecration to truth. She had never thought of it that way before.

The public could not believe a reporter's report of a quarrel if he aligned himself beforehand with one side of it.

When she had a chance she went to Mr. Killian's desk and asked him, her voice wobbly and pleading, whether she might speak to him a minute. She told what she had been thinking, and how she understood the newspaperman's role now, and that she would dissolve her connection to the Independent Citizens' Committee at once. She said she hadn't understood.

He listened to her at length, leaning back in his swivel chair. He looked up at her earnestly. "You know what?" he said finally. "I believe in you."

She thought it stupid of her, when she resumed her work, not to have grasped in the first place what she understood now.

On the weekend Ella Jane was invited by a broker in her office to stay with friends of his on a yacht at Marblehead. He came to fetch her but did not come upstairs, and Ella Jane left with a packed beach bag. Looking down from the window, through the ironwork of the fire escape, Millicent saw her maneuver into an open convertible, cane and all, beside a hatless blond man who sat there.

Millicent had the use of the back bedroom, secluded beyond the bath, while Ella Jane was away. She heard that Charles had been home on a thirty-six-hour pass and that he looked fine in his uniform. But she did not get to see him.

A few days afterward her parents came to Boston to give blood to the Air Force, bringing Patty and Roland for the ride, and called for her so she could give blood also.

They told her that Charles had wanted to drive in to see her, but the family had monopolized him. Grandma Annie and Aunt Celeste's family had come visiting, and Patty had made him walk with her to Yerxa's Pharmacy at Murphy Square so she could show him off to the other kids. Patty had already baked him a boxful of brownies. And Patty had asked to take over his bedroom, which was in the front, and he had said okay, but their mother had vetoed it, saying it would be kept for him just as he had left it.

The blood-bank nurse admitted Ed and Lucinda first, and the three children waited together on the bench.

"It's too bad you can't give fat," Roland remarked to Patty when the nurse was away.

"Very funny," said Patty sourly. "Very funny. They ought to put you on television. For the cerebral palsy campaign or something. As a horrible example."

"Now stop it, both of you," Millicent said. "You could both stand to learn a little kindness."

"I don't want his kindness."

"If you're supposed to be so big-boned," said Roland, "how come you got such big boobs then? They haven't got any bones in 'em."

"You shut up. Or I'll tell Mama you're talking dirty."

"Yes. Roland! For goodness sakes," Millicent agreed.

"What's so dirty about that?" He sat restlessly and crossed his ankles. "You've got the biggest ones in the whole high school," he said.

Patty reddened. "I have not."

"Yeah, who's got bigger ones then?"

"Plenty!"

"Yah, name one. You can't even name one."

"Roland, stop it," Millicent cut in. "I demand that you stop it. Or I'll put my hands over my ears."

He was silent only a moment, and then began again. "They're as big as watermelons. No kidding. Too bad your brains aren't that big."

"I'm not even listening to him," said Patty.

"They ought to have you giving milk instead of blood."

"Boys are just naturally dirty-minded, do you know it?" said Patty.

"Sometimes I think so," said Millicent.

"And I'm gonna see them bare one of these days too," said Roland. "I've got a way to take the lock right out of the bathroom door while you're taking a bath."

"You better not," Patty said.

The nurse came back for a moment and rummaged in a card file near the lamp on the desk.

"He thinks he's such a genius," Patty muttered.

Millicent was sorry for Patty.

Breasts were a nuisance. She had nothing like Patty's massiveness, thank God, but she would rather have had the proportions of either of her roommates, excepting of course Ella Jane's bad leg. They both had smaller breasts than she did, though Natalie was a bigger girl and hippier.

The nurse came back once more and rejected Millicent, because her cold still lingered.

But she waited for her parents, and afterward they all went to her apartment for a little while. A noodle pudding that Lucinda had brought for Millicent and the roommates was squeezed into the little refrigerator beneath the stove.

She began to find the summer dull. Her work was tedious, and she began again to consider whether she should go to law school in the fall. She saw no objection that Mr. Killian could have to it, but if she did decide to do that she would consult him first, to make sure.

Danny McBride still called her Sneezy, and Louie Alpert, the big pear-shaped mustachioed man, had taken it up also. Her cold had largely gone, but colds always left her nose more sensitive for a while after.

She walked over to Aunt Gwendolyn's to baby-sit often, but the way Aunt Gwendolyn did many things irritated her. Aunt Gwendolyn seemed more interested in a clarinetist she had been seeing than in finding a job. Millicent always changed Sharlene's diapers at once, because Gwendolyn often rushed out leaving her wet. And the apartment was untidy. Gwendolyn considered it a great day off to dump the baby with her ex-husband on Sundays and spend the day with her clarinetist.

Natalie talked of giving a party. Ella Jane had had another weekend invitation, but Natalie had quarreled with two boy friends and seemed to have few inner resources. And she hated playground work.

"What happened to your friend Al?" Millicent asked her.

"He doesn't know I exist."

He was certainly aware her clothes existed, that night he was so eager to take them off, Millicent thought.

Once or twice Natalie urged Millicent to come to the beach with her, along with one of the girls she taught with in Winchester and whose car she used for commuting, but Millicent's working hours made it impossible.

Millicent and Ella Jane at first opposed the idea of giving a party, and Ella Jane said no one gave parties in summer, but Natalie said that was all the more reason to. At last they did plan it, for a Thursday evening.

They were supposed each to invite a third of the guests, but it turned out that Natalie knew more than anyone else, beginning with the teachers she had ridden to work with, and there were also girls that Natalie and Ella Jane knew in common from years back. It appeared that women would far outnumber the men, and Millicent was urged to invite any boys she could think of. So she offered to invite her cousin Steve, and to ask him to bring some boys from the College of Pharmacy.

She invited Bob Lyons, when she saw him in the city room, and asked him to invite Tighe. She thought also of Aptaker, the news-agency man at the State House, but decided against him.

She phoned Dr. Leslie Hollander at the Massachusetts General Hospital, her heart in her throat, fearing he would not be able to come. She had not heard from him since the afternoon he slept through the movie.

He said he'd check and call her back. She was almost incredulous when he did call back to say agreeably that he would not be on call that night, so far as he knew. His voice was low, poised and cultured, not like the newspapermen, and like none she had heard for a long time. She described the building to him, with its recessed entry behind a stone arch, and told him the doorbell said Jespersen—McCartney—Gordon.

To Natalie and Ella Jane Millicent suggested that they plan some party games, such as a guessing game based on historical figures. But they said it would fall flat.

Meanwhile Natalie had located a boy, through one of her girl friends, who promised to call other boys, and he called so many that at length some of the boys had to be asked to call girls in order to restore the balance somewhat.

There might be sixty people if everyone came. Millicent asked where they would get enough chairs.

"We're not going to hold a séance," Ella Jane answered.

For refreshments they planned cheese dips and potato chips and peanuts. Millicent thought it skimpy, though she admitted that in such quantity anything more would be prohibitive. The liquor requirements, as Natalie and Ella Jane figured them, seemed enormous, so they decided to provide beer only and send out word to the boys to bring harder stuff. Millicent said she would send out no such word, but the others made some calls. Even so the party seemed a tremendous investment, what with glassware and soda and ashtrays.

Millicent did most of the actual preparation, having the day off. She cleaned, and prepared the dips. Later they took everything from the little refrigerator, including the remnant of Lucinda's noodles, to make room for bags of ice. For the kitten they found a large grocery carton in which he could be confined under Natalie's bed, with his sandbox inside it as well as his green folded bath mat.

Ella Jane wanted to lend Millicent a dress, and at length Millicent took a loose-fitting gray and white one from her, with a collar and buttons and belt, and a slight sheen to the material. Ella Jane wanted to tear the collar and the little sleeves off but Millicent insisted there wasn't time.

She wore the white beads Leslie had sent, and no stockings. She watched Natalie struggle to put a high waist-pinching type of undergarment into place. It was frilled and flowered, and long garters streamed from points in the groin.

Natalie asked her to help with the hooks. The squeeze forced some overflow of clear skin above the blackness.

"How can you wear such a thing?" Millicent said.

"Don't you like it?"

"I think it must be uncomfortable." She would rather have said it was hideous.

"Well, the hourglass goes good with crinolines," Natalie said.

"People just don't look like that," said Millicent. "They're not made like that."

Once guests began to arrive they arrived quickly, at first men mostly but then women too. In a surprisingly short time the living room was quite noisy, with people Millicent didn't know standing about and talking to one another, and girls on every one of the dining chairs that Charles had fixed, and five on the studio couch, with boys at their feet, and another sprawled on a boy's lap in the fat upholstered chair. Millicent kept anxiously busy, at first trying to pass the cheese dip, and putting bowls of it on the mantelpiece and the drop-leaf table and the window sills. She couldn't put any on the big arms of the stuffed chair because people were sitting on them, flanking the sprawling couple. She found her way this way and that through the crowd to fetch some ice. The little kitchen was full of lounging boys. Two of them were rinsing dust and excelsior from the new glassware. Millicent realized she had forgotten to do that. Beyond the sink someone was embracing Natalie, her face smiling without her eyeglasses and half-hidden. His hands were around her black ruffles. Millicent had to ask a boy to move so she could open the refrigerator door, and then she told Natalie they had forgotten to get a bottle opener for the soda. A boy supplied one.

When she returned carrying ginger-ale bottles to the warmth of the living room her cousin Steve grinned down at her, but she felt busy and only said hello without stopping. On his muscular chest was a tight sport shirt of some white clinging stuff, without a tie. At the edges of the crowd people were sitting on the floor, women as well as men, along the walls and the furniture, and the jumble of voices was everywhere. The venetian blinds rose with a battering of slats. She heard a glass break. She set the bottles on the drop-leaf table, which stood unfolded under the crucifix. There were already some squashed limes there, and some ice cubes melting in a dented pot. She asked someone to be careful of the table, as each of the oval wings was supported by one leg only. The door buzzer kept sounding. Men's feet were backed up even on the green tile apron of the fireplace, and she heard someone telling about another party, where somebody had poached some eggs in vodka and caused an explosion.

She greeted Lyons and Tighe at the door as Ella Jane opened it. They looked scrubbed and combed. Behind them came Natalie's friend Al, who introduced himself to her. He had a skinny face, oily hair, and a tiny mustache. She did not like his appearance, nor the way he looked at her, with a kind of smirking admiration. Ella Jane fanned herself, leaning on her cane, and said they might as well leave the door open.

Millicent began to introduce Lyons and Tighe to Ella Jane, ill at ease and hesitant, and they supplied their names. Then across the room she could see that the guests had apparently spread into the bedrooms, and she said she had better get her cat.

She could scarcely get through the crowd, and had not gone far when Ella Jane called after her that a friend of hers had arrived. She looked about and saw Leslie Hollander, smiling down at her and restoring his pipe to his mouth.

"Oh, hi," she said.

She was about three people from him but he maneuvered his way to her quickly. The seersucker jacket seemed to have been cleaned and pressed but his hair was not cut.

"I thought you must have gotten tied up in an emergency," she told him. "I didn't think you'd come."

"Oh no," he shrugged.

"Did you have any trouble finding it?"

"No."

"I was just going to make sure my kitten hasn't been stepped on," she said. "I have a kitten sleeping in a box."

He smiled a little more widely. "All right. Let's find your kitten," he said.

Millicent turned about, waving away some cigarette smoke. "May we get through, please?" she said to someone.

Leslie took the lead, and she brushed after him as he found openings first to the right and then to the left.

"That further door," she told him.

She noticed that some of the men were more unkempt than others. Some talked too loudly. Some stared, and one asked her name.

"Excuse me," she answered him, following Leslie and meaning that she was on some errand. She told Leslie that she had had the cat about a month. "He's a little bigger now than he used to be," she said.

Their progress came almost to a halt in a denseness near the bedroom door. There was a swishing noise as two girls in crinolines squeezed past each other. She heard Leslie ask someone's permission to pass. Someone caressed her buttock. She pulled her hips away and swung a hand behind her to protect her skirts. But the offending hand seemed to come again. She turned angrily and confronted a boy she had never seen before. He was of middle height, with a largish nose and a mild expression.

"Will you remove your hand please?" she said. "And keep it removed?"

He reddened somewhat, and she did too.

"Really!" she said. "If you're so anxious to feel of someone's behind, I suggest you feel your own."

"It's just a friendly gesture," the boy said.

"It isn't!" she contradicted him. She thought his way of explaining it a patronizing outrage. "It's not a friendly gesture. Friendship implies a personal regard. And I can't believe that in that part of the body I'm enough different from all the rest of the world, to make that gesture anything that can be personalized," she told him, staring at his face with all the sourness she could muster. She saw that she had succeeded somewhat in embarrassing him.

But he smiled in spite of it. "Sue me for fraud," he said.

She knew Leslie and others had turned to listen. There was nothing for it now but to justify herself. "That happens to be a very standardized part of the body," she continued sharply. "If you're so interested in friendships I suggest you direct your attention to the intellect, which is where differences occur."

"What do you mean," the boy persisted. "I just touch you and look at the whole beautiful conversation I get. It was like pressing a button."

She thought of telling him she refused to discuss it further, but instead she said nothing, blushing more than ever, and turned away. "I'm sorry you had to hear such a vulgar ridiculous conversation," she apologized to Leslie.

"Come on," he said. He took her wrist and led her further on their way.

"I wanted to put him in his place," she tried to explain further. "I can't stand being pawed. Some people—it's just infuriating. As if I were stuffed with sawdust. A toy dog or something. And he'd just go on doing it again, or doing it to other people, if I didn't say something."

At least Natalie's complex underpinnings were armor—they didn't just hold stockings up, Millicent thought. With her own light pants the boy's fingers had felt as though on skin.

The little bedroom was half dark. A man and a woman lay across the bed, side by side but in no particular disarray, and several men and women sat on it. A yellow brightening illuminated two faces as someone lighted a cigarette.

Millicent knelt, her heart still pounding with embarrassment, and tried to see the box. Under the bed it was quite dark. "Excuse me," she said, trying to push a hairy leg aside.

The carton pulled with a sandy scrape, and she retrieved the kitten. She had expected to find it whining, but apparently she had woken it. She held it to her and it clung to the dress with its claws. Her hand enclosed the fur, and below her fingers she felt the tail wag on her breast. Leslie took her arm and helped her stand. "Can I get you a drink?" he asked her.

"I don't drink," she said. She looked up at him. "Do you want one?"

He looked toward the door. She saw perspiration on his lip and on his forehead. "Well," he said, "it looks like it would be quite a fight to get to the drink table."

She massaged the cat with slow gentleness, still looking at Leslie's moist face. "I'm sorry there's no place we can sit," she said.

"There's still room on the fire escape," a boy on the bed said.

Leslie glanced toward the open window. The broken shade was slantwise at the top of it. "Want to sit on the fire escape?" he asked her.

In the first instant she did not take him seriously but then she saw that there were in fact people out there. She followed him stumblingly, pressing past knees and the knobs of the bureau, hugging the kitten to her shoulder. The girl who lay across the bed held her skirts behind her knees and raised her legs for them. Millicent stepped on a man's foot and excused herself. Leslie's hand half pulled her over the window sill into the exhilaration of the outdoor breezes.

Men and women stood leaning as though on a balcony, the women stocking-footed on the iron slats, and yellowish light from the living-room windows fell on some of them. Others sat higher, on the grillwork stairs, where it was darker, trousered knees leaning apart and silken ones tight in pairs. Voices were soft in the night, and here and there the red of a cigarette moved. Millicent followed Leslie far up, stepping past the other couples and avoiding fingers and the edges of skirts, until they had some stairs to themselves, almost at the grill of the story above. She leaned to blow dirt from the step before sitting.

"Don't worry about it—the rain keeps it clean," he said.

She sat beside him. The gentle winds were good on her face and neck. She still felt somewhat embarrassed, and no conversation began immediately. She looked at her feet in the open flat shoes, beside his big ones. The street seemed dangerously far below. She pretended to be occupied with the kitten on her lap. Leslie took off his glasses and rubbed his eyes.

"I'm afraid the atmosphere at this party really isn't conducive to the best conversation," she said. "I know it's not your kind of a party."

"What?" He began to clean his glasses.

"It's too crowded," she said. "I don't even know most of these people."

"That's okay." He spoke with his pipe in his mouth. "I can't stay too long anyway. I just wanted to drop in." He squinted through the lenses from a little distance and rubbed them some more. He watched the kitten nestling on her lap. Its eyes were nearly shut again. "What's your cat's name?"

"Theodore."

Leslie put his glasses back on, smiling at the cat.

"He's named for Theodore Mieczneslíwy," she added. "You know, the non-machine candidate for Congress? In the Democratic primary?"

"I'm afraid I haven't followed it," he said. He took the pipe, lowering it, and she saw it had no tobacco.

They were silent a moment. She stroked the cat. The tree below her rustled, and beyond it she saw the roof of a car move silently, grayly reflecting the street lamp.

"It's terrible the way we're getting pushed south in Korea," she said. "It's humiliating."

"How's your job going?"

"It's okay, I guess. Only I'm not making progress very fast." She stroked the top of her kitten's head, and played with its feltlike ears and the remarkably short hairs of them. It seemed to doze. Leslie watched. "How's your work?" she asked him.

"Well, good." He seemed to blow slowly through the empty pipe. Then he took it out and looked at it absently, though soberly thoughtful. "I'm feeling a lot better about surgery."

"Did you have doubts about surgery?"

"Well, I'd been thinking of biochemistry—it's sort of closer to the central questions, you know. Of what we are—how it happens—the whole mystery. And spending my life in research." His long fingers played with the pipe, and she could see the hairs standing on them. He had large knuckles, and his nails were cut very short. "So much of medicine is passing out aspirin and cough syrups that won't do any good, and for illnesses that'll cure themselves anyway, and antibiotics for illnesses that the patient hasn't got—and I don't want to waste my life doing that. But on the other hand, you don't have to do that. And I realize more and more that clinical medicine is also research—it's always research—provided you're creative, and you care about the questions. It doesn't matter where you begin. The organism is such a unified thing, and the ramifications always lead you to the same large problems, in a certain sense. Whether you're devising a makeshift for a malfunction of the heart, or whether you're trying to right a chemical imbalance—it's still a question of the creative use of an essentially destructive thing—a knife, or a poison, or some massive compensating unbalance—to nudge the organism back to its natural balance again, where food and work and rest and happiness can work on it. I don't know—am I making sense to you?"

"Well, I think so," she said.

"And there are practical things I had to look at. I owe the Army some time, and with surgery they'll let me take this year at the Mass General first. Otherwise I'd do my interning at an Army hospital. And money's a factor—I've got my brother and my mother to think of. And what's more I like it—I like surgery, more than I thought. In surgery you get in and mess with it and see what you're doing, in a way you can't in any other medical technique."

"I have allergies," she told him. "Sometimes it's grass, but if I don't get tired I don't get it, and if I get tired or if I'm cold I can get it without the grass. And if I catch a cold the allergy sort of takes over, and I sneeze like an allergy instead of like a cold."

"Well, it's like anything else—the factors are endless," he said. "Like take arthritis, which my mother has—there happens to be arthritis research right at the Mass General as a matter of fact. You try to find what some of the factors are, hoping you can find one through which you can tamper with it, and if we find one, then we'll hope we're not throwing something else out of balance through some factor we don't yet know about. The whole body, the whole human person, is like one tangled ball of string. Just as the whole universe is, or all knowledge is. In the larger philosophical sense."

She watched the empty pipe turning in his fingers. He said his brother might end up in research. His brother was doing brilliantly in high school.

He began to talk a little of his family, sitting hunched, and not looking at Millicent. The hair over his forehead was shaggy. He had a soft, hesitant voice. Sometimes he seemed to pause and think before he spoke.

He said that while money didn't interest him he owed it to his mother and brother to see that they got part of their investment back, at least until his brother got through college and medical school, and so that his mother could stop working in her old age. She had never had a vacation. She still kept the store open far into the evening. And during the depression, besides keeping the store, she had ruined her eyes by taking piecework from a factory and sewing canvas bags at home at night. Even now, if he scraped together a few dollars to send her so she could see the dentist, she put it away for Jack. And often he wondered what would become of his brother's education now, if his mother were to die or take ill. College had gotten more expensive.

"Your mother must be a very wonderful person," Millicent said quietly, when he paused.

"Well," he said, in the same, slow, unsmiling way, "yes and no. She's kind of small-minded, actually. Petty. And the total enslavement to her children hasn't been good. For her or for us. I can't stand to be around her too much. But I'd like to be able to provide her with a two-room apartment where she could take it easy, and I could visit her once a month, say. I don't envy Jack being there in the house with her."

"Even so," Millicent said. "To bring up two fatherless boys like that, singlehanded."

"Well, I was fourteen when my father died. But she made men of us, I guess. She had to, or we wouldn't have survived. She made us take any kind of odd job we could get that wouldn't kill our schoolwork too much. I remember Jack had an egg route one time, when he was about the fifth grade, and the kid held onto every penny, and then I got into Yale and she took it all away from him to buy me a suit. And we knew we had to get scholarships, naturally. Second was no good."

"Leslie, she taught you to give of yourself," Millicent said, looking at him, but he did not return her gaze and she saw only his profile.

"Well, that was the only pleasure she could afford to give herself, I guess. To see her boys succeed. We've always had this real feeling of poverty—I don't mean just poor, I mean poverty, because there was never time for anything. Not only no money but no time. Rushing all the time. After school I used to deliver for a grocery. And jobs were still scarce then. I used to have to fight other kids physically to hold that job. And we were expected to get A in everything. If I came home with a B my mother'd go down and ask the teacher to give me extra work. Any waste of talent was a crime."

Millicent heard pleasantries and laughter down the firescape, and the noise of a boy clowning. She marveled at the efficiency with which Leslie used his days and years, and she envied his strength. He made his life matter. All of a sudden her own job, going up and down the stairs, seemed a trivial time killer. Her colleagues, men like Danny McBride and Louie Alpert, were lazy and fatuous.

"I wish I were a doctor," she said.

"Why?" He looked at her.

"Well, you give so much. You're like your mother, Leslie. Really, more than you know."

His eyes smiled through his glasses at her somberness. He struck her knee. "Maybe we can go to a concert sometime," he said. "But I really have to go. I wish I could stay, but—" She saw the lines in his forehead.

"Were you up all night again?" she asked.

"Oh, I got a couple of hours."

"It's horrible the way they treat interns," she said. "It's cruel."

"We'll survive it," he smiled. "We're young."

"I'd love to go to a concert."

"Well, maybe in the fall. When the chamber music starts."

He did not rise. He yawned into his hand, and then talked a little of the exceptional musical facilities Boston offered. She heard him tell how taken he was with the city, as a musical center and as a medical center. He said kings and presidents flew half around the world to be treated at the Mass General or the Peter Bent. Millicent told him it was a great newspaper town too, with four newspaper companies and seven dailies, not counting the Monitor.

"Boston papers stink," he said. He pressed back a yawn. Then he hit her thigh. "I have to go. I'm sorry. Up at five-thirty, and on the wards at six." He rose.

She didn't dare detain him. She got up too, raising the kitten toward her shoulder, and followed. She picked her way down the fire escape, feeling the grittiness of its rail. She thought of how he gave himself to all sufferers there at the hospital, as if his rest and health and pleasure counted for nothing, and yet with all that devotion to humanity at large he did not forget his responsibility to the mother and brother who depended on him. He had told her before that he was still in debt to Yale. And how a man could manage on twenty-five dollars a month to send a few dollars to his mother now and then—he was clearly one of these rare people who could do anything. And he was one of God's saints. She had known boys, especially the political and legal types, for whom concern for humanity was in large part a vehicle for ambition, but with Leslie it was the other way round. His only ambition was to serve. And, perhaps, to know. To learn, and comprehend. She had an urge to tell him he was the most remarkable person she had ever known, if there were a way to say it without embarrassing him.

He did not take the bedroom window this time but led her along the level part of the fire escape, toward the living-room ones. The people standing about made way for them and the potted coleus slipped through the rail. There was no one below and the pot burst with a noise on the sidewalk. Boys began whooping. "That was stupid," Leslie muttered, "whoever left a thing like that on a fire escape."

"It's my fault," she told him. "I had it on the window sill, and I guess somebody put it out to get it out of the way."

Leslie reached through the window and touched the bare shoulder of a girl who sat on the sill. The girl looked about and leaned aside, and Millicent climbed after Leslie through the people who were sitting there. She saw a boy on the floor peer up her legs.

She followed Leslie through the mob. It was stuffy and smoky. More people sat on the floor than before, and there were a lot of shiny round knees. Somebody threw Natalie's stuffed dog at the high ceiling and Natalie laughed. Men carrying a drink in each hand stepped over women. At the door Leslie turned, and she said she would see him down to the street.

They passed a man and woman sitting together on the staircase. Millicent thought of Leslie's childhood. His town of New Britain meant nothing to her, except that she thought it was not large, and she had never realized that poverty existed in such places, the same as in large cities. She had no conception of poverty, she thought. Her family often could not afford what the neighbors had, but her brother had been able to acquire a car while still in high school. And to fail to graduate.

They descended the first flight and rounded the landing without speaking. She still carried the cat.

"I guess what we're here on earth for is to do good for others," she said as they started down again.

"Well, I'd say that's pretty silly," said Leslie. "That type of total selfless altruism. What's our over-all purpose, then, if each of us is here for the others?"

She could not think of any answer.

"Is that what your father thinks?" he asked.

"I don't know what he thinks," she said. "Maybe he thinks we're here to praise God or something."

She almost missed her footing on a step and felt the cat cling tighter.

"Are you religious?" she asked Leslie.

"I can take it or let it alone." He descended looking straight ahead, the pipe in his mouth. "Are you?"

"I don't know. I don't mind it, I guess."

Their feet sounded on the dirty marble of the lobby. He pulled open the heavy door to the recessed walk. Then he took the pipe from his mouth and smiled down at her, without parting his lips. They heard the steady babble upstairs, both from the staircase and from the outdoors. Her thumb stroked the kitten's black fur.

"Do you think tobacco and coffee and tea are bad for people?" she asked him. "I mean as a doctor? I know if I have one cup of coffee it affects me—I lie awake the whole night through. I notice you don't really have any tobacco in your pipe."

"Oh." He was still smiling. "I can't afford it."

"Oh," she said. "I thought maybe you were against smoking. I thought you had the pipe because some patients like a doctor to look older."

He smiled a bit more, although she didn't.

"You might try imbibing some alcohol once in a while," he said. "At least at your own party. If you took a drink once in a while you might be a little less serious and more gay. You know, spontaneous. Open to life."

"Well, people have told me that," she said. "But I feel if I can't be gay while being my whole self, it hasn't really solved anything. I mean, if I can't be gay except by blanking out part of myself."

"You amuse me," he said.

"Why?"

He leaned suddenly to kiss her, his head inclined sideways. She began to draw back from his leaning, one hand clutching the cat, but the kiss struck, with a precise and clean noise upon her lips. His hands did not touch her.

He was straight again, still looking at her twinkly-eyed.

"Good night," he said softly.

17

The fire department was part professional and part volunteer, and Ed was not expected to answer every alarm. But one morning the loud horn started rising and falling just as he finished an early morning prayer service in the temple, so with a word he made other arrangements for the two or three congregants to whom he had promised rides to their homes and drove his car instead to the fire station at Murphy Square. He saw one engine rounding the bend as he approached, its muffler thundering like a machine gun. He threw his jacket and tie to a bench along the wall and swung up onto the second pumper just as it began roaring. He saw a bullet-headed locksmith he knew as Jonas Babcock high at the wheel. The head-blasting trumpet atop the building continued its rise and fall, and the engine paused in the sunlight of the Square, without any moderation in the sound of its motor, while two more men ran to it.

Ed had not realized how fast it was possible to speed down Massapeequit Road until he shot beneath its huge trees, holding tight to a bar alongside the red engine, the wind battering his shirt and shutting his eyes. He turned his face from the gale in order to breathe. The engine paused again, at an intersection amid fields, and a man in overalls ran from an old pickup truck and climbed next to Ed on the running board. In what seemed an incredibly short time he was passing his own house, set far back with its trees up the gentle rise of tall grass. The fire engine slowed a little where the road turned and plunged down through forest. At the duck farm it turned again, and someone shouted to pull in their rear ends when they went through the covered bridge. Across the brook the forest thinned, and the speed and the siren resumed. There was a gleaming bell that someone played with and it rocked skyward. Ed knew almost everyone on the engine—Yates, Pingree and King, and a part-time policeman named Horace Comeau. Someone had told him the woods were burning in Squonkamesset, and already he could see the smoke column that rose white-gray behind the last ridge and drifted in the upper air.

On the dirt roads of the forest they went slower, past fire trucks halted and empty, hose lines, and men in undershirts who walked about already grimy. Once he saw Starkey, his own fire chief, holler at a family group with a baby in a car, calling them rubberneckers and telling them to either go away or get into the woods and work.

Ed was assigned to shoveling dirt where a backfire had been set along a road. He did not see the main fire, that the backfire was meant to control. He worked for hours with many other men, moving down the road and burning out a stretch, and occasionally seeing a tall pine explode like a torch. He heard that seventeen towns had responded, and listened to talk of the drought, and of some cottages being threatened down by the lake. But the wind was not bad, and the fire did not jump from treetop to treetop, the way the men said it sometimes did, but smouldered instead along the ground, now and then shooting up a tree trunk. The woods were hazy with smoke. His trousers became wrinkled and smeared, and when he came near a truck from Wilmerding Mills he put on some abandoned dungarees he found in it. A plump lady in a jersey brought him coffee.

It was after nine at night when most of the Wilmerding men were sent home, and a man with a jeep dropped Ed off at his house. A muscle in his left knee, which he had pulled in a gymnasium many years ago, had tightened up again from too much exercise, and he had to favor it in climbing the stairs. Lucinda had walked to Murphy Square during the forenoon and brought home the car. Lucinda had told him when he joined the volunteer firemen that she thought he could find a less painful way to die, and now she said she wouldn't have time to push him around in a wheelchair.

Besides the firemen he had joined the Muckanaug Lodge of the Ancient Free and Accepted Masons, which conducted its rituals in rooms over the supermarket on Murphy Square. Giles Littleton, the chief of police, was Worshipful Master. There were no meetings in summer, but Ed meant to attend once a month when fall came, especially as some of his parishioners belonged, although for years he had belonged to Cryptic Lodge, which met in the big Masonic building in the heart of Boston, and had not gone very much.

In addition, Congregation Beth El belonged to the Wilmerding Council of Churches, and Ed went to the ministers' meetings, which were chaired by Newton Stillman, the Congregationalist, and attended by all the clergy in town except Father Donahue.

Lucinda had some memberships also; her position as Ed's wife demanded that she join the ladies' groups connected with the congregation, and that she put in an appearance at Sabbath services, which she usually did on Friday evening when the attendance was largest, but she had also gotten into a town club called the Crosswalkers, which was interested in planting flowers at the corners of Murphy Square. She worked too at her own gardens about the house, in whatever time she could, and seemed quite busy; she was tanned and Ed thought she looked extraordinarily well, quite like the girl she had been twenty years before. But she talked often of Charles. He was not at Otis on Cape Cod any more, having been transferred to the deep South, but when she wrote she still asked him to send home his mending. Though he was supposed to be in a mechanic school on the ground she suspected him of joy-riding in planes, as though he would be more tempted now that he was farther away, and if the weather at Wilmerding Crosswalk were stormy she remarked on it anxiously. She questioned Millicent every week or so about the outlook in Korea, or about the possibility of an outbreak in Berlin, as though Millicent as a newspaperwoman were privy to information withheld from the people at large. And she said it was remarkable that every boy she saw in uniform now actually resembled Charles. She had seen a bunch together in Air Force uniforms at North Station, and each one had looked like him—thin, sad and blond.

Ed had expected that his work would be light during the summer, and that he would be able to make progress on his master index of all the commentaries. He was getting to a time of life to concentrate on a few important things. There were also books he looked forward to reading, especially in European and American history, and contemporary philosophers, and some on strange cultures and civilizations, and one by a Professor Simpson on evolution. And two or three times a week he wrote to Charles.

But he had less time to himself than he had figured. The daily service, which he tried to maintain a couple of mornings a week on the theory that it was more important than the Sabbath, took scarcely more than twenty minutes, but it took hours of phoning to make sure that a quorum of ten men would be there. Most had excuses, or trains to catch. Charles's absence had made one less he could count on, although recently the cantor's arrival had made up this loss. Ed had hoped that several members could take turns leading the service, but the only ones who knew the prayers well enough were an old man named Munk and an old man named Resnick. There was also a heavy-set little man named Brill, about seventy years old, with a throaty voice and an accent, who could be counted on to help make up the quorum, and who hung around a lot, especially whenever his daughter-in-law threw him out, but he always changed his seat several times during the service, and kept up a continuous conversation with whomever he was next to, and refused to wear a prayer shawl, which he called a schmatteh, and said aloud that the service was all foolishness and that there was nobody upstairs, nothing there.

Then within a short time there were three deaths among elderly parents of congregation members, and in each case Ed spent a long evening listening to the descendants describe the deceased. Nearly always the life of the person came into being before him, as he sat listening to recollections, and the more easily the eulogy prepared itself the more it weighed on him. These tales of lives were like losing his own parents over and over. In the old days rabbis had had no particular obligation to officiate at funerals—any friend or kin or neighbor might give the eulogy and lead the service. But western civilization was somehow tied up with a notion of death as sacrament, and the notion of clergy, and he could not get out of it.

Meanwhile Newton Stillman got him invited to give the invocation at the horse pull in Furnaceville and it killed half a day.

He had a committee of women who were supposed to get the temple's library into shape, but Amethyst Gilbert was on it, and she phoned him almost every day. It gave her a chance to air all sorts of opinions and personal problems. There were still repairs he meant to do at home, and these calls usually came in the midst of them. He had thought he could fix the gate down at the bottom of the long dirt road merely by changing the position of the hinges, but he saw now he would have to dig out the whole supporting post and wedge it in straighter. He wanted to take down the television aerial. But there were shelves and hooks to put up for Lucinda, doors to be shimmed and planed, and a big hole to be plastered alongside the attic stairs. Lucinda wanted him to repaper some rooms, but he said that would wait until they decided whether to buy. She had bought a new rug for the living room, but instead of giving him the old oriental one for his study she had made him take it to Boston and lay it in Millicent's apartment.

He also gave the cantor and his wife some help in getting settled. They were named Bill and Marilyn Prince, and they were from New York, small, dark, and very young, Bill gloomy and introspective and Marilyn quite shy and timid. There were no Sunday-school or afternoon classes in summer, but there were three boys to prepare for bar mitzvah, each with a separate portion from the Prophets. Besides he wanted to train one of them to give the priestly blessing on the High Holy Days.

He filled in as visiting chaplain at a mental hospital several towns distant while the regular man was away. The Commonwealth of Massachusetts paid him ten dollars for a weekly visit. Actually he went more often, although he was not sure whether it did any good. There was a psychiatrist there who said he liked to work in a team with a religious counselor.

Then for a few days he was away himself, helping to conduct a retreat for teen-agers at a woodsy camp, where he ran some discussions and watched Patty roll and swing in the water, her feet churning the pond like a cauldron, her bathing cap and face all droplets, and blowing like a whale.

The following weekend Charles came home on a pass. He had a ride with a pilot who was ferrying a plane to Bedford Airfield and back. They expected Charles Friday afternoon. Lucinda prepared a roast with mushrooms, celery stalks with liver paste, and a lemon-meringue pie, but he did not arrive until nearly seven. He had gone out of his way into Boston first, to see Millicent during her thirty-minute supper recess, and had hitchhiked from there. He said getting out of the city had been slow.

His lateness disappointed Patty too, as she had hoped to show him off again at Yerxa's drugstore in the afternoon. He assured Lucinda he could have dinner, however, even though he had eaten with Millicent.

Ed carved the roast. He was impressed with Charles's dignity. The gray uniform fitted handsomely.

Patty served the eggplant. "Tuck your shirt in," she said to Roland. "Have you been eating onion grass?" She grimaced. "Wooee, pew." She moved past Roland's chair in a wide arc, giving him nothing, and put a large portion on Charles's plate.

"I thought we were supposed to be not on speaking terms," said Roland.

"We're not," said Patty.

"So shut up then," Roland said.

"Where do you get onion grass?" Ed asked.

"Every place," said Roland.

"And he talks about me," Patty said. "As if I eat too much. He goes grazing in the fields. And I'm not giving you a thing until you tuck your shirt in," she told him. She picked up the celery platter as Roland reached for it and offered it to Charles.

"You're too bossy," Roland said without looking at her.

"Dad, will you please discipline your child?" Patty said.

"Tuck in your shirt," Ed told him quietly.

He tucked it in. "You think you're the whole cheese, but you're only the smell," he said to Patty.

"Yeah, I heard that when I was six years old, and you think it's new," she answered him.

"I heard it when I was one," he said.

Charles throughout the dinner remained pleasant but reserved, Ed thought, much like a visitor. Lucinda asked whether he wanted this or that, and whether he remembered to brush his teeth. He said a tailor on the base did the mending.

Roland told Charles that one of the baby birds had gone from the nest in the porch roof that afternoon. He told him he had caught a perch in the brook, and also how his collection of insect specimens had grown. He said that zoologically we were living in the Age of Insects.

"If I had a bug collection I'd put you in it," Patty said to Roland. "I'd get a prize. For the most loathsome."

"Cut it out," Ed told her.

Afterward Patty announced that Polly Cook and Polly's brother were going to a record hop in Sparkstown, and that she and Charles could go along, the girls dating each other's brothers. Charles seemed indifferent, but Ed said they ought to stay home. He said Charles had had a long trip, and the family had not seen him for a long time, and besides it was the Sabbath.

They all drifted out to the cool of the porch, where the crickets could be heard, but Patty kept pouting. Ed told her they had begun the Sabbath properly, with a candle-lighting and wine and blessings, and it made no sense to have begun that way if a Sabbath didn't follow. Patty said it wasn't fair. She said Charles probably worked on the Sabbath all the time in the Air Force anyway, and Millicent did, and Roland had been allowed to go on camping trips with the Boy Scouts that extended over the weekend, and anyway she had known girls in Brighton who had been allowed to date on the Sabbath provided they walked.

"That doesn't make it right," said Ed. "And you can't walk to Sparkstown."

"Anyway rabbis even work on the Sabbath," said Patty. "When you run a service or give a sermon it's working. Because it's your job."

"Well, I know it," he said. "That's what I don't like about it."

"What's Polly like?" Charles asked.

"Another tubber," said Roland. "Like Patty."

"You shut up," she told him.

Ed walked to the temple alone to conduct the late Friday service, leaving Charles to rest and the family to keep him company. He felt uneasy about refusing Patty. It was true that he had not wanted Roland to be deprived of the Boy Scouts, and in that instance had leaned over backwards, pretending that the actual transport itself did not take place on the Sabbath. And if you gave an impression of unfairness everything could backfire. Still, he thought, as children prepare to leave home, and the time draws near for the family to fly apart, the religious fabric becomes all the more important.

When he got back to the house Patty had changed into the playsuit that she had made herself and was at the piano. He sat and watched her agile fingers. She was skillful, and yet there was something wrong, he thought. It had happened before—she would play something like the Moonlight Sonata to calm herself, but pour her anger into it. Lucinda told him Charles had been very tired and had gone to bed at nine.

He awakened Charles in time for breakfast and for the Sabbath morning service. He shook him by the shoulder, but Charles lay in the sheets, his eyes shut. Outside the window the sun gleamed on the slate roof of the porch.

"Fung gool," Charles muttered without opening his eyes.

"Fung gool yourself," said Ed. "Come on. Don't louse me up. I might need ya. It's hard to get ten guys."

At the temple the way Charles looked again impressed him. He was slim, with fine posture, the overseas cap slanting and jaunty, and he stood looking down at his prayer book, his feet at military attention. The drape of the prayer shawl, with its blue stripe, seemed to do something for the uniform of the

United States Air Force. He was one of the seven called to mount the step to the reading desk in the center of the temple, that a portion of the Law might be read to him by the new cantor, and when Charles said the blessings his voice was soft but deep and clear.

Ed walked home with Charles and Roland, taking a little longer than usual because his knee had relapsed somewhat. The same dogs barked at him along the way that always did.

"Nice dog," he said, extending his hand.

He listened to Charles meanwhile. Charles said that even in the Air Force he was compelled to waste part of his time. There were things like the manual of arms which were of no earthly use. He said he had a couple of inventions in mind, but he wasn't sure if they were patentable, so he had gotten a book on patent law from a town library near the base, to figure out whether it was worth investing six hundred bucks on a patent attorney. He had thought of a screwdriver with a faucetlike handle, but molded to fit the fingers, so that leverage would be greater. A similar device could be used to remove spark plugs. And he had thought of a walk-under bed, to save space in a room. He said you might think it would be too hot, up so high, but there was no reason why it should be hotter than the upper bunk of a double-decker. And in winter the warmth could be an advantage. An alternate version was a bed atop a high chest of drawers.

He also told Ed, as they walked under the big trees, that Millicent was quite upset about Miecznesliwy's defection. He said Millicent had done some volunteer work for the independents in the Democratic primary, which Ed hadn't known, and she was feeling very badly now about Miecznesliwy going over to the regulars.

Who am I, to be these kids' father, Ed pondered, to play such a role in somebody else's life? These individuals, did they choose me to play the role of father? It seemed strange that these young adults were his children. By what quick stages they grow. You've not begun to know their minds at one stage before they're on to the next.

In the afternoon Charles went out to look at his Model T, which Ed had raised on blocks, and then he sat on the bumpy floor of the barn, combing the old dog Roger, while Roland climbed in the rafters with Bobby O'Shaughnessy and Snotsy Vaughn and a couple of little girls named Johnson.

Then he sat a while on the porch rail, talking with his parents, his feet locked in the balustrades. Lucinda told him of the animal that lived under the porch, and which they heard at night, though no one had seen it, and which ate her chrysanthemums. She said Mrs. Davey, whose two old horses pranced in the large pasture diagonally opposite, had told her it was probably a woodchuck. She could get Mr. Featherstone to shoot it, but she was afraid it might have children.

She complained also about the hornets, and told Charles his father ought to get an exterminator. But Ed said Farquhar at the hardware had told him hornets ate the moths that were ruining the crab-apple trees.

"That's right," Charles told his mother. "Actually hornets are like dogs—the chances of one biting you is pretty small. They're not like mosquitoes, that feed on your blood."

"But people exterminate hornets," she said.

"So what?" said Charles. "That doesn't prove they're dangerous. It proves that people are dangerous to hornets."

Ed nodded.

They had wanted to invite Grandma Annie and some of the relatives for Sunday dinner, but it turned out that Charles had to leave in the morning.

They took him to Bedford Airport in the sagging Plymouth, Patty and Roland in the back seat, and kissed him. Lucinda wept a little on the way home, Ed noticed, but she said nothing.

She made a lunch of sandwiches. Afterward Ed went out to mow the yard. He filled the secondhand mower from the gasoline can and checked its oil. His knee was not bad. He depended on the mower and on the woodpile for exercise, and tried to spend forty minutes a day cutting trees from the woods out back, or sawing them into logs or splitting the big ones. Sometimes Roland helped him trim the branches. Lucinda objected to letting the child use an ax, but Roland said the Scouts were supposed to know how. Even with chopping and mowing, Ed felt that his middle was soft. The firemen were supposed to meet for calisthenics, but he had gone to the first class and found nobody there.

He pushed the mower on the broad expanse before the house, its hot racket battering the air, sometimes in breezy openness and sometimes in the speckled light beneath a tree. The big elm looked diseased, he thought. It should have been sprayed.

There was too much land to mow all the way down to the tumbly stone wall and the street, so he had been mowing only around the house and before the barn, letting his dirt road wind through tall grass and bachelor's-buttons further down. But he tended to mow a larger and larger area each time. Across the road he could see the brown horse grazing and the old black one galloping heavily. Past the gray house to which the horses belonged was a white one, where Patty worked three days a week looking after the Hubbard children.

It struck him that he had gotten to know a large number of Wilmerding Crosswalk people in scarcely more than a third of a year, both in his congregation and outside it. He even knew all about the crippled peddler who came every fortnight or so to these out-of-the-way houses, carrying his satchels at snail speed, and whose son was at the University of Massachusetts. Ed and Lucinda always managed to buy some of his household or stationery gimcracks, or some of his wife's knitted goods, even though it was hard to find something they had not already bought, and Ed had gotten him occasional janitorial jobs at the temple.

It felt as though the family had been here much longer. Roland came and went with his friends mysteriously, and delivered papers for several days when the Vaughn kid was sick. Lucinda was growing tomatoes and squashes and talked of watermelons. It was her pleasure, though Grandma Annie mistook it for an economy and said she was nuts to do it. Sometimes she bought milk still warm at the dairy, and new eggs at the eggery, and once she bought duck eggs from Mrs. Godkin down at the duck farm. She rode on Roland's bicycle and had fallen off it. Ed turned the mower and started back. He could see the bruise on Lucinda's thigh now, as she squatted packing the mud about some transplants.

He was glad she was wearing shorts again. She had put them away years ago in Abbottsford, after some ladies remarked about her wearing them to the grocery. She had wept defiantly for half an evening when she heard of it. The ladies apparently had said it didn't look proper for a rebbetsin.

"I'm not a rebbetsin," she had told him tearfully. "You may be a rabbi, but that doesn't make me a rebbetsin."

"Sure it does," he had told her. "What are you upset about? It's a perfectly good Yiddish expression."

"I don't want to be a perfectly good Yiddish expression," she had said.

But he saw all three pairs of her shorts neatly pressed in the closet after that, unworn for years. Until now. And even now she probably looked better in them than the ladies who had complained at that time, he thought. Her legs were still hard. Even though at closer range they showed a lot of blue capillaries.

Yet early that morning, while Charles still slept, he had been quite disgusted with her. She had been complaining of tiny brown lice in the house, so he had searched and traced them to the baby birds in the porch eaves, but he had suggested that the birds were fledglings now and about to leave the nest within a day, since one had already flown, so it might be well to wait till tomorrow before calling the exterminator, especially since you probably couldn't get one on Sunday anyhow. But she bawled him out nastily and at length, saying it was no use talking to him and that he cared for the birds but nothing for how hard she worked. So he telephoned exterminators, but none would come on Sunday. He carefully moved the nest, meaning to take it to the barn if the birds did not flutter away in the meantime, which they did, and he fumigated the porch at once, but she then made him strip naked outside the back door, tossing other clothes out to him, and boiled what he had worn, complaining again that he had no consideration for her. All that was before Charles wakened. And later, when she found a louse crawling on the hall baseboard she still made it his fault.

Explaining only made her accuse you of picking a fight. Sometimes it was good not to talk to her for a day, and take a rest.

He cut with the mower back and forth, widening a swath into a carpet, upon a variety of grasses and crab grass. Despite the breeze he grew warm. Now and then a sluggish little toad, speckled and hardly visible in the grass, leaped away from his mower, but sometimes with such delay that he was not sure.

He cut between the house and the barn, almost up to where the old rusted harrow sat, and lowered himself to the woodpile to rest.

Lucinda came to him. She said Mrs. Davey had offered some rhododendron seedlings and had promised to show her how to make cold frames for them out of old storm windows, but it didn't pay unless they were going to be in the house more than a year.

"Well, I don't know," he said. "I'm still not ready to buy. I'd like to see what it costs to heat the place."

She looked about at where he had mowed. "That mower cuts awful raggedy," she said.

"Well, it looks better from a distance," he said. "It's not the mower's fault. There's too many different kinds of stuff growing. Weeds. The place is a salad. You'd have to sift the whole thing out and start with new grass, to help that. It's a salad. It just needs oil and vinegar."

"And when are you gonna get rid of that damn piece of junk?" she asked.

He looked at the harrow, and the long tufted grass rising through it. "You mean the harrow?" he said.

"Ed, it's an eyesore. Like a junk yard. How are you ever gonna mow there with that thing there?"

"Well, I don't know if I want to mow right there," he said. "I thought I'd preserve that patch as a national forest."

She kept looking at him sourly.

"Did you shave this morning?" she asked.

"No."

After a while she turned, and he watched her legs and the motion of the shorts upon her as she walked away from him toward a garden, through sunshine and shade. Here in the shadow of the barn he could feel the breezes once more, upon his neck, his face, his arms.

In the past few days butterflies had appeared, and a white one and a yellow one fluttered near him now. Lucinda was perhaps right, he said to himself, that it was simplest to buy this house and look no further. She had invested a lot of time into weeding, cultivating, turning over earth. The sun shone into blossoms and through petals until they were like spots of fire. He had helped from time to time, and it was good to reach under leaves, in the face of a humming bee, and put your hand on a fat squash. Spears of asparagus still came up wild in a patch of grass where earlier residents had had a garden, and he had discovered they were soft and tasty uncooked. Raw they were less stringy and bit more easily, with an agreeable pungent bitterness.

Birds alway twittered around here, including a pair of brilliant yellow-and-black ones that swooped over the meadow flowers when the sun got low, and Roland claimed to have counted nineteen species in an afternoon. Even in the woods, which he could see past the clothesline, sprigs of lavender blossoms grew underfoot. Lucinda had had a mild heatstroke picking strawberries in the big field already, and they had found blueberries and blackberries, still ripening. And he knew that if he took a walk to where the brook widened and grew still by swamps he would find carpets of pond lilies. He did not himself have much sense of smell, but Lucinda said she had never known such fragrant air.

Yet, he thought, Abbottsford had been prettier. Their old white house there had had no porch, and uneven wide-board flooring that caught dirt in the big cracks, and cramped bedrooms slanted like an attic under a roof without insulation. The paint had peeled badly. But it had been on a high hilltop, overlooking hillsides where cows grazed and the little town itself, with the river winding through it. On that hilltop the sky had been enormous. It had been a season of fantastic sunsets, and skies of unusual magnificence every day, rays slanting through rolling columns of purple-gray cloud. Driving up to that hilltop shortly before moving in he had seen a complete rainbow, its great arc solid and unbroken, from deep green mountains to the high heavens and down to other green far off—he had never before seen a rainbow from earth to earth, unbroken like that. A week after they moved in there had been another, unbroken like the first, and thinking they must be frequent in the region he had not troubled to get his camera, though there was film for color slides on hand. But he never saw any more rainbows. The strange splendor of the skies was also of a freakish season, unrepeated, and he came away from Abbottsford without pictures of the rainbow, or of those clouds and sunsets, or of the two geese who used to walk in the road. The best shots were always missed. Millicent, as a two-week newborn, had had saucer eyes crossed like Ben Turpin, a unique comical cuteness like none he saw before or since, but when he got around to photographing those eyes they had straightened. And at two years, with her long hair done up in a knot on top, Millicent had had a beauty to make your heart gasp, and he went one noon to snap that picture, when the sun came out, but Lucinda had cut the hair an hour before. Gone, gone, those hilltop skies and the little girl's hair. God and man were alike in their carelessness of beauty.

On the woodpile under him a log moved and he shifted his position. He reached in his shirt pocket for a cigarette but there was none. He was trying to limit his smoking, and it pleased him that he had not craved one until this hour.

He remembered the long grape arbor in his grandfather's back yard, where the city spread south amid wooden houses. His grandparents had made their household wine from those grapes. It's too bad people don't live in a house for generations, he thought. Then you could elaborate walks under grape arbors, paths under trees.

His grandfather, he thought, had understood a religion in which one's books, one's children, and the cycle of the year were all of a piece. And which used agriculture and history, but avoided magic, and researched always into the question of how to be human, in order that man might react to his environment, known and unknown, and belong to society and the earth, while the moon kept track of the calendar.

He wished someone—himself or his sister Rosalind, perhaps—had had the foresight to take some home movies of the old man, so he could be seen again now, walking under his back-yard arbor when he came home from business, in his panama hat, puffing his pipe, taking slugs off the grapes with long tweezers. If he were alive now, how much pleasure the breath of his life would put into a religious tradition. One must in one's person be all of one's dead.

18

Millicent had climbed back up to her party, past the people who sat on the stairs and who stood in the hallway with drinks. At the open door of the apartment her cousin Steve put an arm half about her and spoke softly down to her ear, his face silly and looking somewhat drunk, and asked if her roommate Natalie put out.

She thrust away his arm, too shaken and angry to speak, and fled into the crowd. She was careful all the rest of the evening to stay far from whatever part of the room Steve was in, and even when people began to leave she did not give him a chance to pay his respects. The party seemed long breaking up. A policeman looked in once politely and asked that the noise be held down, as there had been a complaint. Later, after some glassware was broken, Ella Jane asked some boys to leave, and the party did not last long after that.

By three o'clock in the morning the roommates were alone, Ella Jane low in the overstuffed chair with her cane across her lap, Natalie sprawled in her black ruffled gown on Millicent's couch, and Millicent sitting by the little unfolded drop-leaf table. The crucifix hung askew, and Millicent straightened it. There had been a tone of vulgarity in the last hour or two. Some boys had dropped ice into girls' bosoms. The location of Ella Jane's bedroom, with access only through the bathroom, had made for difficulties, because some of the crowd congregated back there and were frequently locked in, and sometimes they pounded on the door and wiggled the knob while the bathroom was occupied.

On the table beside Millicent food was smeared. She fetched a rag from the kitchen and began to wipe it. It occurred to her that she had not been a very good hostess once Leslie had arrived.

"Where do you get such energy?" Ella Jane asked her tiredly.

"I don't," she said. She rubbed her eyes, and sank again onto the creaky little dining chair.

"Let's clean up tomorrow," Natalie said sleepily. "All in favor say aye."

There was a silence, as though they were too tired to answer.

"Where did we ever dredge up such a mob of heathen?" Ella Jane said.

Millicent said the roughnecks were the pharmacy students and frat brothers her cousin Steve had brought, but Ella Jane said no, they were Natalie's. Natalie said nothing.

They began to talk desultorily of a few of the more attractive boys. Natalie and Ella Jane had noticed Leslie. "He's nice," Natalie said.

"The English haircut's an affectation though," said Ella Jane.

"It's not an English haircut," Millicent protested. "He's broke. He hasn't got any money for barbers."

By four they were in bed, but Millicent could not sleep right away. Her eyes hurt from exhaustion, the left eye especially, and its tense raw feeling extended down into the left nostril.

She thought of Leslie. He had been equally welcome at Yale Medical School or at Johns Hopkins, and he had had his choice of internships. Yet with his debts, and mother and brother, she wondered how he could even manage to buy himself a pair of socks. And if he should need a new suit, or a coat, it must be a disaster.

In college he had never had a nickel for a coke.

Near the head of her studio couch she saw the windows growing light. The city was quiet.

She slept, but half awakened when she heard Natalie rise for work, groaning and cursing. It seemed as if the door slammed. She heard Ella Jane telephoning that she had a murderous headache and would not be in.

Millicent next awakened with the kitten Theodore mewing beside her on the wrinkled sheets. The alarm clock on the mantelpiece was turned aside but she could see that it was nearly eleven. Some pussy willows were missing.

After a while she gathered together all the mess. The cat had been into some of it. She swept, still wearing her white pajamas, and put three bags of garbage leaning side by side against the wall of the stair landing.

She saw that Ella Jane had risen, squinty and frowzy in her bathrobe and leaning on her cane, and was preparing coffee. The kitten chased its tail around and around and Millicent sat on the floor to play with it. Then she got an empty spool on the end of a string from a kitchen drawer and sat again, holding it for the kitten to bat.

Ella Jane sat watching and sipping her coffee.

Millicent told Ella Jane she had a kitten once before, a white one spotted black, that she had found bedraggled and sneezing in an icy rain in Chicago. She had picked it up, sick and filthy, and nursed it to health, though she became sick from it herself in the meantime. It disappeared, and she suspected her grandaunt of having got rid of it.

Millicent stood up. She dropped her pajama trousers and stepped out of them, and unbuttoned her top. Then she began her calisthenics. She did not like a waistband when she exercised, but she wanted the jacket on her shoulders for warmth. Ella Jane watched, the elbow that held the cup propped on the table. Millicent touched her fingers to her toes several times, with feet together, and at last her palms to the floor.

"You're cute," said Ella Jane.

With feet apart Millicent swung her arms, one and then the other, out to the side and down to the opposite foot.

"If your friend Hollander could see you now," said Ella Jane, "you'd have him hooked. He'd beg on his knees."

Millicent reddened, still exercising. "He would not," she said.

"No?" said Ella Jane.

When Millicent got to the city room Zucchino was still busy, as there was some overlap in their working hours. Mr. Killian beckoned with a toss of his head, handed her two publicity releases that had arrived in the mail, and told her to see if she could whip them into stories. He waved her away quickly without another word and without having looked her in the eye.

He had never given her anything like that to do before. Once or twice Mr. Hopkins had had her phone the weather bureau and copy down the forecast, but that was all. She sat at a vacant typewriter. The releases were each only a couple of paragraphs. But she worked hard, each word and phrase seeming a decision. Yet she dreaded to appear too slow. She wrote each at last almost in the words of the release and put them on Mr. Killian's desk. She went to her usual duties, and from a distance saw Mr. Killian edit her two little stories. He said nothing. Then Charles phoned that he had flown in on a pass, and she had supper with him at the spa.

Toward eleven, when she brought copies of the city edition downstairs to the city room, she found her two stories in the paper itself, one above the other far down and quite tiny in an inside page, those sentences lovingly familiar now. She clipped them out, to show to her roommates and her parents.

Then on Saturday night quite late, after Mr. Killian had gone, Mr. Hopkins asked her to type a story that Danny McBride would dictate word by word over the telephone. It was difficult. Mr. Hopkins had not indicated one of the special telephones that had earpieces on a separate head bracket, but an ordinary little one, and she had to crook it against her ear with her shoulder while she pecked. She marveled at Danny's skill—standing somewhere in a dark phone booth he seemed to compose his story with ease, orally, exactly as it would appear. But she wished she had continued longer with her typing course. Danny was indistinct, and if she said she hadn't heard he would seem to bellow into the mouthpiece, becoming even less distinct.

Toward noon on Sunday Leslie Hollander called. The drop-leaf table was spread for breakfast, so that the lavender telephone had been removed to the floor, but Ella Jane picked it up and then extended it toward Millicent. "This is Les," he said to her. He asked if she would care to meet him at the Museum of Fine Arts, before a certain small canvas of Corot, which he described.

She was there at one o'clock, wearing her cord dress, and she saw him looking at paintings, holding his pipe and sucking it. They wandered together slowly. She did not know much about the paintings, but he explained how a certain school had developed, pointing with his pipe and moving it in little sweeping gestures. They stayed in certain rooms, which he said were not the museum's strongest but represented a period he found especially fascinating.

After nearly an hour they went to the wide steps out back, where a vista of green stretched into the low expanse of city and a little waterway meandered. They sat on chiseled stone beside the steps. He mentioned chamber concerts that were held at different museums, and said it was too bad she worked Friday nights and Saturday nights, because she would not be able to go to the Symphony in the fall. They did not talk easily at first. She apologized for the vulgarity of her party. Once he called her Mil, and she scotched it immediately, reminding him her name was Millicent.

Yet she told him she had dreamed of him the night before. She had dreamed he discovered that coffee was a cause of cancer, and that he was proclaimed one of the greatest of scientists.

Leslie was amused. They began to talk of cancer. He explained how different varieties of it belonged to different kinds of tissue, and how various organs were therefore prone to different types of it. This led him to a discussion of growth, and how the tissues of the embryo differentiate themselves. He even touched on plants, and said that one upon a time all cells were reproductive cells, and that the appearance among them of nonreproductive cells, of bodies, had been as great a revolution as the appearance of mind.

Talk became easier. When it came time for her to go to the city room he rode with her on the trolley part way. They talked while they waited for it and while they rode, and when she left him it seemed to her that it had been exciting throughout. They had agreed about Senator McCarthy, and discussed her fear of the atom bomb. He had explained his working hours in detail—he had to be dressed, shaved, and in the laboratory by six forty-five in the morning, and made his rounds of the wards a half hour later. Then surgery. He might finish at six or seven in the evening, but every other night he was on call, which meant he could sleep unless needed, though more often than not they interrupted his sleep. Even if he worked most of the night his duties began again as usual at six forty-five in the morning. Yet he seemed grateful that on alternate nights he could sleep undisturbed. She told him he was the most decent person she knew, and that he and Ella Jane were the only civilized people she saw these days.

She worked in the city room quickly but mechanically, her mind reliving their conversation. He said it had been oddly inconsistent of her to choose a college a thousand miles away and then move in with a grandaunt. She had never seen it in that light before.

She was given no publicity releases to make into stories tonight, and no dictation to take by telephone, but only her usual copy-boy duties, back and forth to Mr. Hopkins's desk, upstairs and down, a few times across the street to the spa and back as the night was hot, once down to the sidewalk to chalk bulletins on the blackboard, and once briefly through the city to Heustis Garvey. Nevertheless those little stories of two nights before had given her encouragement, and she felt guiltily that she had done nothing about developing a reporter's eyes, or about really justifying the faith that Mr. Killian seemed to have in her. It was hard on her own to find any news happening. But little items of a feature sort were supposedly everywhere. Maud had told her how she had used to find them as a young girl—curious little stories about a blind man on the Common and whatnot. Millicent wondered if a little feature could be made about Leslie's work at the hospital. Or about Ella Jane's work in the brokerage office, or about Charles's training in the Air Force. Even those seemed difficult. She wondered how one began, or knew what to put in.

The girls were still up when she returned to the apartment.

"How was your museum date?" Natalie asked her.

"It wasn't a date," said Millicent.

"What was it?" said Ella Jane. "An appointment?"

On her first night off Millicent dialed the Massachusetts General Hospital on the lavender telephone about six o'clock, and asked whether Dr. Leslie Hollander were busy. The switchboard lady said she would have him paged. But in a few seconds Millicent grew timid and canceled the call. If he were in the midst of some surgery, preoccupied with a suffering patient, she would seem an awful nuisance. It was risky to phone him at any time, she thought. Even in his off hours he might be on an emergency. She had only asked if he were busy and they had begun to page him right off.

But the next night Leslie phoned, about nine, to invite her for supper on Sunday evening at the home of a friend. A Dr. Mahady and his wife had a tiny apartment where the back of Beacon Hill sloped down toward the hospital, and they were having a few couples for spaghetti and chianti. Millicent accepted tentatively, depending on Zucchino's willingness to swap shifts or work in her stead that day, and on Mr. Killian's permission.

But when she found Zucchino in the city room the next afternoon he had no interest in working Sunday night.

He did not even trouble to give an excuse or to mention commitments of his own. She felt the disappointment bitterly, especially as Leslie had the whole Sunday. A colleague owed him the day. There were so few times when she and Les could see one another. When he was not busy at his work, she was busy at hers. And congenial friendships were so scarce.

Danny McBride passed in back of her at the teletype machines, brushing her skirt. "Hi, gorgeous," he said, and this time his fingers clutched in a probing way. She swung about hotly in an instant, pressing her back to the machines.

"That wasn't just vulgar!" she said almost breathlessly. "It was distinctly lascivious."

"Well, I lost control of myself," he smiled amiably. "The way you sort of wiggled there."

"I didn't wiggle, and you know it! I never wiggled in my life! Now stop this! Once and for all! I won't have it."

She watched him saunter away. She returned to separating the teletype stories with a ruler. She could scarcely swallow her anger. She ought to have asked him, she thought, whether he would care to have his wife and his three little children witness such behavior. Or she should have threatened to tell Mr. Killian. And that was a lie, about losing control of himself, she thought. He planned it.

It seemed to her that Danny McBride went out of his way to be as detestable as possible. He still called her Sneezy, and Louie Alpert copied him.

She had to tell Leslie she could not go to supper at his friends', but they made plans to meet anyway, for a couple of hours early Sunday afternoon.

This time they chose the greenery of the esplanade, alongside the broad river basin, and she found him there ahead of her, waiting on a bench in the shade of a tree. She walked with him along the paths. She saw an aged athlete sculling on a wisp of a boat, his arms and legs white in the sun, and a mother picnicking with two little children. Across the road red brick and shutters rose in tiers up the hill.

Leslie was morose and unsmiling. He told her, talking quietly, that just before coming to meet her he had gone to make his daily visit to a certain baby in the pediatric ward, even though it was his day off. But in the night they had taken him to surgery, and he died. Leslie had found only the rumpled little blanket and the pacifier.

He seemed to have no words to say more, but Millicent felt her own throat tighten. They walked, not looking at one another.

"What an awful thing," she said at last. "To die so young. To almost live, and yet never know."

She felt she had expressed herself poorly. To have looked on this world at all, and have savored none of it. It was horrible.

They sat on another bench. Leslie's mood did not improve. He told her of one of his colleagues, who gave first aid to a child who was wounded with a barbecue fork on the beach at Hyannis, and told the parents to have their own doctor look at the wound again, but they did not, and when it worsened they sued him for malpractice.

For the first time she heard him complain about the heaviness of his schedule. And about the phone that woke him with calls for his roommate even when he was not on call himself. And about the long residencies he would need, which the Army would postpone.

"I won't be married for years," he said.

"Well, I'm with you," she said. "I don't intend to get married for a long time either."

She said she knew it was hard, especially as every penny he spent on himself was as though taken from his mother and brother, but that she admired the strength with which he had planned his life. She told him it would be worth it. "You'd be very foolish to marry before your education's complete," she said.

"Education is never complete," he answered.

They walked some more. They saw a man and woman who strolled holding hands. But Leslie and Millicent walked side by side, their hands not touching. He said his mother was awful. If his mother spent a couple of bucks in a grocery, he said, she would shoplift another nickel's worth. She didn't feel right if she didn't. He could stand her perpetual bargain-hunting, he said, but the petty swiping was too much.

Millicent said her mother was very economical too, and always gave her meat loaves and noodle puddings to take back to the city for herself and her roommates, and bags of leavings for the cat besides, until it became embarrassing to carry so much food on the train.

"It's not the same thing," Leslie said.

Millicent did not go directly to the city room from the riverfront, but back first to change into her denim skirt, and Leslie walked with her toward the apartment.

She asked him what his mother looked like, but could not visualize much from his description, except that she was quite small and not yet gray. She asked him if his brother looked like him, and he said somewhat.

As they crossed a street she told him she thought the work of the hospital must contain material she could use for a newspaper feature. She said she did not want to burden him, when he had more important things on his mind all day, but if he happened to notice something it would be good.

And she begged him to phone sometime on her nights off. He must tire of hospital meals, and could take pot luck with her and her roommates.

They walked on the flagstones where her building indented, and into the musty little lobby of marble. At the foot of the stairs she turned to him.

"How's your kitten doing?" he said.

"Oh, he's fine, thank you."

"I'm sorry about being in a crummy mood."

"No, that's all right."

"I must have been lousy company."

"No, really."

"Well—" he said. He took her hand, almost as if in a parting handshake. Then suddenly both his hands slid about her, to her back and shoulder, and his lips descended on hers, his eyes very near. Now really, is this necessary, she thought of asking.

His arms and his face enclosed her in a pleasant fit, as if he were tailored to her. It crossed her mind that it would be absurd to make a scene. She glimpsed his peaceful brow and closed her eyes. Their cheeks brushed, slowly, almost so that she could feel the down of her own face. The touch of skin seemed very alive. The movement of his hand made her want to move closer and she did. There's no sense in letting him think it's a matter of my being naïve, she thought.

Their lips came together like magnets again.

Just when she feared it might continue too long he stopped. They were still very close. She tried to look blasé and disdainful but he smiled. She avoided the smile, but then changed her mind and took both his hands.

She considered what to say, in the nature of reminding him again to phone, or apologizing again for not being able to go to supper at his friends'. However he kissed her lightly on the forehead. "Okay," he said, with a pat on her arm. "You'll be late for work."

The heavy door closed, with its glass and bars, and she climbed the stairs. We mustn't get mushy, she thought.

In the city room, late at night, her mind returned to him while she worked, and she remembered how he had apologized for being moody and sad.

Les, she imagined herself telling him, I've found one thing. There are people with whom you can truly talk. And they aren't the ones who always have a smile and tickle you with their witticisms.

She thought of the little patient he had lost in the pediatric ward.

During the week she received a picture postcard from Charles. It showed the straight main throughfare of a little Southern town. Hearing from him reminded her that she ought to inquire again about giving blood for the Air Force.

On Wednesday she consented to spend the evening baby-sitting for Aunt Gwendolyn, and had no sooner hung up the phone than Leslie called. She had not expected to hear from him so soon. She explained about the baby-sitting and asked if he could be free tomorrow night instead.

"I'll be on call tomorrow," he said.

"Oh dear," she sighed. Leslie sounded disappointed too. She regretted the hastiness of her promise to her aunt.

But suddenly it occurred to her that they might baby-sit together. She told him she would open some cans there.

They found Sharlene still in the high chair. Millicent tidied up around her while Aunt Gwendolyn dressed in the bedroom, and Leslie waited in the small living room. Millicent glimpsed him there, sitting on the chintzy sofa, his knees wide apart and seemingly bony under the khaki trousers. He was leaning over a low wooden coffee table, turning pages of a magazine past a bowl of artificial flowers. He was perspiring.

In the bedroom she helped her aunt button her dress. The air was sweltering and still. "If you happen to talk to my mother," she asked quietly, "don't mention that I brought a friend."

"I understand," her aunt assured her.

"Or she'll start asking who and what," Millicent explained.

"I won't say a word," said Aunt Gwen.

Leslie rose politely as Aunt Gwendolyn departed, and sat again. Millicent watched him as his eye followed Sharlene's curly blond head. The baby toddled in an undershirt and bulbous pants, shakily erect, her feet softly pounding the floor. She touched the flowers and talked unintelligibly. Sometimes she fell easily, bending suddenly so that her hands smacked the floor and then sitting with a bump.

Millicent prepared a pretty salad of tuna, with radishes for color, and she and Leslie ate at the kitchen table. Part of the time she held the baby on her lap and allowed her to nibble some. She felt the remarkable softness of the baby's skin. Leslie had removed his jacket and opened his collar.

"I'm afraid it's not much of a supper," she told Leslie. "But I didn't think you'd want anything hot on such a night."

"What do you think of your aunt's boy friend?" he asked.

"I really don't know him well yet."

The baby lifted a heavy nutcracker from the table and studied it. Millicent told how Aunt Gwen had had a job for a while and put Sharlene in a day nursery, but it hadn't worked out. And she told about the clarinetist being of Italian extraction, so that she was not supposed to say anything to her family.

When she had put the baby to bed she found that Leslie had washed the dishes.

"You didn't have to do that," she said.

They sat in the living room. He talked of medical things mostly, and told how a wildly angry surgeon had lectured and tongue-lashed a group of nurses outside the operating room for close to an hour on end, because they did not know the contents of various bottles they administered. A piece of surgery could be a masterpiece, a chef d'oeuvre, he said, and an hour later a nurse could kill the patient with the wrong bottle. It was like smashing the Mona Lisa.

It grew dark. The screened windows to the street were wide open and Leslie sat on the sill. They used only the light from the little hallway.

When they had talked a long time Millicent prepared some icy drinks. Then she resumed her seat on the chintz and they talked some more.

She had to interrupt to tend Sharlene, who awakened crying as though from a dream, and Leslie came and watched in the dark bedroom. But soon they were able to return to their places in the living room.

Millicent spoke of how little girls and little boys were the same in the vast majority of particulars, physical and mental. "When Sharlene was six months, she used to constantly keep pulling herself up to standing in the play pen and cry and cry to exhaustion because she didn't know how to get down again. And when Roland was a baby boy I remember he did exactly the same thing." Little girls, just as little boys, she said, had two hands, they explored. When they grew they learned arithmetic together, and climbed trees. Until adolescence forced girls to stop and be something else.

Leslie said she sounded as if she hadn't liked adolescence. She said she hadn't. "Bust development makes it impossible to run, and things like that," she told him.

"I thought little girls looked forward to adolescence," said Leslie. "You didn't like it? I should think it's an exciting time, growing into womanhood."

"I didn't like becoming an object for boys to whistle at," she said. "You'd be surprised. There are girls of eleven, and twelve, and thirteen that have a healthy disgust with 'femininity' and all that stuff. Perfume, and all that. They often do. But in the next several years they get pressured and re-educated into not being themselves any more."

She watched him sucking the ice from his glass. He sat sideways in the window frame, the light from the street palely shining on half his face.

"I don't think of you as a man, Les," she explained. "I think of you as a person. You are a person. You spend your time using your mind and your hands, day after day. Not fathering children. But when a girl is past the age of about nine she's gradually forced into limbo. I suppose years later when she's a mother the responsibilities make life real again, but for a girl those years between nine and marriage are a waste. Lost years. Everything pressures her toward the two per cent of her that's her sex, and the ninety-eight per cent that's a person gets suppressed out of existence. She's pressured into being something that looks nice and smells nice. It's like being removed from the world. Everything is planned to make her think of herself as a reproduction machine. Her clothes. Society."

He was looking at her. On his glass and on the lenses of his eyeglasses there were flecks of light in the semidarkness.

"When I was a kid," she said, "there was this mountain stream, near where we lived that year. Abbottsford. And I showed my brother how to make a dam, like a beaver dam. We worked on it for days. And that was just about the last good year. After that the femininity really closed in."

"Do you resent growing up?"

"No," she told him. "On the contrary. Just the opposite. I've been trying to grow up all my life."

"Do you resent being a woman?"

"I don't resent it itself, but I resent the way it's treated. I think it's nice to be able to bear children. But there's got to be more purpose in the existence of the human race than just a species going on and on. When they make reproduction the central fact of life you're like a vegetable."

"Do you think it's easier for a man?" he asked.

"Of course it is. A boy isn't cut off like that. He winds generators. They don't make him get preoccupied with his body."

"But—"

"Even when they teach a little boy not to cry," she interrupted, "they're already teaching him to be a grownup."

"Maybe it's easier to be a man," he said, "but a man is always asked to be something else besides."

"But that's the whole point," said Millicent.

"Men work like dogs," he said.

"I know," she agreed. "I don't do a thing. But I'd be glad to work like a dog."

"There are women who become doctors. Surgeons even, some of them."

"I know it. And I wish I'd done that. Maybe I still should. But I bet they fight her every step of the way. If you'd ever been a girl looking for a job, Les, you'd know. Everything's stacked against all a girl's efforts to grow up. Of course most girls are such Uncle Toms after a few years that they don't even realize it any more. But if she goes in for being feminine, and housewifey, she's again sort of a child—dependent like a child, on her husband's finances and his way of life, and his place of life, and that's why they have the phrase 'women and children.' And on the other hand if she goes in for doing adult things, like politicking or having a job, it's either regarded as sort of a kid's job or else she's like a kid playing at being a grownup. I've done it, Les. I know how it feels. People see a woman make a political speech and they think it's cute. Trivial."

She wished her voice wouldn't quake so. He was looking at her steadily, not smiling. She wished she knew what he was thinking.

"Your metaphors are mixed," he said. "Uncle Tom doesn't mean children."

"It's the same thing. The Negro slaves were considered like children too."

He looked at her silently.

"It's a whole conspiracy," she said. "Even the words they use for women's clothes, like 'undies' and 'panties.' And if you read something about fashions, or exercises, your stomach is your 'tummy.' They want you to think that women not only make children and take care of children—they are children. Look at the soap ads—a smooth skin. A smooth skin and pretty ruffles, like my baby cousin Sharlene in there. And when a couple goes on a date, the man 'takes her out,' like a baby going bye-bye. And pays her way. 'A man and a girl.' Not a boy and a woman, no. You think it isn't true? And we give a party and it's 'men and girls.' The man's the one that's a grownup. Even if the girl has twice his brains."

There was a twist in his mouth and in his eyebrows. She thought his expression had grown somewhat skeptical.

"What do you think?" she said.

"I think you're a very confused little girl."

"Except I'm not a little girl."

"Baby—" he began.

"There!" she said. "That's what I mean! You've said it! Calling a woman a baby. You were going to call me 'baby,' weren't you."

He shrugged and smirked. "It's an expression. I'm sorry. I just stumbled into that."

"Yes, 'an expression.' "

"It's a term of endearment," he said. "Women call men baby, too."

"No they don't."

"I'll never call you that again, okay? I'll call you 'grownup.' "

"Think of me as a person," she told him. "Like yourself. That'll take care of it."

"Okay, person."

"Just call me Millicent. There's a reason for expressions. Like when an Englishman calls a native a 'boy,' even if he's fifty years old. And another thing, why do they have this tradition that when a man and a woman go out together the man has to be taller? And older? Answer me that. My sister's tall, and none of her friends can be boys that are littler than she is. And why? Because it would spoil the whole stupid fiction, that's why." She changed her position on the couch. She wore her blue cord and it was sticky. "You happen to be taller than I am, Les, but what if you weren't? I'm interested in you as a friend. In your heart and mind."

One of his legs was drawn up before him along the sill, and the other dragged to the floor. He began to unbutton his shirt. "You know, Millicent," he said, "I think you're right. You consider the whole complex of muscles and nerves and organs in the body, blood vessels, and the differences between men and women are highly exaggerated. And it's a stinking hot night, and we should take off our clothes."

"What are you doing?"

"I'm taking off my clothes."

"Leslie!" She rose.

He had thrown away his tie and was undoing his cuffs.

"Are you out of your mind?" she said.

"Come on," he said. "Take your clothes off."

"I'll do nothing of the kind."

He dropped his shirt to the floor and pulled up his undershirt.

"What are you doing! Les! For heaven sakes! Don't be crazy!"

He got up from the sill. A column of hair bisected his chest. "Come on," he said.

"Leslie! Stop it!" She picked up his shirt from the floor and tried to hand it to him. He was already unbuckling his belt. "Here. Put on your shirt. Put on your shirt, Les."

He unhooked his trousers. She turned and fled to the bathroom. She shut the door. When she had found the light she locked the bolt.

"I never heard of anything so ridiculous," she said to the closed door. She felt hot at the neck and her heartbeat had quickened.

She heard no answer. She saw her face in the mirror. She gave her hair a brush or two with her hand. She sighed. Then she closed the lid and sat down. She looked at the walls, and the heavy paint cracking on the riser. From the diaper pail came a faint odor of ammonia. Beyond the door she thought she heard Leslie's footsteps move this way and that. Then there was silence.

"Les—" she said.

There was no answer.

"Les?" she called louder.

"What?" she heard him answer.

She had nothing to say. She wet her lips. "What are you doing?" she asked.

"I'm just lying here on the couch."

"With your clothes off?"

"Sure."

"Everything off?"

"Sure."

There was a silence. She glanced at the bolt to make sure she had locked it.

"I'm disappointed in you," she said.

"How long are you gonna stay locked in that bathroom?" he asked.

"Until you're decent."

"Well, you might as well take a cool shower while you're in there."

"I'll do no such thing."

In her agitation she rose and sat down again.

"Put on your clothes at once," she said.

"Nope."

"Are you really undressed?"

"Come out and look. See for yourself."

"Are you gonna be lying out there naked when my aunt comes home?"

"I might. Why not? I'm cool. I'm comfortable. And I don't see why on a hot night like this two human beings can't continue this discussion with our clothes off."

"You better join a nudist colony," she told him. "It may be hot, but it's not hot enough to affect my mind."

His footsteps came to the door. She saw the knob turn and wobble, but the bolt held.

"Les," she said, "what do you think you're proving? You think you're very bold and shocking, don't you."

"Is there any air in there?" he asked her.

"Les, this is ridiculous," she said.

"Yup," she heard him say.

"You have such a fine mind, and this is degrading."

"Millicent, sweetie pie, you said it yourself. The differences are insignificant. Our toes are the same. Our livers are the same. Even our belly buttons are the same."

She didn't answer him. In her teeth she made a little noise of exasperation.

"Are you sore?" he asked.

"That's not the point."

He said nothing. She heard the floor creak under his feet.

"What if my aunt walked in?"

"She's not gonna walk in."

"She might," said Millicent. "They might have a quarrel and she might come home early."

"A likely story."

She wondered what else to say to him. "I didn't know you were a lunatic," she said.

"Have you ever seen a man in the nude?" he asked.

"Children."

"I mean a full-grown adult male."

"No. Not really."

"Not even your brother?"

"We weren't brought up to prance around in the nude."

"Well, you've been living almost twenty-two years in a world in which half the people are men. It's high time some of the secrecy was ended."

"No thank you."

For a moment or two nothing was said.

"When are you coming out?" he asked her.

"I'm not."

"You can't stay locked in a bathroom all evening."

"I can too."

"I might have to use it."

"Too bad," she answered him.

She nervously tucked some hair behind her ear. The little bathroom was in fact warm and sticky. He seemed to walk around out there.

His footsteps moved away, and for a while she heard nothing. I hope the baby doesn't wake up, she thought.

"Les?" she asked after a time.

There was silence.

"Les?" she asked again.

"Okay," he said from a distance, in a tired tone. "You can come out now."

"Are you dressed?"

"Yes."

"Are you sure?"

"Yes."

She rose and undid the bolt. She opened the door an inch and peeked out, but she saw nothing. She turned out the bathroom light and went as far as the living room. Leslie was in the half darkness on the couch, sitting with knees crossed, dressed as before. Millicent passed to the window sill and sat on it.

"Why did you do that?" she asked, without altogether looking at him.

"I wanted to loosen you up. You're so solemn. Life's a big tragedy with you. Maybe it is a tragedy, but we can't live like that. You have to put some joy in the world. In your own life too."

"Well, you didn't succeed. It didn't make me very happy at all. I thought you must be cracking up from exhaustion, or overwork. A nervous breakdown or something."

They resumed conversation gradually, and he talked of the hospital again. But she was ill at ease, and her mind wandered.

She was glad when her aunt came. Even on the way home she could scarcely bring herself to make conversation. The night had grown foggy, and the tires of passing cars had a wet sound.

In the lobby of soiled marble she turned to him.

"Shall I come up for a while?" he said.

"No. I think my roommates are still up."

"I'd be glad to see your roommates again. I didn't get to talk to them at the party, hardly."

"No, really. They might be undressed, or getting ready for bed."

"Okay." He bent to her, putting his hands to her shoulders, but she leaned away.

"Do we have to kiss every time?" she said. "I kissed you Sunday."

He pulled her to his chest but she avoided his face.

"I don't want to kiss every time," she said. "It's degrading. I told you I don't think of you as a man."

"So it's a kiss between friends. Believe me, when I kissed you Sunday I didn't feel the slightest prejudice against you on account of your being female."

"Don't make fun of me."

He stopped smiling. "If I told you I have yet to meet a woman that wasn't crazy in some way or other," he said, "I suppose you'd resent it."

"I'd consider the craziness very understandable." She broke from him. "And good night."

She hurried up the stairs. During the night she wondered if in fact he had not undressed at all, but had only pretended in order to tease her. She could not make up her mind. She wished he hadn't done it, anyway, whichever it was. She felt resentment, as though a strangeness had descended between them.

She went to the blood bank the next morning. The nurse said her veins were small and deep, and punctured her more than once, with grimaces that made Millicent uneasy.

She lay on the table, watching the slow drip of crimson in the suspended bottle. She tried to think of the injured servicemen to whom her blood might find its way. But the tingling made her edgy.

In the evening Leslie phoned. He said if she wanted to write a newspaper feature about the hospital he would show her around.

It seemed to her a lovely gesture on his part. She felt forgiving about the night before. On the way to the hospital she stopped at a drugstore and bought a notebook with a wire binding.

He had told her he would meet her by the receptionist in Emergency. Millicent explained this to the big, florid-faced nurse at the desk, and then she waited on the molded bench that ran all around the room, built into the wall.

She saw a couple come to the desk with a child, and later a gray-haired man sat a few feet from her holding a hand to an eye. Leslie did not appear, and occasionally she saw the nurse look at her askance. The nurse had a beefy face with small features, and black hair under the tiny folded cap.

Millicent took the notebook from her shoulder-strap bag and folded back the cover. *A Night In The Hospital,* she wrote in her slanting hand. She crossed it out, and wrote *A Night In Emergency*. After a while she wrote *A Night In The Accident Ward* and studied it, biting her lip thoroughtfully.

Leslie came to her suddenly, seeming much in a hurry, and dressed in white. A stethoscope dangled from his neck. He apologized, saying he had gotten tied up and did not know how long he would be, but that if she could wait he would come back. Then he was gone. It was the first time she had seen him in medical clothes. She had never before seen him so quick and busy. His eyes were bright and concentrated, with none of the sleepiness of his off hours.

A heavy-set man sat beside her and told her in an accent about an auto collision. He had no visible injuries but he put his hands to his neck and his back and explained where it hurt. It occurred to Millicent that she had stumbled upon a story for her paper. She told the man she was a newspaperwoman, and then she wrote furiously while he talked. He told exactly how the accident had occurred, and though he spoke slowly she frequently had to ask him to pause.

Then she hurried to a telephone booth in the corridor. Mr. Hopkins spoke to her. "I'll have Heustis check it," he said.

She sat on the bench some more. The man wanted to know when it would be in the paper, and she calculated for him which edition. At eleven o'clock she went home. Leslie had not returned, and even if he still should, she thought, it would be too late to keep him awake any longer.

In the morning she went to a newsstand, but she could not find her story. And when she got to the city room she became busy at once, and did not have time to inquire. When she was sent out on her rounds to the State House and to Police Headquarters, however, it occurred to her that Mr. Garvey would know.

She went to the little room in Police Headquarters where the police reporters sat with their telephones, and opened the door. Heustis Garvey was there, and also young Herlihy, a dark-haired man with a pointed face who worked for one of the other papers. Garvey rose behind his desk, grinning widely but strangely, and she thought for a moment it was some kind of cordiality she should return. She hadn't seen him stand before and had not realized he was so big. Under the white hair his forehead was red.

"There she is now!" he said hoarsely, and shouted a cluster of execrations stunning in their filth. His words seared through her. He raised a brown bottle overhead by its neck and flung it.

"Hey!" said Herlihy, starting up, and in the same instant she felt the bottle's wind as she dodged.

It smashed on the doorjamb like a bomb. She bumped her face on the door, scrambling to get out, and then stumbled almost to the floor in the hallway.

"Run, Scoop!" Garvey shouted, his voice gravelly as though his vocal cords had torn loose.

She ran through the zigzag corridor terrified, putting out a hand to the wall again and again so as not to spill in the curves. She dashed diagonally across the lobby and burst into the street, already weeping, and ran up the sidewalk. It occurred to her that she ought to have called out to the old policeman in the lobby alcove to protect her. She dashed across a street, only half pausing to look for traffic. She heard metal plates on someone's heels and Herlihy put a hand on her gently.

"Take it easy," he said.

She looked back. Garvey was nowhere in sight. She sobbed, her body full of stitches, and allowed Herlihy to lead her back to the sidewalk. He patted her on the back.

"Come on. Sit down and relax," Herlihy said, and led her up an alley toward a lunchroom.

She was too short of breath to speak, and could not stop the shivers and sobs. She felt like saying that that bottle might have killed her. But the words that Garvey had used, and in Herlihy's hearing, seemed an embarrassment that would never wash away. He had called her by an anatomical epithet that was the most atrocious expression in existence.

"Want some coffee?" Herlihy asked her.

"No."

"Give her tea," he told the hard angular woman beyond the counter. "How about an English muffin?" he asked Millicent.

"Okay." She sniffled.

"Make it two," he told the woman.

Millicent turned and looked at Herlihy's face. His eyelashes were like lines of heavy black. His cheeks and neck had not an ounce of fat, as though he were scarcely into his twenties.

"Don't be afraid of Heustis," he said.

"What's the matter with him?"

"Well, that was kind of a stupid trick you pulled on him last night."

"Why?"

"Well, we knew about that accident. It wasn't any good. And I guess he didn't appreciate you calling your desk with a hot tip there."

She sobbed anew. She said she was supposed to pick up the police promotion list from Mr. Garvey and now she couldn't get it.

"No, no," Herlihy said. "Don't worry. I'll get it."

But she didn't see how she could ever come face to face with Mr. Garvey any more. She told Herlihy of the many errands to Mr. Garvey that her job entailed—picking up news releases and various lists and compilations, and every two weeks bringing him his pay check. And now there was nothing for her but to resign. She tried not to blubber.

"Naw, naw, you don't have to resign," he told her.

"But I've never been talked to like that in my life. Nobody ever spoke to me like that."

"He'll let you alone. I'll talk to him."

"You tell him that I've decided to forgive him if he'll never forget himself again. Because he wasn't himself and I realize he was under the influence. And I don't want to report him to Mr. Killian, because I know Mr. Killian has a lot of confidence in him."

Herlihy had begun shaking his head, with a wry face, even while she spoke. "That's just the wrong approach," he said. "You leave it to me."

He patted her hand. Two cups of tea were pushed before them, and a plate of sliced muffins, melted butter soaked in the tiny holes.

"Have something hot," he said.

She lifted the cup, and its warmth was soothing in her hands. She felt a gush of appreciation for Herlihy's kindness. She turned and looked up at him.

"I don't know why you're so good to me, Mr. Herlihy," she said. Her voice was still tearful. "Especially when we work for rival papers."

He looked at her, and then he laughed a little. His whole face showed amusement. She did not know what she had said that deserved to be laughed at.

"You're the second man who's laughed at me in two days," she said.

"I'm sorry. I didn't mean anything." But the laughter was not altogether gone from his face.

She turned from him, and found more tissues in her shoulder-strap bag. She blew her nose.

19

A son of a family who belonged to Ed's congregation became engaged to a girl whose family belonged to St. Timothy's Episcopal, and the girl agreed to take instruction from Ed and be married in Temple Beth El. The boy's parents told Ed about it, and he telephoned the girl's parents. "Well, it's Betsy's decision," her father told him, "and I'm afraid Betsy's the one that's going to have to live with it."

Ed felt the girl should consult first with her family's minister, the young Ralph Briggs. He spoke with Briggs himself. Ed also felt Betsy should take time to reconsider, or in any case delay the wedding until after several months of instruction. But her fiancé, Rodney Weiler, called him up and made threats. "Betsy's bent over backwards," the boy told him. "She's willing to take instruction and everything else. And if you're gonna make difficulties, we've had it. We'll just go to a justice of the peace and the hell with it." While the boy spoke Ed could hear the girl carrying on in the background, asking why they wouldn't let us alone.

So Ed began instructing Betsy Stokes that evening. He had been hoping to instruct Rodney along with her, but Rodney only let her off on the dirt road and sped away. Betsy mounted the porch and appeared at the screen door alone. It was past dark.

Ed ushered her into the room opposite the living room that he used as a study. He wore no jacket or tie and his collar was open. They remarked on the weather. She glanced at the shelves of books and sat in the Morris chair. She seemed to Ed a little blowzy, not at all as he had expected. Her hair was wound about her head in braids. She's the kind who goes in for square-dancing, he thought.

He opened a drawer and offered her a cigarette, but she refused. He sat and looked across the desk at her. She slumped, with her hands on the flat arms of the chair. She wore a wide longish skirt of a drab summery material, with many folds and a tiny pattern.

"Well, I want to make this tradition as attractive to you as I can, Betsy," Ed said finally. "And show you what it can do in a marriage. It can give you all kinds of togetherness, and I don't mean just sitting in a pew together. There's things for the father to do, and the mother to do, and the children to do. Like the children help you collect all the dirt and crumbs before Passover and burn it. And you can send a child out to look for the first stars, so you'll know when the Sabbath's over. Every festival's different. You can hang up grain and the vegetables and sleep in the open, like they used to do when they were gathering the harvest."

"Sounds like fun," said Betsy.

Ed looked at her expression, but it told him nothing.

"It is fun," he said. "To me it's half the fun of being human. If it weren't good it wouldn't have lasted so long, Betsy. Do you realize that of all human institutions—governments, orders, sects, clubs, tribes, anything in the world—this is the oldest thing in existence? Take anything. The nobility of Venice, of Japan. The Dalai Lama. The Salvation Army. The ladies' garden club. Think of all the hundreds of thousands of organizations and associations that exist among people. And this is absolutely the number-one oldest. There's nothing alive and functioning that's older. Not a culture, not even a town. Anywhere on earth. There were plenty of things that were older, but they're all out of business long ago already, defunct. It's the oldest thing going, because whatever started earlier isn't going. Even things that began within a thousand years of it. It's outlived them all. Think about that, Betsy. Nothing lasts that long just out of stubbornness. My kids always knew when there was a new moon, and they knew the time of the early harvest and the late harvest, and the fruit harvest. Even in the city. This is a religion that keeps the country man in touch with history and the city man in touch with agriculture, because it's rooted in the human experience—it's not an unworldly thing grafted on. There's not a human being on earth whose ancestors weren't farmers, Betsy. That's why Congress keeps passing the price-support program, because everybody's got a nostalgia for the farm."

He opened the drawer again, knocked out a cigarette on his wrist, and rummaged for matches.

"Oh, there's no question that a myth can be beautiful," Betsy said.

Ed held the cigarette without lighting it. "Well, our myths are myths to live by," he said. "They're not just decorative. Sure, religion puts beauty into life. But what I ask of a myth is truth. Usable truth, and liveable truth. If the myth is right the meanings should get deeper in every age." He kept staring at her. She parted her lips uncertainly.

"You mean 'beauty is truth, truth beauty'?"

"Well, not exactly," he told her. "I don't think you can seek beauty directly. Just like you can't seek happiness directly. What you have to concentrate on looking for is truth, and if truth is what you want, and if you're lucky, maybe the other things will take care of themselves. You'll know beauty when you see it. But if you seek beauty directly all you get is a nice twenty-dollar corset, you know what I mean?"

The girl's chest heaved and she sighed through her nose. "Speaking of truth," she said, "Rod said soft-soap you and all that, but the fact is I'm an atheist. Rod is too, for that matter. Religion is all right as myth, or decorative as you say, but don't expect me to—I'm not going to pretend to you. It wouldn't be fair to myself for one thing."

"Atheist, or agnostic?" he asked.

"Whichever you prefer—I wouldn't care to argue that point. Just say I'm a nonbeliever."

"Well, you're not required to believe." He had put down the cigarette.

"I'm not?"

"It says you should love God, and serve Him with your heart. That's not just the same thing as telling you to believe."

Her round face was skeptical. "I'm not sure of the difference."

"We don't have any prayer that says 'I believe.' And we don't ask for faith. We ask for peace."

"Isn't there something like 'believe on Me and thou shalt be saved'?"

"No no. Nothing like that. A man believes what he believes—you don't tell a man to believe. Religion is supposed to make life more meaningful, and you don't make things meaningful by insisting on the incredible. What it says is that if we live by the law, the country will prosper."

"What about 'I am the Lord thy God'?"

"All right, 'I am the Lord thy God, who brought you out of Egypt'—it's a statement, no? The beginning of the Ten Commandments. It still doesn't say, 'I command you to believe it.' And why does it mention Egypt? Because it means that the impulse to law comes from the same source as the impulse to freedom. That's how the law is introduced. Law and freedom are connected. A tyranny's a lawless society, a place where the courts don't protect you. And what did the Children of Israel answer there in the desert? They didn't say 'we believe.' They said 'We will do and we will hear.' That's what they said. We will commit ourselves, and the interpretations will grow clearer—we will live thus, and our insights will deepen. If they said 'we believe,' they'd still be sitting on their butts at Sinai arguing about first causes. Betsy, it was sophisticated men that wrote that down—if you go into it you'll find it out. They wrote figuratively, in the language of men and in the language of the time, but every word spoke a volume. They weren't men who thought God was an old man with angels flitting around His head. Why do you suppose they insisted on no images? So that even to a little kid, you don't describe God as an old man with whiskers, or as anything else. That was why. One of my boys, when he was a little kid, he said to me, 'God is nothing.' And I tried to explain, that we can't see, and we're not given to know and so on, whatever you can say to a little kid. But I never told him an old man on a throne. And as they grew older I told them what you'd tell them, that when you probe into ultimates you get to where you can't comprehend. Where you can't even conceive. And what does it mean to ask if you believe in something you can't even conceive? It's meaningless. Isn't it? To talk about something, and ask if you believe in something, you first have to have some conception of it. And idolaters and atheists are alike in one thing, that they both presume that the concept of God can be comprehended."

He pushed back his chair noisily on the hard floor and walked around to the front of the desk. He leaned on it, still looking at Betsy, his hands on its edge behind him.

"The Bible says," he continued, "that Moses asked God 'what are You?', and God answered, 'I am that I am.' That's all we're told. Nothing. Moses asked, please, could he just see God for an instant, just so he could have some kind of concept? And what did God do, according to the Bible? He showed Moses His rear end. You get the point? It's figurative, but there's many meanings there. You try to be a theologian and God says—well, I don't want to use a vulgar expression. Human beings weren't made to be theologians—it's a waste of time. We haven't the capacity." He gestured with one hand. "Our minds don't have the capacity to latch onto anything we can talk about believing. The question is how to live. If the believer and the nonbeliever both act the same, then it's a hair-splitting anyway. All we have is a working hypothesis—to live as if there were a moral law, as if the world were made by God. That's why it says 'love God,' instead of 'believe in God.' Just as light waves are a working hypothesis."

"But if you love God," she asked, "and you do an action because you love God, doesn't that mean you believe in God?"

"Sure. And it's the only kind of belief that means anything. But 'love' instead of 'belief' keeps your eye on what you can understand. Who cares how you interpret your beliefs, as long as you come up with the right action? And you look close, at people that call themselves atheists, and you find them begging the same questions as everyone else, and taking just as much on faith. Anybody that believes the golden rule is binding on him has already accepted a lot on faith—as much as anybody that calls himself religious. And from what I see around me, people that call themselves atheists can still believe in more stuff that doesn't exist than I ever thought of. They believe in neighborhoods, and prestige, and all kinds of things. I don't think people know what they believe. And to ask people to say 'I believe'—it would just make for a kind of intellectual conformity that isn't possible. Every man's a sect, I think. Faces are different, and minds are different. In the whole world no two girls even have the same shape of bosom, did you ever think of that? When I was seventeen already I realized that idea. So why should minds be the same? If people were the same, evolution wouldn't work. Every creature, every individual is different, that's the whole mechanism that makes evolution. Only in order to make a community, then the individuals have to consent to a common practice. But a common practice can still bridge a lot of different theories. And no one who accepts a transcendental moral law is an atheist. Even if he thinks he is. He's accepted in his heart the hypothesis that moral law is real, it's binding. That's all I ask. Whether he says 'God' or whether he has another terminology, that's a matter of what words he's comfortable with. But if he admits that out of that unknown a real law—"

"Law can be a social contract," she interrupted. "Based on practicality, or necessity."

"Well, suppose a man knows he can really get away with something—let's assume it's clear and obvious that he can't possibly be caught, and the crime is to his advantage. But he doesn't do it."

"Empathy for others, perhaps," Betsy said. "An unwillingness to hurt others."

"Why? Who says it's wrong to hurt others? If it's clearly in his advantage? There are people who say it isn't wrong. Criminals, people that aren't bound by anything. Tyrants and criminals who think there's no law above them. And if you say social pressure, how do you account for the man who won't do wrong even when there's no social pressure?"

"His superego stops him then," said Betsy.

"But suppose he's been psychoanalyzed and he knows all about superegos and he still believes some things are wrong. Betsy, you believe some things are just plain wrong, absolutely, not relatively. You believe it's wrong to starve a child to death, don't you? You believe it's wrong in itself, practicality or no practicality. And regardless of what anybody else thinks. And why? Because you're a believer. As soon as you believe there's such a thing as right and wrong, already you've made the same irrational jump that I have. You believe something irrational. You can't prove it—you just know it. If a man accepts no hard core of morality as binding on him, then I'll admit he believes in nothing. And if he thinks that he's God himself, I'll call him an atheist. Two people that I'll call true atheists are the man that thinks he's God himself and the man who commits suicide. But as for the ordinary so-called atheist who's a moral man, as soon as he says, yes, there really is such a thing as right and wrong, then it's as if he said God made the world. It's the same kind of irrational jump of belief, no matter what words are used. Because if God is incomprehensible, if we can't even comprehend what it is we're talking about, what do we mean when we say we believe in it or we don't believe in it? The question is, will you be bound by this law. That's the question. Not what do you think about what your mind can't grasp—that's your own private wordplay. Whether you think it's inspired by God, or the words of men, it adds up to the same thing—provided your thoughts lead to the same actions. No matter how you feel most comfortable wording it. If your behavior's right, you're the same as a believer. I've even known people who come and participate in services and say they don't believe. Purely a cultural thing, that's what they call it. But do you think they don't believe? Of course they believe. Belief isn't what you imagine that you think—it's what you do. And if a man doesn't believe that he himself is God, and if he still thinks life is worth living, then he trusts in something beyond. He's hung his life on that hypothesis. And if he doesn't shoot himself, his heart believes it was good that the world was created. He doesn't know from what it was created—whether he prays or whether he calls himself an atheist, he still doesn't know. Look, not even a physicist can comprehend time, space. We're confronted every day with staggering mystery. And we admit it, all of us, the atheist and the man who prays, except the atheist then proceeds to forget it, that's all." He made a gesture with both hands. "I don't offer you certainty. I offer you doubt, because every intelligent person is faced with doubt. I only hope that with all the doubts, you'll doubt the purely irreligious view as well, that's all I ask. Because if all the universe is just a cosmic madhouse—to believe that all this has no purpose demands an even more fantastic act of belief. Just allow your brain to accept all the ramifications of it and ask if that's any easier to believe—see if you don't have doubts about that also. A God-created universe and a godless one are both beyond grasp. And in the middle of all the doubts, maybe the sum total of all your many doubts will impel you to a desire to create holiness in the world. It was in doubt, and out of my doubts, that I was driven to study. And in an uncertain universe I find that what I need, and what I want, it isn't certainty. What I need and want is the law. The feeling that the world makes sense, because I'm a part of it, and the way I act makes sense. And that's why this religion never even called itself a faith. Because it's not preoccupied with believing. It's called a law, because it's preoccupied with doing."

"Why does it have to have so many laws?" Betsy said. "I mean regulations and everything. I'd agree there's a moral law if you'd limit it to the golden rule or the ten commandments or something, but not a million other little things."

He was resting his weight on the desk. "Well, why can't the Commonwealth of Massachusetts get along on just the ten commandments?" he asked her. "Why does the Commonwealth need volumes and volumes of statute law? I'll tell you why. The same reason. Because it's meant to be lived, practically, not just rhetoric. In all the mixed-up everyday cases, if you take it seriously."

He watched her. She was frowning, her mouth down to one side.

"My grandfather took it seriously," he told her, "and he was a saint. Everyone loved him. Even the people that did business with him. I've seen it with my two eyes."

"Would he have burned witches at Salem?" Betsy asked.

Ed shook his head, with a smile. "No."

"Well, religious people have done some pretty awful things, though," she said. "Look at history and you'll see what they've done. They've murdered and they've slaughtered and they've shackled minds."

"So have atheists," said Ed. "Look at Russia. So what do you prove? Torquemada was a believer, and Hitler was an atheist. It goes back to what I said before—what a man believes might be deep in his subconscious, so you don't ask him to state his beliefs. You see what he does. You look at some of these guys, and you wonder. And you look at Hitler, and by any definition there was a man who thought there was nothing higher than his own will. And in his heart of hearts he truly believed that life isn't worth living. He tried to destroy the world and he blew his brains out."

There was a movement of light beyond the curtains and Ed looked about. A pair of headlights stopped before the house.

"That's probably Rod," Betsy said.

She followed Ed to the hall and he opened the double door. By the porch light he could make out the boy waiting at the wheel.

"Come on in. Join us," said Ed.

The boy came up the steps. He was big and dark, with a certain homeliness, and eyebrows joined—the kind of face that would always look rough no matter how groomed.

"You weren't gone long," said Ed.

"I didn't go far."

"Go in the study," Ed told him. "I'll bring another chair."

"No, we can't stay," the boy said. His voice was deep.

He looked firm.

"Well, all right," said Ed. "Come and have a beer anyway."

He saw them exchange glances, and they went with him past the staircase and down the hall to the kitchen. He bent at the refrigerator and found an unopened quart bottle. He poured three glasses, slantwise. No one said anything. They sat drinking, Rod and Betsy on chairs and Ed on a corner of the heavy unpainted table.

"We're getting along very well," Betsy said to Rod finally. "Mr. Gordon doesn't even care if I believe in God or not."

"Well, I didn't say that," Ed protested. "I said that what people believe and what they think they believe are two different things. And if your behavior's okay, then I have to assume your beliefs are satisfactory."

He took a swallow of beer, watching them, the boy dark and sinewy and the girl light and soft. The glass was cold in his hand, and his feet dangled.

"If there's no God," he asked, "so what is there—a dynamo? Why is there a universe? Why should there be a universe, and all kinds of forces and particles? Who needed it? The void was bothering somebody? It was in the way? A nothingness is unstable? Did there have to be bang and motion, and electrons and forces and particles? You tell me a plain void, a nothingness, wouldn't have been simpler? And did the electrons and the particles have to arrange themselves as a child who smiles?"

20

With a scowling toss of his head Mr. Killian summoned Millicent to his desk. "What's this about you feuding with Heustis Garvey?" he asked her.

It took her by surprise, and she answered only that she was not feuding with Mr. Garvey. But Mr. Killian did not seem quite to take her at her word. He lectured her sourly, telling her not to sneer at Heustis. He said Heustis was a top-notch reporter, the dean of the New England press corps, and had seen reporters come and go.

It left her rather shaken.

Meanwhile Natalie's mother came on a visit from Chicopee and sat in the worn stuffed chair almost the entire weekend, never going out. Her name was Mrs. Frost, and she was elderly and white-haired. It made Millicent aware of how young her own parents were. Mrs. Frost talked dully of inspirational books, and said she had been leaning toward Christian Science. While Millicent did calisthenics Mrs. Frost watched from the stuffed chair and remarked on the benefits of exercise.

Ella Jane watched also. "If I had a shape like that I'd put it to use," she said, almost as though Mrs. Frost were not there, and Millicent colored.

On Sunday Millicent was supposed to go walking with Leslie before work, but he phoned and canceled it. The hospital was short of staff and they had had to take his Sunday from him.

Mrs. Frost slept in Natalie's bed. Natalie slept in the living room, using the long cushion of Millicent's studio couch as a pallet on the floor, as Charles had done, and she seemed glad when her mother finally left, as though a great strain had been removed. She scratched her ribs, sitting on the studio couch in brief crimson shorts, with her knees apart and her feet drawn up, and blew smoke through her nostrils.

"I'm in the mood," she said.

"Well, let's not throw another party," said Ella Jane.

Natalie blew more smoke. Her eyes drifted to Millicent, who sat on a big arm of the empty stuffed chair.

"Where did your cousin Steve get those Tarzan muscles?" Natalie asked.

"Weights," said Millicent.

Natalie's hand hung from a knee, cigarette and all. "Is he Jewish?" she asked.

"Of course."

"Does he go out with Christians?"

"I'm sure I don't know. I suppose so."

"Well," said Natalie, "if you happen to see him, you could tell him if he's not prejudiced I'm not either."

"I'm not likely to see him."

"Well, in case you do. I sort of thought I would have heard from him by now."

"I'm not sure if I'm on speaking terms with Steve," said Millicent. "He happens to be a terrible person."

"Why? What did he do?"

"I don't care to speak of it," said Millicent.

"Gee, it must have been something pretty awful."

Millicent thought of confiding to Natalie and Ella Jane that Steve had inquired whether Natalie put out. But she didn't want to. "What do you see in him?" she asked.

"Oh, I don't know. It's just that I kind of thought he was gonna call, that's all. Maybe I sort of have a weakness for muscle men."

"He's despicable."

"Oh, he's not. Everybody's ashamed of their relatives."

Millicent went home for her days off, since Leslie expected to be on call Wednesday night that week. She helped her mother dig some bulbs. Her mother said she was just as glad the North Koreans were winning, because it meant the war would be over soon.

Her mother spaded in a new place, where she meant to put transplants. Millicent brought the wheelbarrow, which had a bag of prepared manure in it.

"You didn't tell me you invited Steve to your party—I think that was very nice," her mother said. "Aunt Tessie said it was very sweet of you. 'Millicent's so sweet—it's just like her'—that's what she said."

Then her mother asked if she had met anyone interesting at the party.

"I'll let you know when there's anything to report," Millicent said.

"It's too bad that Winkler boy never called," said her mother. Her mother also said Dr. Yarrish's son was a nice boy and was going to teach Sunday school. He was away on vacation, but she was going to inquire if he had a girl friend.

"Mother," said Millicent, "you don't seem to understand. I'm not desperate." They worked side by side in the black soft earth without smiling or looking at each other. "I hope you're not discouraging everybody," her mother said. "And I hope Steve has the decency to reciprocate at least, by fixing you up with some of his friends."

Millicent returned to Boston Thursday afternoon with a meat loaf her mother had given her. Leslie had supper with her and her roommates and ate most of it. Afterward she went out with him to a lecture on migratory birds and bird-banding. He had spoken of a big musical film but she preferred to steer him to events that didn't cost anything. When the lecture was over they sat together on a bench on the edge of the Common, talking. They spoke of perhaps visiting Ruthie Meyers sometime, and seeing her slides of Europe. They agreed that Ruthie was brighter than her husband. They walked around the pool of the Public Garden, looking at the round lights of the footbridge reflecting deep in the stillness. She had never been here at night before. They talked about whether any landscape would not be made more beautiful by the presence in it of reflecting water, and agreed that even a junk yard would look better if doubled in a reflecting puddle.

It was remarkable how they always had something to talk about, she thought.

At last he saw her to the entrance of her building, flicked his finger playfully against the tip of her nose as though knocking an imaginary insect away, and left without entering the lobby.

She thought of bringing him sometime to visit her Aunt Rosalind's apartment near the park and stream called the Fens. They had actually been quite near it the day they had gone to the museum. He would see Aunt Rosalind's watercolors, and Aunt Rosalind knew music, and all the museums backwards and forward, and they would have much in common.

But she knew Aunt Rosalind would make a big thing of her having a boy friend. And if she asked Aunt Rosalind to say nothing to her parents it would become a huge secret. Aunt Gwendolyn was not as bright as Aunt Rosalind, but she could be trusted to take things in stride.

Natalie went off to a resort for the Labor Day weekend, along with the girl she taught with, and Ella Jane was invited away again by office friends. Millicent asked Leslie to a Sunday dinner of chicken with mushroom sauce. She invited him for eleven o'clock, so they could have a few hours of afternoon before she was due at the city room. But there was a pouring rain, apparently the edge of a hurricane, and after dinner they sat on the old oriental rug that had been her parents' and listened to Natalie's portable record player. The classical records were not numerous and belonged mostly to Ella Jane.

"I ought to buy some," Millicent said.

Leslie picked out a symphony by Milhaud, a name she didn't know. It turned upon the machine, the music sounding strange and modern. The black kitten climbed to her shoulder and she stroked it. With her other hand she followed one of the tiny patterns in the rug. The back of the fat chair curved over her, and she could smell the rain in the trench coat that Leslie had slung over it.

She sneezed and the cat jumped from her shoulder. Leslie asked if she were chilly. They could hear the rain on the windows. He asked if the fireplace worked and if she knew of any place to get wood. She said she didn't know of any. She looked at the fireplace. Its glaze of deep green tile looked clean and useless.

Leslie mentioned a phrase in the music and told her to listen for the bassoons. She turned her attention to it.

But in a moment he kissed her on the lips, passing an arm about her.

"You'll catch my cold," she said.

The kiss continued and she allowed him to push her gently down until she lay on the rug, still kissing, one of her arms stretched out, and still hearing the restless music. His eyes were strange without eyeglasses. She closed hers.

She was wearing Ella Jane's gray and white belted dress. His hand found one of her breasts and rested upon it, moving in the slightest massage upon the cloth. His thumb slipped between the buttons.

She removed his hand.

"Isn't that allowed?" he murmured.

"I don't want to be picayune," she said, "but we mustn't be carried away."

The kiss resumed. They lay heavily on the carpet. For a time his hand remained on her arm, but then it sought her breast again. She thought she perhaps should ignore it. But then she thought she had better not.

She sat up. "Les," she began, "if we're going to be seeing each other we have to have an agreement that love play has to be kept within bounds. I've been meaning to say that. I'm not a prude, and I realize we can't avoid a certain amount of necking forever. And I'm not blaming you. It's just as much my fault. But we've got to be civilized."

"I'd say we're being more abrupt than civilized."

"Les, you saw what was happening. When kissing starts to go beyond kissing it means the kissing's gone far enough."

"I didn't think of it as beyond kissing. I caressed you during a kiss, that's all. It's perfectly natural."

"It's still better to nip it before it goes further. Kissing isn't a pastime for rainy days."

"I didn't think of it as a pastime."

"So much the worse then. I hope it wasn't an uncontrollable passion. You know where it would lead."

"Where would it lead? Can't you trust yourself to govern your emotions?"

She looked at him.

"Why should it lead any place you don't want it to lead?" he continued. "What do you think, you have to end up in bed with a guy just because he lays a hand on you?"

She tightened her lips, still looking at him.

"You're not the type to lose your head because somebody touches you," he said.

"Well, since we're being so indelicate and frank about it, suppose I just say I don't like being pawed."

"Millicent my friend, you're a victim of semantics. These aren't paws—they're human hands. My hand touched you. I touched your breast. So what? Why is it any different than if I touched your hand?"

"It is different."

"Why is it different?"

"Because it's sexually arousing."

"Well, just hands touching each other can be sexually arousing. So can just looking. Touching isn't anything, in itself. It's no worse than when lips touch. Why do people kiss?"

"I wish they didn't, actually."

"You mean you haven't enjoyed it when we've kissed?"

She was looking at the turning record, but she knew he was watching her face. Her face felt warm but her back felt cold. The music annoyed her.

"I didn't say that," she said.

"That's what it sounds like."

She leaped up and went to the window. Rain was running down the glass. Leslie remained on the rug behind the fat chair. She could scarcely see down to the street in the grayness. She took a breath. The peeling iron strips of the fire escape all had rounded films of water, disturbed by splashing, and from some points the drip was almost a pouring.

"Les," she said. "I would like to think, at least, that I have too much honesty to have kissed you if I didn't want to."

"Well, that's what I thought."

"What we've done, we've done together. I'm not the type to submit to things."

The music was playing. He didn't answer.

"My lips were freely given, like yours," she said, still staring at the rain. "And so was my friendship."

"You're shivering," he said.

She hadn't thought it was visible. She put a hand to the white paint of the long radiator under the windows. It was cold.

"Why do you wish people didn't kiss?" he asked.

She bent and opened the valve, but heard only the steamless turning of metal.

"Just because," she said finally.

"You're even more of a prude than you admit."

"Why?" She looked around toward him. "Because I believe that friendship doesn't have to be on a sexual basis? I think I do have a healthy attitude toward—physical stuff." Her voice was quavering. "We're not in love, after all."

"I thought you didn't believe in love."

"You certainly misunderstood everything I ever said, if you think that." She sat on the radiator. It wasn't comfortable.

"Have you ever necked before in your life? I mean, have you ever had a real boy friend?"

"I think you're being very inquisitive," she said, with some sharpness despite the quavering.

"I'm sorry."

She didn't acknowledge the apology.

"Am I forgiven?" he said. "Come and listen to the music."

"I'd think good taste at least would dictate some reserve," she reprimanded him, returning not to the rug but to one of the big upholstered arms of the chair.

"Well, I'm sorry. I didn't mean to be asking if you're a virgin or not. It's perfectly obvious."

"Please, Les. I detest that word."

"What—'virgin'?" He had moved on the rug so as to see her.

"I think it's purely a male conceit that a woman's first sex is some kind of a grand initiation," she said, "or that it changes her status somehow. A woman isn't a forest primeval, or a snowfall, or a pie crust."

He was lying on the rug at her feet, looking toward the music rather than at her, but he shook his head. "I wish you weren't so touchy about these things."

She saw him prop himself on an elbow as though to inspect how far the phonograph needle had progressed. Then he lay back again.

"Milhaud—I don't know. I'd rather have started you on Stravinsky," he said.

"If you must know," she began quietly, "I was friendly with a young man in Chicago, and I suppose there was a certain amount of what you could call necking on occasion. But it was never a primary thing in our relationship. We didn't have time for it, for one thing."

"What does this guy do?"

"He's a lawyer. He was going into politics."

"Are you in touch with him now?"

"No."

He was lying with his hands tucked under his head, and he closed his eyes.

She moved down from the chair arm to the rug and sat nearby, as though listening to the music also. She arranged her skirt about her. She felt an anxiety to correct the opinion he held of her.

"What I mean is," she began again, "it seems to me prudery is a mental attitude. What I mean is, I'm not somebody that despises the human body. But sex has to be in its proper setting, like anything beautiful, don't you agree? And a prude is somebody that despises it."

She waited for his reaction, but he just lay with eyes shut.

"And part of the setting is respect," she said. "You weren't respectful that time you took your clothes off at my aunt's."

"I'm sorry about that," he said, without opening his eyes.

"I was very angry. I wasn't sure for a while if I ought to see you again."

"Well, I thought it was high time you saw a man in the nude, if only for the sake of scientific curiosity."

"Please, Les, don't be insincere."

"I'm not."

"I think you know perfectly well that I'm intellectually honest about these things. More so than most people I know."

"Well, you say it's a mental attitude. Suppose you were in a swimming party, say. A mixed swimming party, and everybody took their clothes off. What would you do?" He opened his eyes. "I mean, there you have it. Is the body shameful, or not? Or would you take a walk to the shower with your clothes off? If it were convenient?"

"No."

"Why?"

"Because. And that doesn't mean I'm ashamed of my body."

"Why? Is it wrong?"

"In theory, no."

"And in practice?"

"In practice I wouldn't, because people wouldn't just look at it naturally. They'd take it lasciviously."

"Okay, and what's lascivious? What you mean is, you have nothing against sex except that it's sexy."

She shifted her legs beneath her. "On the contrary. I have nothing against sex except that it interferes with friendship."

"It blends beautifully with friendship. Like bacon and eggs."

"No, Les. Because if we ever let it begin, you'd want to go further." Her voice was low. "And further, and then still further. And maybe I'd want to too—precisely because I'm not a prude. And the trouble with the physical stuff is that once it starts, if it doesn't lead to love and marriage or something it gets to a point where the friendship has to be ended, and I want the friendship. I'm not a hypocrite, Les. And when I told you I want your friendship, I meant exactly that. I wasn't using it as a euphemism for something else."

"Well, it seems to me it's only natural for a girl to want a little necking. And who with, if not with your friends, people you're fond of. Let your kisses be an expression of good health."

"But to keep on kissing a person isn't a static thing. It moves in one direction or the other. That's common knowledge."

"Well, it seems to me that people should just come together. I think you said it yourself once, a friendship should be casual, or something like that. No formal dating or courtship. And I agree. Maybe they kiss, and maybe they go on to marriage, or maybe they try again with somebody else. They find out in good time what course the relationship is meant to take. But when you want to kiss you don't worry about the end of the friendship. You enjoy it. You don't have maps and blueprints."

Millicent arose and wandered nervously to the mantelpiece. "It seems to me that you're the one that has a blueprint," she said. "You have it all figured out." She fingered a pussy willow.

"No I don't. A desire just wells up naturally, that's all."

"Can't you ignore it?"

"I can't exactly leave it at home."

In the mirror she saw him looking at her from the floor. "You can't leave your appendix at home either," she said, "but when it's irrelevant you ignore it. You don't let yourself be a slave to every passing bubble in your juices, or whatever it is."

She walked slowly along the side of the room. He sat forward, picked up the record, turned it over, and started the player again. He sat looking at it, his arms on his knees. Then he found his eyeglasses nearby and put them on.

"You of all people should know that we're not just two bundles of maleness and femaleness," she said. "There are more cells in one brain than stars in the Galaxy."

"Okay," he said without looking around. "We'll ignore sex. And maybe it'll go away."

"I'm afraid you're not being very understanding."

"I'm being understanding. But at the end of a hard week I want to rest in somebody's arms. And so do you, if you're like other people. But that's all right—have it your way. You really can make it go away, you know. I had a spinster aunt who ignored sex for thirty-five years, and then finally it went away."

His phrase about resting in someone's arms struck her with a sudden truth, as though she had not seen it before in quite that light. And whose arms did you rest in, if not your friend's?

But she felt there were other aspects to it. She sighed. She had come to the window, and she put her hands on the wood between the sashes, and rested her forehead on the cold glass. The water was running down.

"One rainy day destroys us," she said.

She looked around. He hadn't moved.

"Les," she said uncertainly.

He didn't answer.

"There's so much for us to talk about," she said, "—so much for friends to learn, and share, in the precious few hours they have together. And there's so little time when we can manage to see each other. When you get a Sunday off I have to be at work at three, and if I'm off Wednesday and Thursday nights you're on call at least one of those nights. And that's all we have. And there's all of art to be talked about, and the whole life of history, even the threat of the bomb. And here we are talking about sex. I hoped this wouldn't be necessary with you. What's all our education been for, if we end up in this same stupid argument? You can have this argument with any moron."

She came and sat in the chair, limply. He looked up at her with round innocent eyes.

"I feel so rotten," she said. There was a break in her voice. "And cheated. If a man is nice he wants to get sexy, or else it's some nincompoop that seems like he's looking for a bride. Why can't a man ever want to just talk to me?"

"Why don't you avoid men if that's how you feel? Stick to women and talk all you want."

"I don't want to be limited to women," she said. "I want men friends in order to transcend sexuality. Not to plunge into it."

"Don't you think all this transcending is gonna leave you kind of frustrated?"

"Yes. I have to be frustrated. And I accept it, as a fact of nature."

"You have to be?"

"I'm not going to get married too soon, or to the wrong man, and I'm not going to let myself in for a lot of automatic love play, and I'm not going to be a tease. So I don't see that I have any choice but to adjust to a certain amount of frustration."

"You do have a choice," he said. "You say you don't want to talk about it. So be casual, and take your necking casually, like a person, and there'll be nothing to talk about or make an issue of. You're the one that started talking. Just relax and let me take care of it. You've practically said you want to, and the only reason you don't begin is fear that you won't stop. And that's the fear that's frustrating you."

"It's a fear that happens to be reasonable."

"Don't you think you're strong enough to stop when you want to? What are you, like an alcoholic that can't take one drink?"

Millicent reddened. They kept looking at each other. He was on the floor at her feet.

"Do you really think you're so oversexed?" he said. "Or that a woman with your character has so little control?"

She parted her lips and closed them once before deciding what to say. "Why invite temptation?" she said finally.

"If it's tempting you must mean you want it."

His hand moved behind her slanting calf and stroked it. She twitched her leg a little and began to remove his hand, but then left it in place and his light stroking continued.

"Suppose we agree to draw a line, and not go beyond it," he said.

"It would be very important that we stick to such an agreement."

"Well, I think we're both people of resolution."

"I guess we are."

"If a girl can't neck and draw a line," he said, still stroking her calf, "she'll never get through these years."

"I suppose that's true."

"Come on down and lean on me," he said. "It's nice to lean on people."

He moved to rest against the front of the chair and she slid down beside him to the rug. His arm enclosed her and she turned her face into the kiss. She leaned her weight on him, but the posture felt neither modest nor sophisticated. She straightened, but moved a hand around his head and into his hair, pulling him nearer and trying to make a show of passion. The dress rubbed slowly upon her bra. Without extricating himself he removed his glasses and put them up on the chair cushion. His fingers returned, with a gentle strength. She lay down with him, stretched upon the rug, still kissing. She opened her eyes, but his were still closed, and she closed hers. He worked at the kiss.

"Don't put your tongue in my mouth, please," she said.

He complied and they kissed some more. He had opened her buttons, and his hand sought her back. She rolled slightly to let him undo a fastening.

"Are you shivering?" he said.

"No, I'm all right."

He kissed the tip of her nose, and then her throat, and she kissed foolishly into the air not knowing when he would return to her lips. Then he did.

Somehow they found a new closeness.

"See?" he said. "It isn't so awful."

"You do have a soothing touch," she said. "It might be good for nervous tension, actually."

"Are you happy?"

"I don't know."

He kissed her again. Despite the rug the floor felt hard beneath her.

"Maybe when the rain's over we'll see a rainbow," she said.

He kissed her again.

"You have a marvelous bosom," he said.

"Let's not discuss it."

He kissed her long and gently, seeming to drink at her lips. Her feet worked against the rug and against each other until she had removed her shoes. The arch of one foot itched a little and she scratched it with the toe of the other.

"No," she said suddenly, and lowered her hand to his. "If a line's going to be drawn, I think the waistband is as good as any. Don't you? It's a well-defined one and there's no question about it."

His hand relaxed.

"I've conceded the breast-fondling," she said, "and I think that really ought to be the limit between us."

"Okay."

"Thank you."

She managed to straighten her skirts under him. His face was against her cheek.

"I think it's a civilized place to stop," she explained, "since you don't want to stop at the collarbone. We do have to be on guard, Les. We live in an immoral age, and especially in times like these, when the world's becoming more and more immoral, I'd think you'd want to be extra careful to act responsibly."

"Okay, okay. Agreed, agreed," he said. He kissed her.

She had not been aware of the music for some time but she was aware now of its stoppage. She heard the record continue to turn idly. The kitten leaped on Leslie's shirt, high on his back, near a shoulder.

"No, Theodore!" she said.

The kitten leaped away.

"Theodore's jealous," she explained to Leslie.

His nose lay at her ear. Her skin seemed to rise to his fingers. It had a liveliness where he touched it that made her want to tickle him in return. But her arm was pinioned by her disarranged clothing.

"There's one other thing I'd like to agree on," she said. "Let's just do this once in a while. Not every time. Because a lot of necking is simply not a healthy thing."

"Let's not put ourselves on a ration. That's not healthy either."

"I didn't mean a ration."

"It can't be mechanical," he said. "Like every third Sunday."

"I know it."

"Anyway," he said, "the opportunities are gonna be so few I wouldn't worry about it. We don't even have a place where we can go. Ordinarily your roommates would be here."

"That's true."

"And what we're doing, it's so elementary, Millicent. People may be virgins and they may not, but this much everybody does. Even high-school kids. Your kid sister probably even does it."

"I wouldn't think so. It's not the way we were brought up."

"Nobody brings up their children to make love," he said. "They learn it for themselves."

She was looking at the ceiling, past his ear. She saw cracks in it.

"Les," she said, "I don't think you understood me before, about friends. What I meant was, a friend isn't something you tickle yourself with."

"You talk too much. Just shut off your brains for five minutes."

"No, it's just that I want you to understand. Can't you see why this isn't practical, really? It means I can't have more than one friend of the opposite sex."

"How many have you got?"

"That's not the point. I still can't do this with everybody."

"No one's asking you to. And it's no crime if you happen to kiss more than one guy, or neck with more than one guy."

"Well, then eventually marriage limits it. Either way the idea of sex limits friendships between men and women. Congenial minds should be able to meet without being hampered. It's just that minds and friendships ought to be free. I wouldn't have any grievance against sex if it weren't for that."

"Shut up and enjoy it," he told her gently. "Especially if we're not gonna do this often."

"Okay," she said.

She shifted her position a bit, and became settled again.

Her fingers rode on the back of his hand.

She heard Theodore sharpening his claws nearby on the fabric of the chair. She heard the rain, and the phonograph still turning without music.

She turned her head a little and looked toward the mantelpiece.

"Well," she said, gazing toward the small alarm clock, "I think it's time to demonstrate the truth of what we said, that we can stop when we want to."

21

For some nights in a row Mr. Hopkins gave Millicent a little story to write, during the slack hours toward the end of her work shift. He gave her an announcement about a children's party to be held at a settlement house, but there was hardly any way to make a news item of it except virtually to copy the announcement. Another evening he scrawled a phone number on a slip of paper and she obtained the details for an obituary by telephone. She saw him edit it, the green eyeshade hiding half his face. And when she took it upstairs to Mr. Valentino she saw that he had scratched away all but her first two paragraphs, but she was pleased that he had left the two paragraphs verbatim, without altering a word.

All the city-room people signed with typewritten initials when they wrote stories, though the initials did not actually appear in print, and Millicent wrote MAG at the bottom of hers. This caused Danny McBride to call her Maggie, and some of the others did also. She did not like it, but she preferred it to Sneezy. McBride particularly seemed to alternate between the two names.

Her stories were always written while Mr. Hopkins was in charge, long after Mr. Killian had gone home, but she knew that Mr. Killian must be aware of them because every day he checked over the preceding night's work, including the initials. She wished he would tell her what he thought of them. However he did not mention them. He rarely spoke to her about anything, and never smiled. But she knew that Zucchino and Dawn never wrote any. And she heard that Mr. Killian preferred to wait for her to chalk the bulletins onto the sidewalk blackboards, rather than have Zucchino do it earlier, because he liked her penmanship.

"What's this 'mister' all the time?" he said to her once, scowling, when she brought his sandwich and his change from the spa. She knew that everyone else called him Dexter, even the other copy boys. Still, she felt she could not possibly call a man that much older by his first name. It would feel disrespectful.

Finally he did beckon her to him and spoke disagreeably and curtly of one of her stories. The smeared carbon copy of it, with her initials at the bottom, was before him on the desk, in both his hands. He told her it was not possible for a burial to follow a funeral service, unless the cemetery and the chapel were both on wheels.

Another time she heard him tell one of the younger men never to refer to a bridegroom as a groom, because a groom meant somebody who took care of horses. She also heard him tell Louie Alpert there was no such thing as a lone bandit, because a bandit meant a member of a band. She looked this up afterward in the big dictionary and found it wasn't so. She wondered if Mr. Killian were somewhat pedantic. But she resolved to try for the kind of precision he seemed to want.

She no longer sent clippings to her parents, but in the apartment she still marked dates on them, and kept them in a brown envelope in one of the drawers that had been assigned to her in Natalie's bureau.

One morning Charles came. She was still on the studio couch half dozing, between the sheets in her pajamas, and the knock and Ella Jane's opening of the door confused her.

"Well! Here's baby brother!" Ella Jane sang out.

Millicent squinted. Beyond Ella Jane he looked tall in the gray uniform, pulling off his overseas cap. "Charles!" Millicent said, pushing herself up on an elbow. "What are you doing here?"

"I'm on a pass," he said, and in the same moment Ella Jane told him to come in. She shut the door.

Millicent sat up, rubbing her eyes and forehead and pushing back her hair and looking at him. She heard Ella Jane ask him if he'd like some breakfast. Ella Jane was dressed, as though ready to go off to work, and Millicent remembered having half awakened when Natalie had gone earlier. She saw Ella Jane sit down again to her coffee at the drop-leaf table, leaning the cane against the edge of it, and push the plate of toast toward Charles.

"You're looking good, Cockeyes," he said to Millicent, and sat down opposite Ella Jane.

Ella Jane asked if he weren't stationed somewhere in the South, and he said he had flown up with a pilot from his base who was coming this way. Millicent rose, thinking she ought to prepare more toast for Ella Jane, and cocoa for herself and Charles. The alarm clock above the fireplace said twenty after eight. In the bathroom she found her blue corduroy bathrobe under Ella Jane's purple flowered one. She thought she ought to be annoyed with her brother for coming unannounced and at such an hour, and for disturbing Ella Jane.

She heard them talking together while she prepared the cocoa and poured the juice.

"Charles, don't eat Ella Jane's toast," she said.

"That's all right," said Ella Jane.

She asked if they would have eggs. Charles seemed to delay answering, and when Ella Jane declined he did also.

Millicent at last brought cocoa and cream cheese and more bread for the toaster, and pulled up a third dining chair. "The chairs have gotten rickety again, Charles," she said.

"I'll look at them again," he said. She thought he was red-eyed, and that his uniform needed pressing.

He and Ella Jane reached for the coffeepot at once. They both stopped short, and asked each other to go ahead, but he allowed her to take it. He drank cocoa, blowing upon it.

"Have you phoned the folks?" Millicent asked him.

"No."

"Do they know you're coming?"

"No."

"Don't you think you should phone?"

"I will."

He told how the plane had brought him to Otis on the Cape, during the night, and how he had thumbed from there on the roads. A salesman had given him a ride to Dorchester, and on the radio in the car there had been a terrible report, about a trailer truck that had rolled backward onto a sidewalk and onto a four-year-old girl who was playing there, so that her legs had to be amputated. In Dorchester he had tried to telephone Millicent, meaning to come in by subway. But the phone had not worked and he had lost his nickel in it, and then discovered that he had no more money at all.

"How did you get in?" said Ella Jane.

"Walked."

"You walked all the way from Dorchester?"

"Thumbing's no good in the city."

"How long did it take you?"

"Oh, a couple of hours."

"And on an empty stomach," Ella Jane commiserated.

"Well, it wasn't that. But do you know what a feeling it gives you to be stuck in Dorchester without carfare? It's very peculiar. It kind of hit me. Very humbling. You realize how important carfare is. You could have money in the bank in some other neighborhood, but if you happen to get stuck without a nickel in your pocket, boy, nobody knows you. The trolley car goes by and you can't get on. You can't even walk up to a counter and buy a doughnut. I thought of it, I thought of asking for credit and telling the whole long story, but I could imagine the look I would have got."

Millicent took bread from the toaster. The kitten rubbed against Charles's leg and he reached down and stroked its fur.

"The cat's getting big," he said.

"How do you like the Air Force?" Ella Jane asked him.

"I don't know, sometimes you get fed up. You know what they did to us? There's this girls' finishing school, and they gave a dance and they were supposed to invite a hundred men from the base. It was for the enlisted men, I mean. So on the night of the dance the officers confined everybody to barracks and went themselves."

"Well," said Ella Jane, "I suppose there are worse disasters."

"You're darn right," he said.

Ella Jane touched a paper napkin to her lips. "How is it out?" she asked him. "Is it going to clear?" She took her cane.

"I don't know. It was pretty raw."

"The forecast was rain, I think," Millicent said. "I'm not sure. Sometimes I read them while I take them upstairs and sometimes I'm not sure if I did or not."

Ella Jane put on a raincoat at the closet and tied a scarf about her head.

"How small an account do you handle?" Charles asked her from the table. "Somebody gave me a tip on Masahbi Iron."

"You haven't got any money," Ella Jane answered. "You lost your nickel in the telephone, remember?" She went out.

He chewed his toast. "Doesn't she ever give you tips?" he asked Millicent.

"No."

"Doesn't she ever try to sell you any?"

"No. I couldn't afford it anyway. I put everything in Government savings bonds."

"Well, you ought to try a growth stock. It's a hedge against inflation, you know. And Ella Jane told me if you took all those quarters and dimes you hand out to bums and panhandlers it would amount to enough in six months to buy a few shares of something."

"When did she say that?"

"The last time I was here."

"It's only gambling, anyway," Millicent said. "And I'm against gambling."

When he had finished breakfast he lay down on the mussed bedding of the studio couch.

He yawned and massaged his eyes. "I'm tired," he said.

"Get up from there and I'll make that," she said.

He pulled himself to his feet, as if with an effort. Millicent folded the bedding and took it away. He stared sleepily at the rug, with a look of confused recognition.

"Isn't that—?" he said.

"Yes, that's the folks' old rug," she told him. She restored the bolster and Natalie's stuffed dog to the studio couch.

He undid his heavy shoes and lay down, dropping them to the floor. Millicent sat on the couch by his feet, leaning on the bolster.

"I'm tired too," she said. "I'm not used to getting up so early."

"I'll get around the other way, so you won't smell my feet," said Charles.

"That's all right."

But he turned and rearranged himself. The top of his head pressed the bathrobe on her thigh.

He sighed. He was staring up at the venetian blinds.

"Sis," he said quietly, "losing that nickel just threw me. I was thinking about that little kid on the radio, she's playing jacks on her own doorstep, right in front of her own house, one fine morning, minding her own business, and all of a sudden she's got no legs. Just as if we were in the stone age and a tiger ate her. As if everybody's always living on the brink of disaster, no matter how well things are going. Anything can happen. And then this phone goes on the blink. That dial equipment is supposed to be so perfect it never makes a mistake. But you can't trust anything."

He looked up at her and she thought there was moisture in his eyes.

"That's silly," she told him softly.

"The world's a pretty scary place, Sis."

"Well, it's a natural feeling." She stroked his hair. "You're in the armed forces, and there's a war going on."

"I don't mean the armed forces. I mean the whole world. Sis, did you ever feel depressed?"

"Yes. Are you depressed?"

"Not now. But I was up all night, in the back of a big old C-47, with a couple of other hitchhikers, and it's so noisy in those things you can't even talk to each other. And I was thinking, here I am in the South, and here I am up in the sky, in a box ten thousand feet in the air, and what am I doing there?"

He paused, and she pondered his words.

"Do you mind if I put my head in your lap?" he asked.

"Do you want a pillow?"

"No, your lap's all right." He shifted and raised his head onto the corduroy of her bathrobe.

It felt heavy to her at first, as though on a bone, and she did not see how he could find it comfortable, but then his face rested against her stomach. He moved his foot, and the goggle-eyed stuffed dog fell to the floor.

"Wouldn't you be more comfortable in the other room?" Millicent said. "Do you want to lie down on Natalie's bed?"

"No. This is all right."

His blond hair was newly cut, very short, and its brushlike fuzziness was pleasing when she moved her hand. The cat climbed to his chest and he stroked it.

"I wonder why I couldn't make the grade," he said. "In school, I mean. I've got brains enough. It's as if I were jinxed or something."

"You're not jinxed. You have to keep remembering that God has nothing against you personally," she told him, stroking his hair, "or you turn into a psycho, or a paranoid or something. There's no such thing as cosmic spite."

"I could have had a commission if I'd gone through school first."

"Dad told you that."

"It didn't seem important then. What gets me is when the officers aren't as smart as I am. It's crazy. The lieutenants aren't as stupid as some of the sergeants, but around major they start getting real stupid again. We've got a major that wouldn't know how to change a tire on a car if he had to. He soaked his distributor going through a puddle and he didn't know what the hell was wrong. He looked under the hood and do you think he knew what he was looking at? He wouldn't know a motor from a washing machine."

"But you're making good progress. Mother and Dad said you're learning all about what makes planes work."

"It's more important to know when they're not gonna work. It could be somebody's life."

The hand that was not stroking his hair lay on the couch beside him. He took it in both of his, and then in one only. The cat went to the floor.

"You cut your nails too short," she said.

"Sis, you're the only one I can talk to." There was a tightness in his face and voice.

"If you could talk to me you would have stayed in school."

"No, you're still the only one. Mother's too stupid, or she's flying off the handle in the middle of a sentence, and how can you talk to Dad? You start philosophizing with him and there's no end of it. He wants to be close to ya, and feel God, and nature, and all that stuff. Right away he's in there over the deep end, all the inexpressible stuff. It can give ya the willies. He thinks the trees are his cousins or something. Because they have a common ancestor in the primordial slime."

"No he doesn't."

"Well, it's a pain having a religious father."

He played with her fingers, silently a while.

"I love them, though," he said. "And I love you, Cockeyes." She felt his head move on her lap and he looked up at her. "I love Fatso too, and Rollo. But I love you the best."

"Don't call her Fatso."

"Well, that's how it is. The people closest to you are the ones you can feel closest to, I guess. Even Grandma Annie. She may be a little lightheaded, but she's the only grandparent we've got left. We've got a close family. Patty writes to me all the time, do you know that?"

"I should have written," said Millicent.

"That's okay. I don't write much myself, and I didn't answer a lot of Patty's. But all the aunts wrote, and Rollo did once, and Jill did."

"I should have. I just didn't think. I assumed Mother and Dad were taking care of the letter-writing."

"They did. They write me everything you're doing. And you're still the best one in the family, anyhow." He had drawn up a foot and raised a knee. His eyes no longer met hers and he rested an arm on his forehead. "If I meet a girl like you, any time," he said, "I'll get married. There's times when I think, what if you'd been Mother. If only you'd been Mother, instead of Mother. Nobody would have had any problems. You have brains, and sense, and understanding, and you'd have known what to do. You know how to talk to people."

His words surprised and warmed her.

"That's very flattering," she said. "I never knew you thought that."

"It's not flattering, it's true."

"I suppose everyone thinks about what kind of person they'll marry," she said. "It's an awfully serious thing, choosing a mate. I guess even if you want a career it's on your mind. It's as if you could choose your parents. I don't mean a mate is like a parent, but I mean, in a sense, you're given a chance to pick your family, rather. Maybe a third or a quarter through life, when you have some experience, you choose a friend and make him your family. It's just as if you were given a chance to decide what parents to be born to."

"I know it," he said. "Maybe there's something congenitally dumb about parents, I don't know. They're too involved from their own angle to know what you're talking about, I guess. But you're different. And you're beautiful besides."

She looked down at his pensive face. "I thought you thought I was cross-eyed," she said.

"They have the most soul of any eyes I ever saw," he told her, looking up again. "They're so deep. They're so filled up with soul, and they look right into me. That tiny bit crossed makes them all the more beautiful. They look as if they're right up next to me. Even if you're across the room. Or right up next to whatever you're looking at. Honest, if a man had eyes like that a woman would think she was penetrated with just a look."

"They're not crossed an abnormal amount," she said. "It's called borderline normal. And nothing can be done."

"It's just like that little shake in your voice. It seems to have emotion all the time. Even if you're only saying 'good morning,' or 'pass the salt.' You must excite guys."

"I do not."

"I mean without knowing it."

She saw him gazing at her eyes.

"How much time do you have?" she asked.

"Three days, altogether. But I should start back a day ahead. I'll try Otis or Bedford for a flight south and I don't know how long I'll have to sit around."

"You better call the folks then. And get home."

"I should." He sat up, sluggishly.

She raised a foot to the couch, massaging her pajama leg where he had lain. He fondled her toes absently a few moments, looking sadly at the rug. Then he rose, and picked the lavender telephone from the floor. He set it among the breakfast crockery and the crumbs.

"It's tough on a guy when his sister's the most terrific girl there is," he said, without looking at her. "He's got no place to go but down." He took the phone from its cradle.

"Call collect," she said, "so I don't have to remember about the bill."

22

Ed said he hadn't had his exercise again, and asked Charles to help him drag some logs into the barn out of the rain. Then he sawed, pausing after every several strokes to rest a few seconds. The big door was still rolled part way open. The rain splattered on its rusty rail, and raw gusts blew in. Charles knelt to massage the old collie between the ears, speaking to it. He inspected the Model T and kicked the tires. The wheels hung free, an inch or two above the flooring. He watched the swallows glide and circle under the rafters, their brown color blending with the darkness up there. At length he took the other saw from its peg and helped his father.

Sometimes the heaving blades were in rhythm and sometimes not. Charles sweated but he did not pause as Ed did, and it occurred to Ed that his son's arm was already stronger than his own. His son was the same height as himself, but if they were to box or wrestle, his son would overpower him. It was a strange feeling.

At the afternoon's end, when they crossed the wet grass to the house, the sky had cleared, and Ed said that often happened at the approach of a Sabbath. Though the sun was low it seemed all the brighter after the day's darkness.

Ed filled the wineglasses at the kitchen table for the Sabbath libation, but instead of conducting it himself he handed the prayer book to Charles, open to the page. He said a visitor ought to be honored.

During supper Lucinda told Charles she was glad he had come home, but she wished he hadn't flown, and that going back she wished he'd take the train.

"I couldn't possibly make it," he said.

"Well, I don't like your flying," she told him. "Especially with amateurs."

"They're not amateurs."

"Well, it was somebody you know. Or a student pilot or something."

"It wasn't a student pilot and it wasn't somebody I know."

"Well, anyway you're in the ground crew, and you shouldn't fly when it isn't necessary."

Charles walked with Ed to the late Friday service, along with Patty and Roland. Lucinda went by car.

Charles attended again in the morning, with Patty and Roland. But in late afternoon he departed for the air base in Bedford, even though the Sabbath wasn't over.

Ed wasn't home when Charles left, as he had been teaching the Ethics of the Fathers to a summer class on Sabbath afternoons, at the long varnished table in the temple's little library, and the final session was meeting then. Betsy Stokes, the Weiler boy's girl friend, had attended the last couple of sessions, and was doing well in her private instruction also, but before her appearance the class had been down to two pupils, Amethyst Gilbert and Marilyn Prince, the cantor's wife. He had told himself that you couldn't expect much community interest in summer, but it was a disappointment to have only women to teach. The men had all dropped out after the first session or two. He was not even sure if the cantor's wife really enjoyed the course, or whether she came out of a sense of duty lest it be a total failure.

When the final session was over, and Mrs. Gilbert and Betsy Stokes took their leave, the cantor's wife seemed to hang around. Ed took his book and buttoned his jacket, but though she had risen she made no move toward the door. She was little, and her skin was nearly brownish. Ed told her he thought her husband had been in especially good voice that morning. He said he liked the way Bill always sang as though the words had meaning, never dragging them out or embellishing. Marilyn acknowledged the compliment with a syllable, without seeming to enjoy it.

"Ed, I wish you'd have a talk with Bill," she said.

She looked troubled. Ed leaned on the table. He had rarely heard her say anything, even in the little summer classes, and in the softness of her voice her New York accent now suddenly struck him. She told him her husband hated being a cantor, that he felt he couldn't go on. He had wanted to be a concert folk singer, or perhaps an actor, but the opportunities hadn't come, and his training and the need of an income had driven him into cantoring.

"Well, it's a job, anyway," Ed said. "He should stay with it until he finds what he wants."

"That's what I tell him," said Marilyn.

She told how she had met Bill, and how Bill's huge family had moved to Brooklyn from the Lower East Side. She sat down again as she spoke. She was not pretty. Bill's family had been poor, but the mother had given piano lessons, and all the brothers and sisters had been trained in music and in religion throughout childhood.

"Partly, we came here to get out of New York," she said. "Sometimes when you're in New York it seems like there's no way out. And he hoped up here he'd get odd jobs on the side, singing around Boston. And now he says he wants to take everything we have and go to Tahiti. We should go there when we're young, he says. Believe me, if I thought it would make him happy, I'd pack up today."

"What would he do in Tahiti?"

"I don't know. He doesn't know. He doesn't even look into anything about it. Maybe he'd record the native songs. Or maybe he'd sing in a night club. I don't even know if they have night clubs in Tahiti. I wish you'd talk to him."

"I don't know what I can say."

"Well, sometimes it's good just to talk."

Ed thought he would perhaps draw Bill into conversation after one of the early morning services during the week, but when the occasion came Bill looked more black and sullen than usual, and at the close of the service old man Brill engaged Ed in conversation, during which Bill slipped away.

The next time, however, Bill remained and sat with Ed in one of the front pews, talking about the curriculum they planned for the children's after-school classes.

The little desks had only yesterday been installed, and they went to the classroom to look. There was no chalk and Bill tried the blackboard with his finger. Then he sat hunched on one of the desks, looking pensively toward the windows and the trees beyond. Ed sat at the teacher's desk.

"I understand Marilyn gave you an earful," Bill said.

"Oh, I wouldn't say that," said Ed.

The blackboard was green. Ed wished they had gotten the black kind. He looked at the faint tracing Bill's finger had made.

"She involved you because she thinks you seem so happy in your work," Bill said, "and I guess she didn't know who else to talk to."

Ed looked at Bill's beetle brows, and the wide nose and wide frown, with lines cut deep around it.

"Well, I don't know," Ed told him. "Maybe it's the wrong job for you. But a lot of guys start off in the wrong job. I started out as a car salesman."

"I know, I heard the story," said Bill.

"Are you gonna quit?" Ed asked him.

"I don't know," he said tiredly. "Ed, let me be honest. The more I search my soul the more I know I'm an atheist. And don't tell me we all go through it—I'm too old. I don't believe in it. I don't believe in the job I'm doing. How long can a man go on? Let's face it. It's a job, yes. But a man has self-respect."

"How old are you?"

"Twenty-six. Don't start telling me you were an atheist at eighteen and a believer at twenty—this I've heard from ten rabbis already."

Ed shrugged. "No, maybe I never was. I used to think my actual ideas were a lot different from my father's, and especially my grandfather's, say, and that I was the modern scientific critical one, and that saying the same prayers together made us feel more alike than we actually were. But I'm not sure now that my grandfather really was so different. I don't know. I think the main thing is the attitude."

"Well, I had too much of it, all my life, and I love it too much to make a fraud out of it. I've been an atheist perhaps since I was eleven."

"You're a good cantor. I think they like you."

"I'm a singer, unfortunately."

"Why don't you open a studio in Boston and teach voice?"

"There's no such thing," said Bill. "Ed, you told Marilyn a job's a job. Is that what you think of your own job? Is the rabbinate just a job too?" He looked at Ed.

"Never mind about me. You're telling me you haven't got belief, so I'm telling you to enjoy yourself, that's all. You haven't got belief—you still have to live. If you can't find what you want, and you're good at this and the money's as good as you can earn elsewhere, so mark time."

"Without belief?"

"You've got a wife to support. Look, it's nice if the cantor has belief, and it's nice if he has big blue eyes, but what he hasn't got he hasn't got."

"I still have to answer for what I've done with my life."

"If you think that, then you do have belief."

"Not in God," said Bill.

"So who do you have to answer to?"

"I have to answer to myself."

"If it's only yourself you have to answer to, so be a little more charitable with yourself. Do you have to answer to Marilyn? Is she complaining?"

"No, she doesn't complain."

"She's a sweet kid."

Bill rubbed his forehead with his hand, looking down. He swung his legs a little. "Another aspect of it," he said, "is that on principle I don't like singing hymns for the entertainment of a bunch of housewives. It feels to me like a pansy's job."

"A what?"

"A pansy's job."

"You don't look like a pansy."

"That's not the point—I mean it's not what a man should be doing."

"Well, join a gym. Build yourself up."

"Marilyn thinks I should see a head-shrinker."

Ed said nothing.

"Do you think I should?" said Bill.

Ed moved his head a little. "I don't know. Now you're asking me a medical question. But I suppose anything you learn that's pertinent to yourself helps to bring you peace. Or wholeness. Whether it's development of a skill, or whether it's self-understanding, or even learning what your religion demands of you. It all concerns you."

Bill was frowning toward the windows again. His hands pressed one another nervously. "Well, I can't quit today or tomorrow," he said. "Not decently. After signing a contract. So I guess I'll be with you for a year."

"That's good."

"Dishonestly," Bill added. "As a hypocrite."

"You're not dishonest. They're paying you to chant the stuff. They're not paying you to believe it."

"But is the service legitimate if it's sung by an unbeliever? Even when I read out of a holy scroll the parchment has to have been copied by a believer."

"You're an unbeliever," said Ed, "so why should you even worry about a question like that? I think you're doing fine. Maybe that's why you sing so beautifully. Because you're burdened. You're disturbed. You hate your job, and that's what brings out that lovely plaintive sound."

"Don't kid around."

"No, I mean it. It says 'happy are those—' you know. Maybe if you were at peace with yourself you couldn't sing so good. You couldn't bring out the anguish."

"The man who prays for the congregation on Rosh Hashanah is supposed to be somebody who's personally blameless."

"So you're blameless," Ed told him. "You're not to blame if you can't believe."

"It doesn't bother you, that your cantor's an atheist?"

"You're getting away with it. I won't broadcast it."

Bill shook his head. "No, Ed. I won't be a fraud. To others, or to myself."

"And what's wrong with being a fraud?" said Ed.

"It's just wrong, that's all."

"Look, when you're reduced to saying 'it's just wrong,' you're acknowledging some authority higher than man. It's a leap of faith already. So why not admit it? I don't say a believer is logical, but I say as soon as you say 'should' you're just as illogical."

"Well, if that rationalization suits you, Ed, I'm glad. It doesn't suit me."

"It's not a rationalization."

He looked at Ed. "I don't understand you, Ed. You're a puzzle to me. I can't make out what kind of man you are. Sometimes you seem like a thinking man, and sometimes you seem like a man that refuses to think. I can't decide whether you really have intellectual integrity or not. And if you are a thinking man, then I can't believe you're as happy as you sometimes pretend."

"Why not?"

"Well, to be very elementary, how do you square your alleged faith with—look, Ed. I've had a thorough religious education, and I find no decent explanation for the problem of evil in the world. I mean the horrible, rotten, filthy, painful, unnecessary things. It's not that the end justifies the means, and God has good purposes in the end, because a God could find other means. A kid is terrified in a concentration camp, and beaten, and the end is that the kid dies. You cannot explain evil."

Ed was frowning also. "Okay, so you can't explain it," he said. "You can be an atheist and you still can't explain it."

"If you're an atheist," said Bill, "there is an explanation. The random hit and miss of nature, that's all."

"If it's random, why do you care? What's evil about it?"

"I care because I care. I don't know, Ed. What do you prove?"

"I'm trying to prove that no matter how you slice it, there's no explanation. But it seems to me that if your heart didn't believe in something, you wouldn't be so angry about it."

Bill shook his head again, slowly. "It's a bum argument, Ed. We're talking in circles. You don't believe atheists are really atheists, and I don't believe believers are really believers. I remember there was an instructor in the extension courses in the seminary, a little pimply guy with droopy pants, teaching philosophy, a young guy, and one day he told the class he believed in God. You know, a class with girls, graduate students looking for summer credits and everything, and some discussion came up, and he said that. And I was thinking that even in a seminary, and even for this young guy just ordained, it took guts to say that. But I didn't believe him. It's wishful thinking, Ed. That's all."

They sat looking at each other.

"Well," said Ed, "so anyway you'll be here a year. Maybe it'll come out in the wash."

They heard the clock on Caleb Folger's church.

"The hell with it," said Bill. "I'm going home."

They went out together. Winged seeds of maple fell on them and littered the sidewalk. For some distance their paths were the same. They walked side by side silently.

Then Ed asked whether Marilyn went to the Crosswalker meetings, and said Lucinda enjoyed them.

They walked up the street that flanked the near side of Murphy Square.

A teen-aged girl came bicycling over one of the diagonal paths of the common. She was in striped shorts. As she circled across the street she smiled and greeted Ed and Bill without stopping, and Ed recognized her as a daughter of a family that belonged to the temple. She rode away from them, her back moving up and down with her pumping, past Colby & Dill's Real Estate and the barber shop and braked the bicycle far up the block, in front of the Eng Hop Hand Laundry. She stretched a leg, and swung the other one off the bike.

"Look how the pants fit on that rear end," said Ed. "Can you tell me life isn't good?"

"While it lasts," said Bill. "And some boy in this town could be hanging himself for that rear end, for all you know."

She went into the laundry.

"Well, the Bible doesn't say God looked on His work and saw it was perfect," said Ed. "It just says He saw it was good."

"And what about 'the Law of the Lord is perfect'?"

"The Law, yes."

"Listen, Ed, I wouldn't treat my children with the cruelty and injustice that God gives his creatures."

"You have no children."

"If I had. And neither would you."

"That's true."

"And if nothing else, we're all condemned to death. The punishment we consider fit only for the worst felons, that's God's sentence for you and me. Can a Creator think so little of His own creation? I don't want to die."

The girl came out of the laundry, with a wrapped package that she put into the handlebar basket. Then she parted her legs, raised herself high on the pedals, and a slow undulation began to move her.

"Never mind looking at girls," Bill said to Ed. "Give me an answer."

"There's no answer," said Ed. "That's why we're commanded to praise God at a time of disaster. It's a recognition that there's no answer. No religion is worth anything if it can't face up to its own confusion."

"Any other advice?"

"I don't know. Did you expect to come to me and find God? Try having a baby."

23

The police chief Giles Littleton was master of the Masonic lodge, and chatted agreeably with Ed after a lodge meeting about how little juvenile delinquency there was in the town, and about how Conrad Bernstein had asked him to provide special traffic cops for the High Holy Days.

Ed did in fact find Horace Comeau, whom he knew from the volunteer firemen, directing traffic in front of the single story of stucco on Rosh Hashanah eve, and the next morning Officer John Yerxa was there, in the middle of the street, with a whistle in his mouth. He touched his hat in a kind of salute to Ed.

The pews were full, not at the beginning but as the morning wore on. It made Ed feel good, after the near emptiness of summer. The ladies' hats were stylish and varied, and their faces were set in powdered frowns. Light reflected on the eyeglasses of the men. He could not help staring at an unusually pretty girl of thirteen or fourteen. A mere child, but with a gorgeous face. Close to two hundred families belonged to the congregation and Ed had visited most of them once in the spring and summer; it was good now just to see gathered at one time so many people whose names one knew, whose interests and homes and businesses and children one knew a little. Some called him rabbi and some called him Ed. He felt a liking for them. He knew large turnouts on these occasions could be deceptive, but the gathering here and now gave him excitement. They could only be here because they cared—because they knew that the past was real, and that therefore the future was real and worth trying to shape. It's those who see the present only who succumb to the values of the ad men, he thought.

He saw Betsy Stokes sitting with Rodney Weiler's family.

The weather was perfect, and he saw the blowing of the trees outside and of the slack flagpole rope. He remembered a little window of blue and clouded glass high under the peaked roof of the pretty little temple at Abbottsford, and how a leafy branch had pressed on it. They had been going to cut the branch away but Ed had asked them not to. Those fluttering shadows of foliage, through the white and blue, had seemed God's way of beautifying the window.

Bill Prince's voice had the quality of a gentle cornet, Ed thought. He could bring melodies to life, pulling the congregation with him, or chant in a way that seemed narrative or expository. Ed stood with Bill and others at the reading desk, which was set back among the congregation on a little platform one step high. The pews on either side of it faced toward the center, so that the high sloping reading desk and its platform were almost surrounded by the congregation, except at the front, where it faced toward the opened Ark of the Covenant, which dominated the room, set into the wall like a tall cupboard decorated with Grecian columns.

> *And Abraham was a hundred years old when his son Isaac was born. And Sarah said, everybody that hears about it will make jokes. Who would have thought that I would give children suck? For I have borne him a child in our old age—*

When it was time for the sermon Ed left the reading desk and went to a small lectern set on a post facing the congregation, to the side of the Ark. He made some announcements, about meetings of the sisterhood and the brotherhood and the Hadassah, and reminded everyone who had not yet registered their children for the Sunday school and the afternoon classes to hurry and do so. He said he hoped also for a good turnout in the adult-education classes, which would start right after the holidays, although the summer had been disappointing. He thanked those whose regular attendance had made it possible for a daily service to limp along a couple of mornings a week, but said it was only a start, and that he hoped many more would sign up to come regularly for a brief quarter hour, morning or evening, some particular day of the week. It wasn't fair that the same men should have to carry the ball all the time, and not fair that they should have to wait around while phone calls were made in last-minute efforts to complete the group.

His eye ran over the attractive clothing of the women and the prayer shawls of the men. Their eyes were on him; yet there was scarcely a face he could read. Even so, it gave him pleasure to address a large audience. He talked a while about the passage from Genesis that had been read, in which a woman of ninety, barren all her life, became pregnant suddenly by a man of a hundred. "Years after anybody would have said this old couple was finished, ready for the undertaker," Ed said finally, "a new shoot is sent up, that nobody would have bet a nickel on, and the future burgeons. And how many times have the experts said our whole people, our whole tradition, was ready for the undertaker? I remember men that gathered morning and evening for a few minutes of prayer. A lot of us remember it. And now is all that ready for the undertaker too? And yet look what a difference it made in human history that Sarah didn't die childless. A tradition, a viewpoint that began with Abraham would have ended with Abraham. We continually surprise ourselves and others by the fact that we aren't dead. A historian writes a book and proves we should be dead. And still it doesn't end. And it won't end, as long as God has use for it. Look, if you think back, don't forget only ten years ago it looked as if democracy and free government were ready for the undertaker. Do you remember ten years ago when France fell? And who could predict what turns history would take then? Suppose Hitler had decided to push the bomb, instead of giving the priority to rockets. And twenty years ago, they were saying private enterprise was ready for the undertaker. And today you hear people say there'll be an atomic war and the whole human species is ready for the undertaker. Or civilization anyway. The real-estate market couldn't be tighter but still they say it. And there's reason to be afraid, too. When you consider that at any instant things could happen that would lead eventually to a fatal chain of events. It's as if the human race at every instant has been snatched from death. And it's always been that way. Now, I'm not preaching resurrection. Abraham and Sarah didn't live forever, and they weren't made young again. They died, like anybody else, and they were buried. But we've read how the old couple shouldn't have had a baby but they did. We're starting a year, and that's the message. In the old age of our history, you still have to believe it's only the beginning. If you believe in the future, that's the same as trusting God. God, the Redeemer. And if you believe there are things you must do about the future, then you believe your purposes supplement His, and you're already getting down to cases and you have a religion."

When he had finished he paused a brief moment, and said on what page the service resumed. Then he returned to his place, near the reading desk.

The curved horn of a male sheep lay on the reading desk, brown in its natural roughness, and Roy Herzlinger, the wholesale drug distributor, took over the blowing of it. He had specially asked to do so. He was a large man, gray-haired and tastefully tailored, genteel and intelligent of appearance, and Ed thought he blew exceedingly well. Once only Roy had to knock the horn against his palm when saliva clogged it, but the rest of the time he brought forth the prolonged notes, the interrupted notes, and the swinging notes steadily and clear, reddening with the effort, while Ed sang out each call to guide him.

Afterward Bill Prince stood before the Ark, his back to everyone, and the tender, drawn-out cry of his voice filled the room with stilling emotion. Bill swayed imperceptibly, so that the drapes and corners of his prayer shawl swung a little. He might have closed his eyes and opened them, and sometimes he clasped one hand in the other. He held no book.

They have delegated me, though I am unworthy. Don't judge them by me—

How can he not believe and yet render it so beautifully, Ed thought. Unless maybe the trouble is that he believes part of the time.

He saw Patty look around at the clock over the door. The service had perhaps another hour and a half to go. But he had tried to arrange it so that as many members as possible had duties to perform, opening or shutting the sliding doors of the Ark, or being called to the reading desk during the reading, or lifting the heavy parchment scrolls or tying them tight, or merely sitting and holding them until it was time to put them away. He called upon those who were heavy contributors, walking quietly to their pews while Bill led the service, and upon those who had attended fairly regularly, and upon others who had no particular claim. The Ark had been built with a light inside, that went on automatically when the doors slid open, but the adjustment was imperfect and the light did not come on until the doors were already parted an inch and went out before complete closing. It reminded Ed of a refrigerator, and bothered him. He decided he would take the bulb out after the holiday. He had also seen a moth fly out of the Ark in the past few days and he reminded himself to spray its interior.

When the time came, while Bill still led the service, Ed took twelve-year-old Paul Brody out to the vestibule and thence to the temple's little kitchen, to get him ready to deliver the priestly blessing. The boy's mother came out with him, and also Mr. Resnick, who happened to be a Levite. The boy extended his wrists, drooping, above the sink, and the thin old Levite poured water over the boy's hands from a pitcher.

"Look out for his good suit," Mrs. Brody said.

Using this kid was really scraping the bottom of the barrel, Ed thought. In a congregation of this size one would by the law of averages expect a half dozen or more families in which word had been passed down the generations of descent from the ancient priesthood, and whose men accordingly would bestow the blessing in unison on the High Holy Days. Even in Abbottsford there had been four or five such men, including a half-witted ice-cream peddler, and they had gone before the little congregation together in due form. An extraordinary shortage like that in Wilmerding Crosswalk Ed had never before heard of. Ed thought there must be some, perhaps untutored, who were priests without knowing it or who did not care to speak of it. Paul's father, in fact, had begged off, saying he had never given the blessing and couldn't possibly learn it. Despite all Ed's urging he had refused, sheepishly and shyly, saying he didn't want to stand up and make a spectacle of himself.

Paul at last stood before the whole gathering, on the low step with his back to the Ark, and Bill Prince stood aside nearby and faced him, leading the interpolations loudly and musically. Paul sang out the blessing in the ancient tongue, one word at a time, as Ed had taught him, his unchanged voice ringingly clear and soprano. The prayer shawl was drawn half over his head and hung over his forehead, its folds falling in a loop there. He turned his upper body a little back and forth, to the right and to the left, his eyes shut, and extended his hands so that they raised the ends of the prayer shawl, his fingers parted in twos in the strange way of Aaron.

When the blessing was finished he returned to his parents. A boy put out a foot to trip him but he saw it in time.

Ed had announced that he planned a little walk in the afternoon to where a branch of Massapeequit Brook flowed under the stone bridge, before the fork just past Murphy Square, and to hold a service there for a couple of minutes in connection with Micah's prophecy about casting sins into the sea. He had talked it up, and buttonholed a few men to make sure they would be there, and in late afternoon, when he went to the temple with Patty and Roland, most of the men who had promised him were in fact awaiting him on the sidewalk, along with several children and a couple of mothers. They walked together, not in a formal procession, down the street and over one of the diagonal paths of Murphy Square, Ed toward the front with some of the children. He heard the men chatting gaily behind him on a variety of matters. At the brook he stepped warily sideways down the steep bank in weeds and high grass. Some of the party came after him, some of the children fooling and others being quite adult, and a number of men being gallant to the ladies. The water was clear and noisy on a shallow bed of brownish rocks. The children were quieted and Ed read some psalms.

Then they parted. But Conrad Bernstein walked a little distance with Ed, and told him there had been a lot of criticism of his presenting the congregation with a priest who wasn't even bar mitzvah.

"Well, the kid'll get older year by year," said Ed.

But Conrad told him many people felt the whole thing had been in poor taste, and could have been left out, and that the morning had been too long anyway.

On the second morning of Rosh Hashanah Lucinda ran her hand at breakfast over the stubble of his cheek. "I hope you aren't going like that," she said.

"I never shave on Rosh Hashanah," he said.

"Well you look like a bum." She told him he might manage to get away with it on Sabbaths, by shaving late the preceding afternoon, but on two-day holidays he really looked a mess.

However, he went to the temple without having shaved. He recalled an occasion last spring, when they were new in the house, and he had taken a vacation from shaving for a few days while he puttered with screens and shelves, and Lucinda had told him the congregation would have a fit. She had told him it was all right for other men to skip shaving but not for a rabbi, because somebody might jump to the conclusion he was planning to grow long whiskers. She wanted him to get along with people and not lose this job, she had said, and if she could give up shorts he could shave.

The temple was not quite so jammed as on the first morning. Ed smiled at Betsy Stokes. He had continued to give her instruction, usually three evenings a week, and she had responded before long with an enthusiasm that made her a delight to teach. Every idea he presented seemed to strike her with newness.

In midmorning Phil Walker lifted the big parchment scroll aloft above his head, each of its sticks in a powerful arm, and turned it in every direction before laying it on the reading desk, that everyone might glimpse the close-written brushwork. Bill Prince read a chapter from Genesis again, this time about the sacrifice of Isaac. His tenor seemed to entwine about the text.

Ed's gaze wandered through the congregation, particularly to the various children who would soon be his pupils, and rested at last on Roland and Patty and Millicent, who sat beside Lucinda. He looked at the faces of each of the three, enjoying their good looks. Looking at those kids, who can deny that my seed is good stuff, he thought.

He looked at Lucinda, her lean face, and the few freckles along that nose, long and low-lying, with a turn-up at the bottom. He regretted that they had not had more children than four.

If Lucinda should die suddenly, in some illness or a car smash, he thought, he would look for some real solid youngster for his second wife, and try to have another seven, eight, eleven children. Pregnant nine months on and nine months off. These four were so fine, so beautiful, so superior. Why had they not done it again and again, exploiting their magnificent genes, until the menopause stopped them, and had fourteen, sixteen? He hoped his children would do it instead, since he hadn't—that Millicent, Charles, Patricia, Roland, each of them, would bear or beget huge families, would each aim for a dozen and have at least ten. The older could help diaper the younger, and they need not all go to college, and could earn scholarships anyhow, and if the world were overpopulated they were still of a folk six million short. If he could live again that would be his ambition from youth, the enormous family. To stud son after daughter, daughter after son, each with new visions, yet bound together by a hearth, and by the tie of having been raised in the Law. Fourteen children, so many sons and daughters, each one of a different temperament, born over twenty years. What fabulous richness. What strength and fortification, for the parents and for the children. What greater trust can God give you? To see the variety of possibility that lay in your sperm, dark ones and fair ones, blue-eyed and brown. Who knew whether your next child might not be the genius who would save the world, or the parent or grandparent of someone the world needed? Mankind's uniqueness, he said to himself, is that one single individual can maybe have an idea that may influence the whole species of billions. Of no other species was this true.

Rodney Weiler and Betsy Stokes had planned to marry during the interval between Rosh Hashanah and Yom Kippur. They were planning a wedding trip of a few days only, and to live afterward in Wilmerding Mills, in two rooms that someone had remodeled in the attic of an old frame house. Rodney was working in his father's real-estate agency in Sparkstown, and Betsy told Ed she would keep on taking religious instruction. He made them postpone the wedding till after the holidays. He suspected they were sleeping together anyhow.

The week of penitence between the holidays seemed to Ed a good time to try for a full program of daily prayers, morning and before and after sundown, and he tried to organize groups to take turns at it, but he was not very successful.

A letter came from Charles. He had been made an acting corporal. He had men under him. He said in his letter that he wanted to know how to repair everything on a plane, not just a section of it. He wanted the feel of how to put fifty tons of metal in the air. The American landing at Inchon in Korea had occurred a few days after Rosh Hashanah and Ed and Lucinda followed the progress of it. Ed told her it looked as though it would bring the war to an end quickly. Lucinda said she hoped so.

Meanwhile she said she was glad she hadn't gotten Mr. Featherstone to kill the woodchuck under the porch with a fumigation bomb, because it had turned out to be a rabbit instead. It sat hunched one morning, half in and half out at the edge, while she hung the wash. Patty told him Roland had hunted quail with a bow and arrow, but hadn't gotten any.

Ed wondered how Charles had managed on the holiday, whether there had been services on the base or whether he had been invited to some town.

He asked when he wrote, and congratulated him on the acting corporalcy, saying he hoped that by the next letter he would be a real corporal. He told Lucinda that the boy seemed to be finding himself.

On Yom Kippur Ed walked to the temple in sneakers, observing the ban on leather, although Lucinda warned him the congregation wouldn't like it. He was surprised that the crowd was a little fewer than before. The Weiler parents were there, and Betsy, but he noticed that Rodney wasn't.

> *You pose as a nation that did rightly, and ask "Why have we fasted and Thou seest not?" Behold, on the day of your fast you run your businesses, drive your employees, extort gain. Is such My fast? To bow your heads like reeds, and spread sackcloth and ashes? Do you call that a fast? Is not My fast to free the oppressed, and break every yoke? Is it not to deal thy food to the hungry, to shelter the shelterless, clothe them that are ill-clad, and not hide from thy kin? Then shall thy light break forth as the morning—*

He felt grateful to Millicent for being there, and for having arranged with her employer to be off on these occasions. She sat as before, between her mother and the other children, primly with a book in her lap, following the reading. The schools in the town had opened in the past week, and he thought Patty and Roland had both made a smooth transition, as though they had always lived here. Last spring they had come to these schools as strangers, but this fall Roland had in the first week of school gone out for the junior-high band, though they had told him he would have to learn the trombone as they had too many trumpets. And at the high school Patty was out for cheerleader and for field hockey.

He had not encouraged the two younger children to fast, but Roland seemed determined to prove he could stand it, and Patty had a notion she could lose three pounds in twenty-four hours.

Early in the afternoon Ed called a recess, but said that for any who wished to remain during it he would hold a study group in the temple's library. Seven or eight did stay, surprising him pleasantly, and he explained the service for a long time, without duplicating his two sermons of the day. But his hunger and thirst were beginning to bother him, and the muscles of his hip had grown unusually painful and stiff, and for the past hour it had hurt even to take a step. He had chopped too much wood the day before. Such rheumatisms ought to make him feel old, he thought, but they did not. Once during the forenoon he had prostrated himself, as the leader of the service was expected to do at that point, and if Bill and old Mr. Munk had not helped him he could scarcely have gotten off the floor again.

A sweltering Indian summer had set in, with no movement of air, and when the service resumed all the windows in the temple were open. Not everybody had come back, and some only socialized out on the lawn, and on the sidewalk under the shade trees. He could see them. A slim young lady in a bright summer dress rocked a baby carriage.

> *After the practices of Egypt where ye dwelt, and the practices of Canaan whither I bring you, shall ye not do. Thy mother's nakedness shalt thou not uncover; she is thy mother. Thou shalt not uncover the nakedness of thy sister, daughter of thy father or of thy mother. Thou shalt not uncover thy son's daughter's nakedness or thy daughter's daughter's nakedness; it is thine own nakedness. Thou shalt not uncover thy father's sister's nakedness nor thy mother's sister's nakedness; she is near kin. Thou shalt not uncover thy father's brother's wife's nakedness; she is thine aunt. Thou shalt not uncover thy daughter-in-law's nakedness; she is thy son's wife. Thou shalt not uncover thy brother's wife's nakedness; it is thy brother's nakedness. Thou shalt not uncover the nakedness of a woman and her daughter or a woman and her granddaughter; it is lewdness. And thou shalt not take a woman with her sister, to uncover her nakedness, to be a rival to the other in her lifetime. Thou shalt not approach to a woman to uncover her nakedness in her period, and thou shalt not lie with thy neighbor's wife. Thou shalt not give any of thy children into the flames, either for Moloch or profaning My name. I am the Lord. Thou shalt not lie with mankind as with womankind; it is abomination. Thou shalt not lie with any beast, neither shall any woman stand before a beast to lie down to it; it is perversion. For in all these things the nations are befouled, which I cast out from before you. All these abominations have the men of the land done that were before you, and the land was made foul, and the land vomited out its inhabitants. Therefore keep My statutes and ordinances, and do not any of these abominations, lest the land vomit you out also, as it vomited out the nation that was before you.*

Ed noticed that Lucinda and Patty had not returned. If Patty had gone for a snack he hoped it was at home, and that she had the sense not to sit in Yerxa's Pharmacy.

When he had a chance he asked Millicent and Roland how they were feeling.

You had pity on the gourd, for which you didn't labor, and which came up in a night and died in a night; should I not have pity on Nineveh, that great city, wherein are more than a hundred thousand human beings too young to know their right hand from their left, and also dumb cattle?

By four o'clock Ed had a headache, and at five it was worse. The poetry of the prayer book grew more intense. Yet it always seemed to him that it was only about this hour, when his brain was half drugged by thirst and hunger, that the meanings of some of the medieval compositions began to take effect, and the repetitions at last hammered their way through to him. He led the service sometimes, rockily, or let Bill, or let it run itself, and prayed with the old men. He looked at Roland, who seemed determined to persist to the end, but he knew the boy felt weak by the readiness with which he sat after each stand, or even failed to stand, resting his head and arm on the back of the pew before him. The poems were of many moods, culled from many centuries and authors. They described their own selves as a jar full of confusion, or expressed stupefaction at the martyrdom of innocents and of creative men, or they pleaded. Sometimes they seemed to write their own music. Bill's voice at length grew hoarse but did not run out of emotion.

On the walk home Ed put his arm around Roland, and the boy said he felt fine. Roland asked him if they would build a sooky this year and whether he could sleep in it with Bobby O'Shaughnessy. Ed said as far as he was concerned Bobby could sleep in it all he wanted, provided he asked Father Donahue.

Ed walked stiffly and for a while silently, stopping now and then to rest his hip, and looking at Millicent, who had walked on ahead gathering a few of the wild flowers from tall weeds beside a low boundary wall of boulders. He thought he would talk to Betsy about that Leviticus passage that belonged to Yom Kippur afternoon. Going to bed with one's mother and sister, women having intercourse with animals, children thrown into the fire. It's all still known, even in our own lifetimes, he said to himself. It didn't end with Moloch and Astarte. In districts of Mexico City or Havana, he had heard, you could still pay a dollar to see a whore perform with a large dog or a small donkey. Tourism, it was. And Nazis had flung children alive onto the burning piles of oiled corpses because there wasn't enough gold in kids' teeth to be worth the time or the bullets to shoot them first. This was the hard-core stuff, he thought; it made you recognize that you did in fact believe right and wrong were real, not just a convention. You could say philosophically you believed in nothing, but this cornered you. You might even philosophize about murder and theft—yet there will remain some deeds that disgust you. Some deeds will make you draw back, and make you call the man who does not draw back depraved. Maybe you would draw a line at a man jumping into bed with his mother. But if you still philosophized, and said even that was wrong only by convention, at least the exhibition in Havana must gag you. Not even those involved would have the gall to justify such use of a woman's flesh. At least when the children went to the flames, you could no longer say with a straight face that all codes were relative, or made by man. Here was the beginning; here, confronted with bedrock, you admitted such a thing as a leap of faith, you admitted a moral axiom as a built-in part of truth, that some core of law is intrinsically binding and given. You could no longer say you had no religion, or that you took nothing on faith; your argument was breached.

Roland asked if the fast was over, since the sun was down. The sky was purple before them. Roland drew a long stem of grass from its sheath and nibbled its soft end.

Ed in the next day or so did begin construction of a sukkah. Planks for the frame, and poles to lay across the top, and plywood for the sides he picked up in a lumberyard. He planned no flooring, but a room about six feet by eight feet, large enough for the Sears-Roebuck folding picnic table and some chairs. He was uncertain whether to hang a door on hinges or leave the entry open, and decided at last not to bother with a door. The top was to be open to the sky.

He got the notion while he worked that it would be good to sleep in it under the stars a few times during the week, if the warm weather continued, and if the mosquitoes did not prove too bad. When he had a chance he drove to Boston and bought a pair of inflatable mattresses at Brine's Sporting Goods.

Roland helped him with the construction sometimes, or sometimes just sat on the covered garbage can by the side door from the kitchen and watched. Roland's friends hung around too now and then, asking questions, walking upon the planks, chinning themselves. Roland's circle of friends was growing, it seemed to Ed. There was O'Shaughnessy and the Vaughn kid, and lately a Speedball Keneally was around a lot.

Meanwhile the O'Shaughnessy boy reported that he couldn't sleep in the sooky. Father Donahue had okayed it, but his parents had found out there wouldn't be any roof.

It was barely built in time for the Feast of Tabernacles, and Patty climbed in knee-length shorts onto a chair that tilted a little on the uneven ground, and helped Ed string fruits and vegetables and bunches of grapes to the overhead poles that lay where a roof should be. There had not been time to paint the wood, and he warned her to look out for splinters. They hung some of Lucinda's tomatoes. It would be nice to grow a variety of produce in one's back yard and decorate the sukkah only out of one's own harvest, he thought.

It occurred to him that next year he might offer to build sukkahs for other families in the congregation, or help build them, in their own back yards, on condition they would use it, at least for a meal or two. He enjoyed carpentry—there was a satisfaction in making something.

A couple of the trees out back had turned red and yellow, though most were green, and Patty suggested he hang a couple of boughs too.

"Good idea," he said.

Lucinda came across the grass to the sukkah and told him Phil Walker had phoned. Phil had been supposed to get palm fronds and citrons in Boston for the membership to wave and hold during the service at the temple that evening, and had brought a station wagon full of palm fronds, but could get no citrons.

Ed continued tying a pumpkin high overhead, without answering. He had better scout around for lemons then, he thought. There wasn't much time.

Roland came out of the side door, slamming the screen.

"Want to come to the A.&P.," Ed asked him, "and help me get some crates of lemons?"

"I have to go on my paper route," said Roland.

"Well, okay," said Ed.

24

Millicent had not come home this time, but Ed, Lucinda, Patty and Roland had supper together in the sukkah, at the tin Sears-Roebuck table beneath the hanging fruits and the open sky. Roland was told he would have to wait till another night to sleep in it. Ed said he had decided to reserve the first night for Mama and himself.

He carried the chairs back to the kitchen late in the evening and when he brought the inflated mattresses he was already in pajamas and bathrobe. The tinny picnic table leaned on a wall, its legs folded inside. He lay down beneath an old patchwork quilt. The sky was clear. He could see stars, and a small hanging pumpkin twisted this way and that before them. On his way across the yard he had noticed a rising moon, outsized and yellow, full as it always was on this holiday, but now that he lay in the quilt a wall of the sukkah hid it. He felt the rubbery hills and crevices under the sheet. They had a peculiar springiness.

The screen door on the house sounded, and Lucinda came across the grass in her robe and nightgown. She got under the quilt without saying anything and without touching him. His eyes were used enough to the darkness to see her lying there, staring up at the hanging shadows.

"Are the kids asleep?" he asked.

"Patty's in the kitchen. She's studying."

He heard crickets. They sounded far off and sluggish. Beyond them he could hear the steady gurgling of the brook.

"This is ridiculous," Lucinda said. "We have a house."

"We also have a sky."

"If ants start walking on me I'm going in. You'll wake up all alone."

"People camp out all the time."

"What'll we do if it rains," she said.

"We'll go in the house."

"I think it is raining, or drizzling or something."

"That's just dew. It's perfectly clear. Look at the sky."

She settled deeper in the quilt. "You're a madman," she said.

Over at the house the screen door opened and shut again, and Roland asked loudly whether he could have some cake. Lucinda told him to take it from the refrigerator. And if he took milk to be sure and put it away again.

But Roland's footsteps came down the wooden stoop and through the grass.

He stood at the entrance of the sukkah, looking down at his parents. He was in pajamas.

"Are you barefoot?" Lucinda asked him. "You'll catch cold."

"How are the mattresses?" said Roland.

"They're fine," said Ed. "Now go have your cake and don't bother us until morning. Tell Patty not to either."

Roland's feet receded into the grass. They heard him go in.

"I wish you hadn't said that," Lucinda said. "Now they'll think we're making love or something."

"It never entered his mind."

"It might. And Patty's certainly old enough to wonder."

"It was a natural thing to say. We want to sleep, that's all."

He turned toward her, and embraced her in silence. She didn't move. He heard her breathing. He felt her softness and her warmth. He adjusted himself against her.

"Don't, Ed. Not out here in the yard."

"Why not?"

"It's not practical," she said.

"Sure it is."

"Well, it makes me feel funny."

He let her alone and rolled to his own side. But he gave her hand a slight pressure. For a while they were quiet. Then when he looked he saw her staring up as before toward her tomatoes and the sky.

"Ed—" she said.

"What."

"Have you had a talk with Charles since he enlisted? I mean about sex and all that? You know, boys away from home. They can get diseased and all that."

"Well, we did have a talk. Not at that time. Not recently, I guess. Maybe I should again."

"How did he take it?"

"Well, he was a little embarrassed."

"Every boy I see in uniform still has this resemblance to him," she said gloomily. "Honest, it's the weirdest thing. There was even a magazine at the hairdresser's, with a picture of boys in Korea."

"Did you worry about me that way? When I was in the North Atlantic?" He spoke softly.

"It's not the same. Sure, I worried."

"He's not even in Korea. What'll you do if he actually gets there?"

"I don't know."

"This Inchon thing has turned the tide, anyway. If you look how that area's expanded in ten days. I don't think he'll even get there."

His hand lay upon her wrist, beneath the quilt.

"Do you really think he'll be all right?" she said.

"Yes, I do. I really do. He's mature for his age. And he has a head on his shoulders. He doesn't get into trouble."

He patted her arm, moving his fingers in a kind of tapping. But she lay still.

"If we buy the house," she said after a while, "the rent we already paid counts toward the down payment, doesn't it?"

"No. A little of it, technically. The down payment would just about clean us out. Empty the savings."

"But it's still supposed to be a good investment to buy, if you're living in a place."

"Not till you know you're going to stay. When they put me on tenure, then it's time to think about buying."

"Well, I'm ready to settle down."

"I'm ready to settle down too, but so what? We haven't been here half a year yet. I think next year I could demand tenure and get it. But in the meantime it isn't prudent to tie ourselves up with a house."

"If it's that sure you'll get tenure we could still buy now, instead of waiting."

"I didn't say sure. I'd say very likely."

"It's the same thing."

"Even if we do stay here, you don't necessarily buy the first house you see. We moved into this one because we could rent it, that's all. Nobody's pushing us to buy. We've got the option here, and in the meantime we can see what else opens up in town. Let's see how it is in the winter first, what it costs to heat the place."

"Don't you think it would be good for Charles if we bought it? I don't want to go changing his address behind his back."

"How long did he live here? Three months?"

"He still has a room upstairs. And when he's so far from home it's all the more important that he knows he has a home, and that he knows where it is."

"I don't want to move either. But wait six or seven months. Until we've got a permanent contract and we're secure."

"I should think you'd want the children to be secure," she said.

He thought of explaining that that was not what was at stake. But it seemed useless.

"And in the meantime," she said, "we can't paint it, and we can't buy things for it, and we can't fix it, and we can't do anything, because we don't own it. Please, honestly, Ed. I don't want to be a gypsy any more. I couldn't stand another move. The way things get busted. I'm not all unpacked yet from the last move. Let's don't wait to see what the heat costs. Look, we've never, never owned a house. And after all I've put into these gardens."

"All right," he said.

"What?"

"Okay."

"What okay?"

"We'll buy it."

"You mean it? Really?"

"I mean it."

"What changed your mind?"

"You did."

He lay thinking about what he had said. There did seem to be some recklessness in owning a home here before the congregation had granted him permanent tenure, signed and sealed. Yet in recent weeks this consideration had seemed more and more a technicality. In the unlikely event of his having to find another congregation elsewhere, the house could be sold, and though it would be a risk and a nuisance, the chance was small enough to be worth the risk. And as for shopping for a better house in Wilmerding Crosswalk, assuming he stayed with this congregation, he sensed that her instinct was right that no difference in houses was likely to justify the trouble.

So let her own, let her paint. She had talked of it all summer. Of the new rug that might not fit the next house, of the narrow lace curtains for the bay window that would be useless elsewhere.

"You're a darling," she said finally. "Thank you."

"That's okay."

"You're sweet, Ed. Sometimes you're sweet."

"How about a kiss?" he said.

She kissed him.

Then he lay thinking about the shabbiness of the house. It would need a lot of repair.

By the time Charles finished his two-year hitch, Millicent might be married. And Patty would finish high school and perhaps live at college somewhere. Even so, if someday there were grandchildren, it was good for a grandchild to have grandparents who were long settled in a house, a big house.

He thought of things he would like to do to improve the house and the grounds.

The moon had risen higher. He could still not see it, but up where the fruits and vegetables dangled he could even make out their colors in the grayness, and their shadows were quite sharp in a long triangle of moonlight on the plywood wall.

He told Lucinda he would like to build a kind of permanent sukkah here, with removable walls so that in summer it could be used as a rose bower.

"You have a one-track mind," she said.

But he explained that it would be an open framework of white, with flooring green or brown in heavy outdoor paint, and all around it white trelliswork would be nailed. He would make a plank table and benches for it, stained redwood, and it would be pleasant to sit there in its openness in summer, among the varicolored climbing roses and the butterflies. Perhaps it could be built instead in the field on the other side of the house, where the ground was higher. A birdbath would be set in line with it. And once a year, for the eight days of the Feast of Tabernacles, vertical boards would be attached from the inside with brass screws, to form the walls and transform the bower into a sukkah. The boards would be in matching white facing outside and varnished natural wood within, and redwood poles would be screwed athwart the white crossbeams overhead, from which to hang fruits and vegetables. Maybe he could buy outdoor candle fixtures of copper, with glass shields.

And then perhaps he might even make a grape arbor too, over a walk, leading that way from somewhere near the house, and stopping equidistant from the birdbath, just opposite.

"Anyway I thought you told me a sooky is supposed to remind us that our houses aren't permanent," she said to him, "and now you want to make a permanent sooky."

As he spoke they had been hearing a train, and now it was louder, just through the woods. The pulling of wheels went on and on.

"Is that the Montreal express?" said Lucinda.

"No. Not at this hour. It's a freight."

One of his hands lay off the mattress and he could feel the vibration in the ground. He looked overhead to see if the train shook the vegetables too, but it did not seem to. A little crook-necked squash turned this way and that.

They knew when the caboose had passed, and the sound grew softer. At length they could hear the brook again.

"Anyway I don't think I like sookies," she added, "if that's what they mean."

"Let's have another baby."

"Oh sure," she said.

"Seriously."

"Are you kidding?"

"Why shouldn't we? While there's still time?"

"It's a disgusting idea."

"What's disgusting about it?"

"Because we have a daughter twenty-two years old. And Roland's twelve—he'd be thirteen. You don't have children thirteen years apart. It would look like an accident."

"What of it?"

"No. I'm too old, and I don't want any more of your crazy tricks. A mother of a twenty-two-year-old doesn't start having babies. I'm too old to have the patience to take care of it. Go through all that again."

"Why should we wait for grandchildren? We're experienced now. We wouldn't have to make so many mistakes."

"I'm just not up to it," she said.

"Patty'd help you. You have a built-in baby-sitter."

"I can imagine what the girls would think. 'Oh Mother, how barbaric.' "

"What?"

"You know how Millicent talks. She'd have some fancy word."

"I bet she wouldn't," he said.

"And we'd be old when the child's in high school. It's not fair to a child. I'd be sixty when the child's how old?"

"Seventeen," he said.

"Seventeen."

"Sixteen," he corrected himself.

"Sixteen. With a sixty-year-old mother. And you'd be sixty-two."

"Well, it's not ideal. We probably couldn't make him perfectly happy. But we could make him happy enough to be glad he was born. I think it's a fine idea. You have to look at the world as if it's just begun. Things are fresh."

"Well you and I haven't just begun," she said. "You have to grow up." Her voice sounded tired.

The conversation stopped. In a little while he tried to sleep. Lucinda changed her position and soon he heard her sleeping. Yet for a long time he did not.

The luminous white moon lifted to where he could see it, small now, between two slats. He saw a moth flutter black across it.

The crickets were weak.

He arose once and went to urinate in the high grass, near the rusty harrow. The entire house was visible in moonlight. All its windows were dark. He wondered what lives had been lived in it before him, and who had loved it. Especially when it was new, so long ago. Other people, other separations. He remembered his grandfather's house—was there also someone living still, far off, who yet remembers this house as a grandfather's house? And wonders who lives here now, what boors now defile it? And would it sadden them to see it now, an old house, no longer stylish, the barn and the great trees rotting, the gardens in changed locations, the yard somehow more barren, and strangers dwelling therein who hadn't known them?

How awful, how useless it must be, to seek out an old house and say to those who dwell there now, I lived here in childhood, I played in the attic with my sister. I helped my father plant this tree. There was a swing there—

He lay down on the mattress, beside his sleeping wife.

Several times he awoke, aware of having dreamed, though the dreams fled at once.

He heard the town clock. There's Caleb's clock, he thought. Does he climb the steeple to wind it, or what?

There was a wind in the trees. He slept more soundly.

The morning was bright and lovely. A few damp yellowing leaves had fallen to the quilt. He looked at Lucinda. The night before she had looked tired, but now she had a prettiness in her sleep, quite like the beauty she had had as a girl in Mattapan, when she had taught swimming, and had been a junior life guard. He lay looking at her.

It was strange, that he and she should have been tied together for a lifetime. Another year and it's a quarter century. A second quarter century still to go.

He could have done worse. She hadn't left him in twenty-four years. And she had never spent more than he earned.

He lay on his back. Beyond the slats, and beyond part of a bough high over them, the sky was a cloudless blue.

And she had even gone along with sleeping here outdoors last night. Yet only yesterday morning there had been a nasty argument. He had installed some pothooks in the pantry cabinets, and she had given him wrong instructions about where she wanted them, and changed her mind, but then she had bawled him out without cause, and talked in a tone she might use to a moron, and accused him falsely of not having listened. Yet her second pot arrangement, which she claimed had been her first, was impossible anyway—she had wanted a pan sixteen inches long to hang from a hook thirteen inches from the floor.

It had always been like that. He thought of their life together. Their courtship had even been in the midst of arguments. Directly after the elopement she had left him in an argument and had fled back to Grandma Annie with the marriage still unconsummated, and they had remained apart for three weeks, until a second ceremony was arranged. He married her twice in three weeks. But Lucinda at nineteen had been unready for marriage. She had been a bitter vixen, shrewish, and her mouth could be foul, so that in the friction of those early years he came to detest the burden of having to make up day by day for the sake of the infant, and with effort renew their unspectacular love, when it would have been more satisfying to go away mad—even a more joyous love to go away mad. And when he decided to sell his interest in the car lot and enter the seminary she baited him for years, in a chilling way.

It always seemed afterwards that the arguments were unnecessary. He had lost aunts, uncles, some of whom he had loved, and some of whom were parents of cousins he loved, and yet he could rarely get Lucinda to pay a condolence call or go to a funeral without an argument first. She said she didn't like funerals. He told her that nobody liked funerals, but that it was a time for the survivors to be together, to be fortified with kin while they asked what it was all about, and to affirm that life was worth living. She retorted that the dead didn't know if people came and sat around or not. Then she argued vehemently that when she died she wanted no funeral, no service, no prayers, no burial, no nothing—she did not want somebody paid to mow the grass on her grave forever. She had gone along with all the damn religion in her lifetime and in her death at least she should be free of it, and have a death in accord with her convictions. He asked her if she wanted to be cut off from her people in death. She said yes, that that was the kind of phony baloney she detested. He told her not to worry, that he'd throw her body in the garbage pail. She said she wanted it given to science. She wouldn't offend her relatives with a cremation, but burials and funerals were out. He asked if she wanted a couple of young boys in some medical school slicing her into bits for their first-year anatomy course. He told her he'd feed her corpse to the animals at Franklin Park. Feeding time was 3:30 p.m., he said, and the tigers didn't get human meat often, and since she believed all life was fair game to be eaten it would be appropriate that she be eaten also. So she had replied that the main thing was that there be no weeping, and he told her not to worry, he'd celebrate.

He had been sorry afterward. His grandfather never would have lost his temper like that.

It was stupid to let her get your goat. Especially as what seemed her most cherished opinions she could forget overnight anyway. Just as she could nag you for the construction of a shelf in some very difficult place, as though she couldn't manage another hour without it, and with no conception of the problems of fitting and support it posed, and accuse you of selfishness, and then, when the shelf was built, never use it.

It seemed to him that they had not begun to get along tolerably well until he had told himself that she would never be fair or rational, she would never admit a point of view that did not tend to prove her own rightness, and that if they were to stay together he must learn to bear with this. As long as he expected justice from his wife, they would quarrel. You couldn't let on that you were trying to be a saint—that would destroy the sainthood and lead to a new quarrel about whose fault some preceding quarrel had been. First you discover, he thought, that she would sooner deny she had said what she said than admit she could be wrong about anything. She would contradict herself and shift the ground of argument, rather than acknowledge a mistake. And then you find she respects you more if your thoughts are a mystery. So little by little you learn to hold your tongue. To dwell and brood upon your spouse, what you said and what she said—it's unbecoming for one created in the image of God. It's not fitting. It's better to try to be dignified. People may still not understand you, but maybe at least they respect you. It goes for your wife among others. And you do bicker less. The early years of regretting that you've tied yourself by children to this alien mind pass on, and little by little you learn to be taciturn without rancor. To let your wife do the talking while you do the thinking. And she had mellowed. Her tongue mellowed. There was a line in the thrice-daily prayer that said, to those who insult me let my soul be silent—and he had told himself sometimes, in those early years, that if he could in time absorb that phrase, in all its force, it would enable him to get along with his wife.

And there was nothing wrong with her, he said to himself. Even in those worst early years he had always known she was a person of good will and of responsibility. And sometimes, he thought, when she was tender, and her mood was soft, you would catch a glimpse in her of that unreal person you love.

It was simply that by the time he had made her pregnant they had discovered that they couldn't talk to each other. He had been a man who loved bull sessions, philosophy, discussion, but to Lucinda a bull session was an argument. She had no hankering for order in the larger sense. Her mind was entirely utilitarian. And if she didn't understand him, hadn't she also had reason to complain that he didn't understand her? Who said they were supposed to understand each other? A wife wasn't for bull sessions. She wasn't a college roommate, he had told himself at last. A wife fulfills a special area, just as a husband does for a wife, just as a parent does, or your dentist does.

Donate her body to science, she said. Science. She had no interest in the simplest principles of physics. She couldn't even comprehend a bicycle chain.

He had tried to explain it to her, but she kept insisting that the faster-turning end must exert the more force. She couldn't read a map. She could not even today stand in the front yard and point which way was the Atlantic Ocean, or which way was New Hampshire. Nor did she have any instinct for law, torts, justice. In Abbottsford she had wanted to tell the landlord that children's crayon markings upon the wallpaper should be counted as wear and tear, but when the landlord's decrepit storm door escaped from her and cracked in a gale while she struggled to lock it she called that her own negligence, and wanted to offer reimbursement.

Such religious obligations as she performed she regarded as a drag—something she had to do for him, like ironing his shirts. She could spend her life married to a clergyman, after growing up with a moderately pious father, and not have curiosity enough to open a book or take a course and see what it was about. As though convinced in her heart beforehand it must be about nothing.

People's hearts and minds aren't close, just because they fall in love and marry, he thought. And perhaps it didn't matter, because real discussion beyond a certain point requires specialists anyway.

It would be good if he could explain religion to Lucinda as he was explaining it to Betsy Stokes. But who knew what Betsy would turn into in a couple of years of marriage? Perhaps the perfect woman for him did exist, but in some other city. Perhaps the girl who would have made him an ideal match would be born on the day of his death.

But there had been a time, he reflected, when people lived in villages and sat at many tables; in those generations, if what filled your mind and sustained your soul was of no interest to your wife it didn't matter—you talked to your cousin or your neighbor. Today, if you couldn't talk to your wife, you were doomed to isolation and silence. The automobile had isolated people, by moving friends far apart, so that visiting was a project, and you lost your companions.

A man can remain at odds with his wife for a lifetime, and afterward mourn her death—he had seen it a number of times. Because by then the isolation was complete.

He saw the sun glisten on the dewy vegetables. Beside him in the sukkah Lucinda stirred, but she did not waken. Her face lay toward him, and still had the prettiness that had pleased him when his eyes had first opened to the morning. He wondered if it would remain with her when she woke. Some mornings she looked drawn, but not now.

You have to see her as a stranger, he thought.

She stirred again. He wanted to touch her.

This is the real meaning of Adam's rib, he thought. A man without a woman hasn't got all of himself. Possibly a woman can manage some kind of completeness alone, but not the male. He's as if with a chunk lost out of his flesh.

She wakened, looking straight at him.

"Hi," he said.

"Hi," she said, not taking her cheek from the sheet. She still had the prettiness.

He kissed her, somewhat prolongedly.

"What's that for?" she asked.

"Fun." He kissed her again.

Beneath the quilt his embrace smoothed her goose pimples, the nightgown seeming to melt before his hands. She giggled.

"That's it," he said. "I'll make you laugh if it kills me." He smiled.

She responded to his hands and his nearness.

"Come on, kitten," he said.

"I'm not a kitten any more," she murmured. "I'm an old cat. I'm an old bag—"

But he kissed her lips, smothering the end of the sentence. A leaf or two drifted down to the back of his neck. He felt her fingers probe.

"What's the matter?"

"I just wanted to be sure," she said.

As though at leisure he brushed some pine needles and some granules of seedling that had found their way beside her head, and pushed away the stray hairs from her forehead. They were of a translucent brown. He kept working her with his gentle thrust, and the whole length of her seemed to meet him with a yawn of pliant lightness. In the midst of a dizziness he felt at the top of his strength. She made her body grip him, and relax, and grip again.

"Hey Dad? Are we gonna have breakfast in the sooky?" he heard Roland's voice not far off, and the dozing smile fled from Lucinda.

He had not heard a door. The boy must have come from delivering papers.

"Damn kid," Ed muttered.

"Ed, he's coming over here," Lucinda said. Her voice was panicky.

Ed's breathing was louder and his embrace had become a clutch. "I can't stop now, baby. I can't stop now."

25

Dexter Killian told Millicent he was sending her to work with Heustis Garvey for two weeks, that she might learn to be a police reporter, and then, during Garvey's vacation, she would be his replacement.

For a startling instant it was scarcely believable, and then it seemed a joyful destiny. She told her roommates and they squealed with happiness for her. She told Leslie also when he came for lunch on Sunday. Of course she would go back to being a copy boy again after Mr. Garvey's vacation, but she had made the break-through. Mr. Killian was grooming her.

She told in detail how Mr. Killian had beckoned with his head, and stood up and bent toward her, resting one foot on a pulled-out drawer. She would work not at the city room but at the press room in Police Headquarters, with her own telephone, desk by desk with reporters from other papers, who would be her rivals. Mr. Garvey would introduce her to the police captains and police inspectors who were his special informants, and even to detectives of the homicide squad.

People thought Mr. Killian was hard-boiled, she said, but actually he was a man of vision and ideals.

Her absence at the city room would be covered by having Zucchino work somewhat different hours, the way he did on her nights off. And when Mr. Garvey actually went on vacation, and left her on her own, she would have a press card with her own name, issued by the police, and she would have to show it to firemen when stepping over fire hoses and going where other people could not go. Because police reporters left their desks and hurried about the city by taxi. In a fantasy she imagined herself reaching across the murder victim for his own private telephone, in order to call the city room faster and scoop her rivals who had run downstairs to the public booth, and a kindly old police inspector warning her to cover the dead man's phone with a handkerchief first lest she leave fingerprints.

She had told Mr. Killian that she just didn't know how to thank him enough, and she asked Leslie whether he thought that must have sounded too gushy to Mr. Killian. But Leslie didn't think so. Mr. Killian had told her there was only one way to thank him—when the big one breaks, to be on top of it.

In a day or so he made her ink her thumb and press it to a card. He kept it, saying it had to be processed. Then he sent her to the photo department to have her picture snapped.

She did not actually go to Police Headquarters until Monday, because on Saturday and Sunday Mr. Garvey was off. It seemed strange to walk to that part of the city, instead of to the usual building.

She went through the zigzags of the corridor and entered with a knock. She greeted Mr. Garvey and the other men, but only Herlihy smiled and returned her greeting. The others did not look up from the card game. Herlihy rose and brought her a chair with damaged caning, that had leaned against the wall. Then he returned to the game. Their desk chairs had all been drawn to Mr. Garvey's desk. Mr. Garvey, florid and his white hair waving into the air, slapped down a card with a graceful gesture of his thumb. Millicent unbuttoned her sweater, and folded it over the back of the chair that Herlihy had brought her, and sat.

Mr. Tilton was a very big man, with a face that had boils or eruptions of some kind, and straggly blond hair. Mr. Cox was also big, but dark and a little fat, and sat with his back to her. Only young Herlihy seemed to have some refinement. She studied his pointed-seeming young face and his dark lashes.

But for a long time nothing happened but the card-playing. They're whiling the time until a story breaks, she thought. The paint on the cracked walls was dirty yellow, and above the sink it was peeling. The absurd calendar was still there, showing a waxy-complexioned nude woman stretched long-legged and unreal upon redness. There was also a new calendar, on another wall, with a color photograph of a kneeling woman who wore only some underpants of an impractical sort. Millicent left her chair and studied the picture more closely. She found its photographic sharpness disquieting. The face leaned toward the camera, smiling demure and large-jawed, clearly feeble-minded.

Behind Millicent the card game continued. She waved away cigarette smoke. A huge street map of the city, showing all fire-alarm boxes, was hung with strips of tape, and she looked at that a while. Her own shadow, cast on it by the room's unfrosted bulb, looked up at her from below. Then she found a little map that showed the boundaries of police precincts, in heavy black, and she studied that too. And there was a yellowing chart with phone numbers, including many hospitals and suburban police stations.

"One more hand and I'm going," said Tilton.

In a while Cox and Tilton left, and Garvey put the cards in a drawer. Herlihy told Garvey he would check around, and then went out also, leaving Millicent alone with Mr. Garvey.

But Garvey still scarcely acknowledged her presence. His manner gave her some feeling of awe, so that she did not know how to begin a conversation. She moved the chairs back to their desks, rolling them on their casters. Then she made neat piles of the newspapers and directories that were sprawled every which way on the other three desks, and picked up the ones that had fallen to the floor. Tomorrow she must remember to bring a dustcloth, she thought, and perhaps donate a broom and dustpan. She might bring a pail and scrubbing brush too after a few days, and a bottle of furniture polish. There was a little bathroom, with its door an inch ajar, and she wondered if there was paper toweling in there she could moisten at the sink. But she was not sure whether the bathroom might be for men only, and she didn't like to ask.

She sat at the other back desk, across from Mr. Garvey's. She wondered about his age. He looked sixty or more. She was glad of Mr. Herlihy, so that there would be another reporter her own age. And she ought to call Mr. Herlihy at least by his first name, she thought, which was John, though it would be embarrassing to begin doing so just like that, since she hadn't begun that way.

She asked Mr. Garvey to please not be afraid to give her lots to do, because she was anxious to learn all she could. He made no answer. After a minute she asked whether he always took his vacation at this time of year. He did not answer that either.

Herlihy returned, and told Garvey that in a certain district a man had stabbed his wife and child. Garvey grunted mildly in acknowledgment, and Herlihy left.

Garvey sat motionless, supported by the solid roundness of his chair.

"How do we get that story?" Millicent asked.

"What story?" He was heavy-lidded, and did not look at her.

"About the stabbing."

His large head turned in her direction, slowly, and looking somewhat irritable. "Honeybunch, I know all about that story. Nothing gets by me."

"Oh," she said. But she was uncertain what he meant. She wondered if he had telephoned the city room about it long before, or whether he wanted to await developments, or whether some policeman was already committed to bring him details. She parted her lips, as if to speak again, but apparently he had read her dissatisfaction.

"It's black," he said. "A bunch of smokes."

"What?"

"Smokes!" he said, a little louder, as though he thought her hearing was bad. "You want it? You think you're working for a smoke sheet? The Baltimore Afro-American?"

"You mean colored?" she asked.

His bulk seemed to relax and settle heavily again, as though the conversation were over.

"Mr. Herlihy seemed to think it was a good story," Millicent said.

"Herlihy's wet behind the ears. And you notice he didn't phone it in."

Millicent didn't reply, but she felt puzzled. Garvey looked at her again.

"You give in a story," he explained, "and they send a photographer, and it turns out it's black. Then what do they do?"

She kept looking at him. He leaned back in his chair and closed his eyes. For a while he seemed to doze.

She felt chilly, and massaged her arms. She got her sweater and threw it unbuttoned about her shoulders and returned to the desk she had sat at before, beside Mr. Garvey's at the back of the little room. She sneezed. The sneeze brought more irritation than relief and she sneezed again. She sneezed a third time, trying to suppress it, but the effort hurt her soft palate and she sneezed again. Her eyes felt hot and sandy. She saw Garvey half open his eyes at her and close them. Her shoulder-strap bag had been set on the window sill, with its strap hanging over the radiator, and she went to it for a handkerchief, still sneezing. The radiator felt cold. She pressed the handkerchief to her nose and mouth and knelt to turn the radiator valve this way and that. She heard no noise but the turning metal. She went back to the desk, shutting the air from her nostrils with the crushed handkerchief, and waited for the exhausting little explosions to stop jarring her.

Garvey's heavy breathing filled the room. Outdoors it was already dark and the window mirrored him palely. The phone on his desk rang, loudly, and he reached out half startled and half asleep, knocking it from its holder. Millicent leaped up and handed it to him, but he snatched it angrily and hung it up.

"Keep your hands off that!" he said. "You want me to get the sneezes too?"

From a drawer of his desk he took a bottle of disinfectant and an opened box of cotton batting. He wiped the telephone all over, carefully, not picking the receiver from its cradle, though the ringing had begun again. The moist wake of each stroke evaporated rapidly and visibly on the black. At last he disinfected the earpiece and mouthpiece.

"Headquarters, Garvey," he said into it.

But his end of the conversation consisted only of monosyllables and grunts, though it took quite some time, and finally a wheeze of laughter. Afterward he sank back and closed his eyes, though she knew he didn't sleep.

She wondered what the phone call had been about. But she felt he might be easier to get along with if she did not pester him.

She unfolded one of the papers that were piled on the desk before her, and looked for items to read. For what seemed a long time no phone rang and Garvey did not speak or move. The police radio and the fire radio muttered half intelligibly now and then, and every few minutes the hammer of the black fire bell high on the wall made a few ticks. The only other sound was the rustle of newspaper when she turned a page.

"Are there nights like this very often," she asked, "when so few stories happen?"

She thought he wasn't going to answer but then he did. "Wait till the full moon," he said without opening his eyes.

She read one newspaper and then another.

"It's gratifying that we're winning finally in Korea," she remarked.

He didn't answer.

She told him she had read some books by Walter Lippmann, and that Lippmann thought reporters were a significant force, because only through reporters could the public arrive at opinions of what it was that government officials wished it to consent to.

Garvey didn't stir, and she felt she hadn't made herself clear.

"I mean, the reporter is necessary to a democracy, as the only possible interpreter between the government and the people," she explained. "And he says a journalist who puts truth first is like a scientist or a scholar."

Garvey said nothing.

She sighed and turned again to her newspapers. Then she rose and looked at the police teletype. It was motionless.

"Would you like me to get you a sandwich?" she asked him after a moment.

"No. I don't like anybody handling my food."

"Well, would you mind if I took my supper now?" She had grown hungry.

He made a tossing gesture with the back of his hand. She buttoned her sweater and took up her shoulder-strap bag.

"I'll be back as soon as I can," she said.

In the neighborhood she found only one dingy luncheonette, in the midst of closing. A swarthy foreign man was mopping the floor. But she bought a sandwich of egg salad, and a small carton of milk with a straw, and took them back to eat beside Mr. Garvey.

When she got back he was cleaning his false teeth at the sink. She thought of asking him if anything had happened, but it seemed clear that nothing had. He restored the teeth to his mouth and sat again at his desk.

"One thing about false choppers," he said. "It don't matter how rotten the toothpaste tastes."

"Yes, I suppose so."

It was the first conversation he had initiated with her and she felt encouraged. But he said nothing more.

She finished her supper. The silence and idleness became more oppressive than ever. She heard his breathing. She thought of asking where he would spend his vacation, and whether there wasn't some work she could do. But she sensed he would rather be let alone.

She did not ask either if the toilet was considered to be for men only. She had noticed that the door was flimsy and that the least sound could be heard through it.

Toward eleven Garvey yawned and rose. He told her she had better get out because he was locking up.

She followed him through the corridor and lobby. On the street she said good night, but he made no answer.

On Tuesday she wore two sweaters. Cox and Tilton were not there, and Herlihy left fairly early. Again the evening was very long. But Garvey was on the phone more than yesterday, and once she heard him telephone a long story to the city room. Yet he scarcely acknowledged her presence. In midevening he went out and was gone a long time, whether to other parts of the building she didn't know.

She worried whether he would want her to answer his phone if it rang in his absence. She decided she had better answer if it rang, but wash it carefully with disinfectant afterward, so she could tell him she had done so. But she felt relieved when he returned without the phone having rung.

He sat as before.

"Don't you think you ought to take me around and introduce me to your sources?" she asked.

She feared he would not answer, and he did not.

"I wish you'd let me try something," she said. "I can't learn if I don't do anything."

"What makes you think you can learn this beat in two weeks?" he asked her. "Are you a ninety-day wonder out of Radcliffe?"

"I didn't go to Radcliffe," she said.

He settled with his hands on his stomach. He closed his eyes.

"I may not learn it perfectly," she told him, "but I intend to do my best. Mr. Killian has confidence in me, after all."

"Make sure he don't get anything else in you," Garvey said, without opening his eyes.

She tried to read a newspaper, but she felt too upset to put her mind to it.

"I know you don't like me very much, Mr. Garvey, but—"

He seemed not to be listening.

"I want to be friends, Mr. Garvey—"

She felt her eyes moisten.

The big hands on his stomach were as motionless as death. The veins stood out on them, and their hairs were tangled and white. Sometimes the breathing became a light snore and sometimes his eyes came half open.

She remembered that Mr. Killian had said Heustis Garvey was the dean of the New England press corps. She thought of trying to ask Herlihy, if he should ever come by again, what it was that Mr. Garvey resented about her—her youth, or being a woman, or whether he was still mad about the hot tip she had phoned from the hospital—and what she might do to make friends with him.

When her days off came she was uncertain whether Mr. Killian meant her to take her usual days, or whether he had meant to switch her days to conform to Garvey's. She was sorry she had not thought to clarify that before. At length she telephoned the city room. Mr. Hopkins spoke to her, and made her wait while he asked Mr. Killian, and then told her to take her regular days.

Wednesday night she saw Leslie and told him about Mr. Garvey. She worried that Garvey's job would be thrust upon her in two weeks with no real preparation at all. She did not know the building's mazes, and had scarcely seen a policeman except the old one in the lobby alcove.

Leslie suggested that she speak to Mr. Killian. She said she supposed she would have to, if she did not manage to work it out alone.

Being with Leslie and hearing his soft, sometimes hesitant voice was comforting. They still necked. When they did he would kiss her much now, and sometimes his fingers could drug her with a sizzling laziness. Once, after a troublesome day at the hospital, he had sought to bury his face in her soft flesh as if in a rush of heartbreak, and she had been quite moved. However she set a time limit of fifteen minutes on these things, which she stretched to twenty, but no more.

And it had not worked out badly. Their friendship had remained primarily intellectual, and once when Ella Jane was away at a hunting lodge her employer's family owned and Natalie was out, leaving the apartment vacant, they did not bother to take advantage of it. Twice they went to chamber-music concerts that cost nothing. At Aunt Gwendolyn's she reclined against him longer than twenty minutes, because baby-sitting was after all a dull way to spend an evening, and his fingers did homage to her skin as though it were velvet, but when at last she called a halt he made no protest. "It would be silly to let love play become a dominant theme in our relationship," she told him once. "It could take over like weeds in a garden." And he said he agreed.

Their talk about Garvey was in a stroll by the river, and they saw couples embracing there on the ground, with only the dark for protection, but Leslie ignored them, as did she. He always remained perfectly dignified in these public places. He talked of borrowing a car but she discouraged it.

Natalie and Ella Jane had offered to arrange to be out, but she had asked them never to do that on her account, and only go out if they had planned to do so anyway. "This is your home," she said to them.

Friday afternoon she went back to the press room at Police Headquarters. She found Cox and Tilton and Herlihy there, playing cards with Garvey again around his desk, and there were also some men she had never seen before, with hats and jackets, sitting on desks and window sills. She supposed them to be photographers because she saw big cameras and leather cases. She sat at Mr. Herlihy's vacant desk to read newspapers.

The phone rang upon it and Tilton seized it. He spoke briefly and put it down. "They're here," he said to the others.

Everyone seemed to spring into activity. Tilton and Cox and Herlihy put on their jackets. Herlihy pulled open a drawer, almost bumping Millicent with it, and took a notebook from it.

"What is it?" she asked him.

"They brought in the car-theft ring. Better get on it."

"Where?"

"Out front. They're bringing 'em upstairs."

He ran out down the zigzag corridor after the others. Millicent rose. Only Garvey remained seated.

"Aren't you going?" she said.

He looked groggy. On the desk before him the cards still lay about.

"Mr. Garvey!" she said. She stepped toward his desk.

His eyes found her.

"We have to get that story, Mr. Garvey."

"Sit down."

"We'll be scooped!" she said.

"I'm an old man," he said. "My legs ain't what they used to be."

"I'll go then," she said, and turned to get her shoulder-strap bag.

"Sit down," he told her, with an edge in his voice.

She looked at him. An anger and redness had come into his face.

"Or I'll slap ya down," he added.

She sat.

"Don't move," he said.

The phone on his desk began to ring. She felt confused and frightened. She had a vision of Mr. Killian holding Mr. Garvey and herself both responsible, and firing them both. But on the other hand maybe Mr. Garvey knew what he was doing. Maybe he was waiting for some bigger story. The phone sat before him, still ringing. He made no move to answer it. She thought of answering it, or of asking him if she should. But she knew what the answer would be, and did not.

The phone stopped ringing. Then it started again. He still ignored it. He did not take his eyes from her.

Oh dear, she thought.

She sat and sat. Sometimes it was quiet, except for the low muttering police and fire radios, and sometimes a phone rang, usually Garvey's, but he never answered it and neither did she. In time voices and footsteps returned to the corridor, and Herlihy, Tilton and Cox came in without the photographers. They pulled chairs together and huddled with open notebooks, comparing impressions and details aloud. There was a quickness in the way they talked.

Millicent listened from where she sat. The criminals had been charged in an outlying district and brought to Headquarters to be mugged for the rogues' gallery and fingerprinted. She heard where they would be jailed overnight, and where the arraignment would take place, and much about their exploits. Garvey sat now as if half asleep. But he took a bottle from one of his drawers and swallowed a gulp. Then he screwed the cap back on and put it away. The other three, with heads leaning toward one another over their books, seemed concerned that their stories be in agreement, and Millicent noticed that the two older men kept deferring to Herlihy. Sometimes Cox and Tilton scribbled busily while Herlihy dictated, pausing every few words for them to catch up.

At last Cox and Tilton pulled their chairs quickly to their desks and dialed their telephones.

"Give it in for me, kid, will ya, like a nice fella?" Garvey said to Herlihy. Garvey dialed his own phone, and Millicent heard him talk thickly to Mr. Hopkins and then to Maud Dickinson. Then he handed the phone to Herlihy.

"Hi, Maud, Johnny Herlihy," he said into it. "Good. And you?"

He proceeded to tell the story, quickly, but with little pauses. He stood with the phone by Garvey's desk. Meanwhile Cox and Tilton sat speaking into their own phones, as if with great urgency. Garvey sat slack-jawed, looking at nothing. I just can't believe it, Millicent thought. These men were supposed to be bitter rivals. Herlihy finished with Garvey's phone and went to his own. Millicent had already moved aside for him.

She heard him tell the story again, this time to his own paper. At last he buckled on his trench coat, and Cox and Tilton put on their hats, and they went out together, casually and jovially.

Millicent looked at Garvey. He yawned. He produced the bottle again, drank from it, and put it away. He gathered the cards, shuffled them, and flipped the deck noisily. She noticed how worn and dirty they were.

"Play gin?" he asked her.

"No."

"What good are you," he said.

He flipped the deck glumly.

"I'd be happy to learn," she said. "If you want. To help pass the time."

"I don't play gin to pass the time," he told her. "I play gin to play gin. All right. Look. Come here."

She pulled Herlihy's chair beside Garvey's desk, facing him, and he dealt.

She found the game difficult at first, but they played the hand, and he helped her from time to time, his voice more kindly than she had ever heard it, and showed her what to do.

He dealt again and they played a new hand. He put a pile of wire clips near her and another by himself, and said they would use them for counters.

He became more talkative. He told her all the different cities he had worked in. He had even worked on the old Boston Transcript. He had had seven different papers shot out from under him. And he wasn't worried about rumors that this one was going to fold either.

"Is that true?" she asked him anxiously. "Is there such a rumor? That the paper's going to fold?"

He didn't bother answering. But he went on to tell her about his power over police officials. One officer had tried to pull a double cross, three years ago, and as a result had not seen his name in print since. Only the other day he had come in and sat where Millicent now sat—an inspector, he told her, in uniform—and pleaded for forgiveness, with tears in his eyes, but Garvey had called him a son of a bitch and told him to get out.

They played some hands without talking.

He took another drink, and this time he left the bottle on the desk.

"Are you sure you wouldn't like me to get you a sandwich?" she asked. "It would do you good. That's not very nourishing, just whisky."

"It's nourishing," he said. He played a card, with a slapping sound.

"No it's not."

"Honeybunch," he said, "you went to college, but you don't know everything. Alcohol happens to be the safest food known to man."

"It is not. How could it be? What do you mean, 'safest'?"

"Because a God damn germ can't make a living in it. You get a cut or a scratch, and what do you clean it with? Alcohol."

"That has nothing to do with it. You still have to eat."

"Eat what? Milk? Do you happen to know that microscopic organisms start multiplying in milk the minute you open it to the air? That's why milk sours. The sour is nothing but the crap products from all these small little microbes. Or take meat. Bacteria. By the million, in a dinky quarter pound. Or bread. Bread collects all the dirt, don't it? Like a sponge. You keep your eye on a piece of bread and you'll see mold start to form. Spores. All right, vegetables," he said. He gestured, not with the hand that held his cards. "Where do they grow. In the dirt, right? Manure. Which happens to be a carrier of every disease known to man, and that includes polio. You think you can wash that off? It grows right up in the inside, it's absorbed. And all the bird stuff on it, and dog stuff. Right with the farmer's dirty shoes. You can even boil it, and as soon as the temperature goes down the germs go right back in again."

She stared at him. But he was looking at her with frowning intensity.

"You ever walk in a store?" he said. "A fly comes out of the garbage and walks on the tomatoes. And every customer handles it. And the store guy handles it, and how do you know what kind of disease he's got."

"Don't you ever eat?"

"Sure I eat. Of course I eat. And I smoke, too. And do you realize what crap collects in the big colon, the small colon? It's a breeding ground. That's why the whole stomach and intestines should be completely sterilized at least once a day. The alcohol kills all that. Ask any doctor. They age whisky twenty years, right? And it's better than ever. Why? Because it can't spoil. But would you age a ham sandwich twenty years? It stinks in twenty days. I got a weak stomach and a weak liver, and I can't risk it. I got to keep clean."

"Alcohol is bad for the liver."

"Oh no." He gestured. "Don't tell me about sclerosis of the liver. What's pickled in alcohol never spoils. You go in a medical school and they show you an appendix, or a foetus with two heads. In a bottle. And what's it preserved in? Alcohol. It'll last that way a hundred years. That's what they did to Lenin in the Kremlin. Dead twenty-six years, and all his organs in perfect shape. That proves it, don't it? I'll prove it again. You ever go to a dentist, to look at your teeth? And you brush your teeth and you get cavities anyway, right? And what did the dentist tell you causes decay? Food particles, right? Rots the bone. But did a dentist ever tell you alcohol rots the teeth?"

She gave no answer, though she knew he waited for one. She concentrated on her cards.

"Did he?" Garvey insisted.

"No."

"No. If I understood that thirty years ago I'd have my teeth. A guy's got dandruff, losing his hair, and he goes to the barber for some hair tonic. What's in hair tonic?"

She was determined not to go along with this.

"Alcohol," he said. He played the card that ended the hand, and counted some clips from her pile. He shuffled the cards and gave her the deck.

She dealt, methodically back and forth. "You can get along perfectly well without vitamins, I suppose. Or minerals."

"Minerals are rocks," he said, taking up the cards she dealt him one by one. "The body can't burn them. That's why you get gallstones."

"And vitamins?"

"Vitamins spoil too. You don't know how long that stuff's been on the shelf. There's only one safe vitamin, and that's sunshine."

"Are you married?"

"Divorced," he said. "Been divorced seventeen years."

"Did you have any children?"

"No. Why?"

"I just wondered."

"Sunshine. That's the only one you can trust," he said. "Because sunshine's a germ-killer."

She gathered up her hand and spaced the cards.

"Honeybunch," he said, "all religions are based on alcohol. The Catholics, the Jews, everybody. God's blood turns into wine, with alcohol in it."

They played a long time without discussion. Then he told her she owed him twelve dollars and fifteen cents.

"Oh dear," she said. "Were we playing for money?"

"What'd you think? Marbles?"

She sighed, and rose from the chair. "Well, I suppose it's all right, this once. If that's the only way you enjoy it." She got her bag from where it sat on a window sill, its strap curled about it. "I really can't afford it."

"That was your lookout."

"Is it all right if I pay you in installments?" She looked into the bag.

"Sure."

"It would make it a lot easier." She rummaged, and took some crumpled bills. "I'll pay you three dollars now, and I promise I'll pay you the rest as soon as possible."

He put the money in his trousers.

She sat at Herlihy's desk, thinking of the money she had lost. She wanted to get Ella Jane a birthday present this week.

She sneezed, and then had to sneeze several times, against the crushed handkerchief. It seemed to exhaust her eyes.

"Is it possible to get some heat from that radiator?" she asked finally.

"We don't get no steam at night."

She breathed through her mouth, against the handkerchief.

"Whisky's the best thing for a cold," he said.

"I know, my father takes it. But I think I'll pass it up if you don't mind. It's not really a cold. It's just an allergy I have. Dust and things."

"There's no dust here."

On Saturday she did not see Mr. Garvey, as he was off, and she worked instead at the city room, doing her copy-boy duties. The same was true on Sunday. During Sunday evening Mr. Hopkins told her to report to the city room again the following day, instead of to Garvey. She asked why, and he said he didn't know, that it was Killian's orders.

When she came in Monday Mr. Killian beckoned her. Then he stood and leaned on his arms, his hands on his desk, and looked down at it, wrinkling his forehead and his face. He said Heustis had told him she was not catching on quickly, and he had decided she was still too young and inexperienced to take over a beat like Headquarters. He waved her away.

She walked toward the teletype machines at the far end of the room. Stories hung from them, spilling in rolls on the floor. Her face tightened and she sobbed. But she sniffled and made herself suppress it. There was a long night's work ahead of her.

26

Millicent had sometimes to go to Maud Dickinson in order to take Maud's stories a page at a time to Mr. Hopkins, and also passed Maud's desk often on the way to rip stories from the clacking teletype machines. Quite early in the evening Maud asked her why she looked so miserable.

Later on Maud told her she thought Heustis must have been upset mainly by the suggestion that he could be replaced by a mere copy boy, with no reporting experience at all. Maud seemed to feel that it had in fact been an unthinking and tactless arrangement for Mr. Killian to make, and that Mr. Killian ought to have known better. She kept referring to him as Dexter.

Millicent was a little comforted by the thought that her failure had actually had nothing to do with herself.

Then on Tuesday Mr. Killian beckoned her with his head and handed her a press card, saying only that she might need it sometime. He gestured her back to work with his thumb, scarcely looking at her.

She was surprised. There it was, the card he had meant for her to use during Garvey's vacation. Apparently the machinery of city government had just now processed it. Yet he need not have given it to her. Apparently he did still intend that other opportunities would arise.

When she had a chance she displayed it to Maud. She loved the warmth of Maud's smile. It showed bridgework and all but shut her eyes, wrinkling up the whole skinny powdered face.

Millicent read the card's tiny print many times during the evening. An impressive municipal seal had molded hills and valleys into the lettering and even into her tiny photograph. She was quite certain that Zucchino and Dawn did not have press cards.

She resolved to keep it always tucked in her knee sock, ready for emergency.

The first of her nights off was one on which Leslie was not scheduled to be on call, so during the day she bought a roast, in order that he might dine at the apartment with herself and her roommates. She also bought some enormous mushrooms, and then artichokes, avocados, capers, imported Scottish marmalade and British tonics, spending more than she had intended. She had eaten with him in the hospital cafeteria and knew the drabness and sameness of its fare.

She discovered only in midafternoon that Ella Jane had to work very late and would not join them.

Toward five, shortly before Millicent was to put the roast in the oven, her mother came tiredly up the stairs with large oblong bundles. She had not known her mother was in Boston.

Lucinda put down the bundles, kissed Millicent, and greeted Natalie, who was in underwear, working at the ironing board. She explained that she had gone to the sale at Filene's to look for a dress for Patty. Patty was joining the Rainbow, she said, and needed a white dress for the initiation. She let herself fall to the studio couch and pushed off her shoes.

She looked worn. She said she hadn't found what she wanted at Filene's and had walked to several other stores, and had seen a coat that was perfect for Millicent.

She asked where Ella Jane was. Natalie said she was working late.

"Would you like a cup of tea, Mrs. Gordon?" Natalie asked her.

"Oh, you're a darling," said Lucinda.

"I'll put the water on," said Millicent.

She wanted to start the roast, and to begin preparing the mushrooms, but she hesitated. Her mother would involve herself in it, and would ask why such a large fancy dinner was being made for two girls, and she would have to explain that they were having a young man for company. She knew the questions her mother would ask. She even knew her mother's discreetness, and just how she and Leslie would appear through her mother's eyes.

So she delayed putting on the roast, and kept away from the kitchen, trusting that her mother would stay only a moment. She heard her mother running water in the bathroom.

But her mother came back and sat with her tea a long time, not drinking it but blowing on it gently. Millicent asked if she would like some milk to cool it. But her mother said no and talked on in a leisurely way, about the awful crowds in the stores, and about Patty, and started to explain to Natalie what the Order of the Rainbow for Girls was, but Natalie said she knew. They had had it in Chicopee also. Lucinda said it met in the Masonic lodge over the A.&P. in Wilmerding Crosswalk, and told Millicent that it would be very good for Patty. Polly Cook and almost all the girls were in it.

At length she rose in her stocking feet and untied one of the oblong bundles. She lifted up the white satin dress and showed it to Millicent and Natalie. It was long and sleeveless, with tiers of ruffle about the skirt.

"Oh, that's lovely," Natalie said.

Lucinda talked about how she would alter it, and how Patty was tall, and big in the hips and bust, and how she would take in some in the waist. Natalie nodded politely.

In any case dinner won't be ready in time for Leslie's arrival, Millicent thought.

She had the feeling that her mother's visit had been brought on in part by her own failure to visit Wilmerding Crosswalk since the holidays.

Her mother sat in the worn stuffed chair sipping tea, and massaged the toe of one foot against the sole of the other. She gave a start when the cat brushed her stocking. She talked amiably with Natalie about school and asked what grade Natalie was teaching. She said the trees in Wilmerding Crosswalk were red and yellow now and very pretty, and told Millicent that Daddy said to remind her to come home and register, so she could vote in November.

Millicent suggested that her mother had better watch the train times if she hoped to get to Wilmerding Crosswalk in time for supper. But Lucinda answered that if she were not home Patty would prepare something, and that she had told them she might be late. She said she thought she might catch the seven o'clock.

Millicent wished she had mentioned casually in the beginning about Leslie. It was harder to bring it up now. It seemed to her that a delayed mention now would only make it apparent that for some reason she had hoped earlier to keep it secret.

Her mother looked drawn from the fatigue of shopping. She had noticed that her mother for the first time lately looked a little oldish.

She could not decide how to bring up the subject of Leslie and dinner. She resented the easy cordiality between her mother and Natalie. She expected that at any moment the doorbell would ring and Leslie would appear, with her mother still in the chair and Natalie half naked at the ironing board. She thought Natalie must have forgotten Leslie was coming, and she felt furious at her. The cat played with a brassiere of Natalie's that dangled from a chair. Lucinda talked of making drapes to replace the busted shade in Natalie's room.

"No, Mother, for goodness sakes," said Millicent.

"Why not?" said Lucinda.

"You've got children at home to make drapes for, if you want to make drapes."

"What's the matter?" said Lucinda.

It seemed now to Millicent it had been madness not to have started preparing dinner when she had first intended, and to have announced innocently she had invited a young intern. But it was more impossible than ever to blurt it now, so belatedly, as though trapped by the hour's approach.

"Now look what I bought you," Lucinda said, and went to the studio couch again to open the other box. She lifted up a coat in a rich blue. "Try it on," she said.

Millicent put it on.

"A perfect fit," said Natalie.

"Oh, I know her size," said Lucinda.

It was not what Millicent would have chosen, with its velvet collar, and rather too trim and tailored waist, and the flare to its bottom.

"I'm self-supporting," Millicent said. "I wish you'd let me buy my own clothes."

"But you don't buy anything," said Lucinda. "You need something for fall."

"I still have my gray coat."

"That shmutty?" said her mother. "It wouldn't last another season. It's a winter coat anyway." She caught Natalie's eye. "That means rag," she explained.

She asked Millicent to turn around. Millicent turned. Her mother gave one of the sleeves a little tug.

"It doesn't need a bit of alteration," she said.

It was true that Millicent had bought scarcely any clothing for a long time. She did not like to wear new things before Les, since he could not afford any.

She hung the coat and went to the kitchen to pour cream for the cat. When she returned she noticed by the alarm clock on the mantelpiece that it was past the time that Leslie was due.

She thought of mentioning that her mother had better run if she hoped to catch the seven o'clock. But she was afraid it would sound as if she were trying to get rid of her. She wondered if her mother now planned to stay for dinner.

But her mother went on talking about various things. She said Charles was going to be transferred to a base in New York State, which would be much nearer home. She also said two different ladies had mentioned young men and asked for Millicent's phone number, and that Millicent could have a better social life if she transferred to the day shift. Millicent said it was quite impossible.

Her mother even sat a while with eyes closed.

But quite suddenly she rose, said she had to be going, straightened her hair in the big mantelpiece mirror, kissed Millicent, took up the dress box and some smaller bundles, and left. Natalie had gone to her bedroom to put on a dress meanwhile.

Millicent started preparing the dinner at once. Natalie came to help her and asked where Leslie was.

"He's late," said Millicent. "It's a good thing, too. He's probably delayed at the hospital."

Soon afterward they did hear his tread on the stairs, and Millicent ran to the door to let him in.

He napped on the studio couch nearly an hour, and when dinner was ready they woke him.

Millicent had hoped to go with him after dinner to Cambridge, where an open lecture was offered on Political Trends in Postwar Germany, but dinner was so late that there was no time. She was quite disappointed.

Instead they walked by the river. The rippling water shone like ebony. There were some dead leaves beneath their feet, pasted to the walk by an earlier rain. Far off the string of lighted windows of a subway train wormed silently up over the bridge.

"My mother's a noodnik," she said.

"All mothers are noodniks," said Leslie.

They moved slowly the whole length of manicured embankment, back and forth, talking of one thing after another. Suddenly Les seemed so easy to share ideas with that there was nothing she could not say to him. She was almost moved to tell him so. Even the silences were easy.

The autumn damp made her sneeze, and he massaged the back of her sweater vigorously. She thanked him.

Sunday morning he came by again, fairly early, with a black Volkswagen he had borrowed from a colleague named Murphy. Millicent felt vaguely annoyed about the car, and reminded him that she had told him not to borrow one, but he said he wanted to drive in the country and show her the autumn foliage. She went with him, but she told him again that it was not good to borrow other people's cars. You could have an accident and damage them.

They drove far. At a bend in a road a big maple as yellow as the sun stood against a background of evergreen. They went through hamlets and past woods and sloping fields where corn shocks stood. In some places the leaves made so fine a stippling of yellow and orange, or red and orange, that the forest shone like brass or copper, with touches of green like gleaming rust. By fences there were shrubs that must have been scarcely noticeable green, yet gaudy now like bursting rockets. One scene after another seemed to have a blend worth memorizing. She realized she had not really noticed New England at this time of year for a long time. At least not since Abbottsford. In the city the trees were for some reason less colorful. She wondered how it was now in Wilmerding Crosswalk, whether the arching trees of Massapeequit Road were a thick solid tunnel of gold, and what the woods and the swamp and the weeds by the covered bridge now looked like.

They calculated together how long they could drive if Millicent was to be at the city room on time. He told how molecules of cholorophyll fell apart in the cold and their remnants made the autumn dyes, and how one of the dyes was related in turn to a vitamin in the human body. He knows everything, she thought. He's the kind of man who relates his special medical knowledge to an interest in the whole universe.

She talked to him of all sorts of things, including Korea, and her mother's notion of taste, but returning again to the scenery. The Communist capital had been captured, and she said that while at first she had not thought it wise to cross the parallel she realized now it was best after all to unify the country.

She told of Mr. Garvey's rumor that the Coddington interests might close the paper and sell its assets, and said she hoped it wouldn't happen, because prejudice against women was so fierce she didn't know where she would find another such job. She lifted a knee in her brown corduroy skirt and turned back her sock to show him the press card.

Leslie parked at last on a curve of a hillside road. There was no traffic, and no one about. He said they were only a few miles from New Hampshire. Through the windshield the mountain opposite was a jungle of hues. There were oaks in a deep wine color, and trees like garish rosy lipstick, bushy and nearly fluorescent, and even lavender trees she had not seen elsewhere. The green firs were the dullest, but added to the mixture.

They gazed, saying nothing. He let her out of the car. She stood beside him. The hot colors lay in bracing air under a blue sky. She herself was dressed somberly, in the drab brown corduroy and a heavy sweater of darkest gray. Deep in the valley they could see the bend of a stream, with colored trees reflecting.

They began walking. He took her hand, lightly, but she did not want to hold hands and pulled it from him. She walked on a little ahead, smiling, kicking at leaves where they were bunched at the edge of the road. She pushed a long stick before her in matted leaves until it broke.

They returned to the car. He reached across her to pull the door shut, and then behind her as if for a lock button. But instead of straightening up he suddenly leaned upon her passionately, his lips to her neck, and his hand rose up in her shaggy dark sweater.

She pushed at him irritably, but his pressure returned. She pushed more angrily.

He straightened, and his eyes looked questioning through his glasses. "What's the matter?" he said.

She straightened her sweater. "It's not what we came here for."

"What of it?"

"So stop it. I'm not in the mood. I'm sick of that stuff. Let's just do without it for once. It's not a necessity."

He opened his mouth as if he would answer, but closed it.

"I never intended for us to make a habit of it," she said. "I told you that. I thought I made that clear."

He still looked at her. She folded her arms.

"Les, really. I'm sick and tired of all the kissing and smooching and I'm sick and tired of you rummaging around in my clothes."

He gave a barely audible sigh and tightened his mouth glumly. He started the car, backed around, and set out downhill the way they had come.

She still felt anger. She had suspected all along that the use of a car would lead to that. The whole borrowing of it seemed now a plot. There seemed a cheapness in going to such a length.

He took a somewhat different route and found other scenery, and consulted with her whether it was as pretty as the other place. It wasn't quite. She knew she had dampened his spirits, though he tried to put a good front on it.

He meandered back toward Boston, again on a scenic route. But neither of them spoke, and she began to feel he was sulking. Then she felt that perhaps he was only feeling the same strain that she did. Still she felt it was all his fault.

The continuous sound of the motor without conversation became depressing. The trip was long. They had walked saying little or nothing, but now the absence of talk seemed a bristling no man's land, a desolation between them. She wished she had rebuffed him with a little more grace, so that he would not have become more offended than he had a right to.

They came into the urban outskirts. She felt it had been a small quarrel to cast so great a pall.

He stopped and paid for gasoline.

She felt she had over-reacted somehow. After all, they had not necked the other evening, when Natalie had been home and they had walked at the river. She had been right in wanting to protect the principle that they need not neck every time, but the occasion of his borrowing a car seemed now a poor time for a test case.

There were such long intervals between the little times they could be together, and he had perhaps gone to considerable trouble and initiative to arrange this, and make a nice half-Sunday. And it was for them both. Even the necking was. It's a way of blowing off a little steam in our bachelorhoods, she thought.

The little car crept in traffic, amid horns. She watched his profile, the glasses, the brown hair hanging in a curve on his forehead. There was still no conversation. It took a long time to reach the center of the city. Surgeons live always under great tension, she thought. He could seem calm, which was why he was a good surgeon, but the nature of the work must create frightful tensions within.

She did not want to apologize, only to say something casual. But she could think of nothing.

He halted the car double-parked near the newspaper building, and he looked at her for the first time in a long while.

"Okay, here you are," he said.

She could not read his expression. "Thanks," she said. She opened the door.

"I'll be on call Wednesday night," he said. "Off Thursday."

"Oh. Will you come to dinner again?"

"Okay."

27

The newlywed Betsy Stokes Weiler was far and away the best student in Ed's adult-education courses.

The fall enrollment had turned out so disappointing that he would have found the whole program unbearable without her. Jewish Homemaking got no takers at all, other than Betsy, and Hebrew for Adults only one dowdy matron in her fifties. The Talmud class was a handful of ladies, and Amethyst Gilbert sat forward on her chair hanging on his words, but despite her agreeableness the questions and discussion she offered always showed him she had just barely missed the point.

He had announced a course on the Prayer Book too, especially for men, hoping it would encourage participation in the weekday services, and had promised it would be as rich, as bottomless, as many-faceted as Shakespeare, and that he would give the course even if only one person took it. One fourteen-year-old boy did show up, but quit when he saw he was alone.

Ed had even meant to offer a course on American Colonial history, based on a couple of good books he had read, and open to all residents of the town, on the theory that a temple should foster all branches of learning, but the executive board had discouraged the idea as pushy and show-offy.

The young convert, however, was a joy to teach. Betsy had a quick intelligence and an openness to ideas, with no ax to grind. More and more when he addressed the little class, around the oblong seminar table in the temple's library, he was in fact talking to Betsy and wishing the others would shut up. It was not just that she was fifteen or twenty years younger than the others. Actually she wasn't even pretty. Her bosom seemed limp and her clothes lacked style.

In class she took notes with breathless speed. Once Ed told them that the Talmud forbids you to give more than twenty per cent of your capital to charity, lest you go broke and become an object of charity yourself, and Betsy's left hand at once arose fluttering, while she was still writing with the other and bending over her notebook. As always she asked the right question—when they had distinguished between those righteous actions that one could do without end or surfeit and those that must not be overdone, had he not said the Talmud classifies charity with the unlimited ones? Furthermore, didn't it say that charity should be generous enough to enable the recipient also to give charity?

Ed answered that there was no inconsistency. The limit on capital giving did not limit your total giving—you could give out of income. Moreover charity could be in deeds, giving your time or energy, even a loan, even a word in the right place. And helping a man to get a job or setting him up in business was the best charity of all. The goal was not some unreal and spectacular renunciation, but the practical building of a good society.

She turned a page, still taking notes. He saw how these things fascinated her.

Or she smiled, with a slight nod, as he explained something to someone else. Once a lady asked how one teaches a child such a thing as thou shalt not bear false witness—her child had caught her praising her sister-in-law's strudel, when in fact they had thrown it to the birds, and she felt like a hypocrite. Ed answered that the Bible did not forbid lies, but only false witness against thy neighbor—in other words only lies that were against someone, that could hurt someone. He found himself more and more addressing his explanation to Betsy rather than to the lady that had asked. He said the Talmud on this point cites a passage in Genesis, wherein the angels told Abraham a white lie to keep him from getting sore at his wife. The Bible had been written with careful attention to every word, and deserved to be read with careful attention to every word.

Ed had begun the course by saying that man was a moral animal; something told man that there were things he could do that he nevertheless should not, and things he might avoid doing that he nonetheless ought to do. So why should not the particulars of this moral impulse and the effective implementation of it be studied, like any other science? He said the tradition extending from the Bible through the Talmud and beyond was the most massive, thoroughgoing, detailed, advanced, sifted, sensitive, huge-scale, serious and practical attempt to do this that mankind had ever known. Man studies trigonometry, and psychology, he said. Man studies bugs. With whole careers, and endowments. Why should not man study his shoulds and his oughts? It's as huge a study.

Human situations were complicated, he said, and effective ethics took expertise. Doing the right thing in human affairs was a science, to be practiced from morning till night, in a myriad of situations, with knowledge and finesse. That's why the literature was so voluminous. Saintliness took background and cultivation, not just slapdash impulse. You couldn't study those pages without becoming a more decent person. Not if you studied with love.

A religion that consisted only of an injunction to love thy neighbor would not be sufficient to teach you to love thy neighbor.

He had seen at the opening class that the whole idea was congenial to Betsy. And she seemed to approach each session and each problem with an excitement of discovery, as though she had always wanted religion if only it could be approached in this way. The other ladies cluttered the talk with irrelevancies but Betsy always saw the point, so that he could see her world enlarge, and he planned the classes in terms of her. Once he told her that the Talmud should not be studied alone but in the company of a fellow student, and that it even contained a rule to that effect, because it was meant to be discussed and debated and tossed around line by line, by people in touch with people, not like an isolated scholar or a meditating monk.

He liked teaching. He enjoyed the afternoon children's classes. Many of the children seemed remarkably bright and were fascinated by history, and by an exotic alphabet, and by learning the elements of a foreign tongue. Ed found pleasure in the way ten-year-old girls arrived ahead of time and clustered about him affectionately and locked arms with him when he arrived to unlock the temple. And another pleasure in their classroom laughter. Bill Prince had some of the children, but the schedule was juggled somewhat to give Ed more than his share, because Bill went to a clinic in Boston twice a week now for psychoanalysis and had also found a part-time job on the Sparkstown radio station as announcer and relief disc jockey.

It all took a larger portion of Ed's time than he had expected, because within each age group some children had had previous training and some had none, so that he tried to give the best pupils and the worst ones extra tutoring, if their parents permitted, even at their homes.

He heard that Betsy's piety was irritating her husband and especially her in-laws. She would not let Rodney watch television on Friday evenings, which happened to be when the best programs were, and would not answer the telephone on Saturdays, allowing it to ring interminably, and had even refused to eat at her in-laws' because they did not observe the dietary discipline. The elder Mr. Weiler at last phoned Ed angrily.

"You did a fine job converting her and we appreciate it," Mr. Weiler said, "but enough's enough. You know? You're gonna bust up the marriage—the kid can't even get cream in his coffee. He didn't marry a fanatic. So lay off the food business, will you? Nobody keeps that stuff. I don't know, a rabbi's always unrealistic."

Mrs. Weiler got on the phone too, and told Ed her son was used to variety, and interesting meals. She said you could do wonders with leftovers if the meats could have cream sauces.

Ed knew that most of the congregation sided with Rodney and the in-laws, and that the situation was something of a scandal. Conrad Bernstein's wife also spoke of it and told him he had taken advantage of Betsy's innocence.

But Ed admired Betsy's steadfastness. When her in-laws had told her it was all just a rationalization of a bunch of primitive taboos, she only stiffened, because he had supplied her with rebuttals beforehand. It seemed to him that Betsy had come upon these disciplines with newness and freshness and did not find them difficult, though her in-laws found them impossible. Her enthusiasm for the parts stemmed from her enthusiasm for the whole.

He became aware gradually that some of the congregation were more bitter about the Betsy matter than he had realized, even some who didn't know the Weilers socially, and some had said he was a sinister person.

Yet it seemed possible to him that Betsy, with God's help, could win out, and even be a good influence on her in-laws. There would be an irony in it, but perhaps the devotion of this convert would in time stir others of the congregation too, especially when they saw it was not just a passing thing. Attendance at the temple was terrible, and in their homes he knew that most had no longer any habit of religious observance at all.

To back up Betsy, and to encourage others, he posted some recipes in the temple's entrance hall and called attention to certain cookbooks he had placed in the temple's library. But he heard of no reaction, except that some of the ladies had said to one another that he ought to mind his own business.

He also conceived of a new type of restaurant, which would keep to the religious rules, but feature the highest-style Continental cuisine, not the old East European stuff. He made an appointment with Roy Herzlinger and urged him to do it as an investment.

Nantucket plaicefish en chablis, cervelle de veau sautée en margarine—you would need a top-notch chef to work it out, he said, but the principle was sound. An atmosphere of candlelight and fashion, beautiful waitresses, modern art, high-fidelity music. Meat and dairy kitchens, each with distinctive cloths and crockery, would serve a single dining room, and free leaflets containing the Grace After Meals would be brought with the finger bowls. He said Wilmerding Crosswalk had need of a good restaurant. There was nothing in town except Bingle's German & Yankee Cookery, which was a dump.

But Roy was not interested. He said Bingle's was long established, the original Sebastian Bingle having been lieutenant of the town's company in the Civil War, and members of the congregation preferred to go to Boston when they dined out, or to eat Chinese. Anyway restaurants did badly in dry towns. Ed argued that the idea would catch on and a chain of restaurants would stretch from Maine to California, earning a fortune, but Roy shook his head.

It occurred to Ed afterward that a kosher Chinese restaurant should be especially easy to work out, with a little imagination, because the Chinese used no dairy.

Ed had for some months been on a round of visits to his parishioners, one family at a time, and now and then he touched on diet on these occasions also. He meant to confer with each family as to how it might, without inconvenience, increase its religious consciousness, or its religious activity—perhaps one family might begin with a sentence of blessing before meals, or another would take to the suggestion of Sabbath candles. Or a bedtime prayer. He could say it helped give children a sense of security. Or maybe somebody could be induced to enroll in a class. He wanted to approach each family as a special case. He did not expect much success, and he tried to be especially on guard not to antagonize, or to seem a busybody. But he felt there must be a few who were waiting for encouragement. Now and then a young woman or an old man tried to bait him, but usually the evening passed as a polite social call.

In one family there was a tubby little bald man named Abe Morgan, whose cigar rolled around his mouth when he talked, making him pronounce R's like L's, and who harangued Ed all evening to the effect that a man's relationship with God was a private, individual thing, a personal matter. A man named Gottlieb told Ed that the services were just exercises in nostalgia, so Ed asked him what was wrong with nostalgia. Nostalgia tended to be selective, Ed told him, and to remember things as better than they were, so it was a mechanism by which the better elements in the past may influence the present.

He could find answers like this to silence people, but he knew they remained unconvinced.

In another family a housewife told him she had let her children go to school on Yom Kippur, though he had not realized it before, so he told her that if kids could stay home from school on Columbus Day they could stay home on Yom Kippur.

"But Columbus Day is a legal holiday," she said, pouring tea.

"There's nothing illegal about Yom Kippur," he said to her.

He told himself that people did influence one another, even when it seemed there was no agreement. It struck him how not even two unbelievers thought alike, and the feel of each home was different. In a way each family, each person, is a sect to itself, he thought.

He tried in these visits to find recruits for the Sabbath and especially the weekday services, which were the worst disappointment of all. They had promised him, when they had brought him to this town, that members would sign up in advance for certain days, so that several times a week a group of ten would be available, but it had not worked out, and he had found that to scrape together a fifteen-minute service he sometimes spent two hours on the telephone.

The worst was when he got nine, and could not scrounge a tenth, and some of those who had come would complain about being called out on a wild-goose chase.

He would find himself missing Charles then, and remembering that Charles had often made the tenth. But it was not right anyhow, that a community should depend on the rabbi and the cantor and the rabbi's son for three of the ten. How could anyone say no when asked to help form a minyan? When guys are waiting around to pray, and ask you to complete their number? Ed had never said no to such a request, at any time in his life. He had used to shut down the car lot for twenty minutes, half an hour. It was true that your relationship to God was personal, as they say, but your people's need of you was more than personal.

It was easier on the anniversary of a death of some member's parent; then the member would often call his friends, that prayers might be said in the manner of a congregation, with mourners rising at the appropriate time. So Ed kept track of the anniversaries.

It was apparent that the congregation had wanted the weekday prayers out of deference to the few old men who lived with married children in the town, and felt that such services were for those old men alone. Friday evening was the only time he could expect a big general attendance by the congregation at large, but even then the bigness was only relative, and seemed made up of women and twelve-year-old girls.

Two straight weeks passed without a single weekday service, and the few men who had come had to say their morning prayers as though alone, not in the congregational style. Ed promised coffee and scrambled eggs on a hot plate in the entrance hall after morning services, and announced it in the mimeographed newsletter. A flagpole had been erected outside the temple, and Ed had raised the Stars and Stripes on Labor Day and on Columbus Day, but he threatened now to fly it at half mast unless attendance improved. He had always believed in cold snacks and an occasional shot of whisky after Sabbath services, and now he put Bill Prince's wife in charge of Saturday morning refreshments and had the library seminar table covered with a variety of cakes, breads, smoked fish, caviar, ginger ale and coke. But the main result was that teenagers came around in time to skip the service and get the eats, and their parents complained about the old men and their whisky.

The various social organizations connected to the temple all seemed active and busy, but prayer and study were nearly a vacuum.

One man after another would promise to come to services, and show up once or twice, only to buzz in conversation without actually participating or looking at the book, and return no more. It was a rebuff. In Brighton, as someone's assistant, he could have his own little knot of cronies in a congregation large enough to run itself. But here he felt the loneliness of the pulpit.

He did not want to feel apart from the congregation. He wanted to be a scholar within the laity, not a priest standing between God and man, not a prophet cursing the community.

That they avoided dirty jokes in his presence, that was nothing. But their disinterest, the shallowness of their interest, made an obscurantist of him, and the tradition deserved better. He wished he could get them to look at it, with open minds. Instead of so lightly assuming that the generations that had gone before must be stupid.

He began to hear that members had complaints about him. Some did not like his not wearing garters, so to please them and to please Lucinda he put on garters. Conrad Bernstein told him there had been some disappointment at his buying that ramshackle farmhouse in the sticks, instead of something in the center of town, and also that it didn't look good for a rabbi to lie under a car. Barry Fox's parents were insulted because his sermon at the boy's bar mitzvah was so brief. Ed told them his sermons were always brief, and that if they came around more they'd know it. Anyway he gave a longer sermon at Paul Brody's bar mitzvah, to avoid trouble with the Brodys, and that made the Foxes madder. He had trouble with the volunteer Sunday-school teachers. One of them, Dr. Yarrish's son, showed up always sleepy-eyed and very late, with a half-asleep young woman waiting in his car, and finally showed up not at all. Another teacher, a Mrs. Kramer, resigned in a huff because Ed criticized her for just reading aloud dully. He made some calls, but couldn't find another teacher. He thought of asking Millicent to come to Wilmerding Crosswalk Sunday mornings and do it, at least temporarily.

Patty told him there was a rumor that he had run out to a volunteer firemen's alarm in the midst of a morning service, and that he had ridden on the fire engine with a phylactery still on his forehead and his prayer shawl flying in the wind. It wasn't true. There had been only that one time, and he had left his prayer shawl and phylacteries in a pew.

They even heard some disapproval of Patty's being a cheerleader, but some other members seemed to approve. Lucinda asked Patty not to jump so high, and wanted to lengthen the hem of her uniform a little, but Patty said none of that could be changed.

Ed had hoped to have time for his own studies, and perhaps to make a start on his project for a master index of all the literature, or at least of such a part of it as he could know something of in a lifetime. Even if it was more than a man could do before he died, a promising enough start would still be of some use and might be completed by better men. But he had little time to himself. Preparing his classes took at least twice as long as he had planned, plus the private tutoring, and Bernstein and Walker made him come around on some fund-raising visits though they had promised they wouldn't. Roy Herzlinger pledged a lot of money, and so did Dr. Yarrish and Dr. Tobias. The fund-raising was complicated by an argument among the members as to whether they should first build the superstructure, what some of them called the main sanctuary, and turn the present substructure into a recreation hall, or build a recreation hall onto the classroom wing first. Ed tried at least not to take sides in that. He helped organize the teen-agers' club and spent much time on it, and the couples' club and the Hadassah each called him as a speaker when they were stuck. If any member was sick he was expected to visit the hospital, whether in Sparkstown or Boston. He had built the library up to three hundred titles, new and secondhand, and spent less time now on it, but Amethyst Gilbert was running the mimeographed newsletter and telephoned him long and often about that. Moreover the welcoming friendliness that other clergymen had shown him had spread to the town at large, and he was now the fashionable man for invocations. He was invited by the Kiwanis and the Rotary and the Young Republicans, and gave a one-minute thought on the Sparkstown radio. And here as anywhere else funerals cut into his plans when he least expected them. He buried parents who lived elsewhere and whom he had never met.

If he tried to work in his study at home Lucinda found things for him to do. Even if she went out she would phone him that the car had broken down, and he would have to take Roland's bicycle and find her and fix it. Once it was only a wire off a spark plug, and once it was nothing at all—the motor started the moment he tried it. He tried to work some mornings at the temple's library, but the little old man Brill found out and kept coming there to bother him. He did not want to hurt Brill's feelings, because the poor man was constantly being turned out by his daughter-in-law and had no place to pass the time, and besides was sneered at by everyone else, as a jerk or a lunatic. But Brill was a nuisance. He wanted to build a bomb shelter under the temple, for the sake of the children, and wanted Ed to ask Roy Herzlinger to give the money for it. He said Herzlinger had more money than God. He would talk sometimes in Yiddish, which Ed understood only partially, and even in English his accent was so heavy that he was hard to follow. He would run on in his phlegmy voice about screwls, breecks, lombair, stil bims, plens. Ed told Lucinda that the man was a pest.

"Well, one of the occupational hazards of being a rabbi is that you have to get involved with Jews all the time," she told him. "I warned you that when you went to the seminary. But you wouldn't listen."

In the midst of all of it he never had the feeling of giving real spiritual or moral guidance to anyone. In Brighton he had, and he thought that in two cases he had perhaps helped prevent a suicide. But not here. Father Donahue had said something about being tired of being Dorothy Dix, and it had sounded to Ed like a different world. Ed's people did not come to him. He told himself that the sick and the marginal were not his main object of interest anyway. His main interest still had to be the healthy ones, as a community—the creation of a spiritual atmosphere in which a good society would follow.

It constantly surprised him that the other clergymen in town, such as Caleb Folger and Ralph Briggs, thought of Ed's congregation as especially vigorous. It amazed them that he could get children to come not only on Sunday but after school during the week. They didn't know that some of the parents humiliated him even as a pedagogue, by letting the children skip often, so that the curriculum became anarchic.

Actually the communal spirit and the state of observance here were no better than in Abbottsford; it had only seemed so because the population was larger. And it was hard to instill habits in people late in life, and hard to give children a feel for customs that their parents didn't follow. When you considered the state of the tradition it seemed a shambles.

They were good people. Many attended the Boston Symphony. Yet it was hard to find a case for religion that convinced anybody. Perhaps the trouble was that in a town and a congregation in which most people were reasonably decent, it did not really seem to them that religion could make people specially decent. They were not in touch with evil much.

Of course most people these days were pretty good anyway. But in a lifetime you met only one or two who were unusually good, who were warm and saintly. Ed had known some. His grandfather for one. And because he had known his grandfather he had recognized it in others, and believed in the possibility of still others, of whom he had read or heard. It was this cultivation of saintliness that the people here didn't understand. It was a cultivation that took study.

Betsy was absent from the weekly Talmud class. It was completely different without her. He missed her at services also, and the following week she was absent from Talmud study again. He wondered if she were sick, or if she and her husband were away. He feared that more likely it was a delicate situation at home, or with her in-laws. Because of the possibility that it was he hesitated to telephone, lest he embarrass her further. He thought he would wait a week and inquire then if she had not returned.

But he bumped into her one evening in the supermarket, when Lucinda had sent him for eggs. She seemed flustered at seeing him.

"Oh," she said. He did not have time to say anything. "I'm afraid I lost my faith again," she said, with a sudden widening of her mouth. She turned and quickly lost herself with her shopping cart down an aisle of cans.

He stood dumbly, and then remembered to get his eggs. He would have understood, he thought. She did not have to give him that phony smile. Especially she did not have to speak in a phrase so alien to everything he had taught her.

He wondered if he would ever again have a student who took notes.

28

Leslie dropped her brassiere off the studio couch, down by his folded glasses and the shoes, and she felt the warm tight rubbing of his long hands upon her back and her arms. The wrinkles of his shirt sleeves pressed her skin. She had worn a shirt dress of Ella Jane's, of a handsome blue-gray stuff, but already the buttons had been undone to the belt line and her arms taken out. The drawing of the line had not been done in quite so vivid and absolute a way before, she thought, but still, if they were going to have this fondling, it made sense to have the fabric cleanly out of the way. Their mouths stayed joined a long time, puckered and slowly exercising, as if they drank at one another. One of his hands seemed to support her, as if to ensure their nearness; the other was never still. It coaxed and shaped a breast, or dragged lightly, and played upon the bumps of her backbone, or moved in a hug about the smallness of her waist down next to where clothing lay about her like debris. It rose again to her neck, behind her ear, and played a long time with her hair. She saw the smile of his lazy eyes. His belly rumbled.

She heard the ticking of the little clock over on the mantel, and the window above their heads rattling in the wind. Her eyes were scarcely open, but in the yellow half-light she saw the dirty dishes and chop bones on the drop-leaf table. She saw the black kitten watching from across the room.

"Theodore knows you now," she murmured to Leslie.

But his eyes were closed. She heard the gentle breath in his nose. One could doze like this, she thought. Only the shaded little fixtures that flanked the fireplace mirror were lighted, and they cast crazy shadows about the ceiling one.

The graze and lick of his fingers had followed her skin down into her clothing, and she felt his hand take a buttock with a slow kneading motion that continued. It was beyond their agreement, but the loosening of their belts after dinner made it understandable. Their lips met again, sleepily. His hand smoothed, rounded, reached, held, and kneaded again. She was aware of an airiness, and that her elastics were not where they ought. The underpants about her, in their readiness to fall away, to melt aside, seemed a party to the excitement.

His fingers lost themselves, sandwiched in her flesh.

"Will you look out?" she said. "My pants are half off. Watch what you're doing."

His embrace tightened.

"Hey," she said. She pushed off the heavy arm and struggled from him. "Where's the bra?" She reached over him, clutching her front with one arm, and retrieved the brassiere from the floor. She dressed, still on the studio couch, but sitting as if on a carpet and with her back to him. He lay with half-closed eyes. "It's no good," she said, buttoning the dress. "It's just not practical. I get carried away for five minutes and you've got me practically nude."

She swung her feet across him and stood. She smoothed her dress, and walked slowly upon the rug in her socks, not looking at him.

"I should have stopped you sooner," she admitted. "When you went below the waist. But I thought it was your turn to police yourself for a change. I never bought the idea that it's up to the woman to do all the policing." Near the further window she turned. Pale strips of glow from the venetian blind played on her. "I shouldn't have to do all the policing," she said. "It's not fair. We had an agreement. I have to be able to count on you."

He still lay on the couch.

"If I didn't get up," she said, "we'd end up having intercourse or something."

"Possibly."

"Oh, and that would be perfectly all right, I suppose. Let's just jump into bed while we're at it." She turned away, and looked down through the slats of the blind.

He sat up, almost as though rising from a nap, and put his feet to the floor.

"Are you sore?" he asked gently.

"I'm quite annoyed with you." She watched dry leaves turning in the night.

He came toward her in his stocking feet and put his hands on her shoulders from behind. She moved slightly, uncertain whether to shake him off.

"I'm sorry," he said.

"Are you?"

"Yes. I'm sorry. Come on. Let's kiss and make up."

She turned into his embrace. He stood with her, holding her near and firm.

But then she exerted a push and looked at his face. "And that's another thing," she said. "You're all aroused and I can feel everything and I don't like it. It's indecent."

He let her go.

"And it's not the first time," she said. "It's just a little shameless, don't you think?"

He turned from her, looking bent and patient. "I'm sorry my physiology doesn't suit you," he said. He sat heavily on the studio couch with a little bounce. "Maybe I should take a cold shower."

"Don't you dare." She leaned against a fat arm of the stuffed chair and half sat on it. "Les, what's the matter with you? For goodness sakes! There's a certain side of your nature that I don't much care for and I wish you'd stop it."

"Well I'm getting slightly annoyed with a certain side of yours," he said. "It all gets a little unrealistic after a time. You can't turn it on and shut it off like the gas."

"You know perfectly well what would happen if we didn't shut it off. That's why we agreed to draw a line at the waist."

"That's no good. All that does is just get your reactions all jangled. It's sick. You don't start and stop. We never should have started this stuff."

"Well that's what I said!" Her voice rose. "Isn't that what I said? I never wanted to start."

He didn't answer but kept looking at her. He was sitting carelessly and round-shouldered, his hands hanging across his knees.

"Are you still aroused?" she asked. There was an anxiousness in her voice.

She saw him smirk.

She felt herself color. "I was against necking from the beginning," she said. "I told you I didn't want to be a tease."

"Staying at arm's length wouldn't have avoided the problem," he told her, somewhat more gently. "The frustration would still be there. We can't sit like a couple of wooden Indians."

"Oh, we should just go right ahead and have an affair, I suppose."

"Well, normal sex would have one advantage. The advantage of being normal. You have to admit that."

"Is that what you want?"

"Why not? Of course I want it."

She stood nervously, and then put her face in her hands.

"Damn," she said, half in a whisper.

"Bury your head in the sand," he said softly.

She sat back limply in the chair.

"You said we could go so far and no further," she told him. "You said we were strong and could stop when we wanted to."

"We can, but it's not good."

"That's not what you told me when we started." Her voice shook. "Why are you changing your argument?"

"Because you're ready for the truth. I've been fooling around and indulging you, but sooner or later it's got to be said. Physically it's taken care of, in one way or another, but emotionally the prolonged frustration just isn't the way we're made. It certainly can't do any good. And it's unnecessary."

"In other words," she said, her voice quaking worse than ever, "I have to begin because it would be too prudish not to even kiss or anything, and once I begin I have to go the whole distance so my responses won't get jangled."

"Well, in a sense. That's why morals are changing."

"I thought you were honorable," she said.

"What's dishonorable about sex?"

"I mean I thought you were honorable about agreements. I didn't think it was a case of give an inch and take a yard."

"I did it your way," he said. "We started, we stopped."

"But you want more."

"Am I dishonorable for wanting? I was created to want."

"I'm sorry I started. I knew better."

"I never said I didn't want to sleep with you. I said we'd go only as far as you were willing. But now you raise the question, do I want wholesome, healthy sexual release, and a normal relationship, and the answer is yes. Naturally."

"I didn't raise the question," she said. "Les, I've heard every one of the arguments. It's natural, and it's normal, and it's beautiful, and it only makes you feel dirty when you don't go the whole distance—I've heard all that. Petting and stopping is dishonest, and to be together and not pet is also dishonest. I'm not as naïve as you think. I've been through college, and I've talked with my contemporaries, and I've read the usual literature, and I don't think there's much I haven't heard. But I thought you were above that baloney."

"Have I made you feel dirty?" he asked her.

"Have I said that?"

"I don't know."

"Well I didn't," she told him. "I didn't say any such thing. I know it's not dirty. But you made a tease out of me, that's all. There's such a thing as having respect for yourself, and respect for sex. And the last thing I wanted was to get you all aroused and jangled. I told you that weeks ago. My idea was to put our minds on other things."

"Any girl who makes herself attractive and doesn't sleep with men is essentially a tease," he said.

She looked at him sternly but unhappily. When she spoke there was a coldness in her voice despite the quavering. "Maybe we'd better stop seeing each other in that case. Because I can't be responsible for having such a troublesome effect on you."

"Are you asking me to leave?"

His eyes were questioning her, without glasses.

"Can't we just go to museums," she asked, "and listen to music, and discuss things?"

"Sure we could. But in addition to thinking of you as a person, don't you want me to think of you as a woman too? You are a woman, after all. And basically a normal one."

"Can't you think of me as a woman without wanting me sexually?"

He paused, looking at her quizzically. "Now really," he said. "Just ask yourself what you mean by that. And tell me if you're not muddleheaded."

She sighed a little. "Well, maybe I am muddleheaded, but at least my behavior isn't muddled, and I plan to keep it that way. Or it wasn't, until a few weeks ago."

She tried to read his face. He was gazing at her and seemed completely calm and self-assured.

"Sex is a damn nuisance," she said. She saw his lips curve. "I know it should be beautiful," she added, "but the boys that are always talking about how beautiful it is are just the ones that are intent on making it a nuisance."

Leslie rose up, with the tired little smile, and came to her chair. He sat on the arm beside her, and started to tousle her hair, but she removed his hand gently.

"I'm sorry," she admitted, gazing before her at the rug. "It was my fault too. You work very hard, and you're under a strain all the time, and it's natural to have desires. But we have here a perfect example of how sex mars an otherwise fine relationship."

"How can something perfectly healthy mar anything?"

"All this arguing. It makes us fight."

"Well, if it took its normal place in our lives it would stop bothering us," he said. "When needs are met they don't obsess you. Whether it's food, or sleep, or sex, or esteem in the community, or whatever it is. It's a need that's denied that becomes a nuisance."

"Do you think it makes you more manly?" she asked. "Because it doesn't, in my opinion. There's nothing reprehensible or unmanly in a man staying a virgin until he marries."

"Millicent, it's such a natural thing, I don't know what all the fuss is about. When you're in the midst of an act of love, it's as if you belong there. You'd be content to do nothing else for the rest of your life, if it were possible."

"I don't know if that's a recommendation." Her fingers played with the frayed upholstery on an arm of the chair. On the other arm he towered over her. "Anyway I've started teaching Sunday school," she said.

"So what. You could still teach Sunday school."

She watched her thumb and forefinger twisting frayed threads.

"Is it a matter of what your parents think?" he asked.

"No. I feel free of them. And I'm not going to run my life according to them. But it's silly to say you don't even care what people think. I care what they think, just as I care what you think. And I know they think I wouldn't. And there just seems something rotten and soiled and pretending, in letting them think that, if I would."

"Think you wouldn't what? Sleep with a man?"

"Well, live like that. Go to bed with a man. Have an affair. I know I've led them to think I'm the kind that wouldn't."

"Why did you?"

"I don't know."

"I suppose your father being a rabbi has a lot to do with it."

"No. That has nothing to do with me. But I'm not going to jump into an affair just to prove my independence either. I'm going to live my own way, Leslie Hollander. And if you don't like it it's too bad."

"Am I persecuting you?"

"No."

The kitten was squeezing between her ankles. She lifted it to her lap, and fondled it, but with such absent-minded motions that it scratched her. She let it go.

"There are moral considerations," she said. "Don't you think so? I have a responsibility to my family, and an even greater responsibility to the child I could bring into the world. We could have a child, Les. Do you think of that? It's not just a matter of I want this and I want that. It's wrong to the child and it's a wrong against the whole society we live in. To conceive a child we're not ready for."

"There's such a thing as contraception."

"And accidents. And I can't believe that the invention of these little rubber things should make such a difference in what's right and what's wrong."

"The history of man has been changed by smaller things. And people who don't want accidents don't have them, Millicent. Not that kind. And morals have changed. Or norms have."

"To some extent."

"To a great extent."

"That doesn't mean I approve."

"Why do you think Harvard College allows women in men's rooms? You know they do, don't you? And why, Millicent? Because they're enlightened, and they know people need it."

"That isn't why."

"Why then? Why else? They can't state it in so many words, because all the ministers and bluenoses would raise a stink, so they do it discreetly. But every intelligent person recognizes it."

"Well you wait. As soon as there's a scandal they'll change those rules."

He shook his head. "They'll never put the lid on it. It's gone too far. Go over to Cambridge, and look at all those girls walking along the sidewalk hanging on a guy's arm and smiling up at him. They're all getting it."

"Oh sure. That's why they're smiling, I suppose."

"Don't you think it's true?"

"No I do not."

"Well, it's not a joke. It's assumed." He slid off the arm of the chair and walked about a little in the dim light as he spoke. She drew her feet up. "They do it," he said quietly, "because if they didn't people today would assume they did anyway. Couples study together. A girl takes her books to a guy's room on Saturday."

"I know all about it."

"All about it?" He stood before her, not walking.

"Well, something about it. I haven't been dead to the world."

"You don't think they're just sitting there all Saturday afternoon with their clothes on."

"Well if that's what things have come to why doesn't everybody just go around naked." Her voice still had a quake. "Why bother buying clothes."

"Well, you know the answer to that," he said in the same quiet tone. "Clothes have various uses. But it's accepted that when you're alone with your lover you don't just sit with a book."

"You don't have to assume the worst. You have a dirty mind."

"I have a clean mind, Millicent. And so have the university administrations that permit it. They assume the students are mature."

"Les, in Chicago I helped a boy with a political campaign. And it was just that. We worked on a political campaign. We didn't jump into an embrace just because we were alone together."

"Maybe you didn't." He had wandered behind her chair, and began to massage her shoulders. But she hunched, so he withdrew his hands to the back of the chair. "I don't know," he said. "I don't know what the circumstances were. Or how involved you were. But by and large, Millicent, when a girl of your intellectual level gets close to a guy emotionally over a period of time—it's the usual thing. They have an affair. What do you think? Studying together, and going out together, going up to his room together—sexual fulfillment is a normal part of the relationship between a man and a woman."

"I still don't believe they all do." She felt she was blushing again, for no good reason, and was glad he was behind her and that the light was dim. "I'm sure there are still some that don't."

"Sure, I suppose so," he said. "Of course. A small percentage."

"The small percentage still has to be made up of real people."

"Sure. Do you know who they are? Maybe there are girls with so little on the ball, and so little self-confidence, that they keep their virginity because they think they've got nothing else to give a guy. And then you have to include the girls that never go out. The girls that don't know how to make themselves attractive—the dogs. And the girls that have never gone steady or been close to a guy. The children."

"And me."

"And you. You don't want to be one of them. They're not your type."

"I'm my own type."

"Well, if you're a person worth living with, then virginity's irrelevant. Just like you told me your parents bought an old house—they don't insist on being the first ones to live in it, do they? And girls who go with guys, and know guys, and make friends with guys, go to bed with guys. It's that simple. In your heart you know it's true. Don't you?"

Her face felt hot.

"I suppose there's a fad," she said. "Or a trend."

"It's more than a trend. I don't know about Chicago, but in an eastern college you'd never have gotten away with it for four years."

"You'd make it a requirement for the bachelor's degree, I suppose."

"Well, at Yale you have to swim fifty yards. I'd say it's as important as that. Men are real, Millicent. You have to live in your own era. And you've got a problem. You want companions who are enlightened and aware, your intellectual equals, and of your own class educationally, and at the same time you want them to have the moral codes of a much narrower and lower class. You're looking for a rare bird. It's like looking for a Wall Street banker who supports Henry Wallace. It doesn't exist."

"It does exist."

"Millicent, anybody seeing you for the first time would just naturally assume that at age twenty-two, for Christ sake, you've at least known what it is to enjoy a healthy sex relationship. I don't mean they think about it—I mean they just assume it, the same way they'd assume you've read Camus, and like they'd assume you must have supported that Douglas-Stevenson ticket when you were out there in Chicago, and the same way they'd assume you're in touch with what's being done now in art and music. Because your whole manner puts you in that class. The whole intelligence and refinement in your face and your voice. It types you."

"I haven't read Camus."

"But you're aware of Camus." He walked around toward the couch, his socks silent on the carpet. "I mean the way anyone would know immediately that you're a graduate of a top university, for instance. The mark of the enlightened intellectual is all over you. The way you don't wear paint, and the natural hairdo, and the socks." He sat. "You look intelligent and informed, in other words. And intelligent people know it's good for the organism to live as it was intended. It's better to breast-feed than bottle-feed, and better to work than be idle, and better to have sexual intercourse than be celibate."

"You think this trend is a great liberation, don't you. The enlightenment."

She saw the kitten touch some lint on the toe of his sock, and he moved his foot without looking down. "Well, I think it's a fact," he said. "And I also think it's an improvement in the social order, yes. It's certainly questionable whether Victorian morality was a good society. With its repressions, and its maiden aunts, and its whorehouses. People went places and did things they couldn't talk about. And today the whorehouses are dead, for the first time in history, because in our generation people get their sex in a healthier way. And instead of a split in the psyche there's a wholeness."

She was curled in the chair, frowning, clutching a foot she had tucked up.

"But I still can't agree with this whole idea that sexual intercourse is life's big moment," she said. "Gee, Les, for goodness sakes, if it is, if that's true, if the greatest joy is sex, then we're just trapped, like any other species, and our purpose on earth is just to go blindly on, producing the next generation, and the next, and the next. Just God's fools, like antelopes, or zebras. Pumpkinheads in nature's big laboratory. And I won't be so stupid—I can't feel so little and so caught—I can't believe that's all there is to it. We were put here for something besides just producing more of ourselves. At least I was. I don't believe it, that that's the big marvelous thing. The sex drive, and that moment of union, or fulfillment, or whatever you call it. That can't be the biggest thing. There has to be something bigger than that." She felt moisture in her eyes and tried to fight it.

He was studying her somberly from under his brows, his head a little down, and looked quite handsome. The light was on his forehead and his eyes were in shadow. His hands hung loosely clasped, one across the other.

"I don't say it's the one big thing," he said.

"We're not just bodies around seeds. Like plants or something."

"It's part of the composition," he said. "Let's say sex is one little dash of red in a corner of a large canvas, with lights and shadows, but it belongs, in the integrated effect of the whole picture. You don't make it central but you don't exclude it."

"They make it a habit and they think it's a need," she said.

He gave his head a little shake. "One thing doesn't substitute for another," he said. "You want to enjoy the best of life. You want work. Creative, if possible. And exercise, education, the arts, marriage, children. It's all part of a full life. And a man's fortunate if he can help to push back the frontiers of knowledge someday, as I hope to do. And do you think I should be deprived of sexual release in the meantime? For years? Until I'm in a position to marry? Just do without? Why should I? It would be completely pointless. The girls are willing, thank God. And society understands and expects a normal sex life, finally. I don't live at the South Pole."

Millicent rose and turned nervously. She stood again by the blind and stared down absently at the street lamp.

"How many girls have you slept with?" she said.

She waited for his answer.

"What do you want? A biography?"

"Two?" she asked, her voice growing shaky again. Her fingers pinched the cord of the blind. "Three?"

"Approximately."

"And I'd make four? Three?"

"You don't ask that. Every relationship stands on its own."

"And how many affairs should a girl of my status and education have? One? Two?"

"How many marriages should she have?" Leslie said. His voice was subdued.

"One, preferably," said Millicent. "And I'd say three is far too many."

He gave the slightest sort of nod. "Well, as for affairs, if she has more than one, it's still no sin."

"Two?" She looked at him. "Twenty?"

"I'd say twenty's a little sick in the head."

"Well, is three sicker than two?" Her hand made a wave travel up the blind cord. "Where's the border line between sophisticated and a trollop?"

"It's not a set number."

"Well, that's it. How does she know?"

"It depends on the individual."

"But what's right for this individual? And how much does she have to love him? And at what age does it become okay? Is it right when she's twenty-one, and wrong at sixteen? It can't be right at thirteen, can it?"

"No, it isn't right at thirteen. It's a matter of emotional maturity."

"But when's that? When does she get emotionally mature? For driving a car there's a set age."

"What can I say? Seventeen years and eleven months, provided her periods are regular and she's home by midnight? What do you want? The new morality hasn't got a Talmud, for Christ sake."

"I want a code."

"Do you know what I think? I think you think too much."

"Well, from what I've been able to gather of this new morality it's the kind of thing that keeps shifting under your feet all the time. It can't make up its own mind about any criteria or anything." Her hand swung the cord, knocking the tiny knob at its end against the woodwork. "It isn't regularized. Nobody's sure what the ground rules are. If it's a morality people understand it, and they know what they're supposed to do."

"You have to trust your heart a little bit."

They continued looking at each other. She kept swinging the cord against the wood as if scarcely aware of it. Some of the blandness seemed to have left him.

"If you want a rule," he said, "I'd say I believe a woman's entitled to the same personal freedom I expect for myself. Nothing else is fair. You ask me questions like how much. How much is too much. For a well-adjusted person it answers itself."

She hit the cord harder and dropped it. She looked down out the window again. He came toward her. He stood behind her, and she let him put his hands on her shoulders.

"It's not a matter of everybody that asks you," he said. "But certainly, if you expect to spend a lot of time with a guy, and provide most of his female companionship, it just isn't good form to refuse to let him take your pants off. Don't you think a guy needs a woman's private parts in his life? You can't be a dog in a manger. Nobody can afford to devote all his time to people who don't satisfy him sexually. And you'll find you can't either."

She said nothing. He fondled the dress upon her shoulders.

"Do you want to keep on being a kid?" he asked gently. "Don't you want to be a woman? Don't you want the pleasure of giving yourself to someone? Of undressing, and letting all your beauty come alive, and excite someone, and sharing his excitement?" His hand moved warmly down upon the dress, and then clutched her boldly like a G-string.

"For goodness sake!" She resisted with a thrust of her whole body. "Don't! I'm not going to be bullied!"

She sat on the window sill, her back flattening the tilted slats. She leaned a little forward again from the blind.

He sat back on the arm of the stuffed chair, looking at her and seeming calm.

"Well, I've got other things to do than be sent home full of cramps and aches," he said, still gently. "Life's too short."

"Young men don't need women," said Millicent. "It's a myth."

"They don't?"

"Not if they're constructively occupied. If they're busy."

He was staring as if with a mild curiosity. "I don't know if you're ignorant, or what. Look, I'm not going to indulge in emotionally sick behavior, and I haven't got time to spend all day under a cold shower either. So what's left? Women. Normality. That's all. What my body was meant for. What do you recommend? To enjoy each other's company, and shake hands and part, and go our separate ways, and masturbate separately? It's absurd."

"Why don't you sleep with nurses at the hospital?"

He renewed the curious stare.

"Maybe I should," he answered, "but that's neither here nor there."

"Why don't you?"

"Well," he said, "the circumstance usually doesn't arise. I haven't had that much to do with nurses socially."

"But there must be lots of nurses around, and student nurses. Even when you were only in med school."

"Well, I guess they were around, but I was busy. I never did too much of that. I was holding jobs. And usually I never had a dime for coffee, or decent clothes, or a haircut. I just didn't have time for being with people, and making friends. Or maybe I was somewhat shy, even if you don't think so. I think I was."

"I'm sure you could find somebody of loose morals."

He studied her without answering immediately, and she colored again slightly.

"Do you mean that?" he asked. "Would you really rather I slept with others?"

"Yes," she said. "If you're so obsessed. I just want you to get over this preoccupation. All you think about is sex."

"I think it's pretty obvious that it's not all I think about."

"Well, with me, anyway."

"You should be flattered."

"I'm not."

"And we've talked of a good many other things, as far as that goes. We've talked music, we've talked art, and we've talked McCarthy, and we've talked Korea and the U.N. and we've talked how to win the uncommitted peoples. And we've talked your job and mine."

"Yes, I guess that's true."

"And we've talked about our families. Your kid brother and my kid brother. Over and over again. And sex, all right, sure. And you tell me about student nurses—it just hasn't happened that way, that's all. Life isn't a big sex party. I'm talking about balance. And about a meaningful relationship. Do you think that would be a healthy arrangement, to have one girl for companionship and talking, and a different one to sleep with?"

She left the window sill and wandered to the mantelpiece. She played with the vase of pussy willows, watching her fingers turn it slowly at its base. The two wall fixtures made strange double shadows.

"Les," she said, "what about those friends of yours, where I was supposed to go for a spaghetti supper one time."

"What about them?"

"Are they carrying on affairs?"

"They're married."

"But they had other men there that brought girls, didn't they? That weren't married?"

"One or two did. Some came alone."

"And do those couples sleep together?"

"I don't know. We haven't talked about it."

"If it's so all right and okay and accepted, why don't they talk about it?"

"It's a personal thing."

"Oh sure. It's so okay they don't dare tell anybody. They have to be furtive."

"Well, if it came up legitimately among friends I'm sure there'd be no secret about it. You don't go telling everybody about your bowel movements either, but it's assumed you have them. Married couples don't go broadcasting their acts of intercourse either."

"If I had been there," she asked, her eyes focusing on the lines of the vase, "would all those people have assumed we're sleeping together?"

"I don't know. If they saw us several times in succession it'd be taken for granted, I suppose."

She took her hand from the vase and sighed. "Oh dear."

He turned to see her better, and straddled the fat arm of the chair. He put a foot on the cushion.

"Millicent," he said, "I was talking the other night with the assistant resident—he's older than me and he's been around a lot—he was in the war and everything—and he mentioned that there used to be this expression 'easy lay,' that everybody used all the time, and it just dawned on him that he hasn't heard it in years. Just as if the whole expression has gone out of existence. Because the concept has, it's disappeared. He said every girl he's had an affair with in the last few years, it happened the first night. Without exception. And decent girls. I don't mean he necessarily slept with every girl he went out with. There must have been blind dates where they didn't click, and didn't make love, and never saw each other again, but the point is, if it happened, it was right away. In every single case. At his place or theirs. And that's increasingly the fashion. He said he was out with a girl the other night, and they ended up at her apartment, and she told him she never goes to bed the first night out with a guy, only the second. She promised him for the second. And he said to her, 'that dates you like an old song.' And it was after that that he remembered that concept of 'easy lay,' like something out of the past. From ten years ago."

Millicent had walked alongside the wall toward the door, and she clicked on the wall switch of the ceiling fixture, whitening the room. She turned to him with her eyes moist. "I don't believe it! That things have come to that. I know it can't be true."

"It is true."

"Well I can't believe it. And I wish you hadn't said it. Your argument would be stronger. Such as it is."

"Millicent, that's how it is now. The criterion is, if a girl likes you, and she wants you to know she'd like to be friends, and you make the pass, that's it. And why not? If they strike each other that way? If they're mature? It's the normal thing to happen between a man and a woman. What do you think, they should wait for six months? Why? Out of guilt?"

"Look," she said, "I don't know your friend and I don't know if he made it up or what. But do you think all this would be socially sound, if it were true?"

"I say this—it fits in with everything I hear, about how things were and how they are, and with what little direct experience I have."

"And do you include me in what little direct experience you've had?"

"Well, you're the exception."

"No, I'm living in the wrong epoch, I suppose." She was circling the room slowly, past the inlaid cabinet and the doors of the bathroom and the kitchen.

"Well, you are something of an anachronism," he said. "You haven't quite caught up with your times."

Her eyes were still wet. "No, I should have jumped into bed as soon as possible. I'm one of those girls ten years ago trying not to be easy."

"Well, you haven't been easy."

"Thanks," she said tearfully. She sat on the studio couch.

"Millicent, ten years ago a girl that let a guy take everything off but her pants was still considered slightly more moral than if she let him take everything off. Today that kind of behavior is considered sick. Now I ask you, which is more wholesome?"

"I don't know."

"Eight or ten years ago people felt they needed a whole phony subterfuge and excuse about each separate piece of clothing that came off. But today two people just get undressed."

"That's true—I know of the kind of thing you mean," she said more calmly, with some warmth of recognition. "You mean all the coyness, and a girl making believe she doesn't see that the boy's undressing her."

"That's it."

"I detest that."

"You should detest it. That's why the country had this big sick-in-the-head breast fetish before the war, because a lot of people used to stop at that point. But people who have healthy sex don't go in for all that feeling up we've been doing. That breast stuff was prewar."

"What did you suggest it for then?"

"Well, it was the kid-stuff approach of my youth, I guess. And I thought maybe you needed that immature kind of approach. But breast-fondling is for twelve-year-olds."

"It is not! Did you do that when you were twelve?"

"No. When I was sixteen. Seventeen maybe. I was a little retarded."

"Well, that's a relief."

"And when I was twenty I was still doing it, when there was less excuse for it. And actually it's only bad if you don't go further, anyway. What's gone out of fashion is the prolonged love play. Like for instance, you say you hate dating. Do you know what a girl of your class means when she says that? She means she likes to begin an affair quickly, without the nonsense."

"It's not what I meant by it."

"I know it's not. But it's what it means, and it's what people are gonna think you mean, if you keep saying it."

She had reddened. "I don't know," she said. "I suppose it's all true of a good many people, but I don't think it's true of everyone."

"Look, I don't mean they go bed-hopping. A girl might even go a couple of years between involvements, with no affairs and no sex. But her affairs begin cleanly and simply, the way a love affair should begin. Especially among people of taste and breeding. She tries to do the right thing with the right guy, and it's permanent or semipermanent. It's a normal part of the search for a mate."

"Oh, I know it's what people say." She rubbed her brow. "I've been hearing things like this for years, and I think it's very exaggerated. I think you'll find a lot of cheap journalism has something to do with it."

"How would you know?"

"They exploit these things."

He shook his head a little. "It's not journalism. It's a matter of understanding that what's normal and healthy is respectable. Not the other way round. And the how-far-shall-I-go game is passé. It came in with the rumble seat and went out with the war."

"Why don't they just get married then? All these couples that are faithfully sleeping with each other?"

"Well, why complicate things? If they're not sure—or not ready to raise a family—or if they're very young? When two people finally realize they want to spend their whole lives together, that's when they get married. Knowledgeable people don't just start talking marriage with no sexual history."

"They don't?"

"Of course not. Without knowing if they're compatible, or if the other party's frigid or something? If a guy started talking marriage to an intelligent girl without having slept with her she'd think he was nuts. Or impotent, possibly. Today an intelligent girl expects sex. She wants it."

"Aren't they supposed to be in love?"

"Well, there's certainly a connection. I suppose a woman differs from a man in that before she's in love she doesn't desire sex specifically, as much as she just desires to be desired. But one thing leads to another. And love is a desiring. You don't love in the abstract. It's an attraction that continues."

"Oh, baloney."

"You'll find out."

"Are you in love with me?"

"Well, you wouldn't expect me to stay in love forever with a woman that's unattainable."

"So are you in love with me? Or not?"

"Maybe. I'd like to find out."

"Really, Les, I'm not a child. Love isn't a crazy mystique. And anyway you said it's not love. You said people just sleep together between friends."

"Many a friendship has progressed to love that way. It would be strange if love didn't grow in a good relationship."

"And then they break up again."

"Sometimes. Love isn't always permanent. Life isn't permanent, for that matter."

"And what if a girl sleeps with a guy thinking it's going to cement a bond of love, and it turns out he doesn't even come back any more. Or he was only fooling around in the first place."

"Well, that happens. That's usually what's meant when you hear a girl say some guy is a bastard."

She sat not moving. Their eyes were on one another.

"Les, I'm not feeling well. I think you better go."

"What's the matter?"

"I'm just not feeling good. Sort of a bellyache." Her voice was soft. "I'd rather you'd go."

"Okay."

He came near where she sat to find his shoes. Then she watched him go to the closet. His topcoat was a large-grained tweed of black and white yarns. The ends of the sleeves looked worn.

He opened the door to the staircase landing.

"Les—" she said.

He turned.

"Do you really think it's respectable?" she asked him.

"Well," he answered, "it's pretty obvious that all the girls that are getting laid these days aren't exactly ending up in ruins. They settle down and get married, and raise families, like anybody else."

"Things can't change that fast."

"I don't think you'll say that when you're ninety. Look, other things change. Medicine changes. Politics, science—remember back ten years ago and look at the changes."

"Even so. If it's really so widely accepted, then why do these things still have the power to shock?"

"It's a question of who's shocked. We're in transition. But this notion that you have to be married first just gets lip service."

"But you see? They still make sure to give it lip service. And you don't do one thing and give lip service to another thing, unless you have a bad conscience."

"No, it's cultural lag. Everybody gives lip service to obsolete mores for a while. But they do less and less. People are getting more honest and open about it. I mean, you ask why isn't it public, but give it a little time. Some year soon this'll all burst out from underground, into the light of day. You're witnessing a classic case of how a historic era begins. For years minds change privately, and suddenly the new age is here. You're watching it."

"Les, I don't know. I'm all confused."

"Today to be properly dressed even, is to be sexy," he said. "Look at a good tasteful dress, or look at a well-cut pair of Bermuda shorts, on a girl of the best upbringing. If it doesn't beautify her body, on the body's own terms, it's not well designed. There's not a thing they put on the well-tailored girl today that isn't designed to make boys want to take it off. They cut one thing just close enough to bring out her shape, and the next thing hangs so that a bulge just pushes it when she moves, you know, just loose enough to make you want to slide it around, in other words. And every season they perfect it more. They milk every wrinkle. You can't look at a knee without your eye going up, and you can't look at a neck without your eye going down. And it's good. When I walk down a street I'm glad I'm living today, and not twenty years ago. And I'm glad some things are finished and gone. Like this business of holding out, and marrying someone whose body you haven't even seen."

"It seems to me there's plenty of evidence that unchastity isn't the road to happiness."

"No one thing leads to happiness. You know that. But what are you gonna do, Millicent? Stay a virgin until you're married?"

"Maybe."

"And don't you think that's just a little ridiculous?"

"I don't know. Possibly. It's my life. I have a right to be ridiculous if I want to. I don't care. I'm not in any hurry. I think life is good enough to be worth living slowly."

"Okay. But don't let it get too slow. Because where there's no activity there's no life."

She wet her lips. "It's against everything I've been taught."

"There wouldn't be much hope for mankind, if people never knew better than they'd been taught."

"You have an answer for everything, don't you."

"No. I don't. I wish I did. But I think you should look into yourself, and ask yourself precisely what it is that you're afraid of. Put aside your father, and your mother, and just be yourself."

"I am being myself. I'm trying to be. You won't let me."

"I'll let you."

"I get to where I think I've got it thought out, and I have a reasonable adjustment, and—I don't know. I wish I could just stop and think and think and think."

"You can't stop and think. You have to think while you're living. Life goes on."

"The Sabbath is to stop and think," she said. "I need a Sabbath."

He was still standing by the door, across the room from her, and she still sat on the couch. Her gaze had drifted to the rug, but she looked at him again.

"I'd really like to be alone, if you don't mind, Les." Her voice was a little weak. "I'm coming down with something."

"Are you feverish?"

"No."

He held out his hands, as though appealing for a good-night kiss. She went to him. He clasped her. For a moment they were silent in each other's arms. His lips moved on her face, and then she rested her face on his collar.

"Another thing that's gone out in the last decade," he said. "This business of a guy trying to persuade a girl, like I've been doing to you. Today they don't have to."

"Why do you bother with me then?"

"I like you. I think you're worth it."

He was holding her in a low-slung embrace.

"Mad at me?" he asked.

"Do I seem mad?"

"You're so deliciously female," he said gently. "It's too bad you don't appreciate it."

His hands lifted her skirts behind her to the smoothness of her underpants.

"Don't, Les," she requested softly.

He let the skirts fall into place.

"I want to hold you tight," he murmured, "and touch you everywhere, and I'm not ashamed of it."

"I know," she said.

"And if you feel about me as I do about you, you shouldn't be afraid to be undressed. It was bringing us closer, wasn't it? When we were lying there?"

"If it doesn't separate us first. Les, there's a time for everything, and the time for sex is marriage."

"The time for sex is youth. It'll never again be like now. How long do you think your breasts are gonna stand up like that, and have the capacity to drive a man wild that they have now? Now's the time to enjoy it. How long do you think your face is gonna have that baby smoothness like that?"

"Les, please, I don't want to hear any more."

She stayed in his arms. His hands moved with fondness and gentleness. She leaned on his chest and his shoulder.

"I don't know," she said, hardly above a whisper. "I need more time."

Their cheeks touched.

"Do you think I'm immoral?" he said.

"No."

"You sure?"

"I think you're very moral, Les. And intelligent, and kind, and good."

She had taken her cheek from his. She saw him look down into the wedge of her dress, above the buttons, where the collar curled away.

"Sweetheart, do you know what breasts you have? They reach out to me. They do."

"Don't say any more, Les."

She looked up to his eyes. Her hands were before her, on his chest, and his embrace loosened somewhat.

"Please go," she said. "I really do have a stomach-ache. It's worse."

"If you're sick let me examine you. I'm a doctor, after all."

"No, please. You're not my doctor. I want you to go. Be nice."

His little smile began to fade, but he brought it back.

"Okay," he said. He released her.

"Thanks," she said, as he went out. She caught another glimpse of his smile as he shut the door.

29

Roland and Patty had a fist fight, from which Patty emerged crying with pain and outrage. Lucinda confined Roland to his room for the remainder of the afternoon, until it came time for his paper route. Ed was told when he came home, and lectured Roland about not hitting a girl, even a girl who was bigger and taller and older, and especially not a girl who was really physically a grown woman as Patty was. He spoke to Patty too because it seemed that she had provoked it, by tampering with Roland's bugs again and also taking some stamps from his bureau that were intended for a friend's collection and flushing them down the toilet.

It seemed to him that Patty could still be awfully childish, considering her size, and the womanly hams that swelled that girdle now. She had been doing foolish things all week long. She ate three candy bars in Yerxa's Pharmarcy and told her mother afterward she didn't even like candy bars. And when Lucinda asked her why she had eaten them if she didn't like them, she said she always forgot. She still baby-sat for the Hubbards, who lived in the white house beyond the Davey house, and she had been giving the perambulator little pushes away from her as she walked, catching up to it again, but it had gotten away from her over a little rise on Massapeequit Road and coasted far down the hill, tumbling over and spilling the baby out. The baby cried some, but Patty said nothing that day to the Hubbards. She worried privately for three whole days that some internal damage had been done and that the baby would grow up crippled or feeble-minded, and at last telephoned the Hubbards, near midnight. The baby was fine.

And at fifteen you'd think she would no longer pick fights with a brother of twelve, Ed said to himself. In years past she had often beaten Roland up. This was the first time she had lost.

The quarrel flared again at supper, because Roland had discovered belatedly during his confinement that some botanical specimens had been thrown out also, and Patty said they were still only weeds and he could get lots more, and there had been only one bug and the stamps were canceled anyhow. Roland ordered her to stay out of his room. "You just remember that, Patty-cake. I'm warning ya."

"All right, genius. You ought to clean your own room," she said, "and I wouldn't have to."

"I do clean it."

"You're big enough," she continued.

"I do. Nobody asked you to clean it."

"I don't have to be asked to do things. And I don't like to live in a messy house."

Lucinda and Ed both reprimanded them, but in a moment the bickering started again. Patty said it was no punishment to confine Roland to his room because his friends came under his window and entertained him. She also said his friends were a bad influence, especially that Snotsy Vaughn, who never tucked his shirttails in and used language that was absolutely unprintable.

"I didn't know you knew what it meant," said Roland.

"I said that's enough," Ed repeated.

He noticed that a day later they were still coolly hostile to each other, and when Patty got home from the football game Roland taunted her because Wilmerding had lost.

"Rollo dear—" she said finally.

"What."

"Please wend your way somewhere."

At the close of supper she remained at the table to read the grace with Ed and Roland, as she sometimes did, with a boy's skullcap balanced on top of the red hair.

Then she reminded her mother that it was Roland's turn to do the dishes and fled up to comb and to change, because she had a date with Junior Garafalo.

She wore her hair long now, and it made the color especially striking, Ed thought.

She had told this Junior Garafalo that she couldn't become engaged because he was the wrong religion but that she would go steady. Ed knew this, and knew that Lucinda had bawled her out about it and forbidden her to go steady with anyone. But it mattered little, as apparently no one else asked her out.

Ed went out to the barn to put antifreeze in the car. The dog, lying by its supper dish in the near darkness, made a sound of recognition, almost like a mewing, and he bent and stroked it. The dog must know people now by footsteps or smell, he thought; he was sure it was nearly blind. He reminded himself to make a place for it to sleep in the kitchen, before the weather got cold.

He propped his lantern so he could see under the hood of the car, and checked the hoses. Deeper in the barn he could make out the tall erect Model T, raised on blocks, its spare tire toward him. He thought he might saw some pine logs when he finished, even though night had set in. The moon had risen early, and the kitchen windows also shone on the woodpile. He had had no time to exercise all week long, and Saturday night was usually one of the few when he had no duties at all, with no committees of the congregation or of the town.

He took the saw outside, his jacket half zippered, and left it by the woodpile while he went past the rusty harrow to drag a cut tree from the tall grass and out of the mess of branches he had already stripped from it. He raised one end at last over a crate near the woodpile.

After every several strokes of the saw he stopped a few seconds to rest. It had occurred to him he might save oil by keeping the registers in the living-room floor closed all winter and heating that room entirely by the fireplace. He had bought a cord of wood for the winter to come, but the trees he cut and weathered would be good for the year following.

The frosted square of glass upstairs was lighted, and he knew Patty was there.

He was glad she had joined in the grace. A half hour before supper, when she had rushed in from the game, he had asked her to assist him in a libation to mark the Sabbath's end—he would have gone to the yard with her to search for the first stars, and given her the filigreed silver spice box to hold, and the twisted two-flamed candle. But she had declined; she had to go directly to iron some things or she'd be late. And Roland was out delivering papers at the time.

You couldn't have a decent Sabbath. Not when Patty was a cheerleader and had to be at the games. And you couldn't forbid her, now that Roland had his own daily paper route morning and evening.

The route was good for responsibility, and he had allowed it with the understanding that Roland would arrange for a substitute on Sabbaths and holidays, but the substitute rarely materialized. He remembered how he had used to think the Sabbaths would be when someday he would own a house like this. A fire would be kindled an hour or two before sundown, with a fat log atop the smaller ones, that it might blaze untended far into the night, and there would be such warmth, and such melody, that no one would have need to go elsewhere. He thought of the Sabbath as a liberation. But you couldn't tell Patty that. She didn't want to be liberated from football games.

The two children who had not yet left home were extraordinarily busy—it seemed to him they never rested. Especially Patty. Muckanaug Chapter of the Order of De Molay, and Louisa M. Alcott Assembly no. 156 of the Order of the Rainbow for Girls, each of which met biweekly in the Masonic lodge room over the supermarket, were jointly sponsoring a dramatic play, and Patty was to have a part in it. She had also become the organist at the Rainbow meetings, and lately had even gotten a job playing the organ at St. Timothy's Protestant Episcopal Church. A young lady named Miss Perkins, who had played the organ for the Rainbow and for the church, had gotten married and left town, and as she had heard Patty's skillful fooling around at the keyboard after the Rainbow meetings she had recommended her in both places. The minister Ralph Briggs had telephoned Ed somewhat apologetically to ask if it was all right, and told him the stipend, and how Miss Perkins had praised her, and assured him that at the organ bench she would not have to pray or kneel. Briggs even made some joke about not holding her as a hostage for Betsy Stokes. Patty loved the choir robe, even as she loved the cheerleader costume. Ed had not seen it, but she described it as wine color with cream trim.

If she wasn't busy doing something she was busy doing nothing. If she double-dated with a boy from another town she might spend half an hour on the kitchen phone giving street directions. He had seen her there gesticulating rights and lefts and telling some stranger to take a left at Colby & Dill's Real Estate, and over the stone bridge, not the road past the cinder-block shed and the old Pigs Gusset Indian Reservation. It was a large field that was called that, although it had a ball diamond and tennis courts.

Or she sat around with Denise Saint-Onge and Polly Cook, talking about boys, or about Doris Avery being in love with Christopher Slaney, or singing and playing records. They knew all the newest hits. He would hear them sing one song after another—the whole hit parade. Why Won't You Say You Love Me; Yesterday's Tears; I'm a-Ting Ting Tingle Tangle Tingle; Sweetie Sweetie I Want You Bad; Mama Von't Know De Difference; Flouncy Bouncy; How True; I'm a-Datin' I'm a-Matin'; Buckety Bum; Why Didn't I Know; Come Into My Igloo; Gimme Gimme Jimmy; I'm Gone On John. The songs were awful, but he liked their voices. He asked once if they would sing some old songs, like Drink To Me Only, or some Stephen Foster, but they didn't.

He thought it remarkable that Patty had been accepted as a cheerleader. Polly Cook, who was hefty like Patty, could not have been. But Patty, despite her overweight, had an agility and a spirit that apparently were just what was wanted. Denise, who was slight and slinky, was also a cheerleader, and sometimes he heard Denise and Patty go over the cheers together. For a long time Polly was never around, and Denise and Patty seemed to talk about her, but he was glad when they became friendly with Polly again. He thought she was a good influence. It was Polly's long straight hair that had inspired Patty to wear her own that way, and it kept Patty out of the beauty parlor. And Polly had also backed up Ed and Lucinda in an argument they had had with Patty over a tight sweater, or had at least seemed to back them up.

Apparently Lucinda had not known the sweater was still around, but Patty had dug it out of her undersized things of an earlier year and wore it at the organ bench in Briggs's church before Lucinda found out, and planned to wear it to school the next day. Lucinda was horrified at her having worn such a thing before Briggs's congregation in the church service. Patty said the robes covered everything anyhow and that girls in the choir wore all kinds of peek-a-boos and see-throughs under them. But Lucinda had insisted on throwing it out anyway.

"Aw, my bust measurement is the only advantage I get out of being fat," Patty had protested.

"It's not an advantage," said Lucinda. "There's such a thing as making yourself ridiculous."

Ridiculous my eye, Ed thought. Didn't the kid have any sense? Didn't girls know anything about boys?

He paused in his log-sawing, because a pair of headlights were turning in and bouncing gently far down on his dirt driveway. The car approached up the big curve and stopped before the house. Ed put down the saw and walked toward it. He heard the storm door slam and Patty crossed under the porch light and descended the steps, her coat on her arm.

Polly Cook had gotten out of the car and in again and Patty had slipped into the back seat beside Junior Garafalo by the time Ed got there. A strange boy was at the wheel and Patty introduced him. Ed saw that Patty had eyebrow pencil and eye shadow. He had not shaved since before the Sabbath and he wondered if his stubble embarrassed Patty. The children told him they were going to the movie at Sparkstown, and that they would probably stop afterward at the More-On Sandwich Shop. Ed was standing by the closed door and lowered window of the car, nearest to Polly. Despite her heftiness her face was quite striking in an Anglo-Saxon way. He knew she belonged to St. Timothy's Episcopal.

"Let's go, daddykins," Patty said to the back of the driver's head.

"What's this daddykins?" Ed said to her. "He's not your daddy. I'm your daddy."

Then he looked past Polly to the boy at the wheel, and asked him if his brakes were good. The boy said they were, and Ed asked about the brake lights, and the directional signals, and whether the horn was working. The boy tooted it.

"How are the tires?" said Ed. He kicked a tire and ran his fingers on the tread. "All right, drive carefully, will ya?" he said.

"You're just making the driver nervous," said Patty.

The boy told Ed about a front-end noise. Ed lifted the hood and the boy turned the engine a few times. Ed bent over, listening. "Do you think it's the generator?" the boy asked him.

"It sounds like the fan belt," Ed told him. "But bring your car around in daylight sometime. I'd like to check it over. You'll learn something."

The children drove away at last. He watched the taillights.

He decided not to return to the sawing. He had been sweaty in his open jacket and now he felt cold. He went back to put the saw in the barn.

Then he entered the house. He drank some cider in the kitchen. Lucinda was in the dining room with some mending. "What were you doing out there so long?" she said. "Sawing wood? In the dark?"

"Well, I put antifreeze in the car, and I sawed some wood. There was light from the windows."

"You waste more time fiddling with that car," she said.

"That's fiddling? Antifreeze?"

He had meant to write to Charles this evening, so he went to his study and sat at the desk. But he kept thinking of Patty. All that beauty, and you have to lend it out.

He had been brought up with his twin sister Rosalind, and having a sister was good training—it taught you to keep your distance. But as best he could remember he had had a keen appreciation of girls' figures as a high-school kid. He hoped there were still boys who could just think and let it go at that. He found it hard to talk to the boys who came around. Everything they said to him, even if about the weather, had a dullness that seemed evasive. Even the girls became hard to talk to if the boys were there.

Even when they were little, long before they were shaped yet, you feared the future, when they would have to travel off into the night, sitting next to somebody's trousers.

His elbows were on the desk, and his chin and mouth rested on his folded hands. What potential rage lay within him at the idea of any molester or tempter, he reflected, and how strange it was that it was naturally there, despite his having been on the other side in his youth. How keenly he had felt it with Millicent's adolescence. At twelve, thirteen, Millicent had seemed especially sacred and untouchable.

How exciting a girl was at that age. And how incredibly beautiful. You could wish it were permitted to go on being Daddy, and clasp that babyness to you. He had always been glad he had had daughters. And it was a loss, in a way, that the budding of one's own daughters could not be witnessed in the family circle, as part of the child's growth, and thereby a growth of the parent too. Perhaps there were households where there was not such privacy as here. But modesty, bathrobes, locked doors were Lucinda's way, and she had imparted it to the girls so early that the children's own embarrassment had imparted itself to him—he had learned to know that if he stumbled upon a nine-year-old in shirtwaist and panties her discomfort would be unbearable. This flesh of his flesh. They were scarcely out of babyhood before they were hidden. Perhaps this was how all mothers brought up daughters, and in the long run the only way, if you wanted them to be modest outside.

This past summer the Conrad Bernsteins had invited him and the family to their waterfront cottage for a day, and he had watched Patty in her bathing suit. It was amazing that his infant daughter had become all that.

At last he put it from his mind and took pen and paper from the drawer, and wrote to Charles, congratulating the boy on his promotion. Mother had written the day before and Patty had baked special brownies, he told him, but he wanted to send his own congratulations separately. He said he was happy not only about the promotion but especially about the usefulness of what Charles was learning about aircraft engines.

He thought of mentioning what fine background it would make for engineering college after his hitch. But he decided not to. It was probably what Charles had in mind anyway, and the boy had been feeling sensitive about references to his schooling.

He also suggested to him, toward the end, that he not get out of practice with his prayer book and phylacteries. Ed had packed them among Charles's things at the time of the enlistment. He did not actually inquire, however, if they were being used. It seemed not discreet, like one of those things you don't ask.

But he wrote how important it was that Charles should learn to do his job perfectly, because nothing less than perfect was good enough in the maintenance of aircraft. Men's lives could depend upon Charles's attention to those planes and his thoroughness. Just as much so as if he were a physician. It was no light matter to hold someone else's fate in your hands. There comes a time, he wrote, when you realize that every task you undertake is either God's work or a boondoggle.

He told him again to take care of himself. Your loving father, he wrote, and signed it Dad. He didn't seal it. He thought Lucinda would want to add her love, even though she had written yesterday.

He rose, enjoying the image in his mind of Charles wearing corporal's stripes. He knew Charles had not yet been trained to know a whole plane, but only part of it. Yet he would have confidence in whatever Charles checked over and okayed.

As he left the room the sight of the double front door, curving up to a point, and its engraved glass and the night beyond made him think of Patty again. The talk, the coquetry. To see your son becoming a man was different. Unless he rejected you totally, he enlarged your house. Even if he made his mistakes, and angered you here and disappointed you there, his physical being made you proud. What defeated you was your daughters becoming women.

30

Mr. Hopkins, harried and busy, sent Millicent out on a real reporting assignment. The biennial election campaigns were now at their height, with a great many candidates, and Mr. Hopkins explained that Dexter Killian had told him to use her in a pinch if he found himself shorthanded.

"Oh, I'd be delighted," she said.

Maud Dickinson had already written the whole story in advance, he told her, but Millicent was to go to the scene and watch, just in case the candidate should happen to fall ill and die in the midst of delivering his speech, or in case the story should otherwise fail to occur as planned. She set out carrying a pencil, a small wad of blank paper taken from the city room and folded in half like a makeshift booklet as she had seen the reporters do, and also a rolled-up copy of the mimeographed speech that the candidate was to read. She felt a warmth toward Mr. Killian. He had twice now demonstrated confidence in her, without her having brought in any feature articles on her own yet, or having done anything to deserve it. It made her feel guilty about her inefficiency and inertia. She resolved to make better use of her mornings and her days off.

She found the hotel just as the dinner party was beginning, and someone directed her to a special table reserved for representatives of the press. It was close to the dais. Her card was ready in her sock but no one asked to see it.

At her table there were reporters from two of the other papers—a silent courtly gentleman who looked nearly eighty with a wrinkled neck in a high collar, and a big, greasy, jowly young fellow who clearly liked her looks and who tried to be gallant and charming toward her. She made herself as cool and discouraging as was possible short of actual rudeness, scarcely listening to him, and once or twice reminding him that she had to pay attention to everything that took place.

She was brought a dinner, like everyone else, but it was rather too sumptuous and after the pea soup she did not eat much. The old reporter hung a napkin in his high collar like a bib, and the big jowly one grew quite helpful, pointing out public men to her and explaining various political alliances. When at last the candidate spoke she followed in her mimeographed copy with great care and attention, touching her pencil tip to every word. He read miserably. When he had reached the end of the closing sentence she hurried to a telephone booth and called the city room as Mr. Hopkins had instructed her.

Mr. Hopkins transferred her call to Maud, and Maud asked her a few questions. Millicent answered excitedly, her voice shaking. Then she described to Maud how the candidate had stumbled over words, how he had mistaken them and misread them appallingly in a confused monotone, as though he had not seen the text before and had no comprehension of what it meant. But Maud told her the story could not include such a description; it must give only the news, without slanting.

"But a candidate for attorney general of the Commonwealth," Millicent said, "and he can't even read? Isn't that news? He can't read a simple English sentence."

"No, dearie, that's not news," said Maud.

Millicent held the receiver while Maud inquired of Mr. Hopkins what Millicent was to do next. Then Maud told her to return to the city room and spend the rest of the evening at her usual duties.

When she got there Mr. Hopkins told her there had been a phone call for her. He gave her the name of Dr. Hollander and the number of the hospital on a scrap of paper.

She had to go down to the sidewalk to chalk bulletins on the blackboard. But when she had a chance she called Leslie back. She used a telephone on a vacant desk near the back of the city room, and held a hand cupped about the mouthpiece. Leslie began to tell her his schedule for her nights off, which night he would be on call and which one he would have free.

"Les," she cut in, "I've decided on a moratorium on seeing each other for a while. I think we need a cooling-off period."

The moment of silence told her she had surprised him.

"Well," he said, "let's get together and talk about it."

"No, I don't want to see you," she said. "Not for two weeks." She spoke softly behind her cupped hand, glancing with her eyes to make sure no one overheard. "Les, men invented morality, and now they want to take it apart. And I think it's time we both did a little thinking."

He began some protest but she cut in again.

"I just want time to think, that's all," she said. "That's fair enough, isn't it? After all, men decide that morals are changed, that there's been a sexual revolution or something, and women take the brunt of it."

"You seem to want to deny that there are two sexes," his voice said at her ear. "Life will be richer when you admit it."

"Leslie, I can't argue on company time. You call me in two weeks."

She hung up the phone and returned to her work. Some edited pieces lay in the basket on Mr. Hopkins's desk and she took them up to Mr. Valentino. On the stairs she realized she had forgotten to tell Leslie about her first reporting assignment.

On the way home also she thought more about Leslie than about the reporting assignment. She walked part of the way, but the heavy sweater was insufficient in the cold, so she took the underground trolley. She waited a long time in the nearly empty station.

She felt that all the arguments and all the reasoning had somehow changed nothing. And she felt a little mad at him for giving her guilt feelings about being a virgin.

He talks about me being immature—what about his wanting what he can't have? Chastity still exists, she said to herself. Even if he doesn't think so.

She felt quite certain that neither fear nor frigidity was at the root of her self-denial. She thought that in admitting frustration she had proved she had normal desire.

I'm not Victorian, she told herself. It's not as if I thought sex was sin or something. She felt certain she would prove quite capable of enjoying sex competently and confidently, when the time came, within the context of marriage. It seemed to her that her ability to talk uninhibitedly about it, and discuss sex, and argue, was proof that she was open-minded—and therefore her choice of virginity was free and rational.

The whole friendship with Leslie had started out as a lovely relationship, she thought, with real sympathy and communication and with independence from the physical, but lately he had gotten worse and worse.

Of course his theory was that if they were each other's intellectual equal, and if they had frequent enough sexual release, then sex could not possibly become central. Instead of hours of tension and bitterness over a sex argument, there would be a few insignificant minutes of intercourse followed by hours of talking about something else, with sex relieved and therefore far from their minds.

Yet putting it that way made such an ultimatum of it. Men were so arrogant.

But Les was such an intelligent boy. And people with brains were not easy to find.

So many boys took that attitude. Excepting Eugene it included most she had met at the university. She remembered one disagreeable young man who had warned her that if she didn't change her attitude toward love play she would have very few dates and would find herself isolated. She had told him off, and never saw him again. Mr. Hackelman, she had said, since I'm not interested in you, I'm delighted that you're not interested in me either. She had of course never called him mister before, and she was pleased with the way it put him in his place.

And a girl she had studied with in Chicago told once of even being assured by a boy that if he should abandon her afterward she still would have been enlarged by the experience. Millicent remembered being shocked by the story, and by the boy's gall.

This notion, this line, she thought, that what a man does to you fulfills you as a woman. What a detestable male conceit. It takes more than that to fulfill me as a woman. That's not what initiates me into being a woman, or makes me a grownup, or any of that. Physical intimacy with some patronizing male. It doesn't make men out of boys and it doesn't make women out of girls. If you have an infantile mentality you can have sex from now until doomsday and it won't help any.

When she had climbed to her apartment and unlocked the door Charles was there, in his gray uniform, rising from the worn stuffed chair and smiling at her.

"For goodness sakes," said Millicent. She frowned.

"Hi," he said. His stuffed round barracks bag was on the floor by the studio couch. Ella Jane sat by the table in her robe. Apparently Natalie had already gone to bed.

"You haven't called the folks I bet," Millicent said to him. "You shouldn't come here first every time you have a furlough."

"Oh, leave the kid alone," said Ella Jane. "He likes it here."

"But it's nervy, walking in on you," said Millicent.

"Don't be silly," said Ella Jane.

Millicent looked at Charles. He was even childlike in his slimness.

"I got a flight into Otis," he said. "It's a lot nearer to come here."

"Well, you can still get home. I don't think you should sleep over. Mother and Dad will be anxious to see you. I'll see you there Sunday anyway. I teach Sunday school now."

"I'll go in the morning," he said. "Mother wouldn't want me on the roads at night anyway."

"Dad would come and get you."

"Well, no, I've missed the last good train and I don't want to bother him. I'll go tomorrow." He put his hands on her shoulders. "Sis, you're beautiful," he said.

She freed herself with a slight squirm. She looked at Ella Jane. She was embarrassed by the way Ella Jane seemed amused at her effort to boss Charles.

She sighed. Then they removed the long cushion from the studio couch and prepared it on the floor for Charles to sleep on, as they had done the other time. Ella Jane said good night and went off with her cane to her bedroom.

"Good night," Charles answered her, and in the next instant raised a curving hand to his mouth. A great silent belch seemed to shake him. Millicent had apparently looked at him askance, because he caught her eye and explained that he had had a sour stomach all evening. He had stopped at a little delicatessen and eaten a whole quarter-pound slab of Danish blue cheese in a pumpernickel sandwich, and the dry cheesy aftertaste had given him an insatiable craving for orange juice, so he had drunk a whole quart of it from a carton until it made him sick.

"I'll make you some warm milk," she said. "That'll be good for you." She went to the kitchen and began to wash a pot. She made a disapproving noise with her tongue and her teeth. "Don't you know how to take care of yourself better than that?"

She poured milk into the pot and lighted the gas. He watched, leaning sideways on the doorjamb.

"Maybe I should make you some bicarb," she said.

"No, I hate bicarb."

"What did you talk about to Ella Jane all night? Stock tips?"

"No, just sitting. Waiting for you."

"What time did you get here?"

"Nine."

At length they lay side by side in the darkened living room, Millicent upon the couch and Charles down on the floor.

"You seem to get a lot of passes," she remarked.

"It's not a pass. I've got a delay-en-route. I'm being transferred."

"That's right," she remembered. "Mother said you'd be in New York somewhere. And she said you're an acting corporal."

"I'm a bona fide corporal. It came through."

"Oh. Well, congratulations."

"That's nothing."

"No, really. I think it's wonderful, Charles."

"Twenty-two more bucks a month, that's all."

For a while there were only the soft noises of the night, a turning upon bedding or the sound of passing tires.

But in time Charles began talking, slowly and quietly, almost as if he were lying there not to sleep but to pass the time of night. He spoke of the Southern towns near the base where he had spent the past few months, of their people and their girls, of one of his buddies, and of one or another of the family and relatives. "Dad's a guy that talks with God—you have to give him that," he said at one point. "Even if God couldn't care less." He talked also of the housewarming party their parents had had last spring, and said he wished there could be more occasions like that, that would bring all the cousins together. Then he talked a while about Patty.

In the morning they slept late, neither of them arising until Natalie and Ella Jane had gone.

She did her calisthenics with both parts of her pajamas on and the buttons closed, and then shut herself in Natalie's room to dress.

She boiled eggs, after inquiring about Charles's stomach, and set them in eggcups. She looked away from the tight fullness of his underwear.

"Get dressed for breakfast," she said. "That's terribly sloppy."

"Okay." He was wiping his face with a towel.

She finished unfolding the drop-leaf table and laid out the breakfast. When he sat opposite her she found herself watching him pensively. He was occupied in peeling bits of shell from the first of his eggs.

"Charles—" she asked. She felt slightly red-faced.

"What?"

She didn't know what had brought her to what she was about to ask. Perhaps it was the recollection of some of his talk during the night about loneliness.

She swallowed her embarrassment.

"What do you do with girls?"

"What do you mean?"

"You know what I mean. Do you make love to them? How far do you go."

If the question made him uncomfortable he hid the fact behind a kind of blankness. "Different distances," he answered. "I don't know."

She kept looking at him.

"It depends," he said.

"What does it depend on?"

"I don't know."

"Do you go pretty far?"

"Sometimes I go far, and sometimes not so far."

"Can't you tell me about it?"

There was a momentary pause and a pensive lifting of his brow. "You'd disapprove," he said.

"If you can't tell me, don't you ever again say I'm the only one you can talk to."

He gave a slight shrug. "Well, I've been laid, if that's what you want to know."

She knew she had not really believed that that could be the answer. It jarred her at first out of any reply. She watched him take a spoonful of egg.

She wet her lips. "What kind of girls were they?"

"Oh, just the local talent down there. Girls. I told ya."

"How do you meet them?" Her voice did not have much force behind it.

"Oh, some you hear of, and some you just meet."

"Do you sleep with every girl you go out with?"

"What do you think I am? A Casanova or something?"

"I mean do you try with every girl? Or what?"

"Not if they're decent."

"What percentage are decent?"

"No special percentage."

"I don't mean exactly—"

"You just size them up."

"And you can always tell?"

"Oh, they can fool you."

He ate unconcernedly.

"Are your eggs too soft?" she said.

"No."

"They're better for you soft."

He spread butter thickly on toast.

"Tell me about some," she asked.

"What."

"Some of the girls."

"What do you care?"

"I just want to know."

"Well," he said, "you meet all kinds."

"So tell me."

"Well, there was one that was a Holy Roller. There really is such a thing, you know."

Millicent ate too, slowly, watching her spoon and trying not to seem overly concerned. "Did you sleep with her?"

"No. I couldn't get to first base with her. Kissed her, that's all."

"Was she intelligent, at least?"

"No. She was pretty stupid. And all full of talk about the niggers have the mark of Cain, and asking me who's my pastor, and all that kind of stuff."

"Was she pretty or what?"

"No."

"What did you go with her for?"

"I don't know. I just went out with her a couple of times. There was nothing else doing, and she was sort of in love with me."

"And what about others?"

"Well, there was one you couldn't even understand what she was talking about. The accents of some of these people down there—the way they say some things, it could take ten minutes of talking back and forth to explain what they mean. I keep saying 'what?—what?' I ask her what she's been doing all day and she says 'airnin'."

"What?" said Millicent.

" 'Airnin'."

"What's that?"

"Well, that's what I said. I finally found out it's ironing."

"Oh." She was finishing her egg. "What are they? Hillbillies? What do you call them in that part? Crackers?"

"No, no special name. They're just stupid."

"And did you sleep with that one?"

"No, she sort of had a sister that kept tabs on her."

"What about the others?"

"What others?"

"What I asked you. That you slept with." Her hands were in her lap, and she looked at him across the table without flinching. Her face maintained a steady tone of color.

He tossed his head a little to the side. "Well, there was this one I met right in front of the library. It just goes to show you. She just looked like a sweet, nice girl—I didn't figure there was anything there. And I was just killing time, and she was sitting there by the steps reading this big book, so I said 'what's that book about?' and we started talking, you know. She told me about the book."

"What kind of a book?"

"Oh, about a holy relic or something."

"A novel?"

"I guess so. Ya, a novel."

"And then what happened? With the girl, I mean."

"Well, we took a walk, and the next thing I know we were kind of walking with my leg stuck to her leg, if you know what I mean, and we were holding hands, and she's holding my hand tight, sort of pressing against her, so I said, 'where can we be alone,' and she steers me to this woodsy place, and we get there, and all of a sudden she pulls her dress up and says 'let's get it over with.' "

"Just like that?"

"Just like that."

"I don't believe it."

"So help me."

"I bet you bragged all over the barracks about it."

"No. I might have told a couple of guys."

"Did you ever see her again?"

"Sure."

"And is that where you go with them? Outdoors?"

"Or in their houses, if nobody's home. In the back of a truck once. I wouldn't have believed it, Sis. The kind of people you meet. There was one I had to tell her I had nigger blood to get rid of her. That's how ignorant she was."

"You had what?"

"Nigger blood. She was calling up the base all the time, so I told her it didn't show but I was one-sixteenth nigger."

"You're blond."

"I know, I told her it didn't show, but it's still black blood. I told her my grandfather was a slave on a cotton plantation in Virginia."

"Virginia was tobacco country."

"Well I don't know. I told her Virginia. She was in love with me. She thought she was gonna marry me or something."

"How did she take it?"

"Cried. She said she didn't care, but I told her we'd have all these black nigger kids and it was against the law and everything else."

"Why didn't you just tell her you're a Jew?"

"Well, I thought of that. But it didn't seem right to use religion. I don't think it would have meant anything anyway. I don't know if she knew what a Jew was."

"Why'd you have to get rid of her?"

"Well, she was calling the orderly room. She thought we were getting married and all that chazerei."

"Did you tell her you were getting married?"

"No, I never told her. She just talked it into herself. She was crazy. And I was afraid of her making a stink because she was jailbait. Fifteen years old."

"Fifteen?"

"Ya. Statutory rape. She looked older, you know. Big. And she told me she was eighteen, and then it comes out she's fifteen. When an older girl brings charges you can get all your buddies to testify she's the town pump or something, but when she's under age that's no good. The whole gang of you would go to Leavenworth."

"That's awful."

"Leavenworth?"

"The whole thing."

"You know, I wouldn't care about Leavenworth—I'd get put in charge of the motor pool or something. But I'd care about the dishonorable discharge. I'd lose all the G.I. educational benefits, and no moment of pleasure is worth that."

"What are these girls? Crazy? Or what?"

"They're everything. Sis, you wouldn't believe the things. There's girls that can tell you all night long about some guy they're mooning for, because he hasn't written to them for a couple of days or something, that they're supposed to be in love with. Even while they're doing it with you, practically. And girls that use dirty language. I was amazed. Gee, there was one I was sitting in the living room with, and we were fooling around, you know, and she lives with her old grandmother. And then the grandmother walks in the door, so she stands up and introduces me, and she doesn't even cover up. I mean she stands right there with her whole dress open, and her breasts hanging right out, actually, and she's introducing me to her grandmother. And then I realize the grandmother's blind. I was so shocked—I'm telling ya. I'm standing there saying 'how do you do.' That poor old lady, trying to bring up an orphan. I'll never forget it as long as I live."

"And you went right back to fooling around?"

"No. I couldn't. What do you think I am? Her skin felt like it was made out of soggy rubber or something. God. Honest, Sis, I'm telling ya. I could write a book."

"Why don't you."

"Nobody would believe it. There was even one girl down there that was pregnant. I mean really far gone pregnant. And she was still out walking around with her girl friends, looking for a pickup or something."

"And did you go with that one?"

"Of course not. What do you think."

"Charles, it's horrible. Don't you think it's horrible?"

"Ya, it's horrible. That's what I'm telling ya."

"It's just squalid. I wish I hadn't heard it."

"You mean the pregnant girl? Or the one with the grandmother."

"Any of it. All your looking for women."

"Well, I'm sorry," he apologized.

"Can't you see it's squalid?"

"Well, that's why girls don't ask their brothers things like that. You shouldn't ask."

He blew on his cocoa.

"Well, I wanted to know," she said. "I don't want to live in ignorance either. I can't be ignorant forever. Just because I belong to an evil generation."

She was looking at him. She could scarcely move.

"Why do you do it?" she said.

"What do you mean, why do I do it. I like it."

"Wouldn't you rather live cleanly, instead of so squalidly?"

"Well, sometimes it gets pretty squalid."

"What do you think Mother and Dad would say?"

"Oh, they'd hit the ceiling."

"It's just sickening."

"I know it."

"If you realize it why do you do it? Why don't you give it up, stop it? If not for Mother and Dad then for me. I don't believe in a double standard. I believe it's just as bad for a boy as for a girl."

He looked somewhat badgered. "I wish I hadn't told you," he said.

"I asked." She tried to look at him firmly.

"Well, maybe I'll try, but I can't promise a thing like that. You don't understand, Sis."

"I don't mean as a promise to me. I mean for your own good. Charles, you're so young."

"I'm eighteen, for God's sake."

"You may be bigger than I am now," she said, "but I can remember when you weren't."

"What's that got to do with it."

"You enjoy it, don't you," she said.

"Sure."

"It never disappoints you?"

"Well, sometimes."

She sighed. She pushed back her chair and started clearing the table. Charles began to follow her with dishes to the kitchen. He half tripped on the cat.

"Pour some of the cocoa in a saucer for Theodore, will you?" Millicent said without looking at him.

Then she worked a while without speaking to him.

"Help me wipe. Don't be so lazy," she said finally, still without looking at him.

He wiped dishes and utensils while she washed. The sink had an accumulation in it from the night before.

"Were any of these girls ever virgins?" she asked.

"One," he said.

But she sensed that he searched for more to say, as though the exchange could not be left there.

"It was sort of sad," he said. "I don't know. I guess some girls sort of try awful hard to be gay, or feel enraptured or something. When they're getting it for the first time."

"What do you say to them?"

"Different things."

"Tell me. If they say no, how do you talk them into it? How do you get a girl to go further?"

"Oh, there's different lines. What comes into your head."

"Give me an example."

"Oh, like I might say, 'gorgeous—' "

"What if she isn't gorgeous?"

"You say it anyway. Or you say, 'sweetheart, let's try each other out—maybe we were made for each other.' Or I might say, 'I want you, baby. Let's not get all this close and just go apart again.' "

"How can you mouth such stuff!" Her wet hand rubbed a pot with steel wool.

"Well, it's according to the type of a girl. Like there's an old slogan that says treat a queen like a whore and a whore like a queen."

"What?"

"It's just a slogan. Like a folk saying. A proverb."

"Boys say that to each other? Now that I resent. I really resent that. You think women are some kind of fools to be manipulated, don't you. To be flattered and taken advantage of." The movement of submerged crockery became louder. "The conceit of men is just unbearable. You don't even think women are real."

She washed something with a splash. He backed away a step, still wiping, though she faced the sink, not him.

"Charles, I'm furious."

"I shouldn't have told you."

"Not just you. I mean at the whole male sex."

"Well, that's why you shouldn't ask things like that."

"All these girls, lying down like that with men who care nothing for them, and demanding this fraudulent pretense of affection, and knowing it's fraudulent, and you supplying these lying words, and you know she knows it's a lie, and yet she accepts it— It doesn't upset you? Wouldn't you rather just say, 'I despise you and you despise me, but my glands are bursting'?"

"Well, hell, you can't do that. They need some pretense."

"Why?"

"Out of self-respect."

"It's so ugly," said Millicent. "I wish I lived in a moral age." She grimaced almost with a shudder, the corners of her mouth bending down, and bit her lower lip. "What's so wrong with human beings, that self-respect has to be based on pretense? How can it really be self-respect?"

"Sis, you don't know that type," he explained. "These kids, it's drek."

"That's fine gratitude for their favors."

She stacked the last of the dishes, clean and dripping, beside the sink, and snatched the towel from him to wipe her hands.

"They're human beings," she said. "They're no lower than you are."

"It's Saturday-night stuff. If I didn't knock them over they'd do it with somebody else."

"You said some of them were in love with you." She gave the towel back to him.

"Well, some of them," he said.

She went to the living room and slumped in the worn stuffed chair. She spread her hands on the arms of it. On the carpet the cat was trying to poke at a sunbeam. She could see Charles still wiping dishes.

"And another thing," she said. "Straighten up your bed in the morning after you sleep here. Put that cushion back. Fold the blanket and put the sheets away."

He continued with the dishes. She saw him try to distribute them in their cabinets.

"Can't you see what a shame—what a disgrace—degradation it is for you to seek out the company of nitwitted women?" she said. "To feel compelled, like that? To have these brainless women for companions? Foolish, mindless, stupid women? Do you want me to respect you? Then live so I can respect you."

He came to the living room and yanked the sheets and blanket away. She watched him restore the long cushion to the studio couch.

"I don't know where you get such crazy girls. They should be in lunatic asylums. And you should, too."

"Where should I put the sheets?"

"In the wash. In the hamper."

"What hamper?"

"In the bathroom."

She was still in the chair when he returned. His face looked sad and chastised.

"Do you think Patty would let a boy get familiar?" Millicent asked.

"No. I don't think so. Do you think she would?"

"No," Millicent said.

He sat on the studio couch.

"However," she added, "there's a man that wants to have an affair with me, actually. For your information." She noticed the way he stared at her. She crossed her knees and folded her hands.

"Don't you do it, Sis."

"I have too much sense. Believe me," she said to him. "And you're not to tell anyone what I told you. About that somebody wants to, I mean."

"No." He kept staring. "Who is he?"

"A friend."

"Well get rid of him."

"Why?"

"Because you're too fine. He's got no right even talking to you that way."

"He happens to be a fine person. At least in some ways."

"You've still got no business going with a wolf."

"He's not a wolf."

"Well, whatever he is."

"What do you expect, when men's minds work like yours?"

"I wouldn't try to seduce anybody decent."

"You really want it both ways, don't you."

"What do you mean?"

"Nothing," she said. "I just don't get it." Her loosely clasped hands moved on one another.

"Tell me honestly, Sis. Is this guy making any progress?"

She felt herself color. "None whatsoever."

"What's his name?"

"None of your business. I'm not being rude. It's just none of your affair."

"Have Mother and Dad met him?"

"No."

"Is he a guy they know about?"

"No."

"What line of work is he in?"

"It's honest work."

"How'd you meet him?"

"A blind date. Through a friend."

"How often do you see him?"

"Well, right now, zero. I told him I didn't want to see him for a while."

"Will you see him again?"

"Probably."

"Don't give in, Sis."

"A lot you should care. I feel like telling girls not to give in to you."

"Tell the son of a bitch to buzz off. As a favor to me."

"It won't be as a favor to you."

She rose and wandered and gazed at the street. Some brown leaves were circling, some almost as high as the window.

"I can take care of myself," she said. "Better than you can. You're really disgusting."

When she looked at him he had leaned far back across the couch, his head against the wall. The packed barracks bag was on the floor near his foot, the cords tied.

She felt a gush of sadness, as if she might cry. But she did not. She went to the couch and sat on the other end of it, facing him, one foot half under her. He looked thoughtfully before him, not at her, his chin on his chest.

"Charles," she said. There was some pleading tearfulness in her voice. "Listen to me. Do you know what the Bible says? 'Drink waters out of thine own cistern.' Do you know that? 'And running water of thine own spring. Let the streams pour out like rivers flooding the streets, but let her be only thine own.' Or something like that. 'Have joy of the wife of thy youth, a lovely hind and a graceful doe—let your fountain be blessed, and be ravished always with her love.' And something about her breasts, I forget. It's very beautiful, Charles. And it says, 'My son, then why wilt thou be ravished with a strange woman, and embrace the bosom of a stranger?' "

She remained looking at him. She could see his breathing, and once or twice his lips seemed about to form words.

"I don't know," he said. "When people are older, and married, I suppose they can say you should wait till you're married, but when you're young, and marriage is a long way off, it's just too much fun to say no to it."

"Isn't it supposed to be reserved for someone you love?"

"Well, sometimes there isn't anyone around you can love, and you still need it."

"Oh, you and your old need. Don't they give them saltpeter in the Army?"

"Air Force."

"There are plenty of men and women that do without it and nothing happens," she said. "What if you were overseas, in some jungle place, or on an island, and there weren't any girls?"

"Well, so I'd do without."

"Of course you would. And Charles, don't you know that if you keep associating with girls of low morals that's the kind you'll end up married to?"

"No I won't."

"Yes, Charles. Because it's hard to find someone with the right qualities you want—it takes an awful lot of searching, and you just can't afford to waste time. And if you squander time with girls you detest, just because they go to bed with you, or because they might, it doesn't leave time enough for the real search. You don't have time enough for it as it is, what with getting ahead in your work, and you may have school again. Maybe you'll even fall in love with one of these girls you go with, because by then you'll get to think that that's what girls are like, and that that's what you have to accept." She swallowed, still looking at him. His eyes turned to her. "When I get married," she told him, "I want the best possible marriage."

31

Lucinda had been going to sew the corporal's stripes on Charles's blue-gray shirts, but Patty insisted on doing it. She took them to the hassock by the fire. Ed found her working there alone, and shut the French doors of the living room behind him.

He pulled together the scattered sections of the Sunday newspaper, from the floor and the sofa and the dining room. A section of Old English type had been torn from the front-page banner head to show that Roland had gotten it without charge. It was the first chance he had had to look at any of it, except for Millicent's having shown him a little item she had written.

"Will you please remind your son not to leave the refrigerator open?" Patty said without looking up.

"Which son?" said Ed.

"Rollo. Which do you think?"

"Tell him yourself."

"I'm not speaking to Rollo."

"So write him a letter. Send him a telegram."

He looked again for Millicent's tiny item, but found only a neat oblong hole. Lucinda must have already clipped it for the scrapbook.

Charles had borrowed Ed's car and had gone for the evening to meet his cousin Steve. During the day he had explained something to Ed about the relation of a plane's engine thrust to the type of wing, and Ed now relived Charles's little lecture warmly, and from the sofa watched Patty meanwhile. Her fingers worked quickly, as though the sewing came naturally. He saw a few inches of black thread each time she lifted the needle. The firelight was on her cheeks and her hands. He saw her check the buttons also, to make sure they were tight.

Charles had wanted all the relatives to be invited for Sunday, but the idea had upset Lucinda, as though Charles had been moved by a fear of never seeing any of them again. He assured her that this was not the case, and that even if he were sent overseas he would be given a furlough first. But the idea was dropped.

After the weekend, however, when Charles's stay was coming to a close, Lucinda did ask some of them to visit, and when Ed returned from teaching a children's class he found Grandma Annie there and also Celeste with Jill. He recognized Grandma Annie's car before the porch steps, with its smashed fenders, and in his study he could hear all the voices from the kitchen. Lucinda's voice was emotional, as if it were the tail end of some argument. He knew that his mother-in-law interpreted every country art that Lucinda acquired, such as the making of preserves out of the crab apples that grew in the yard, as a deliberate economy, a shocking drudgery that must arise out of poverty, and that if Lucinda denied it his mother-in-law interpreted the denial as a covering up. She had put this same poverty interpretation on Lucinda's buying milk right from the dairy farmer, unpasteurized in a big can. He knew his mother-in-law tried to sneak ten-dollar bills to his wife and that his wife tried to shove them back. Apparently it had arisen this time because Lucinda had mentioned that Mrs. Davey, who kept the two horses diagonally across the way, baked her own bread. And from the way Lucinda was defending him with such a tone of half hysteria Ed knew that Grandma Annie's criticisms of him had affected her.

It was all the worse because he and Lucinda had had some nasty words about the budget in the past few days. She had wanted to decorate the windows with shutters, and he had said it wasn't practical with storm windows, and it had all turned into an argument about how much they could spend on the house.

He honestly considered his mother-in-law to be not entirely of sound mind, but he knew she had the same opinion of him. To her a clergyman was someone who believed in spooks and heard voices. And even before he had talked of going to the seminary, even at the time of the elopement and before, she had considered him a nut.

Yet, if he had a twenty-thousand-dollar-a-year pulpit in Boston she would have admired him as a successful racketeer.

He disliked her handsome automobile with its smashed fenders, and he disliked her mascara. He thought the mascara was a bad influence on Patty.

Grandma Annie's own parents had been traditional people. And yet with a fine disregard of tradition she had insisted that her first granddaughter be named after her, in her own lifetime. They had compromised on the middle name finally. Audrey stood for Annie.

Even the designation Grandma Annie was the result of a compromise. She had wanted her grandchildren to call her simply Annie, by her first name alone, but Ed had forbidden it. Lucinda had argued that it was only a small thing, that would make her mother happy, but Ed replied that he could not stand children being taught that kind of familiarity with their elders. That kind of thing—kids who didn't call their parents' friends Mr. or Mrs., and who didn't say Aunt or Uncle, and who even called parents by first names—it had always seemed to him a disrespectfulness that at heart was a disrespect for everything. He had answered that sometimes small things imply big things. And calling your grandmother by her first name was just too damn dry-martini goyish.

When he went in to supper he was of course cordial, but during the meal he scarcely said a word. He told himself there was no need to, with five women at the table—Lucinda, Celeste, Patty, Jill, and his mother-in-law.

Charles had packed his barracks bag, and a short while after supper the visitors offered to drop Charles at the station, or at the airport. But Ed said he would take him. It was not in their direction, and he wanted to be with Charles as long as possible. Charles had made phone calls to Otis Air Base and to Bedford Air Base, and knew that a plane would leave Bedford for Griffiss in New York, where he was to be assigned as a mechanic.

Ed drove to Bedford with Charles alone. Lucinda would have come, but Patty was preparing to go out to Polly Cook's Hallowe'en party and needed her assistance. And Roland was already out with his friends.

At the base the guard did not allow Ed to pass. Ed gave his son a quick kiss and a handshake, and asked when he thought he'd be home again.

He rode back in the night. He remembered that Lucinda had asked him to get some corn candy, in case the Hubbard children or other children rang the bell, so he stopped at Yerxa's Pharmacy.

Kids were already on the streets, middle-sized ones and little ones, in their witch and spook and gypsy costumes. He drove slowly from Murphy Square, over the stone bridge and taking the left at the fork, and recalling how in other neighborhoods he had used to take his children on Hallowe'en walks. He remembered Millicent at the age of three, with her dime-store jack-o'-lantern and funny-face mask and sheets dragging down to her feet. He had still been in the car business then.

Suddenly, along the beginning part of Massapeequit Road, where it was still thickly settled, he thought he saw Roland by the light of the high street lamps racing down a sidewalk almost toward him, chased by a tall man. Ed almost jammed on his brakes and then actually did so when he saw it was in fact Roland.

"Roland?" Ed shouted at the closed window, turning.

The boy had not seen him or recognized the car. Ed glanced around and prepared to back up to get ahead of him again, lowering the window, but Roland had dashed into the street behind him.

"Roland?" he shouted again, leaning, one hand on the wheel.

Roland paused in the middle of the street to look at him and his pursuer grabbed him by the collar. It was an old man, quite big. He shook Roland violently with both hands.

"Hey! Take your hands off him!" Ed commanded.

The man stopped, seeing Ed for the first time, but did not quite let go. He was taller and broader than Ed but looked at least seventy. "Who are you?" said. He panted heavily.

"I'm his father," Ed said angrily. He got out and came to them quickly. "What's the matter?"

"He put garbage in my vestibule," the old man said, letting go of Roland at last. He had a nervous, bumbling way of talking. "And cut my clothesline, that's what."

"We just tied the door," Roland began.

"We'll hear your story later," Ed told him. "Let's look at the damage," he said to the old man.

The man indicated the direction of his house. They crossed the fallen leaves of the gutter. Ed passed around some little costumed kids, feeling agitated.

"Did you just happen by, or what?" the man asked him.

"Yes, I just happened by."

Roland began again to explain but Ed told him to be quiet.

The old man cut a poor figure. He was hulking in shiny pants and a torn sweater, and his walk was elephantine and flat-footed. It surprised Ed that he had been able to chase a boy, even a short distance, and catch him.

"There was another one," the man said, still breathing hard. "His cohort got away."

It was almost the nearest property, a high square house decorated with old-fashioned ironwork. The yard around it was narrow. Ed saw that the door handle was entangled with rope.

"And there's a pin in my bell," the man said. "Using up my battery."

"Take the pin out," Ed said to Roland. "And untie the door."

"Let me show you out back," the man said.

"And meet us out back," Ed said to Roland.

They found the back door still open. The little entry hall inside it was a smelly mess. A big metal garbage barrel seemed to have tumbled across the threshold, and the flooring before it was strewn with eggshells, coffee grounds, bones, rinds, and slimy putrefying stuff, as though the barrel had been full and not emptied for a long time. A wrinkled, slovenly woman in a shapeless brown dress appeared from the kitchen and smiled at Ed without saying anything. He nodded gravely.

"You say my son did that?" he asked the old man.

"Oh, they did it all right."

"He'll clean it," said Ed. He straightened up the barrel and began picking up scraps.

When Roland came back with the rope he said he had only leaned the barrel on the door, but Ed set him gathering up garbage. He asked the man and woman for a pail and soap and a scrubbing brush and for a while supervised Roland's working. Roland said the man had stolen Bob O'Shaughnessy's football but the man said he didn't know anything about that. The man wanted to be paid the cost of a new hundred-foot clothesline, which he said cost a dollar, because they'd cut the old one, or broken it. Roland, squatting in his work, said it wasn't broken, but Ed paid the dollar.

"I'm just laying it out for you, Roland," he said. "You'll pay me back out of your paper route."

"That line was no hundred feet, either," said Roland.

"We won't argue about it," said Ed.

The old lady was sometimes there and sometimes not, though she never spoke, but the big old man remained and watched.

"I'm owed something for the aggravation, too," the old man said. "It's not proper, for a man my age."

Ed told him Roland would also come another time and do some chores for him, by way of making up for the aggravation.

When the floor had been scrubbed clean, even the cracks between the uneven boards, and the filled garbage barrel restored to its place in the yard and covered, the old man said that if the boy was going to be sent to do a chore there was some work to be done in the cellar. He would show them if Ed had a match, as the bulb was out down there. They descended a few planks of dusty stair and a match was struck. It was the dirtiest, the most jam-packed and crowded cellar Ed had ever seen, though its dimensions seemed endless in the dark. Piles of newspaper were stacked atop glass china closets and scraps of wallpaper rolls atop those, all so dust-laden it seemed none of it had been moved in years. Near the stairs coal had spilled into the junk from a broken bin. The cold air in Ed's mouth tasted thick with gas and mildew and he felt cobweb on his face. He could scarcely see a path to walk down there. The old man said in his bumbling, agitated voice that the boy could come every day to shovel the furnace and carry the ashes and also clean the cellar little by little. It was not what Ed had had in mind. He had thought of Roland perhaps raking the leaves one afternoon.

"Well, I'll let you know," he said.

The old man said he was owed three cents for the soap Roland had used cleaning the vestibule. Ed was surprised, but the man looked serious. Ed found no pennies but handed over a nickel. The man said the doorbell battery had probably used up a penny's worth so that was about right. Ed apologized again for Roland and made Roland apologize.

"Come on," he said to Roland. "Your Hallowe'en's over."

In the car he told Roland he was surprised at him.

"Am I gonna have to work in that cellar?" said Roland.

"No. But you owe him something. Like tidy up his yard once."

"It's not fair to make me do all the work, you know. Just because I got caught."

"Who else was in on it? Bobby O'Shaughnessy and who else?"

Roland didn't answer.

"How many of you?" said Ed.

"Four."

"You could ask some of the others to help you."

"I'm not a stool pigeon."

Ed asked what they had picked on that particular house for and if they knew the people. Roland said the old man's name was Houghton, and that some of the junior-high-school kids crossed his yard every day as a short cut, and he had gotten Bob O'Shaughnessy's new football when it spiraled into the bushes, and refused to give it back. Bob O'Shaughnessy's father had even driven around and spoken to him, and old man Houghton had said he'd have to get a lawyer.

"Even so," Ed told him. "I suppose he was in his rights, even if he was mean about it. And you know better than to plague an old man like that. And his wife. The Bible says you shouldn't carry a grudge. You know that."

"It's not his wife," said Roland. "It's his sister."

Roland told how they had untied the clothesline carefully, leaned the garbage pail quietly against the back door, tied the line to the front door, and jammed the bell with a pin. The idea was that Mr. Houghton would go to the front door to stop the ringing, be unable to get out, and go to the back, whereupon the garbage would fall in. They had even hoped he would cut his own clothesline before he realized it was his.

"Who thought all that up?" Ed asked.

"I did," said Roland.

"You thought all that up yourself?"

Roland said Houghton and his sister were crazy and that they sat in the dark to save electricity. Ed said they were perhaps on a small pension.

But the children's strategy interested him, and he asked Roland to tell it again. Then he told Roland of a prank he and his friends had once played on a neighbor they were mad at, in Dorchester, at the age of thirteen. They had broken a cellar window while the man was away, and run his garden hose into it, and turned on the water full. And that wasn't even Hallowe'en. He laughed involuntarily as he told of it.

"Did you get caught?" Roland asked.

"No."

Ed brought the car into the barn and walked with Roland toward the house, carrying the little bag of corn candy. He told of a Fourth of July when he and a friend had blown up a lady's rainpipe with a twelve-inch cannon cracker. It was a triple-decker house, and the lady had stuck her head out a top-story window right beside the rainpipe and shouted at them in an accent when the bottom of it exploded. Her ears must have rung for a month.

"Boy, those were the days," said Roland.

In the house he gave Lucinda an explanation of his bringing Roland home, without much detail, and told of seeing Charles off, and asked if Patty had been picked up for her party.

He heard Roland telephoning in the kitchen, to find out if Bob O'Shaughnessy had gotten home, and then Roland went to his room. In a moment Ed knocked, feeling uneasily that he had not given Roland the right idea, and entered. The boy sat at the little table he used for a desk, with his books. The green-shaded desk lamp that curved over the books gave the only light. All about, on the table and on the shelves, were books, knives, pieces of leatherwork, pieces of carving in wood or soap, a compass—on the dimly lit walls were two framed displays of butterflies and four huge Audubon Society charts of North American birds.

"Is your homework done?" Ed asked.

"Yup."

Ed sat on the quilted bed. He said he regretted those pranks. "And if old man Houghton is crazy, and his sister, crazy and lonesome, that's their burden, and they have to live with it. We don't know their problems. And kids shouldn't tease them. Don't you agree?"

"Sure."

"Why do you want to tease them? Old people. Especially a lot of old people are crazy. I shouldn't have done those things either. And you shouldn't. You come out of a pious home, Rollo. And especially because you're known as a religious boy, and if you do things like that, then it brings discredit on religion. That's called a desecration of the Name. Just like, for example, it's a sin for a scholar to let himself look like a shloomp. It says it in the Talmud. Because it would make people think scholarship was unworldly, if the professor's pants weren't pressed. Do you see?"

They were looking at each other, but he didn't wait for the boy to answer.

"And if you're outwardly pious," Ed continued, "and people know it, and you're nasty to others, your whole life becomes an advertisement against being pious. You have to so behave, and so act, that the people around you will think to themselves, 'this guy is a mensch, so maybe his God is also okay.' You have to be a public-relations man for God, in the whole impression you give to people. That's what we call sanctification of the Name. You have to always live in such a way as to create God, and make your religion true. And we mustn't conduct ourselves in such a way as to give God a bad reputation. Or religion, or scholarship, or your people a bad reputation. If you're a scholar, it's especially incumbent on you not to look like a jerk with egg on your vest. And God forbid if you're a martyr, you die like a man, so people don't get the impression your religion isn't worth so much, or that it hasn't made a man of you. Even at a man's death, he should try to give the spectators a good impression of God, not a bad one. And if you're a rabbi's son, you don't dump garbage in old man Houghton's vestibule, so people don't think that's what your father taught you. That's why it says Name. What you're sanctifying is a Name, a reputation. And when our God has a good reputation among men, that's when history will change. I believe it, Roland."

He remained looking at Roland, and Roland sat looking at him, with round eyes. He resembles Millicent, Ed thought.

He rose, patted his son's shoulder, and looked away. He wandered to the bird charts and studied them. Roland came and stood beside him. Ed remarked on the illustration of the snowy owl, and Roland told him how the species had gotten that color.

The next night Ed happened to drive past the Houghton house and noticed that it was kept in darkness, as Roland had said.

Then in a few days Mr. Houghton died in his bed. Ed read of it when the weekly copy of the Wilmerdingian came. The story said he and his sister were the last descendants of a certain Colonial governor of New Hampshire. He was to be buried from the First Parish Church of Wilmerding Crosswalk, with Caleb Folger officiating.

Ed thought he had best wait till after a decent period of mourning and then send Roland to the man's sister, to rake the leaves or perform some other such task.

32

A boy at school told Patty she ought to be declared a National Monument, and she came home weeping and started a program of reducing exercises. She took an old medicine ball from the attic, that had belonged to some previous occupant, and got her mother to practice with her in slacks on the living-room carpet. They sat feet to feet, each in turn catching the big heavy leathery ball, lying down with it, sitting up and tossing it back with a two-handed thrust. They had just begun when Ed came home and he enjoyed watching them. It was heavy and rocked them as they caught it. But Lucinda quit soon. "I'm not as young as I used to be," she said, dragging herself up. "I can't do that any more."

Patty said that Denise Saint-Onge ate anything she wanted which showed it was all a matter of glands, but Lucinda insisted that diet was the main thing.

"I'm gonna put you on a diet and you just have to stick to it, if you ever expect to wear cute clothes," Lucinda said. "You're tall, and you have a big frame, and if you're fat besides you're gonna turn into a horse. I don't know where you get all that lard from. Nobody else in this family was ever fat."

Patty did seem to keep to the diet Lucinda planned for her, as far as Ed could tell. She often rehearsed her lines for the De Molay play around the house, and said she wanted to lose twenty pounds by spring so as to look good on stage. She was to play a decrepit old lady, and she practiced hobbling about the house, hunched up, as though her joints creaked. She told Lucinda she would need an old-fashioned dress with a high collar and high-buttoned shoes. Even at the table, if she asked Ed to pass the salad, she was likely to practice speaking in a cracked, feeble voice. "Patty, you're old before your time," Ed said to her.

Patty said she might ask Grandma Annie for pointers on how old people feel, but Lucinda said it wasn't a good idea. "It might hurt her feelings," she told her.

"She's liable to slug ya," Roland added.

Despite rehearsals and learning her lines Patty still managed time for her other activities. She played in a field-hockey game Friday afternoon that lasted into dark, so that Ed had another lonely Sabbath, and it fell to him to take the dog's dinner to the barn. She was in a piano recital at the high school, performing a difficult piece from memory with more virtuosity and nimbleness than ever before, except that she could not find the ending and repeated the middle portion several times, as though trapped inside, going into the whole repetition every time she got to the repetition point. At last on the fourth or fifth time her fingers recalled the way out and slammed along to the spectacular conclusion, but she told Ed and Lucinda she had thought for a while she'd be playing round and round forever, unable to get out.

And she seemed to enjoy the organ these days even more than piano. She told Ed how she enjoyed making a great swelling sound. It could pipe so reedlike and little, and then fill the whole world.

Her job at Saint Tim's, as she called it, required her to be at choir practice, and the minister Ralph Briggs happened to meet Ed on the streets of the town twice within a short time, and told him how marvelously Patty played, and how the choirmaster had called her a real pro, who ought to go far in music. Ed told Patty. Then Ed met Briggs again, this time at a meeting of the Wilmerding Council of Churches, and Briggs told him how he had come early to an Evensong service and found Patty already there far ahead of time, playing I'm a-Datin' I'm a-Matin' at the organ. Ed reported this to Patty too, and she replied that Briggs was a nut and that everyone said so. His sermons were wild and he ought to settle down. He was dating about five different ladies, and she didn't see how he could kiss any, with his broken neck and the big surgical thing.

Caleb Folger had chatted with Ed at the same Council of Churches meeting, and listened to Briggs's story about Patty, and told Ed that he and May wanted to ask him and Lucinda over for an evening.

Folger, not Briggs, was the minister Ed bumped into on the sidewalks most often. He lived in a white Victorian house with a tall narrow front, a cupola, and a porch at the side, set behind a well-kept hedge at the beginning of Massapeequit Road, just past the fork, so that Ed passed that way often, and Caleb always spoke if he saw him, and sometimes engaged him in conversation. Caleb was a tall, gaunt, balding man with serious eyes, and even when he wore no glasses the mark of some showed on the bridge of his nose. He was sixtyish, but without a trace of a pot. He would talk to Ed across the hedge, or at the juncture of the walk, speaking of politics or of the world situation, and would frequently tell him things about the town, in the way one might to a younger newcomer. But Caleb was not patronizing and seemed to welcome Ed as a person to whom he could talk. He told how the town and the parish had been founded together and had remained identical for a century and a half, until the parish voted to become Unitarian, and how Newton Stillman's church at the other end of the common had been founded by the Congregationalist rump that seceded at that time. He told how during the Second World War a town meeting had changed the name of the common to Corporal Kevin Aloysius Murphy Square, after its only son ever to win the Congressional Medal of Honor. He thought the name change a lot of foolishness himself, and said most of the older people still just called it the common. And he told how some of his ancestors had been related to Ben Franklin, through the Folgers of Nantucket.

Once Caleb told Ed he had heard that Ralph Briggs's mother had been Catholic. And once or twice they even discussed religion, but Ed said that your beliefs are like your emotions—you don't really know their true nature, and they're not always the same, and you can't express them with exactness. "Don't ask me to define my beliefs," Ed had told him. "Whatever I tell you I'll think of a better answer when I've gone to bed."

"What if you do?" said Caleb. "That's worth while too, isn't it?"

In a day or so May Folger did telephone Lucinda, and she and Ed went over one evening to visit. Lucinda brought a jar of her crab-apple preserves. They sat chatting in the living room, Ed leaning in the settee with the calf of one leg resting on the other leg. The furniture recalled his grandfather's house to his mind, especially the circular dining table, heavily carved, with lion's feet branching out from its stem, that he could see through the arch, and the brown square brocaded cloth whose corners hung from the table's round edge.

May had thick glasses, round cheeks and white hair, and rocked a little in a wicker chair. She had quick smiles that sometimes disappeared nervously, and her voice was somewhat loud. She remarked during the conversation that Ed's call to the ministry must have been a clear and unequivocal one, to cause him to leave an established business like the automobile business. "It must really make you feel the choice between God and Mammon," she said.

"Well, I never thought of it that way," said Ed.

May asked Lucinda if she preferred being a clergyman's wife to a businessman's wife.

"Well, the clergy," Lucinda answered. "I think it's basically more dignified. Don't you? I mean it's a profession, after all."

May nodded. It crossed Ed's mind that at times he had heard Lucinda say quite the opposite.

"And I thought there'd be money in it," she went on. "But so far it hasn't worked out that way especially. Not considering the way prices have gone up since the war anyway. But the car business—used cars, on an open lot—it's not good, really. It's up and down, and sometimes you can go two weeks and don't sell a car. And Ed wasn't cut out for it. He's not a businessman."

"No, that's not so," said Ed. "I made a living out of it."

"Well, you know, no businessman's completely honest," Lucinda explained, "and Ed's not that practical."

"I was practical," said Ed. "Look, it was a rough business. Some poor guy needs a car to make a living, and he comes to you with money he borrowed from his brother-in-law, and from the bank, and you sell him a car, and in three weeks the car's kaput, and he comes to you crying. He's broke, he's got nothing, and he's deeper in debt. And you feel terrible, but what are you gonna do? You can't take all the risks yourself and let your children starve, but if you didn't tell the truth as to the nature of the gamble you couldn't live with yourself. I think I did all right considering. Nobody was making money in those days."

"Well, you have to be a businessman too, I suppose," said May. "But I suppose honesty is good business too."

Caleb nodded.

"But people started making money in it right after he got out of it," Lucinda said. "The war came and there was money to be made. People bought and sold old cars like crazy."

"It wasn't right after. It was several years after."

"That's what I mean," she said. "You weren't a businessman. You picked the worst time to get out."

"Yeah. If you could get the cars to sell, and if you violated the O.P.A. ceilings. Took money under the table. I'm glad I got out before that."

"And what about after the war," she said. "Boland's done beautifully. He's got the Chrysler agency and you should see how his place looks now. And you gave it away."

"I didn't give it away. I got a good price at the time."

He resented Lucinda's saying that it was impossible for businessmen to be honest. He wondered where she got such notions. His grandfather had been proverbial for his honesty and yet had gotten to be pretty well-to-do. His grandfather had had a big house and had assisted a raft of relatives.

But the conversation turned to other things. Caleb expressed satisfaction with the progress in Korea, and so did Ed.

Caleb talked about tax deductions. He mentioned that clergy were allowed to deduct the cost of country-club memberships, and said he was also in the habit of writing off practically his whole car expense and had never been challenged on it. He asked permission to smoke, and lighted a pipe, and asked Ed if he could get him anything to smoke. He looked for cigarettes in some drawers under a built-in cupboard but found none.

Caleb remarked, as the conversation went on, that if he could live his life over again he would have become a broker. He enjoyed following the market, and he felt there were more bull years ahead.

After a while he asked Ed if he would like to see his study upstairs. They went up, leaving Lucinda with May.

At the angle of the staircase there was a little window of colored glass. Caleb's study had the rounded cupola windows in one corner, and a fireplace, like the living room below it, and Ed was pleased by the extent and fullness of the bookcases.

Ed looked at titles in the oblique lamplight from the desk and walls. Some books were soiled with age. The arrangement wasn't orderly and there was a mixture of centuries, sects and viewpoints. There were shelves and shelves, floor to ceiling—books on philosophy, classic and modern, and sociology, politics, psychology, education, marriage, Gandhi and whatnot.

"Borrow anything you like," said Caleb.

Ed took down a volume. He read part of a page. When he looked around Caleb was sitting in the cupola, where a rounded bench was built under the windows, and smoking his pipe.

"Do you find the pulpit satisfying?" Caleb asked.

"Oh, on the whole, I guess," said Ed.

"I'm the fourth generation in my family," Caleb said. He puffed the pipe again.

"That's a lot," said Ed.

"Well, I guess there was a time when they expected the millennium sooner than that. But by the nineteenth century it was fairly typical."

Ed restored the book to its place and looked at more titles. Here and there he saw one or two that he himself owned, or that he intended to read. But the books in Ed's study thus far took only one wall and part of another—hardly a third as many as here. He complimented Caleb on the extent of his library.

"Are you orthodox or reform?" Caleb asked. "I've forgotten."

"Well, Beth El is unaffiliated, actually," said Ed. "We have too many factions."

"Some of your flock have one credo and some have another?"

"Well," said Ed, "I don't know. We squabble about procedures, rather than credos. I suppose we'll split if we get big enough to afford it."

He looked at Caleb. He had taken another book, and sat down in a chair that was near him as though to thumb the pages, but instead he looked at Caleb's face again. The angles of the light made shadows in all the wrinkles.

"I was surprised to hear you say you'd go into brokerage if you had to do it again," Ed said to him.

Caleb sucked the pipe a few moments, holding the bowl. "Well, Ed," he said, drawing the pipe out and looking at it, "maybe I should have quit when I was ahead. About the age of twenty-five. Or thirty. It was fun to be a young minister, and I feel kind of foolish as an old one. I haven't grown in it." His eyes moved from the pipe to Ed. "It kind of came to a head for me about a month ago. I gave an invocation over in Sparkstown, at the Chamber of Commerce luncheon, and I tried to word the prayer in such a way as to make them think, you know, about their social responsibilities, and—well—I'd done it before. But this time—well—Ed, it was just something in the clatter of dishes and silverware the instant I finished. The sight of them digging into the fruit cups, chewing the grapefruits, the minute I stopped. As if to say, 'that's over.' I wish I'd kept my eyes shut a minute longer. Because I asked myself, whom had I talked to in that prayer—God or these men—and all of a sudden it struck me—I'd always known it but all of a sudden I saw it—how little I influenced anyone. How little influence we have. Starry-eyed youths plunge into the ministry, or politics, or even music say, and they think their lives are going to be meaningful. And thirty years later they find it so drab that they might have found more challenge in business. Nobody listens to us, Ed. They're prejudiced against the whole idea of listening to us. They look at us gravely and politely, that's all."

"Maybe we're living in the wrong century," said Ed.

"Except that for a churchman there can't be such a thing as a wrong century. The wronger it is the righter it is. You don't go into the ministry to find satisfaction." He paused, looking dolorously at Ed. "You don't expect happiness when you choose battle. And maybe that's where I've made my mistake. Maybe

I should have been the social-action kind of minister. And pushed the idea of the church as the vanguard of social improvement and all that—the opportunity's always there. Before the war we had the labor unions, and the farmers, and now there's the U.N., and the bomb, and the race question not solved yet. And conscientious objectors—I've even had a few right here in town. Or urban renewal—there's no end of city problems. A minister can do social work, or get into politics—there's no politics in Wilmerding Crosswalk. But even if I did those things, even if I had—I'd accomplish something, I'd do good, and I'd get some notoriety, but I'd still have a feeling of only selling the common wisdom of the race. Your wife called it a profession. But a professional, a doctor or a lawyer, he's got a knowledge and skill that the layman doesn't have. I look at these social-gospel ministers, and they accomplish something—they do—they deserve credit. But I ask why a minister—I think of taking up settlement-house work down in Boston, say, and then I ask myself if it's a question of busywork—well, maybe that's not fair. But Ed, I preach on Sunday, and try to needle them, and relate religion to the morning newspapers, and even when I needle them, sometimes I have the feeling of being a quack, in the sense of selling only common knowledge. I've had a feeling of being small in the pulpit. As if I don't have any insights that the people I'm preaching to don't have. And the old people looking for some convincing assurance that their lives are justified—what have I got to say to them—what phrase of assurance can I give them, that won't evaporate into doubt again an hour later? And the young, that come to church socials, and never seem to question. And of those that never question, it seems to me that with most it's really because they assume I couldn't possibly give a worthwhile answer. I don't even know more about ethics than they do. Ed, do you ever ask yourself why they pay you a salary? Does a twentieth-century American community truly pay a man to teach them righteousness, to chastise them, to lecture them on the Golden Rule?"

Ed didn't know what to say. "Well, what's your answer?" he asked finally.

"I don't know," Caleb said. "In my better moods I say, they support the church—they listen to the minister, and they send their children—so they must certainly have faith, after all, some residuum of true faith. But I also know that they spend time and money on many things that they never really use, so I'm not sure."

He looked down at his pipe.

"Pipe's gone out," he said. "I've talked so much that my pipe's gone out."

He felt with a thumb in a pocket of the vest that hung on him leanly, and then rose as if to go to the desk and look for matches there.

But before he got there he turned. "Do you know how people consider a clergyman?" he said. "Like a half-wit son of the oldest family in town. Treated respectfully, but not respected. The youngsters even—they're on best behavior when I'm around. But not because they think I know more about the good life—it's because I'm supposed to know less about the evil life. I'm supposed to know less than my parishioners, not more. Do you know the feeling I mean?"

"Have you ever been a chaplain?" Ed asked him. "In the armed forces?"

"No. I never have."

"Well, I have. And when you're part of a military force you see it even sharper there, I think. You're like a mascot. There are good moments, but most of the time a chaplain is just a good-natured joke."

Caleb smiled sourly. "Yes," he said. He was standing pensively in the middle of the room, one hand hanging with the unlit pipe, and a thumb of the other in a pocket of his vest. "That's it. They think men who go into the clergy are like men who go into teaching. Only worse. I've got a few years on you, Ed, and in time it'll affect you. My son said to me, 'Frankly, Father, I'm an atheist.' And what could I say, except commend him for having a mind of his own. For his independence. He didn't go into the ministry. And my daughter. When she was a child an angel of the Lord actually appeared to her in a series of dreams, do you know that? And spoke to her—she asked questions and the angel answered. What more could you want? And what wouldn't I give, for that to happen to me. But if it happened to her today she'd go see an analyst about it."

May shouted from downstairs that coffee was ready in the living room. "What are you men doing up there?" she added.

Caleb sighed. Ed had been holding an unopened book. He leaned to put it on the desk, and rose. They started down.

"Well, I've talked your ear off," said Caleb. "I'm an old man, and I've got things on my mind."

"No, I enjoyed listening to you," said Ed.

They sat with May and Lucinda. May had put out a fruitcake as well as tea and coffee. Caleb sat cross-kneed, holding his saucer and hot cup and blowing.

"It would make sense," he said, "if I were reaching new people every year, but I don't. If I reach anybody, it's the same ones I reached last year."

"Oh dear," said May. "I know the whole conversation."

"I rarely shake anybody up," said Caleb. "I try to persuade myself that I've talked a rich man into Christianity when he hands over a large sum to charity. It's a pageant, you know. Church and town and village green. It's a fool's paradise."

"Why don't you tell them that?" said Ed.

"Oh, I have."

"The old folks like an old-time minister," May said, "but to get the young folks you've got to have a young one." Then she asked if anyone wanted cider instead of tea or coffee.

During the short ride home Lucinda said she didn't know who was the worse slob, Caleb with his garters showing or Ed with no garters.

Ed drove, following the glow of his headlights between the great trees, saying nothing. Caleb's depression troubled him. He too felt that, living his life over again, he would not again choose to be a clergyman.

The trouble with clergy, he said to himself, is that the clergyman becomes the representative of religion, a man of God. You can take him apart too easily, while remaining loyal to your family, and too often he's some maudlin nonentity perhaps, or some guy who didn't have the facility with math to become an engineer. But in the old days, when congregations like your grandfather's just got together and functioned without a rabbi, then the natural vicar in your heart and home was your father. Or one of your grandfathers, so that his shortcomings didn't destroy him, and when he died it devolved on you.

Who should know God? Father and grandpa should know God. A clergyman is only some ass in town like the mayor or the hardware man. And earns his living on the Sabbath.

33

Millicent learned that Ella Jane had been having an affair with a married man; the facts were tossed out with bitterness on a Saturday morning, almost as if they had never been secret. And Natalie apparently had known all along.

Ella Jane's mood subsided from careless anger into controlled despair. Millicent at first felt incredulous shock, which seemed only to bring Ella Jane's quiet contempt.

Then Millicent sank into misery. Ella Jane shut herself behind the door of her room, beyond the bath, and Millicent heard the cane fall. It had been that same blond man who worked in Ella Jane's office and who had sometimes taken her away. It had been going on when Millicent first met Ella Jane, and the whole length of time that Millicent had lived here.

Her mind could scarcely grasp it. Ella Jane was someone she believed in as a person. This crippled girl, that she had helped naked out of the bathtub so many times.

Natalie tried to calm Millicent's confusion. "When a girl goes with a guy she wants to marry she usually sleeps with him," Natalie said. "It's as simple as that."

"It doesn't sound so simple to me." Millicent was red-faced.

"Where have you been the last twenty years?" said Natalie. "You're not a little child."

"And how could she hope to marry him? He was married."

"She still hoped to marry him though," said Natalie.

"You mean break up his home?"

"He wasn't living with his wife. Not all the time, anyway. He is now—he's gonna try to make a go of it for the children's sake."

"Didn't she know he was married?"

"What do you mean, didn't she know. Of course she knew."

During the weekend Ella Jane seemed in an agony of mourning, keeping to her room much of the time, so that Millicent felt some sympathy for her, but she could not express it. It was as if Ella Jane had turned into someone strange, and she hardly knew how to speak to her. Ella Jane made her uncomfortable, as though Ella Jane thought her embarrassingly stupid.

She spoke little to Natalie, to Ella Jane scarcely at all, and devoted herself to her cat.

Sunday she rose early and went to Wilmerding Crosswalk to teach Sunday school at Temple Beth El. She had been enjoying it. She taught the littlest tots, several of whom were exceedingly beautiful and strikingly intelligent. They were well-behaved, and sometimes their questions charmed her.

After dinner she returned to Boston.

In the city room that afternoon a stranger in an open raincoat entered and she directed him to Mr. Hopkins, who sat at Mr. Killian's desk on Sundays, but in a moment Mr. Hopkins turned him back to her and asked her to write a little story out of his material. She sat herself at the nearest vacant desk and the man pulled a chair to the side of it. He had some mimeographed notices about the award of gold-plated buttons to members of the Gray Ladies for five years of volunteer work in one of the hospitals. He was smooth-faced and smiling, with dark hair, in his middle or late twenties. She asked several questions, until she felt she understood it all, and then he left. She pecked out a brief item, which she handed to Mr. Hopkins, with her initials at the bottom, and returned to her copy-boy duties. It was the first story they had given her in ten days or more, and she wondered unhappily if he had given this one to her because it had to do with women. If that were going to be the policy it seemed a kind of jim crow.

In about an hour there was a phone call for her, and she took it at one of the back desks. It was the publicity man, of the smooth face and open raincoat, calling her by her first name. He invited her to a cocktail lounge.

"No thank you," she said.

He offered dinner, naming a cabaret with some pretension to elegance, whose ads she had seen, and mentioned alternative evenings.

"No thank you," she said, and hung up.

When she returned to the apartment Ella Jane was still up, in her bathrobe, sitting red-eyed at the unfolded table. Millicent said only routine things to her. The strain was still there, and she could not venture into conversation. But when Ella Jane had gone off to bed Millicent talked again with Natalie a little.

"I wouldn't sleep with a man just because I was hoping to marry him," Millicent said. "And I don't think I'm inhibited. Or if I am, I accept it that there comes a time when you have to throw your inhibitions into reverse. But it seems to me the best time to do that is marriage."

"If you wouldn't want to sleep with him why would you want to marry him?" Natalie asked her.

She could not sleep. She lay in one position and then another, trying to be still. At the foot of her studio couch the door to Natalie's room was open, and she could hear Natalie's sleeping breath. She tried not to wonder what time it was. Ella Jane must have unstrapped her leg irons in order to do it, she thought. Or else he unstrapped it for her.

That poor, straight, thin leg, like skin upon bone, so fragile, beside the healthy one. She supposed they must have been careful of it.

Yet she found she could not imagine their feelings at all. She wondered if that withered, deformed leg had marred the beauty of it for them.

It can't always be beautiful, she thought. It certainly was never beautiful for Aunt Celeste, with that bumbling, incompetent, grizzle-haired Uncle Ira.

She wondered if Grandma Annie still had intercourse, with that lined little man she had taken for a second husband. It was repellent to think of it.

She lay on her side, fingering a corner of the pillow, her eyes open in the dark.

Was Natalie a virgin? She had always assumed that Natalie must be, though perhaps she went pretty far at times. But you couldn't trust anybody.

Had Ruthie Meyers and Justin slept together before they were married, she wondered. The possibility had never occurred to her before now. She hoped not. It was too awful to fight this battle all alone. It was terrible, grotesque even, to think of Ruthie giving herself to that pompous boob. That self-satisfied fluffhead. Not when she didn't have to—marriage was another story.

They must long since be back from their European trip, and she had never thought to phone them, all this fall. She ought to call tomorrow and say hello. No, Ruthie was Les's cousin, and would ask about him. It was even possible that he had been in touch with them, though it was unlikely.

She had heard nothing from him, though the two weeks had passed and more. At first she had thought he might phone even before the two weeks, requesting that their separation be shortened. But when it became apparent he was taking her at her word she counted the days, expecting he would call promptly at the fortnight's end. She would consent then to a fresh start, on certain conditions.

She was unsure whether he had interpreted the two weeks as meaning from the last time they had seen each other, or from that night when she had told him on the city-room phone not to call. She had in fact meant the former, though she knew she had said the latter. She counted the days both ways, and both dates had passed.

And another day and another. Probably he was so busy, so tired, that he simply hadn't yet gotten to it. It could even slip his mind for a few days, if he were overworked enough.

It would not be like him to delay phoning simply to unnerve her.

She thought of phoning him to find out if something was the matter. But if nothing was the matter, her phoning would weaken her position. She hoped he would clear it up soon by phoning and explaining. It even crossed her mind that he had found a new girl, even a nurse or a student nurse, and had no time for another, and meant to drop her without a word. She told herself it was useless to bother herself with such thoughts. There seemed little she could do except wait for a call.

These sexual exercises that boys beg of you, that lead to no pregnancy, for them it is perhaps the physical fulfillment of the body's need, she thought, as they claim, because their gonads do all they're meant to do. But they forget that your ovaries remain as nonfunctional as ever.

It was all too bad. We're so congenial. If we had both been men, we could have been such good friends.

That act of sexual union, was it really such fulfillment, as they claimed, so all-surpassing, or did it just seem so to men, because it was as near as they could ever get to the real reproductive process? Who knew? It's the viewpoint of males that colors everything. Men write the books, preach the sermons, establish the authorities, and make the rebellions. And they've just about put across the view that the act of begetting is a bigger thing than childbirth.

She lay on her other side, and rearranged the blanket. The heaviness in her eyes was already uncomfortable.

How was one to live then? There must be a way to kiss and go no further, without feeling philistine about it. Or to be with a man and not kiss, without feeling prudish about it.

Presumably it was also possible to live without finding life such a problem.

Patty was following the normal course expected of girls—bending all her energy to learning to walk the tightrope between coquetry and virtue. Stupid. Enough coquetry and primping and you'll begin to see yourself as men see you. Be beautiful so that a man may cherish your beauty, as he cherishes the beauty of an automobile.

I'll be a wreck at work tomorrow, she thought. She lay with eyes shut. She tried to relax her face, her arms, each muscle of her body.

She wished she had a clearer notion of what the new morality really stood for, what its guiding principle was. Ella Jane had taken a married lover—would Les approve of that?

She wished she knew. Or could the reasoning here be that the marriage had become no longer a marriage?

She slept much of the forenoon but awoke unrefreshed, with a headache. Not for an hour and a half did she find the will to begin her calisthenics. She frittered time and idled in the apartment, angry with herself for it. She sat reading Sunday's New York Times, which was still scattered about, and did not begin the laundering she had planned for the day. An article in the magazine section about the moral attitudes of the young caught her eye at once. She read it but it told her nothing.

At two-thirty she set out for the city room, already looking forward to the hour of going to sleep.

She went to bed as soon after midnight as possible, explaining to Natalie that she had had a headache all day and had to be up early the next morning to vote. Ella Jane had already retired.

Yet once the apartment was darkened, and the blankets lay upon Millicent, she found herself as wakeful as ever. The trouble with the new morality, she thought, is that it doesn't tell you at what point you become a trollop. Does it say that there are no trollops, and that it's quite all right to go to bed with anyone, whenever the impulse moves you? Or does it say that it's all right only if you're in love? But what does in love mean—that you want to sleep with someone? If that's all it meant, the rule evaporated in a redundancy.

She had tried during the afternoon to find some light in the city room's big dictionary, but it had been useless. It said in love with meant enamored of, and enamored meant inflamed with love, charmed, captivated. So was it okay to sleep with anyone who charmed you, in other words anyone you felt a desire to sleep with? She wished she could understand it.

Maybe, she said to herself, the principle is that it's all right as long as you're not promiscuous. That must be it. Or does Les really believe in promiscuity too—is promiscuity really the ultimate liberation? And do they believe in promiscuity in Sweden and is that really the wave of the future?

Anyway, she wondered, how many affairs constitute promiscuity? Or maybe it's not the number. Maybe you're not considered promiscuous as long as you have affairs with only one man at a time. So long as you make each affair last a reasonable time and are faithful to your lover during it. Was there a logic in drawing the line at one place rather than another? And where do they draw it—is there any general agreement about where to draw it? And if there is, what is the general agreement?

She sighed and put her face in the pillow. If it's the wave of the future, I can see what a fine world it's going to be, she thought. All the boys worried all the time about whether they make out or not. That isn't love. It's selfishness. I don't like the new morality. I like the old morality.

She lay on her back again. Well, doing things the old way, the virginal way, how many real crushes does the average person have before getting married? Two to five, say? Is that the answer then?

It occurred to her that Leslie could not be called a libertine. He was not like one of these pseudo-artistic irresponsible rebels. He was in the soberest of professions, and in dead earnest about his work.

And he had taken the position that it was just as much a want and need of hers—that it would not constitute a submission on her part. His position was that a right-thinking boy could have only a high opinion of girls who give in, because how could he think badly of them for having the same ideas that he had?

Les did not see himself as lax, but as the possessor of a higher truth. She realized that. Which was why she had to find a still higher principle, that would transcend his position and hers and iron out the differences. Because you can't win a debate just by urging your adversary to return to what he considers benighted.

Moreover she felt she owed Les some answers. Girls who pretended not to notice when boys unbuttoned them she considered dishonest. But was the total shunning of sex dishonest also? I must still resolve that to myself, she thought. And the compromise answer, the disjunction of love play from the sex act, hadn't avoided the problem. It had led to it.

In the Victorian days, she thought, in the days of chaperones, it was assumed that a girl who began at all went the whole distance. And that at least made some sense.

So is that how a friendship between a man and a woman has to be? Bed every so often, so the sex thing will go away and let us alone? He had said he wanted a wholeness in the friendship.

Just the sight of a good-looking woman makes a man think of sex. There's sexuality everywhere. And our sexual equipment is with us all the time. And he has the advantage in argument when he claims such extreme pleasure for it, because he's experienced what he's for, and I haven't experienced what I'm against.

But if it's all right for unmarried couples to sleep together, then what is marriage?

Well, marriage is the building of a home to raise children in. Does sex have to wait for that circumstance? Sure, marriage was fine, but it didn't help you when you were unmarried. And how do I know that the deepest love must precede sex? Maybe it follows it.

She tried to bring to mind the arguments she had used against him, but could only recall her insistence that chastity still exists. Anything that has to insist that it exists is in a pretty bad way, she thought.

Am I really out of step with the times, with my generation? Maybe they're right. Maybe it's no use, and sex can't be avoided. I wish I lived in a simpler age.

It's silly to wish that. I might as well wish to be a child again.

But it's confusing, and that's why it's not a code. A code is clear.

Well, I told him I wanted time to think, and at least I've done that, as promised. I've thought and thought about it. Even if I haven't gotten anywhere.

Maybe the answer was to think less, and not try to understand the principle, but to be an animal more. Yet that was no solution either, because she was not sure how to behave as an animal. Her strongest impulse had been to say no. Animals are cautious.

Passion is for savages, she thought. It gets civilized people into trouble. Or at least into situations they were well out of.

She sneezed. The next sneeze hung in her, as though getting ready several times to jump and not finding the wind. She breathed through her mouth until the irritation grew less. I've just got to overcome this insomnia or I'll get sick, she thought. I can't go on lying awake night after night like this.

She rose, thinking some hot milk would help her. She turned on the kitchen light. She saw the sleeping cat, a black circle. She found a pot.

In the living room the Sunday paper was still scattered, and she could see her alarm clock dimly over on the mantel. She thought it said three.

That Times article came to mind. There were phrases in it she wanted to examine again. It was all a constant agitation hammering at her.

She turned the blue flame as low as possible. This stove needs a cleaning, she thought.

Les had asked what she was afraid of. Maybe she should go to a psychiatrist.

She had heard girls talk of going to psychiatrists, to be helped to get over their inhibitions. Or of boys telling girls they should. But that was begging the question—you had to believe it was right in order to do that. Or at least want to change your beliefs. If it's wrong, you should be afraid.

And she did not feel she really was afraid, anyway. Not of sex in itself.

She tested the milk with her little finger, and when it was warm enough she took a glassful to the living room and clicked on the overhead light.

While she sipped she reread the article, sitting on her disarrayed bedding. At last she put it aside and settled down again in darkness.

The article had been words and words. A university psychologist opposed relations among young people who were unready. But it didn't say whether he was for it if they were ready. And it didn't explain how you knew when you were ready. It quoted a college dean as saying the current generation was basically moral, but there was not a clue as to what he meant by that. Nowhere could you penetrate the vagueness. A dean of women said no girl should do anything that would bring discredit on the school. Another dean said not many young men had abused their privileges.

They yak and yak, all around it, and what they mean between the lines they haven't guts enough to tell you. You're supposed to have a healthy attitude, whatever that means. It's as though they don't dare tell you because they don't know themselves. If only somebody who seemed to have some knowledge and authority would give a plain answer. Les gives a plain answer.

She sat up, sighed, went to the bathroom and came back.

At the university she had known girls she had thought were virgins and many who admitted they were, though in conversation they might proclaim some ideology of the right of lovers to sleep together. The whole debate seemed to proceed so confusedly, so inarticulately. You were supposed to be for healthy sex, and against unhealthy sex, and you were to talk of it with emotion, but nobody ever defined anything, least of all premises or norms. She remembered girls' conversations at the university, discussions of sexual situations of which one had heard, and it seemed that while there was always vague unanimity the mood varied—the same crowd could speak disparagingly one day of sleeping around, and disparagingly the next day of chastity. You couldn't pin it down, either in private discussion or in public attitudes. It gave you the feeling that society wanted to keep it amorphous. Anyone who defined his position clearly was considered a nut, no matter which position he took.

One bull session in particular among a little group of university girls had stayed with her. With scarcely any dissent they had nearly all held that the rule, the principle to live by, was that being in love made it right. She had been impressed by their vehemence and she had known no way to challenge them—especially as a marriage ceremony was just hocus-pocus, and her mind could find no other rule. But after all the talk, walking to her grandaunt's, it had occurred to her that these same girls had defined being in love as desiring to sleep with him, so that it canceled out, and left you still with no rule. Whatever rule you devised, some flaw blew it up. Unless you had no rules at all. But one and all agreed that if you had no rules at all you were a slut. Never had anything been so hopelessly confusing. Even the metaphysics in her philosophy courses was not so confusing.

True, metaphysics wasn't like sex—you didn't have to live with it. But in metaphysics you didn't try to solve a problem by putting a ring on your finger and claiming it changed determinism into freedom of the will.

Was it true, as Leslie said, that times changed, and now the contradictions had been ironed out, and men married girls with sexual experience because they assumed all girls had sexual experience?

Had easy lay really gone out of the language, because there was no more need for such a word? If that were a linguistic fact, it seemed significant. And if it had, had slut and whore also gone out?

She had set her alarm clock, in order that she might go to Wilmerding Crosswalk and vote, but the rising of Natalie and Ella Jane wakened her. She rose and breakfasted, about the time that Ella Jane was leaving for work.

When the brown bus from the Sparkstown depot passed her own house she did not get off, but rode it all the way to Murphy Square, thinking she would get the voting over with first and walk to the house afterward.

The polling station was in the basement of Caleb Folger's church, and the black-and-gold steeple clock was striking the hour as she got there. The sun gleamed on the whiteness.

A middle-aged lady seated at a card table penciled through her name on the list, and another smiling one gave her a ballot.

She took her time in the makeshift little booth. She had half decided to vote throughout for candidates of the Prohibitionist Party, as a protest, and now she did so. She had gotten a poor impression of Republicans and Democrats in the Commonwealth during the brief Mieczneslíwy campaign. As far as Washington was concerned she considered the Democrats the lesser evil, but the Democrats had put up no one for Congress in this district.

In the local liquor referendum she voted to keep the town dry. It interfered with no one's personal rights, she thought, since anyone who wished could buy it in Sparkstown.

She came out of the church. The trees were gray and bare. She walked slowly on the common, her shoulder-strap bag across the flared blue coat her mother had bought her. Then she crossed the roadway again, to Yerxa's Pharmacy, and ordered hot chocolate at the counter.

In the rack the magazines were displayed, and a ladies' magazine with a glossy smiling face offered an article about morals. It was not the lead article, but was listed further down, about opposite the cover girl's nose. Millicent stepped over and picked one up.

She returned to the counter with it. Her chocolate came, and she folded back the magazine and read.

The article said nothing she disagreed with. It ended in a banal enough way, with a statement that sex was no good unless it was meaningful.

She continued looking at the final paragraph. She was certain that a few years ago a routine article of this kind could only have ended with a clear endorsement of traditional morality.

Yet here was the kind of large-circulation magazine that was said to avoid offending its readers, to have no policy except to step on nobody's toes, and it hesitated to endorse chastity. As though the nonoffensive common denominator had become instead the meaningless assertion that sex should be meaningful. The climate must be changing, as Les had said.

For five thousand words the article weaseled and pussyfooted. It said you should be able to handle yourself alone with a man, behind closed doors. The problem of what to do behind the closed door—give in, put him off, hold him at arm's length—was not even hinted at. And the ending was hair-raising, not because of the empty thing it said, but because of the empty thing it didn't say.

Apparently things had come to such a pass that chastity offended people. A nice family magazine, with recipes, and articles on royalty and home decoration, and it doesn't dare to come out flatly for virginity any more.

She felt tears in her eyes. She glanced at the white-coated boy behind the counter, and about the store, to make sure no one had noticed the oddity of her weeping.

She leaned on her elbows, holding her hands to hide her face.

In a moment she put down the money for her cocoa and her magazine and slid from the stool.

She bought some articles she needed at the opposite counter. Then she left the store quickly, trying to hide the wetness of her eyes as much as possible, and set out toward her house. Where the street of the stone bridge departed diagonally from the Square there was a big sidewalk can for trash, and she tossed the slick magazine into it. She did not want her family to think she had taken to reading such drivel.

Among the big trees of Massapeequit Road her step slowed. The air was cold, though the high wintry twigs did not hide the sun any longer. Milkweed pods were brown and dry, bursting with fluff.

Apparently by a healthy approach they meant when you were in love. Or at least part of the time they did.

But Les and I don't claim to be in love, she thought. And once you've admitted that it's a need, what do you do about the need when you're not in love? If you need it even though you're not married, maybe you also need it even though you're not in love.

Between friends, is what Les had said. Maybe that's it. When you're not in love, two friends make a deal to take their needs out on each other.

I must examine that—now I'm getting somewhere, she thought.

But her brother Charles's little affairs, they were then a bunch of little short-term deals. And how many little short-term deals were you allowed?

There had to be affection, that was the difference. Between Les and herself there was affection.

No, that's not the answer either. You wouldn't even hold hands if there weren't affection, so if affection is the criterion, then going to bed is okay whenever hand-holding is okay. Maybe it is, according to Les. But then you need a definition of affection that will carry all that. If you feel affection for everyone you want to sleep with, the equation cancels out again. All you've got is that you shouldn't sleep with anybody you're mad at.

Or do you have to feel it all without definition, just as you don't define what constitutes a friend?

She picked up a crooked stick that lay at the roadside, and as she walked she peeled dry bark from it.

Charles anyway must be wrong. Anything is wrong that makes you lie to people, and makes you associate with people you have contempt for.

He's probably seen more girls in the nude than I have.

How do boys still manage to concentrate on careers and schooling when their thoughts are so occupied that way?

I'm glad I'm not a boy, she thought. It was better to be a girl, and have your body all of a piece.

Clearly there could be no rationale for this aimless seeking of intercourse, for its own sake, where children are not desired. But if you ask a boy for the rationale he'll tell you some garbled tale about the psyche requiring it, and so on, which was patent nonsense. It was inescapable then, that men were tyrannized over by this instinct. It taxed their minds and it taxed their time.

They all ought to be gelded, except for a few studs eugenically chosen, and then men and women could be friends together. It would free men to be decent and human.

She let the forward branches of the stick touch the roadway, where they scraped and shuddered along the irregularities in the paving. She felt the vibrations in her hand.

The brevity of men's role in the reproductive process she had once considered enviable, because it seemed to free them for other things, for careers, but apparently it was not true. The truth was that men were slaves of their bodies even more than women. She had used to think women were relatively tied down, but the way men had it was worse. Their glands never let them alone, never stopped clamoring for relief. Their freedom in the higher sense was limited thereby. Secretions made minions of their thoughts and feelings—just as it was with birds, and the whole world of subhuman creatures. It was tragic. Their glands kept filling, and they had no automatic release like a monthly discharge. For a wild species it made sense—it could not survive unless the males sought out the females. But for civilized men it must be a horrible nuisance, to live always with hunger, craving, distraction, and have such bothersome things hanging off you. They lived in torment.

The miracle was that people so distracted could have created so much.

The stick caught in the paving and shattered. She flung it aside.

Women are slaves to men, she thought, and men are slaves to an animal urge. Like Macbeth is a slave to witches, and the witches are slaves to a frog. It's just awful.

34

On Sunday she went to Wilmerding Crosswalk again, and taught her class of children at Temple Beth El. They colored pictures showing Moses and Aaron talking to Pharaoh.

At noon she rode to the house with her father and Roland. Patty was already back from her organ job and opened the door for them. "Hello, brat," Patty said to Roland.

Millicent went upstairs and left her coat in Patty's room. In the bathroom she chanced on the direction slip from the tampax box she had left there on election day, and she found herself looking again at its familiar diagram. Its soft lines showed a cross section of a woman's body, with her internal parts. It was all so delicate, so tender.

That diagram ought to be shown to boys, she thought, that the delicateness, the tenderness might be brought to their understanding.

She came down to the kitchen and helped set the big unpainted table.

During dinner her mother mentioned that a lady in the congregation knew of a boy in Boston, in case Millicent was interested. He was supposed to be good-looking, Lucinda said, and a nice dresser, and in business for himself, and doing very nicely. "And even if he's not a college man," she said, "he can still have friends who are."

"It's not too likely," said Millicent.

"Well, I give up on you," said Lucinda.

Millicent had noticed that her mother had grown less insistent lately about these things, especially if non-college men were involved. It was as though it had gotten across finally that she was too serious for mere dates for the sake of dates. And she had found too that it didn't pay to goad her mother by arguing, as usually the boy never called anyway.

Before dinner was over Denise Saint-Onge came around to the back door, which opened into a side of the kitchen, and knocked. She had a greenish raincoat of a smooth fabric, which she folded and placed across the top of the washer, along with a loose package she had brought. Lucinda asked if she had had dinner.

"Yup," said Denise.

Then she sat on a chair in the corner and watched the family eat. Lucinda offered her dessert and a place at the table.

"No thanks," said Denise.

Her cheekbones, eyes, and eyebrows all slanted in a way that made her look like a cat, Millicent thought. She was small and thin, in a heavy black sweater, and had slender hands.

Patty pushed her chair back and asked Denise to come to the sewing machine in the dining room, but Lucinda told Patty to wait until others were finished, and said she would have to show them how to use the machine anyway. Ed asked what they were doing, and Patty said they were going to put gold stripes on their cheerleader costumes.

Millicent helped clear the table.

"Whose turn is it to do the dishes?" Lucinda asked.

"Patty's," said Roland.

When the girls had gathered around Lucinda at the sewing table in the dining room Millicent wandered to the dining room also, and sat and half watched from a little distance, for want of anything else to do. She idly picked up a section of the Sunday newspaper that Roland had brought earlier, and which lay at her elbow on the lacy spread. Roland lay on the floor reading the funnies. The machine whirred a few seconds and stopped. Ed came in, and picked a walnut and the nutcracker from the centerpiece. The crack was loud.

" 'Wilmer, Wilmer, Ding, Ding, Ding,' " Patty sang. "You never saw me in my uniform, did ya," she said to Millicent.

"That's all right. I don't want to."

"Why?"

"I've seen cheerleader costumes before."

"You didn't see ours," Patty said to her. "And it's your town now. Just as much as ours."

"I'm sure it's as ridiculous as any other."

"What's ridiculous about it?" Patty said.

Millicent didn't answer right away. Her nose moved. "Well, I'd think you'd feel silly," she said. "A spectacle out in front of everybody like that. And everyone else fully clothed."

"That's what I thought," said Lucinda. She wetted an end of thread in her mouth and probed it down through the machine, her face close.

"It's not so short," said Patty.

"What do your parents think, Denise?" Lucinda said.

"They don't mind."

"And the whole idea of it," said Millicent. "The boys play the game, and the girls stay on the side lines and sing their praises."

"Well!" Patty looked at her. "What a prune you are." She made a cross-eyed grimace. "Don't pay any attention to her," she said to Denise. "She's always like that."

"We have more on than the boys on the basketball team," said Denise.

"Not football though," said Patty. She stepped over Roland on the floor and took a chair.

"It makes a decent approach to the knee," said Ed.

"It happens to be a very conservative uniform," said Patty. "If you want to know." She reached for a walnut.

"Well I don't know," Lucinda said. "I heard a certain story about the Pepperell game I didn't like too well."

"What story is that?" Denise asked.

Patty ran her tongue out in disgust. "It's just stupid," she said.

"I heard about you getting down on your stomachs and pounding on the ground," Lucinda said.

"That was because we were losing," said Denise.

"Well," said Lucinda, "I know a lady that was there, and she said you could see everything."

"What's the everything?" said Patty.

"Well, legs and everything. Thighs."

"Oh, pish tush," said Patty.

"The pants are supposed to show, like when you jump or anything," said Denise. "That's why they're that color."

"Well, you should wear a girdle at least," said Lucinda. She ran the machine a little, her face close to it.

"You couldn't do those stunts in a girdle," said Patty.

"No, that's right, you really couldn't, Mrs. Gordon," Denise said.

"And I hope you make sure you have a good strong bra when you do that jumping," said Lucinda.

"I do," said Patty.

"I still think it's ridiculous the way they encourage them," Lucinda said. "Millicent's right. High-school kids."

"Well, that's not the kind of thing that worries me," Ed said to her. "A couple of turns on a field. In front of a couple of hundred people, that have their minds on a game. On a cold afternoon."

"I still don't see the need of it," Lucinda said.

"Well, maybe not," he said neutrally. "I suppose it makes it more festive. Pretty girls. People like it."

"Yeah, you'd like it," Lucinda said, running the machine. "You're an old letch, that's what you are."

"Well, I enjoy looking at pretty girls. Or a cute pair of knees. Why not?"

"And a rabbi yet," Lucinda continued. "He has to be a rabbi yet."

"Look, that's not lechery," said Ed. "Girls are nice to look at, that's all. Like babies. Girls dancing, girls walking. There are pretty girls in this town and I'm glad there are. I walk down there, and I walk across the Square to the shul, and a pretty girl comes walking down the street—it makes the whole world brighter."

"Oh, is that so," Lucinda said.

"Sure it's so. Young girls and beautiful babies are ambassadors from the springtime. All the rest of the year. And you should apologize for calling me a letch."

"You're crazy," she said.

"What does our religion teach about sex?" Millicent asked him suddenly.

"What?" said Ed.

She was already sorry she had asked.

" 'Thou shalt not commit adultery,' " Roland muttered on the floor.

"What do you mean?" Ed asked her.

She colored near the ears. "Well, just what does the Bible say exactly?" She felt conscious of everyone in the room. Her mother's back, and Patty and Denise looking at her from different directions, though she did not look at them.

Her father was standing with his hand on the back of a chair, as though he had been about to sit at the dining table while talking to Lucinda. "Well," he said to Millicent, "like any other part of life. It's to be enjoyed, and made holy."

Roland had not looked up from the funnies. His feet swayed in the air, behind and above him.

"Why don't you come in the study," Ed said to Millicent. "We'll look up a couple of references if you want."

She rose. There was nothing to do but follow him through the living room and across the hall to the study.

When she had entered he shut the door.

"I just meant for purposes of discussion," she said. "I was just curious what the view of sin is, and all that. Like Roland mentioned 'thou shalt not commit adultery.' Does that cover just married people, for instance, or unmarried, or what?"

"No, it refers to a man with another man's wife." He sat on a corner of his desk.

"Is that all?" She had sat below him in the square cushions of the Morris chair, the back of which was catercorner to the bookshelves, and she spread her hands on its flat arms.

"You mean the sense of the word in the original," he asked her, "that's translated 'adultery' there. I assume that's what you meant."

"Yes."

"Well, that's what it means."

"Just married women?" Her voice was shaky. "What about a married man with an unmarried woman, for instance? Does it cover that?" Her embarrassment was mixed now with her curiosity, and with her awareness that she did not in fact know the text, and it seemed as though she might as well make the most of it.

"No." He was looking at her with a mild expression she could not read. His gaze was steady. "Have you been propositioned by a married man or something?"

She felt her blush darken. "No!" she said angrily. "Of course not! I wouldn't ask you if I thought you'd think something like that! Can't I ask a simple question?"

"Sure. I'm sorry. I appreciate your interest."

"People have discussions," she said. "Academically. Intellectual discussions."

"I know."

She paused a moment, as if uncertain whether to talk to him any more.

"Roommates and whatnot," she explained further. "And you've always said these things can't be translated exactly."

"I understand. Well, that's what the word means. Intercourse with another man's wife. It refers to the woman's status."

"That doesn't seem fair."

"It's just as much a crime for the man, you understand."

"If the woman's married, you mean."

"Or betrothed," he said. "Betrothed to someone else."

"But it doesn't refer at all to a married man cheating on his wife? Or to unmarried girls, or premarital sex or anything like that?"

"No."

"That's surprising."

"Well, that's just as far as that particular commandment goes. There are commandments about unmarried girls." He left the desk, and stepped past her knees, and took an English Bible from a place in the shelving quite near her.

He thumbed it.

At last he handed it to her and she saw it was open in Deuteronomy. He pointed out a verse. She read it on her lap.

> If a man find a damsel that is a virgin, that is not betrothed, and lay hold on her, and lie with her, and they be found, then the man that lay with her shall give unto the damsel's father fifty shekels of silver, and she shall be his wife—

"There's also a law that if he gets a girl pregnant he's got to marry her," she heard her father say over her. "But you don't mean that."

"No, that's a special case," she said without looking up.

She kept studying the passage.

"That still leaves a lot unsaid," she told him, still looking at it. " 'Lay hold on her'—does that mean rape?"

"It's without consent, yes."

"Well, suppose she consents? And it says 'if they be found.' What if they're not found?"

He took the book from her. She saw him turn to another part of it and flip pages. At last he put it on her lap again. The page was in Exodus.

> And if a man entice a virgin that is not betrothed, and lie with her, he shall surely pay a dowry for her to be his wife. If her father utterly refuse to give her unto him, he shall pay money according to the dowry of virgins.

"See?" she heard him say. "They're not talking about sin. They're talking about responsibility."

Millicent glanced at the subsequent verses but they dealt with other matters. Her eye returned to the verse. She could see her father's hands in his pockets, before her, and knew he was watching her read.

"What if she doesn't want to marry him?" she asked.

"The same law applies. She doesn't have to. She gets the money for her hope chest."

She kept looking at it a while. "Well, I don't know about this either," she said. "What if she's not a virgin? What then? What if the first boy pays the money and she doesn't marry him and now she's sleeping with the next boy?"

She glanced up and saw her father smile wryly.

"Or what if he didn't entice her?" she said. "What if she enticed him? Or what if she did it just to get him to marry her?"

"You have a good mind," he said. He put his hand out for the book. She gave it to him and he turned pages again.

"Isn't there any law in the whole Bible that just says flatly to stay a virgin until you're married?" she asked.

He turned pages quickly, as if looking for something in particular.

"And anyway those passages are about getting married afterward," she said. "Nothing about that they shouldn't have done it in the first place. You mean there's not one single law against fornication in the whole Five Books?"

"Here, look at this." He gave it to her open once more. "'Profane not thy daughter, to make her a harlot, lest the land fall into harlotry, and the land become full of lewdness.' There's a midrash on that, that it means a father shouldn't give his daughter to a man to sleep with, except in marriage. Also that she shouldn't do it on her own without marriage. There's other contexts that bear it out."

She looked at it, frowning.

"Where's that interpretation?" she said. "In the Talmud?"

"I think it's in Sifra. I could locate it for you. The oldest commentary on Leviticus. Older than Talmud."

At last, without rising from her chair, she pushed the book into its place in the shelves.

"Does that cover it? There's other laws too," he said, walking around the desk and sitting down, "for different circumstances—the general intent is clear. The Bible was meant for a real society and it tries to get the girl married off. Not chuck her on the junk heap. We're known as a sober and a home-loving people, you know that. And your mother and I have tried to give you kids a solid upbringing, so you'd know where you're at."

"I know, but I can be interested in the Bible, can't I? I just wondered how it relates to morals, exactly. That's all. There's so much written and discussed."

"I didn't mean anything," her father said. She saw that he blushed a little.

"Every time you pick up a newspaper, practically," she told him. "You can't avoid talking about it."

He nodded, not quite looking at her, and leaned back in his chair, rubbing his lip. For the moment he looked ill at ease, and she wondered if she could end the conversation now. But he began talking again.

"There were special rules for the priests," he said. "In Leviticus there. Kohanim can't marry a non-virgin, for instance. Just like Kohanim can't go to funerals. The altar was to be honored by a distance from fornication and death. But the Leviim and the ordinary people can marry a virgin or a non-virgin.

You get the point?" He looked at her. "It's a fact of life that these things happen, and it's also a fact that socially it's not good. The Bible isn't always creating laws—sometimes it's just looking for a way to live with the common law of all men, or the laws of that time, or human nature. And they knew then just like now, that a man thinks it's something special to be the first to touch a girl. It's worth something. And that's why the guy who took it from her had to increase her attractiveness by putting a dowry in the hope chest. Millicent, I think it's one of these universal things that cuts across cultures, no matter what a guy tells you. I don't care how sophisticated he is. Even if he has nothing against non-virgins—let's say he's understanding, fair, intelligent—still, his heart attaches a special grace to the girl who's untouched until she's spoken for. Like an extra bonus. A girl betrothed in freshness, that you can teach yourself. To have her to yourself, and be the only man she's known. That happens to some men, and they're glad, no matter what they tell you. It's a fact of life. Just like the fact that a lot of them aren't so fresh, which also has to be lived with. And if she's had one or two guys before, all right, so it isn't fifteen or twenty. A man doesn't dwell on his wife's premarital guys—he puts it from his mind. But don't let him tell you he's happy about it. I don't care if he's a college professor or a truck driver. Look, a girl's been knocked over right and left, and a guy wonders, how come I'm the one that picks up the tab? This can be had for free by the smart guys and I pay through the nose? All right, maybe he does. And I'm sure girls have slept around and settled down anyway eventually and made a man happy. But personally, other things being equal, I'm glad nobody had your mother. Even when the going was rough, I never had to say to myself, I should have just had an affair with her and dumped her. That kind of second judgment I was spared. Because I knew it wasn't possible." Without taking his eyes from Millicent he fumbled in the drawer for a cigarette. "A man wants to take his mother seriously, and he wants his children to take their mother seriously. He doesn't want his children to have been born through a birth canal that every man has gotten into. Any more than he himself wants to have been born through a birth canal that every man has gotten into. He wants the birth canal he was born through to have been his father's private preserve." His hand held the cigarette on the desk, unlit, behind the black telephone. "Suppose you're being courted seriously by two men," he said, "and you can't make up your mind. What should you do? Sleep with them both? And you want to know something? Even in this liberal sex crowd, for all their talk, you'll find in practice the same old double standard. Because even there they think less of the girl that does it without love, for instance. They fall back on saying it's okay if you're in love. But for men they don't have that requirement. They may tell women they do, but in their hearts and among themselves they don't." His fingers played with the cigarette. "You know what I used to tell the teen-agers in Brighton? I used to meet with the boys and the girls separately and this is what I told them, I told them both the same. That it's not consistent, and it never will be. Because look—no matter what these smart young kids tell you today, they're obviously not going to advise a girl they care for to sleep with some other guy. Not a girl they're thinking about for marriage. So what about that? Even when I was a young guy, you know, boys used to tell girls these things—they'd say they'd never consider marrying any girl who wasn't experienced, or a girl that hadn't gotten her wild oats out of her system, and they'd say they wouldn't marry a girl without trying her out to see if they were compatible, and all that sort of stuff. All that. And then they'd go and talk to each other in a completely different vocabulary. Whether they scored, and first base, second base, third base, and all that."

Millicent suddenly gave a sob, involuntarily. It seemed to startle Ed. She wept, half hiding her face. He watched her without saying anything.

"I'm sorry. It's just depressing," she explained tearfully. "The attitudes men have. If they think that. They must think they use a virgin up, like a chocolate bar, bite by bite, until there's nothing left. And I think it's just horrible. They want to seduce a girl in the first place and then downgrade her for it. Like the Nazis forcing women to be prostitutes and then shooting them if they got a disease."

"Well," her father said, "I think you're being a little extreme."

"I'm not being extreme."

"Men still aren't Nazis, for the most part."

"Men stink."

She gave a shudder.

"Millicent—" His voice was lower.

"What."

"What happened?"

"Nothing happened," she said irritably. She felt in the pocket of her dress for her handkerchief, but she had left it in her bag up in Patty's room. "Have you got any kleenex?"

"No. Want my handkerchief?" He pulled a crumpled rag from his hip.

"No." The crying had stopped but she still breathed through her mouth. "It makes me sick," she said. " 'Facts of life'—you always get a man's-eye view. 'Human nature.' Men wrote the Bible, didn't they. I mean, women didn't. Why is God always He? Oh, I know, it's figurative. But why not She half the time?" She sniffed, and pressed her nostrils, wiping their moisture on her fingertips.

Her father seemed to have forgotten the cigarette on the desk somewhere without having lighted it. "Millicent," he said, "do you remember what we ask forgiveness for on the High Holy Days? Over and over again?"

"I don't know."

"Yes you do."

"Lots of things."

"Not the technics of this and that commandment violated," he said. "But crimes against your own dignity as a human being. Being mean, hard. Loud, foolish, vulgar, cheap. You remember? Isn't that so? Anything that reduces what it is to be human."

She met his eyes. They were sad, and his forehead was wrinkled.

"Don't hold yourself cheap. Don't give yourself without a promise that he'll take care of you."

"Promise?"

"The contract, that we sign at weddings. I know, these days you're bound to get invitations."

"What do you think? I'm on my way to get seduced or something?"

"No. I'm not worried about you. You're solid, and you have a head on your shoulders."

"All right, all right. I've got to get to Boston. I've got to be at work at three."

"There's time."

"No there's not."

She rose. He started up also, and offered to drive her to the depot, but she refused. It seemed necessary to flee out of here as soon as possible.

"I can get the bus if I move," she said.

"I don't mind taking you."

"It's silly. I can get the bus."

"Well, it's up to you. I think Mother has some things for you to take. Chicken, and crab-apple jelly."

She hurried upstairs to Patty's room. Her coat lay across the extra cot.

She put it on, and fastened the buttons. Maybe her father had an old-fashioned dirty mind, she thought, and what the new morality was really about was the abolition of the double standard. Maybe in the new morality boys would not be promiscuous, and would only sleep with their best girl friends.

But she was not sure. One thing her father had said, about the different vocabularies, had rung true in a sour way.

She remembered how it had seemed at college, how the talk had sounded. Girls said, if I loved him enough. Or even, if I were attracted to him enough. But boys said, I'd like to make that. She had overheard them. Boys did not say, if I loved her enough.

35

Ed did not tell Lucinda how the discussion had gone, and she didn't ask him. Perhaps she assumed that he and Millicent had rummaged idly in obscure books together, or perhaps she had just forgotten.

Denise had gone away even before Millicent had left, and for a while Ed helped Patty memorize her lines for the De Molay play. He held the book and gave her cues. He thought she spoke them well, with comprehension and a sense of timing. It struck him that she had some talent as an actress. Often it had seemed as if the children were in many ways extensions of parts of himself—Patty for example had his knack for drawing—he had used to draw in his youth, though not nearly so well as his sister Rosalind, and had done pencil portraits with good likenesses. Yet the children also had talents and worlds that were not his, he thought, as he watched her play this character role. He had none of her skill in music, for example. It was strange, how quickly beings who had lived such a short time found themselves things to do. Like Roland, awake before his parents and out on this paper route, and planning his afternoons so he could deliver at five.

Ed listened to Patty for more than an hour, and then left for the Concord Reformatory. He went to the barn for his car, discovering it had begun to snow. The crab apples that had fallen had rotted and then frozen, and snow lay on them thinly. It could not last, so early in the season, but he was glad of it anyway, because the volunteer firemen had been worried about the dryness.

He had an appointment at the Reformatory with a boy and his mother, and there were two other boys he wanted to drop in on. He had been filling in for a regular chaplain who was away. But so far he had not found it rewarding. The boys seemed to have little interest in religion, except insofar as a pretense of it could help get them out.

On the way home it was dark, and the wipers pushed sleet. His thoughts were of Millicent. He had discussed morals with youth groups in his congregations, on various levels, but no one had ever pressed him for answers with Millicent's preciseness.

It had been odd for her to stumble into such a conversation with him, but it reassured him rather than worried him. She would scarcely have blurted so, if she were considering saying yes to some pursuer. Girls did not put their fathers on the scent. In the past, especially if tired, he had had gnawing anxieties about the secrets his daughters might come to have, and the clues were few and vague, and he had clung to the remark that she had once let drop, that she had liked a boy in Chicago because he was above necking. It had seemed obvious today that these conversations and talks she spoke of had not all been just idle ones, without reference to herself. Yet what she had seemed to want of him was an understanding of the moral instinct that came so naturally to her. To know with her mind the morality she felt.

And what a mind, he thought. To inquire after the original text, always aware that a translation was only a translation—this was the mind of a scholar. Orderly and curious. This was one of those rare women. He understood her better than Lucinda did. Lucinda would berate her for declining invitations or for "discouraging everybody," but it seemed to Ed she was doing fine—she didn't want to waste time with a lot of men who were beneath her, for the sake of dates, and was waiting for the right one. From the first weeks of life she had been a darling. Never had an infant had such aplomb. Never had an adolescent's beauty been so breath-taking, so clean. And it was lousy to be a father and entertain the young men that came to take your daughters out, and hope that a worthy one would like the goods, and that they would not just paw the merchandise. How many more years of that did he have ahead?

But it was good to have daughters who could be trusted. Patty too, just this past week, had had an encounter in which she behaved admirably. She had left a boy's car and telephoned from a farmhouse and Ed had gone to get her. At home she had gone upstairs, still a little breathless, to where Lucinda lay in bed, and sat on the bed and told them the story. It was a boy named Doug Watts, who played the hired man in the De Molay play. He had taken her to the movie in Sparkstown and on the way back he had gotten fresh. But she had said, I'm a mailbox. And Doug Watts had said, what's a mailbox, and she had said, three hundred dollars fine for tampering. And Doug Watts had said, it's just animal spirits, and she had said, I'm sorry but I didn't know it was Be Kind To Dumb Animals Week. But he had begun again, apparently, so she had told him to quit it because she was the rabbi's daughter and besides she was the organist at Saint Tim's, and he had said, if I believe that, I suppose you'll tell me you're the Pope's girl friend. And that was when she said, I'm getting out. She had tried to walk home, but he had followed in the car, apologizing, so she had run to a farmhouse and asked the old couple to lend her their phone.

And today, Ed thought, one of his daughters had actually come inquiring what the Law said. Of course that didn't mean she believed, any more than he had at that age, but the inquiry itself was good.

The Temple Beth El Sisterhood had asked him to address their November meeting, which fell the Tuesday after his conversation with Millicent. Usually they followed the business session with some miscellaneous entertainment, such as a skit, or a review of some popular novel, or films of somebody's vacation, and once this fall they had spent twenty-five dollars for a lady who came to lecture on Japanese flower arrangement. But it was also their policy that at one meeting during the year the rabbi should be the entertainment. The Hadassah, which included most of the same ladies, had had Bill Prince once, and he had played the guitar and tapped his foot and sung folk songs that made them titter.

Ed thought of addressing them on the laws of marriage and divorce, as a likely subject to entertain a bunch of housewives. But on the way there, walking in the night, he changed his mind. His aim in this community was to bring them closer to their religion, and to help raise their observance of it, and it was foolish to lose any opportunity to do this. Better to let marriage and divorce go till another year and talk now of something more practical.

The meeting was in Dr. and Mrs. Yarrish's house, on the hill up past Murphy Square where the fine new homes were, and which sloped down on its other side toward Wilmerding Mills. Lucinda had gone ahead of him with the car, as she was on the refreshments committee.

He found a splendid living room filled by about seventy-five ladies and their folding chairs, and Amethyst Gilbert already standing at a card table and presiding with a little gavel. He sat on a folding chair reserved for him near

Amethyst and crossed his knees. From a table at the side he could tell that they had had their coffee and social hour beforehand. He watched Amethyst and half listened to the discussion of plans for a pancake supper, which was supposed to raise some money. She looked as trim and stylish as ever, even from the angle at which he sat. Her nervous hips made him think of the photographs that advertised girdles in ladies' magazines. At last she turned and smiled down at him, dimplingly, with her pixyish glasses.

He rose, with a hand in his pocket. He told the gathering that he wanted to give them some notion of what the Sabbath was about, and perhaps knock apart some superstitions about it.

He saw the tilt of varishaped hats as faces in the back moved to get a better view of him. He said the Sabbath did not prevent you from doing what you wanted, because you could do those things on other days, but it freed you from what you didn't want to do. As he spoke his eye wandered over fur pieces and tailored clothing, and he was struck anew by the fashionableness of this congregation.

He said you were supposed to work six days, and if a man's job only took five he could spend the sixth puttering around the house, or on the golf course, or shlepping the kids to the beach, or throwing a party—those things were work too. But on the seventh day he didn't shave, and his wife couldn't ask him to put up the storm windows. Nor could his wife be asked to sew a button on. An afternoon nap was especially recommended, and so was sexual intercourse.

He said the literature did not describe the Sabbath as a day on which to be more pious than other days, but as a day on which to be like princes, like gentlemen of leisure. On the Sabbath you did not see the bills, because you couldn't rip open the envelopes. You could read, study if you wished, but you mustn't take notes. It was a time to be fallow, to permit your mind to wander free. You didn't touch your car or your tools, because your car and your tools would sooner or later lead to headache situations. The ban on travel was designed to keep you in the bosom of your family, and make you available to your children, but you could not on that day shlep your daughter to dancing class or the dentist. On the Sabbath no rotten movie could rob you. One evening out of seven you could read without having to shut out the racket of television turned on by some other member of the family, and the family did not have to endure the stink of your cigars. The ban on writing and telephoning made even a scholar relax, and made his interests pleasurable. A woman didn't cook, as the meals were cold, and if company dropped in she had a perfect excuse for not brewing coffee. A fire in the fireplace was perfectly fine, provided all the work of making it was done beforehand. It was good to have one day a week without cigarettes and coffee. You had whisky instead.

When he had talked about half an hour he asked if there were any questions. His eye moved from one motionless face to another. No one said anything.

"No questions at all?" he said.

Amethyst rose beside him, as if about to ask for questions also, but then a short fortyish woman he knew as Mrs. Dembitz stood up in the audience and slung back a furry tail of fox that had slipped from her shoulder. She had a beak of a nose, and eyes near together. She asked Ed if he had read a certain best seller about a young woman who returned from the dead.

Ed could see no connection between the question and what he had talked about. He knew of the book, as it was having a vogue. It was supposed to be not fiction but a true documented case. However he had not read it and he said so. He said as far as he was concerned it was nonsense. People didn't return from the dead.

Then Mrs. Dembitz asked about life after death and Ed said he didn't believe in that either. There was a murmur through the room, and though it wasn't loud it startled him. He hadn't meant to shock anyone. Mrs. Dembitz had seemed to be referring to some clear-cut survival of her present consciousness past the grave.

"Do you believe it?" he asked her.

"Well, I don't know," she said. "It seems to me that's what we pay the rabbi to believe. If the rabbi doesn't believe it what are we here for?"

"That's right," said another lady. "If the rabbi doesn't believe I can't even believe in the rabbi." He heard some murmurs of approval.

He rubbed his forehead, pushing back a lock of hair. "In the whole Bible there's no reference to immortality, or afterlife," he said, "and it seems to me the omission was on purpose. I don't think it was just because nobody had thought of it yet, because they must have known the Egyptians believed in it. It's just not in the Bible. And in the Psalms, for instance, it says 'in death there's no remembrance of Thee—who will praise Thee from the netherworld?' Look, if you want to believe in it, it's very human. I can't tell you no. But it's in the area of the unknown, and our whole tradition avoids spelling it out. And I never heard pious people of the old generation mention it. I asked my grandfather once. I asked him because he was sad that he didn't think he'd live to see me married, so I asked if he didn't believe the soul would see what came after, or something like that, and he shook his head and said, 'that has nothing to do with this.' And that's all he ever said to me about life after death. His only reference to it. All the religion he taught me was for this world. And to me it seems, when the Talmud talks of having a share in the world to come, that's figurative, like owning shares of stock in a company you never see. When the good society is achieved, even long after our death, that's our world, if we believed in it, and if we lived for it. If you worked against it, if you did nothing and cared nothing for it, then when that world comes it's not yours. You have no share in it. Your life will make a ripple, and it'll have its influence. Like when we say in our prayers that 'God keeps faith with those who sleep in the dust.' If you keep faith with those who've gone before you, then you become the agent by which God keeps faith with them. Or when we say 'He gives life to the dead.' It means if it weren't for God we'd all be dead. We've all had escapes from death. And it means that without the ties to mankind that God gives you, you're the walking dead anyway. Just like 'He gives sight to the blind.' "

"Do you believe prayers are answered?" another lady asked. It was Mrs.

Kramer, the one who had quit as a Sunday-school teacher. Mrs. Dembitz had sat down, and Mrs. Kramer asked the question without rising. Ed felt a hostility in the audience and it made him uneasy.

"Well, yes, in a sense," he said. "I'm not sure how you mean that—you don't mean a Santa Claus proposition. We only pray for things that can actually be affected by prayer. Like insight, knowledge, healing in general, the rebuilding of Jerusalem—"

"But does God actually listen to prayers, or what?" Mrs. Kramer said. "Aren't you praying to God? I mean, why do you pray three times a day if you don't believe anybody's listening?"

"Well, I didn't say I don't believe anybody's listening. Look, sometimes I give a sermon and I don't know if anybody's listening, or if I'm getting through to anybody, but I give it anyway. If we believe there's a purpose in our having been created, then there's an impulse to get closer to it, and to express that wanting, and ask aid, and the impulse doesn't have to wait for the reduction of the unknown to the known. Like the other day Mr. Brill asked me to prove for him that God exists. That's not my job. What I offer you is commitment. And I believe prayer works, if it works at all, through natural phenomena, but I don't know how God orders natural phenomena. Do I know? Do I know these ultimates? God said to Moses, 'no man may look on My face and live.' That means, don't even try to be a theologian. You say God is this, God is that, and you end up with fairy tales. You want religion to be real, and you have to face this fact of life, that it's in the nature of things that when you talk about God you don't know what you're talking about. We haven't a clue. You discuss God, and all you do is argue and argue about something you can't even define. That's why Abraham had to start off negatively. He was the first ever to draw a distinction between religion and superstition, as far as I know, and he did it on the most modern level. And that was the starting point of this whole movement. He starts with what God isn't—with what not to believe. And when the Temple was built, what was in the Holy of Holies? An empty room. That's all. That room contained everything we know about God. Nothing. A blank. And the injunction against images implies also that we shouldn't even make a definition of God. It was to keep the people reminded that we don't know, so they wouldn't invent beliefs about things we don't have a glimmer of, because a serious religion has to admit we don't know, and shouldn't be cluttered up with bunk and unreality. That's the reason for insisting on God's unity, because once you break something into parts you think you understand it. Listen, we don't even understand the physical universe, that we're a part of. There are planets that the human race will never have an inkling of, because it would take too many billions of years for the fastest signal to get there. Do you know that? All our knowing is a drop surrounded by an ocean of not knowing. And we struggle so hard to learn so small a fraction about something so remote—a fraction so small it still tells us nothing. You learn that the universe oscillates or that it's a single bang—then what do you know? I remember when I was a kid, I used to read The Book of Knowledge, and it said the universe was shaped like a big watch. And then ten years after that they said a spiral, and then in a few years they said all that was just a galaxy at one end of a galactic system and the galactic system was drifting among a trillion others, and another few years and they said space is curved, and the universe is shaped like an expanding balloon, and you want my theory? I think when they figure it out, it'll turn out the universe is shaped like a question mark. A big question mark. That's what I believe. And you want to draw a little picture, or write down an idea on a piece of paper, and call it the God of all this? Even the empty room was destroyed. But we're forbidden to utter the Name, which amounts to the same thing. We don't even know how to pronounce the Name."

"That seems like a pretty cold kind of religion," said Mrs. Kramer. "An empty room."

"No," said Ed, "there's family, there's community, there's festivals—it's not a cold proposition. But religion, to be real, it can't be based on pretending you know what you don't, and I don't offer you that kind of faith. All right, I'll guarantee you something. If you want belief, and if you live the Law, belief will come. That's a promise. I promise you that the more you practice the Law, the more it'll grow on you. And things will happen, and even if you don't know God you'll start to have a suspicion sometimes that He knows you. Because I started off myself with more or less of a secular attitude, but I studied, and by the time I was in commentaries I'd seen the decisions and attitudes of this tradition hang together so well, and make sense so often, and so consistently, that after a few years I began to trust it to make sense. Even notions that put me off at first impressed me with their subtlety later on. It's remarkable, but the more you study the more divine it looks. It doesn't come apart. And you'll pray. And you'll notice how our prayers are worded—we don't ask to be brought nearer to God, but to be brought nearer to the Law. It's through the sweating effort of mankind that God will bring the millennium about. What we ask for is our own creative capacity. We don't even ask for daily bread. We ask water for the earth, so we can make our own daily bread. You know, knowing God and knowing the divine imperative, it's two different things. It's for us to know what we should do, and study and research what we should do. Not to know God. It's when people insist on knowledge of God that we haven't got that belief becomes an issue."

He paused, and his glance searched about among the faces for more questions. Then he asked if there were any.

At last Amethyst arose and thanked him smilingly, referring to him as our gracious guest speaker of the evening, and there was some applause.

Amid the confusion of finding coats and putting on boots he said a word of small talk to one member and another, and found Lucinda.

"He sounds kind of atheistic to me," he heard one lady mutter to another behind him.

He drove home with Lucinda. He felt the evening had gone badly, and he made no conversation at all until well onto Massapeequit Road.

"I guess I didn't go over very well tonight," he said finally.

"Well, I don't think you geared it to their interests," Lucinda said.

He did get some word during the next several days that he had made a bad impression, but not so much for the reasons he had supposed. Apparently one of the ladies had brought her eleven-year-old daughter to the meeting, though Ed had scarcely noticed the girl, and the feeling was that it had been quite irresponsible of him to mention sexual intercourse.

36

Toward noon one day, while gray rain beat on the windows, Millicent received a phone call from a man named Malcolm Stack, who wanted a blind date. He said he had been told about her by a neighbor of his, a Mrs. Blink, and had then gotten her number from telephone information.

"Mrs. Blink?" said Millicent.

"Yeah." He said Mrs. Blink had a friend called Mrs. Lebensalt, and Mrs. Lebensalt had a sister who was in Millicent's father's congregation. The sister's name was Mrs. Kiss.

He mentioned a restaurant he wanted to take her to. His diction was terrible.

"I'm sorry," Millicent told him. "I work nights."

"What about your nights off?"

"No," she said. "I'm sorry." She ended the conversation.

Then she proceeded to do her calisthenics.

She had been answering the phone with promptness lately, usually before the first ring was complete, hoping it might be Les. It never was. Usually it was not even for her. Once Mr. Killian called and asked if she could come to work early because the other boy was sick, and today there had been this blind-date person. But most often the call was for Natalie. There was a stupid-sounding boy who would manage to call just after Natalie had left, or could not remember that Natalie did not get home till four.

Millicent watched the rain, and then fed the cat and had her brunch, and spent some time tidying the apartment, and lay in a hot bath.

Then, just as she was readying to set out for the city room, Leslie did call.

"Oh, hello," she said. His voice took her by surprise. She was standing with the phone, her lined raincoat hanging unbuttoned and a kerchief over her head.

He asked blandly whether they could get together this week.

She hesitated. "Les," she said, "I've decided we should stop seeing each other."

His hesitation was only an instant. "Okay," he said.

She had expected him to argue.

"I mean, Les," she explained, "it's all been made very clear. I mean, it's dishonest to be together and not start, and it's also dishonest to start and then stop—"

"Do you realize what you're saying is that you want to?"

"Really, Les, I'm not going to argue about it."

"Okay. I said okay."

"Well, okay."

"So long," he said.

"So long," she said confusedly. She hung up the lavender phone.

She walked to work. The rain was cold.

She had not meant the conversation to go like that.

She wished she had made it clearer that she had only meant, unless they had an understanding, unless he agreed not to argue any more. She had not meant, not see him under any circumstances.

But she saw no way to call him back and explain this. To call back would weaken her position even further.

Anyway, he probably understood, she told herself. And if he thought better of it he would call again.

His delaying so long beyond the two weeks had weakened her position, and she had had to be sharp with him in order to strengthen it. But she wished now she had rehearsed it, or that she had waited until they were face to face.

She did not dare to hope for a new call, even though for several days she constructed fantasies about how it might have gone differently.

Then she told herself that it didn't matter anyhow—it would have gone badly no matter how she had worded it and it was best to have ended it now rather than later. It was better for him too—if he was going to be so bothered during the years of bachelorhood ahead of him, it was better that he be free to use the few hours he had to himself to pursue girls who went to bed more easily.

Yet there must certainly be congenial, intelligent men in the world. Young Mr. Herlihy the police reporter, or Mr. Lyons on her own paper—they were not suitable as eventual marriage partners, but they were intelligent and congenial. Only there was no way to approach them, or to approach any man. It was bound to be taken for courtship, on one level or another.

She taught her Sunday-school class again. Then at home she heard her mother bawling out her father because he hadn't cleaned away the dried-up hollyhocks. Her father said he would do it when his leg and his back weren't tied up with muscle spasms. Then Lucinda said he wouldn't have spasms if he had done it when he was supposed to instead of fooling around the car, so Ed said putting on snow tires and waxing it wasn't fooling around, and Lucinda said that piece of junk wasn't worth it, and Ed said a woman can't understand that to a man his car is like his house. They have such stupid arguments, Millicent thought. She and Les had at least argued about something important, like sex.

While she wiped the dishes she asked her mother if there was a Mrs. Kiss that belonged to the temple.

"What do you want her for?" Lucinda asked.

"I don't. I just asked if there is such a person. I just heard the name."

"What did you hear about Mrs. Kiss?"

"Nothing." Millicent was beginning to be red. "I just saw it on a list or something, and I thought the name was odd."

"Yes, it is sort of odd," said Lucinda. She stacked some dishes high in the cabinet. "She's a regular kocheleffel. She's in everything."

So, Millicent thought, those ridiculous names were real people. He hadn't made them up.

Her mother asked if Ella Jane and Natalie were going home to Chicopee for Thanksgiving, and Millicent said that Natalie was but Ella Jane wasn't. So Lucinda suggested that she invite Ella Jane to Wilmerding Crosswalk.

On the train ride back to Boston it occurred to Millicent that she ought to have asked Leslie, when he phoned, to have Thanksgiving turkey with her and Ella Jane at the apartment. She would have prepared it, and it would have been fun.

Now he would probably eat his Thanksgiving meal alone, a slice of dry bird and a slop of floury gravy on a metal tray, amid the blue-white fluorescence and echoing tile of the hospital cafeteria. It was such a waste.

She extended her mother's invitation to Ella Jane, and the two girls rode to Sparkstown together. Ed met them at the depot.

At the table Millicent noticed that when Ed said the blessing Ella Jane shut her eyes. It seemed to her that the family were all cordial to Ella Jane, and except for her father a bit excessively so, apparently because of the cane and irons and shrunken leg. Roland even helped her with her chair. Patty was deferential as though to one of her elders, in a way she had never been to Millicent. Ella Jane was relaxed but quiet, seeming to enjoy being made so at home. Millicent saw her mother smilingly give Ella Jane more stuffing and ask Ed to cut her more turkey. She'd have a fit if she knew about Ella Jane's affair, Millicent thought.

The evening train ride back to Boston was quite silent, except for the clacking wheels. It began to seem to Millicent that she and Ella Jane had no more to say to each other than an old married couple. The turkey leftovers and stuffing her mother had given them for the apartment was in a package on the seat between them. She felt in a rut. It was her own fault for not having shown more initiative in her career. Some timidity or something seemed to keep her from knowing how to get started.

Millicent climbed to the apartment slowly beside Ella Jane, who pulled herself a step at a time. As they got to it they heard the phone ringing.

It was Malcolm Stack again. "Maybe you're busy and maybe you're not," he said to Millicent, "but you still got to eat. So what can you lose?" She ended by tiredly agreeing to have dinner with him on Wednesday the week following.

"I don't know why I accepted," she said to Ella Jane when she put down the phone. "He sounds awful."

"Why did you?" said Ella Jane.

"Well, I thought he's probably lonesome."

During the week she took some walks in the hours before work, her press card in her sock, with her eyes open as Mr. Killian had said, in hopes of stumbling across some happening or circumstance that could make a news item. She also looked through all the Boston papers daily to get more of a feel for the kind of things reporters discovered. Once she even wandered far southward into the slums. Usually it was blustery cold, though without snow. But she found nothing more unusual than workmen busy at a manhole. There must be something wrong with her approach, she thought.

One afternoon Mr. Killian told her to go over to the Parker House, where the Federation of Women's Clubs was in convention, and to see if she could get advance copies of certain speeches. She was to read them to him from a phone booth and he would tell her whether to remain and cover the meetings or not. He thrust into her hand a packet of such press releases as he had about the convention.

Descending slowly in the newspaper building's elevator cage she found a convention program in the packet, and a ticket for dinner at the press table, and other items.

Making her way to the Parker House she wondered if it was only a coincidence that she had again been assigned to a women's event, or whether she was really being jim crowed in this fashion. However when she had read Mr. Killian what he wanted from the phone booth he told her it was not worth coverage.

On the way back to the city room she gave the dinner ticket to a shivering old beggar and told him that if he went to the Parker House at six-thirty, to the ballroom indicated, he would have his dinner. He looked at it bleary-eyed. She had seen this old man about the sidewalks many times in the past, and had usually given him dimes or quarters.

She felt uneasy afterward. She had thought a ticket and a dinner should not be wasted. But it seemed possible, when she thought about it, that the convention people might be upset about this derelict tottering in, with his dirty clothes and white stubble. They might get in touch with Mr. Killian and complain. Or they might think the old man had stolen the ticket, and have him arrested. It seemed more and more a foolish thing to have done.

For a few days she worried that Mr. Killian would receive a letter and that she would be bawled out. But nothing happened. He did, however, beckon her to his desk and criticized her for having submitted an expense form for five cents, the amount of her phone call. He told her always to make out her swindle sheets for at least a dollar, because the treasurer's office didn't like to make out checks so small.

She said nothing, but she didn't see how she could put in a dishonest claim. She resented his calling it a swindle sheet.

On Wednesday evening she was ready early and waiting for Malcolm Stack to ring the doorbell. Her coat and scarf were beside her on the studio couch. Natalie had returned from Chicopee, and from the sound of Malcolm's voice she did not care to parade him before her roommates. She met him on the stairs.

He smiled, confirming her identity and his, and doffing his hat with a slight bow of his head. He was quite presentable-looking in his way. He was of more than medium height, with a certain skinniness and a long triangular face, light-complexioned under a high forehead and wavy hair. The smile showed even teeth and closed his eyes nearly to slits. He had drawn off a soft gray glove, though she did not offer her hand. His clothes looked new and well fitted, and she felt underdressed. A heavy silk scarf bound his neck with exquisite neatness.

"Okay, so let's go," he said, taking her elbow.

"Don't take my arm, please. It's not necessary."

He let it go. He said the restaurant was only a couple of blocks from her apartment and that it didn't pay to use the car. But when they got to the crossing it was quite windy.

"You ain't cold, are ya?" he said.

"No."

"I noticed on the stairs you got knee socks. I could have brought the car around, but it's just two–three blocks. I figured what the hell, you know."

"I don't mind walking."

At the curb he took her elbow, not absent-mindedly, but lifting his brows and looking down with a querying little smile. She permitted it.

He released her elbow at the opposite curb, and as they walked he asked about her job. He does have an admirable posture, she thought. Then she saw their shadows lengthen on the uneven darkness of the brick sidewalk as a street lamp receded behind them.

The restaurant had a quiet entrance—two great urns by the door of what might have been a residential building. Millicent had seen its green canopy before without paying it particular attention. Inside the walls were cream-colored and paneled with delicately carved molding. "Good evening, Mr. Stack," a bald man in black said, and they gave him their coats. Another man in black, somewhat European-looking, also addressed Mr. Stack with a little smile and a suggestion of a bow, and they followed him.

The ceilings were high, also paneled with molding, and there were great chandeliers. The room did not seem large, as it was not wide, but it had considerable length. They were taken to a raised part at the rear, beside tall many-paned dark windows and velvet curtains. The man assisted Millicent with her chair. "Cocktails?" he said when they were seated.

"How about it?" Malcolm asked her. "You look like the dry manhattan type."

"Do I? No. I don't want anything, thanks."

Malcolm waved the man away.

The tablecloth was a satiny brocade of white on white, with curlycues and monograms. Malcolm handed her a tasseled menu. She noticed that he wore French cuffs, with cuff links of silver and black. "Well," he said, "like I said, you got to eat."

She asked what he was going to have. He recommended the grapefruit stuffed with grapes, avocado soup Chambord, the pompano aux amandes, asparagus Beauharnais, petites champignons sauce Neuilly, and mousse Mirabeau.

"Well, I guess that'll be all right," she said.

He made a slight motion of his head and another man in black came quietly to the table. Malcolm ordered the same dinner for them both. He told Millicent he would recommend a smoky wine of the Loire.

"I'm a teetotaler," she said.

"Skip the wine," he said. The waiter bowed and stepped away.

Malcolm took a roll from a silver dish, buttered it, and handed it to Millicent. His fingernails looked manicured.

"What's this with the liquor?" he asked. "You on a special diet or something?"

"No. It's a matter of principle, I guess."

For an instant she thought they were about to lapse into an awkward silence, but he began to talk, quite easily. He said he owned a factory. He made paper hats, crepe-paper decorations, honkers that unroll when blown, noses with spectacles and mustachios. It struck her as strange to be here with him. Comic noses and mustaches—she had never known anyone who would think to make such a thing.

"I'm the second biggest in New England," he said.

"How many people does your factory employ?" she asked him.

"Twenty, forty, depends on the season. I got a whole floor. It's growed a lot since my old man kicked the bucket. I'm branching out already. Other interests. Short-eared racing rabbits. I got a farm in Vermont."

"Short-eared what?"

"Racing rabbits. You don't know what short-eared racing rabbits is? They use 'em in South America, Argentina. But they don't breed so good there. They breed 'em in Vermont. I just bought into this place. It's practically got a monopoly."

She had begun to feel incredulous about his whole tale. Her face must have shown it.

"You want a pair? I'll get you a pair. You got a kid brother, don't ya?"

"I don't think we want a pair of rabbits."

"All right, I understand. One rabbit. Okay? I'll get you one rabbit."

He buttered another piece of bread. Around his eyes she saw the beginning of crow's-feet. He was perhaps thirty, she thought. The oldest man she had ever gone out with.

His eyes met hers. He remarked that he and she had the same initial, and that he was superstitious about things like that.

"It's only the first initial,'" she said.

"That's all right," he said. "But I'll tell ya. Once I had a dream, about a certain piece of property, and the next day I went out and bought it. And today it's worth double what I paid." He handed her the buttered bread.

"No thanks," she said.

"I don't mean I'm a gambler. I don't want you to think that. I look an investment over." He tapped the tablecloth. "Real estate's a good thing in Boston now. This town's down so far it's got to come up. But even so, I got to know before I buy. I go into it. The location. The zoning. The everything. I don't go off half cocked. On the other hand, when I see it's good I don't horse around. You know what I mean?"

"You mean you're decisive, but you're not impulsive."

"That's it. That's exactly it. I see you got a flair with words."

He talked on, about taxes, and then about Senator McCarthy, whom he called McCarty, and food was brought meanwhile. The soup was of a perfect warmth, without hotness, and so was the fish. Everything was soft. Even the colors were mild. She was surprised how one flavor after another could be so delicate, so simple-seeming. Nothing was sharp, nothing was strong. And no mouthful left a taste once it was swallowed. But Malcolm's approval of Senator McCarthy began to irritate her, and at last she cut in angrily, telling him McCarthy was a contemptible, meretricious adventurer, without regard for the national safety. She said she had little enough regard for the President, as far as that went, and his letter to the music critic had certainly put his fitness into question, but the President at least was a patriot, with some principle in his own fashion, while McCarthy was a charlatan and an opportunist. She was shaking. Her emotion embarrassed her, and she thought Malcolm would be angry. She called McCarthy a vulgar impostor.

But Malcolm was quietly attentive and did not take his eyes from her. At length there was a silence. She ate again. He asked what she thought of the Korean situation.

She answered more quietly and timidly than before. "Well, I'm sorry now we went into the northern part," she said. "And it's too bad the Chinese came in. China and Russia sort of seem to have us in a squeeze."

"You read a lot, I bet," said Malcolm.

"Well, I try to. Mornings, and my days off. Not half as much as I should, actually. And I've given up on fiction. What they're doing now just isn't worth reading any more. I think the novel's pretty dead as an art form. I read history mostly."

He seemed to value her judgments, even though he didn't comment. At length, when dinner was finished, he took a tiny crooked cigar from his jacket. But he caught her eye and paused.

"You'd rather I wouldn't smoke," he said.

He put the cigar away before she could speak. He drew a pair of red theater tickets from a pocket and held them up, forming a V.

"Well, I think I may be a little allergic to smoke, actually," she said belatedly.

"Guess what we got," he said. "Surprise. Belly Buttons And Bows. Eighth row center."

Then she saw him count three ten-dollar bills from his wallet and place them on the tablecloth. She knew of Belly Buttons And Bows. It was said to be a tremendous smash, the most sought-after musical in years.

She followed him to the cloak racks, unsmiling. A man in black was waiting with their things, and assisted them.

At the curb, almost in front of the restaurant, was a large white convertible, and Malcolm opened the door of it. She was startled.

"Is this your car?"

"Down to the ground," he said. "I don't go for installments."

It was long and wide, glittering with chromium, and the rear was sculptured into high fins. She sank down into upholstery of dark blue leather. He shut her in and went around. When he was beside her he showed her how shiny little switches made the windows go down and up again, with a hum of machinery. Then with a different mechanical droning the whole roof slowly reared, gaping and rising, until she saw the cloudy night sky above her reflecting the city's reddish glow. The roof folded down behind them, and then rose whirring again and closed. She was annoyed by the demonstration and by being maneuvered into the car. His hand turned the starter switch. The wide polished dashboard had an imitation wood grain. She could feel the quiet motor come to life.

"I didn't know you were planning on theater," she said with irritation.

"You in any hurry to get home?"

"No, not necessarily, but you might have had the consideration to consult me at least before making a selection."

He switched off the motor. "You seen it already?"

"No, I haven't seen it," she said. "But I don't particularly care for musicals. I don't see anything especially gay, or cheering, about women marching around half naked. Or seven-eighths naked. On a public stage, while other people pay to sit and watch."

He pouted his lower lip and looked thoughtful.

"It seems to me," she said, "if you want to look at skin so badly you can lock yourself in your bedroom and look at your own. I mean, what are those poor girls selling, actually? It's depressing."

"They ain't selling nothing."

"They're selling their dignity."

"Well, what would you rather see?"

"Well, just about anything rather than that. A city like this offers a whole broad range of worthwhile entertainments. And if you want theater there are things like To The Angel Of Death I'm Not In, for instance. At least it's serious drama."

"Okay," he said.

Methodically but quickly he tore the tickets to bits. It hadn't occurred to her that he would do such a thing, and she feared she had angered and wounded him deeply. But when she looked at him it did not seem so. He buzzed the window down with its automatic switch, scattered the tickets out, and buzzed it up again. She could think of nothing to say.

The car started smoothly, with a sinking and lift, and the radio began playing with loud bell-like tones. They turned a corner and halted at a stop light. She was not sure where they were headed. If he intended now to take her to the play she had mentioned it seemed too much extravagance and indulgence, and she was aghast at herself for having pricked him into it. The more she thought of her behavior the more unmannerly it seemed. It seemed wanton.

"You shouldn't have torn up the tickets," she said apologetically, as the car started again. "I'd have gone."

"Princess," he said, "this is your night. What pleases you makes me happy. And what don't please you don't make me happy."

"They'd have sold the tickets for you at the box office."

"And make you wait around while I peddle tickets?" he said.

It occurred to her that he must have paid a fantastic premium to get those tickets on such short notice, or else have enormous know-how. It was after all a sell-out, and eighth row center had sounded like the best seats in the house.

"I only meant it would usually be better to ask first," she tried explaining, half in a mumble.

"That's right," he said. "I should have. It serves me right."

They left the car in a huge garage near the theater where To The Angel Of Death I'm Not In was being staged. There was no difficulty getting tickets.

While they waited for the curtain he looked about in the half emptiness, and said she was the most beautiful woman there.

"You could say so what, who's here," he added. "A couple of hundred ordinary people, and that puts you in the upper tiniest little fraction of one per cent. Okay. But there could be a pile of good-looking ones here and you'd still be the best looking."

There was nothing to say to such stuff. She shrugged.

The play opened with bad lines and dismayed her almost at once. It was clearly trying, in a pretentious way, to appear somewhat experimental, but it had no cleverness. She made herself hope for a while to find some merit as the scenes dragged. But she could not help but despair of it. It made her feel even worse about having ruined an evening into which Malcolm had put such expense. She told him she was sorry. But he said he liked it. "You got good taste," he said. "It's about time I took in some of this intellectual stuff." He applauded after every curtain.

When they came out, after three hours, she was miserable and wilted. She apologized again for having suggested such a third-rate production.

"Naw, naw," he said. "What do you mean, third rate."

He suggested a tearoom, but she said she was quite tired.

They cruised in the big purring car toward her apartment, though it was scarcely more than a half-dozen blocks. Her scarf spread over her coat.

"You off tomorrow?" he asked. "Suppose I show you the plant."

"No, I have some things I want to catch up on."

"Okay. Well, I'll tell you what. When you go to work Friday I'll stop by and drive ya to work. What do you do, walk, take the subway? Why should you do that? I'll give you a lift."

"I'm afraid it's not possible. I don't start work until three."

"I'll pick you up at two-thirty."

"Don't you work?"

"I work for myself. I don't punch no time clock." They had reached her apartment building. He braked the car and turned to her. "Princess," he said, "here's the pitch. I fell for you in the first ten minutes. And like I told ya, I don't horse around. Now you figure I'm nuts. What the hell, a guy proposes the first date, you don't even know me. All right, take your time. Go ahead. Don't say nothing. Look around. Compare. You don't know me yet, but I know you, and you're a jewel. A gem. I been looking for you all my life. And I never proposed to a woman before, and that's the God's honest truth."

She had been turning crimson. "Malcolm, will you stop it?" she cut in when she could. "You're being ridiculous!"

"Millicent, listen, I ain't just clapping my teeth. You ain't seen the last of me. I'm gonna be around all you let me be around, and if you make up your mind in six months that I can make you happy, I want you to know I made up my mind the first night. Because you are absolutely the most luscious thing on this whole round earth. I seen you and I didn't have to think twice. I never seen nothing like you. I'm telling ya, I'm overwhelmed. I look at ya and all I can say is wow. All my life I dreamed of something like you. You got everything. You're like a queen. And everything I got's at your feet. You name it, you got it. No cigars, no liquor. You want a career, you have a career. Anything you want. You want a kosher house, we have a kosher house. Live in the city, live in the country, it's all up to you."

"I think I'd better get out," she said, reaching for the door handle.

He got out quickly on his own side and went around and opened her door.

He walked with her through the stone arch of her building, his hat in his hand. She turned to him.

"I'm afraid I sha'n't ask you up," she began. "My roommates—"

"That's okay." His narrow face smiled in the way that showed his teeth and nearly shut his eyes.

He moved a bit nearer, almost as if to kiss her, but she drew back and he stopped.

"Sure I'm nuts," he said, still smiling. "I'm nuts about you, that's what I'm nuts."

She thought of saying something like go soak your head. But she could not. He unlatched the heavy door of glass and iron. She stood in its opening and gave him her hand briefly.

"Well, I must thank you for the evening," she said. "I think you've been most courteous and gentlemanly."

"Good night, Millicent." He was still smiling, but not showing his teeth any more. He raised a hand shoulder-high and waved it a little. "Sleep tight. Don't let mosquitas bite."

37

There was frost on the windows Friday, and when she went down to shop she found it had gotten much colder. She came back up with groceries and the earliest afternoon newspapers, shivering, and massaged her numb fingers and warmed her back at the gas stove. Then she sat with her cocoa, reading the papers, and saw a report that To The Angel Of Death I'm Not In would close at once, without completing the two-week Boston tryout, and that the New York opening had been canceled. It renewed her remorse about the tickets. But in a little while, when Malcolm phoned and offered her a ride to work, she refused him.

"I really prefer to walk," she told him. "I enjoy the walk."

"In this weather?"

"Well, it does me good," she said.

"Okay," he said resignedly.

She did actually force herself to walk it, bundled and miserable. But after work she returned by subway. When she got to the apartment Natalie and Ella Jane showed her a crouching furry animal in a satchel-shaped cage of mesh, on top of the inlaid cabinet, and told her a delivery man had brought it for her in late afternoon.

"What is it?" said Natalie.

"I think it's a short-eared racing rabbit," said Millicent, looking at it. It seemed the largest hare she had ever seen and did have rather short ears, which lay back in the fur.

"A what?" said Ella Jane.

"They race them in Argentina," said Millicent. It had somehow turned around in the tight space so that the greens that had been put in for it were behind it. The nose kept moving. She felt pity for it.

"You're kidding," said Ella Jane.

"No I'm not."

"The short ears cut wind resistance so they can run faster, I suppose," Ella Jane said.

"As a matter of fact," Millicent told her, "that happens to be the truth."

She took the cage down and lifted the rabbit out. Her hands could feel its fright. It crouched where she put it on the floor. Then she set a saucer of water before it, but it did nothing.

"Don't be jealous, Theodore," she said, lifting the cat.

"You clean any messes," Natalie told her.

"Don't worry," she said.

The rabbit at last ate some vegetable she put down, and she explained to her roommates that the man she had been out with bred them.

Roland was greatly pleased with it, when she brought it to him at the house before Sunday school. And during dinner he discussed with his parents where the hutch would be built. Millicent told them only that she knew someone who raised these rabbits professionally. She watched her mother for any sign that word of her having gone out with Malcolm had gotten back to her, through Mrs. Blink and Mrs. Lebensalt and Mrs. Kiss, but apparently it hadn't. She was glad that her mother seemed to be learning not to ask questions.

That night at midnight, when she came down to the sidewalk from the city room, Malcolm was waiting with his car to chauffeur her home to her apartment.

"Maybe you like to walk in the daytime," he said, "but the streets ain't that safe at this hour. And the subways are no bargain."

She was grateful not to have to take the subway. She disliked the loneliness, the wind, and the dirt of those platforms late at night.

"Call me Malc," he told her.

They arrived at the stone arch, and she thanked him at the glass and iron door.

"I'll have you up sometime, and introduce you to my roommates and my cat," she said.

He phoned three mornings later, on Wednesday, and said he felt like chatting with someone and was wondering how she was.

He told her he had had a fight with his brother. He was planning to expand into rubber masks, only they would be made of plastic. Also into the toy line. People that couldn't even buy themselves clothes would still buy toys for the kids, and kids busted things, so there was turnover. He'd be big enough soon to have his own sales force. Now he did most of his own selling, though some of it was handled by jobbers who carried other lines. It was all cutthroat, dog eat dog. He also had a chance to get into a third business, that would make films for television commercials, but was afraid to get overextended.

Finally he said he noticed in the paper there would be a cultural lecture tonight at Harvard about Venice, open to the public, and asked if she would like to go.

"Well, all right," she said.

He said he'd come by at six and they'd grab a bite.

This time the restaurant was a Scandinavian one, dark and low-ceilinged, with carved scrolly wood and little stained-glass windows. Their table was near the fire, and she watched the low flames that licked sometimes bluish from the glowing remains of logs. She could see the fire's redness on the side of Malcolm's face and feel its heat on her own. It was good after the bitter outdoors.

He began to lean toward her, staring at her face, his elbows on the table, and the table wobbled, shaking its little candle. But then he sat back decorously.

"You know what?" he said. "The stores ought to pay you to wear all their best minks, and the latest Paris creations, because you'd make them look better.

You know that? You could give them something, but they couldn't give you nothing. You could be in a big nifty spifty by Dior, and Russian sable, and diamonds, and you couldn't look no better than you look right now. It's the diamonds that need you."

She gave her head a little shake. "Really, don't say things like that. You embarrass me."

"You're modest."

"Well, the fact is I wouldn't make them look better because I'd be miserable in them. I don't like all this decoration of the physical. I'm not a little plumed horse in a circus."

He looked at her silently a moment. He nodded a little. "Is that why you don't wear no paint?" he asked.

"Well, I'd say it's one of the principal reasons."

"And I notice you don't wear no stockings either," he said. "I don't have no objection—the socks look perfectly good. But I never met a woman that didn't wear stockings, that's all."

"I wear them when I have to," she said. "But stockings are a plague. They keep falling apart for one thing."

"Yeah, runs and everything. And you have to buy new ones. It's a waste of money."

"Well, I think they design them to fall apart, on purpose," she said. "It's part of the whole cult of fragility, I think. But this whole business of jewelry and furs and gowns is of a piece with all the corsets and foundation garments that go underneath, if you want to know, and with make-up and beauty parlors, and even with all the spangles and G-strings like in that show you tore up the tickets for. Because all of it's designed to transform a woman into some figment of the male imagination." The shake was in her voice.

He wrinkled his brows, smiling a little. He seemed to understand.

"Don't you go into beauty parlors?" he said.

"Just to get it cut."

"Your hairdo looks to me like the latest and the greatest. One of these natural jobs."

"Don't call it a 'hairdo.' I just comb it. But do you see what I mean? Whether they're wrapped up in Dior gowns or exposed on a stage in frilly garters—it's all to make a woman unreal—make her something men dream about. That's why I don't care for these shows like 'Lady Godiva Clad' and 'Belly Buttons And Bows.' I really would have had an awful time sitting through that the other night. Especially that song, 'Nancy Fancy Pantsy'—ugh. And they start this whole degradation awfully young, Malc, if you notice. Even little girls' underpants are made to show part of the time. But you don't see a little boy's underwear. A boy is given that much dignity."

He still looked at her in the same intense way, with a trace of a smile. "You got something there, you know?"

"I know perfectly well I've got something there," she said quakily. "I wouldn't have said it otherwise."

The smorgasbord was brought to them on a wagon.

"You're thinking all the time, aren't ya," he said to her.

"Aren't you?" she said.

The evening went quickly. The lecture turned out to be on the Republic of Venice at the height of its power, with slides showing details of paintings. There were magnificently expressive faces of commercial men and aristocrats, one after another, young and middle-aged, their eyes showing all sorts of temperaments, which the lecturer tied brilliantly to the spirit of the time. The fifteenth century and the concerns of its people came to life, and held her spellbound. Malcolm turned out however to know nothing of history, and she had to explain it to him in the car afterward. But he listened. She wondered aloud whether paintings like those could be done today, and decided they could not, because there were no longer processions or public events which so expressed the life of an entire community.

At the heavy door of her building Malcolm said that the following evening there was to be a Greek play at Harvard, performed in ancient Greek, and asked if she would like to go. She declined.

On Friday morning he phoned and told her he had gone to the Greek play alone. What floored him, he said, was that the audience actually knew when to laugh.

Then he asked if she'd care to see his factory. What a strange man he is, she thought. It occurred to her that his factory might be a subject for a newspaper feature.

"I'd like to," she said.

He called for her within the hour. The factory was all on one floor, halfway up a narrow dirty building a few blocks below Chinatown, near where the elevated came out of the subway. With a great leaning effort of his body he slid open a heavy metal door that worked on rollers. There was a long room with lights burning, and windows admitting daylight at both ends. Perhaps thirty women, young colored ones and aged white ones, worked in rows at benches with piles of parts before them. At one end there were machines, mostly idle, but one stopped and started every few seconds with clanking noises. It was run by a savage-looking man with a complexion spotted in pink and brown.

Malcolm swept his hand toward a wall he said he would knock out when the lease expired next door. He took her into a varnished little office and introduced her to a very fat woman named Ethel, who sat behind a desk, and to his brother Yitzy, who was sprawled tieless in shirt sleeves beside a table littered with papers and corrugated cartons. Yitzy rose. He was dark and brooding and sallow, entirely unlike Malcolm except for his skinniness. He had unkempt black hair and wild eyes with black pockets under them.

Malcolm examined his mail. Meanwhile he told his brother to run out and bring Chinese food. He named off the dishes. Yitzy muttered.

"Yitz!" Malcolm said. "Move! You work for me, you got to jump!"

Yitzy turned scowling and put a long gray overcoat over his shirt. Malcolm opened a door in a partition and led Millicent among rows of racks. He showed her samples of his manufactures. She was impressed by the variety of party hats, of every color and design, some of soft crepe paper and some of shiny cardboard. There were also paper cocktail napkins printed with drawings and jokes, mainly of a sort of bathroom humor. Malcolm told her Yitzy had done the drawings. "The kid wants to be a cartoonist, but he doesn't have no self-confidence."

Millicent said she would like to have a collection of the paper hats, one of each kind, but that she disliked the napkins. She asked if he really felt right about purveying vulgarity of that kind. "Aren't there enough clean jokes?" she said. And she suggested that napkins could be decorated in other ways. With drawings of Boston scenes, for example, such as the Old North Church, or with modern nonobjective art. His face was thoughtful and grim. "That's a good idea," he said.

Yitzy returned, and they ate at the desks on paper plates. The radiator valve hissed.

"Ethel," Malcolm said to the fat woman, wiping his mouth, "we're discontinuing the napkin line. Write a letter to every customer that's got any on order and tell 'em it's discontinued."

"Ya crazy?" his brother shouted at him, staring. His mouth was full of food, but for so thin a man his voice was strong and bellowing.

"Yitz," Malcolm said, "we're getting rid of it. We're going in for high-class stuff. There's a market for modern art—the nonobjective stuff. You ought to see how many people go to Greek plays and lectures on Venice and stuff. Those are the people that use cocktail napkins."

It occurred to Millicent that he was a sound businessman and that there might really be such a market. Yitzy chewed a little and stopped. His eyes kept staring at Malcolm. "You know how much dough you got tied up in there?" he said loudly.

"All right," Malcolm said sharply. "So it's a no-good investment. That stuff is uncouth. It's cheap. It makes us a cheap outfit. And you want to know something? It ain't even funny. Miss Gordon looked at them and there wasn't one she could crack a smile at. Not one in the lot."

Yitzy's dark eyes went to Millicent.

"That's right," she said to Yitzy. "They're not even amusing. They're not only filthy but devoid of any humor. Of any genuine redeeming humor."

"You hear that?" said Malcolm.

Yitzy looked at Malcolm long and sourly. "She gives out with the big words and you flip," he muttered. He shook his head with exasperation. "Riding high, aren't ya. Got a dame with class."

"Watch it," Malcolm said. "I'm telling ya, watch it."

"Look at him—he's got an educated dame and he's in the clouds," Yitzy said to Ethel.

"Yitz, ya jealous?" Malcolm said sharply. "Now jump! Go on! Go in there and clean 'em out. The whole back room there. All the napkins. Everything goes in the barrel. The cuts too."

Yitzy stood in his stooped way, looking at him. He looked at Ethel, spreading his arms in a gesture of appeal and frustration.

"Ya gonna make me do it myself?" Malcolm asked. His voice was threatening and quiet.

Yitzy went toward the back room, slumping and with a dragging step.

"When you get through with that," Malcolm said after him, "fix up Miss Gordon a collection of hats. One of everything. The whole line."

Yitzy said nothing.

"And then go to Korea. Get in uniform, ya slacker," Malcolm said after him.

"How about you," Yitzy said without turning.

"I was in the other one," said Malcolm.

Yitzy slammed the door.

Malcolm looked at Millicent with a toss of his head and shrug, as though his brother were impossible. "Come on," he said, taking her arm. "Let's get out of this dump."

He took her to a building a few blocks away, and into a large room where rows and rows of men's suits were hanging. It was poorly lit, except for one side where tailors worked under fluorescent tubes. He looked at a number of bolts of cloth, accompanied by a bald potbellied man in shirt sleeves who had a tape-measure hanging about his neck, and asked Millicent her opinion of some. At last he told the man to make him several suits of clothes.

At three o'clock he brought her to work, opening the door of his car for her. And toward midnight, when she finished, she found him waiting again, to drive her home. He had a paper-hat collection for her in a big corrugated carton in the back seat. In front of the stone arch of her building he sat with her in the car a few minutes, talking sadly of his brother. Then he turned to her, and the pale light from the street made shadows in the angles of his face.

"I'm thinking of a good-night kiss," he said.

"Must we?" she said, frowning.

He looked disappointed. The expression of his face touched her. She leaned and kissed him on the cheek. She thought it was quite spontaneous of her, and when the sadness left his face she was glad she had done it. She let him hold her hand.

In a few minutes she went up, and he followed, carrying the big carton. She went in ahead, to tell Natalie and Ella Jane to put on bathrobes, and then Malcolm put the carton into a closet. They had to move shoes. He went down again without having removed his coat.

She slept well, but in the morning she lay thinking of him. It was good, she thought, to be able to be a friend with all kinds of people. He was of a world she had never known and might never know again. And it was broadening to see how an entrepreneur used his energies and how he expanded his business. Her own little world after all had become a narrow one.

He would interest Charles, she thought. Charles hoped someday to exercise initiative like that, and could learn from him. It took courage to go and compete in the market place like that, with no resources but your wits and your self-reliance. It took ability, and it took an energy such as she wished she had.

But she was doing something for Malcolm too. She was broadening his cultural horizons. He wanted that. There was a symbiosis in a friendship with someone so different.

And there was no denying that companionship was a necessary thing. He had a kind of bounce, and a certain glowing brightness, full of agreeable self-confidence and jerky motions that sometimes amused her, but buoyed her moods. He seemed at times to have a sense of complete fun—at the play he had been the perfect audience, enjoying and uncritical. She needed such a tonic, at least for the time being, until new friends were made. The pattern of her life had become an awful emptiness. Ella Jane had never talked a great deal, and lately was silenter than ever.

And he was so resilient that she had no fear of hurting him. She had even begun to correct his speech, and he welcomed it. Even once or twice when she thought she might have gone too far, he had shown his knack for setting her at ease. In his way he was never without poise. And anyway it would be snobbish to refuse to associate with a person who was interesting and kind, simply because of his grammar.

He was not stupid. He understood her feelings, and he was considerate even in his awkward compliments. She sometimes found him staring at her face, as though it were startlingly beautiful, but he would not do it too long. Les had never once given her a compliment, that she could recall. And when she had told Les he was a fine person, he had just taken it as his due. Apparently he thought his wish to sleep with her was compliment enough.

In a day or so Malcolm took her to a movie at noon, a well-reviewed one. But the movie immediately turned out to have an extremely sentimental tone, and after only ten minutes he insisted that they walk out, though the tickets were two-forty each, and took her instead to the movie across the street. She thought it quite a cavalier thing to do. And she felt less badly after that about the Belly Button tickets.

The day after that he brought her a huge bottle of Arpege perfume. She had not considered the possibility of gifts from him and was flustered.

"Don't be embarrassed," he said. "It's just a small little token of my esteem, that's all. And if you don't want to put it on, just enjoy sniffing it. Take a whiff of it under your nose for the fun of it once in a while, if you don't want to wear it."

"But it's so big. I never saw it so big."

"It's cheaper that way. Anyways I don't do things by halves."

Then for a few days she did not see him so regularly, because her Aunt Rosalind died, and she went to the funeral and spent her days off with her family, and felt also that she should be less active for a few days as a kind of mourning. She had noticed at the service that her father was the only one who wept. Her uncles, the two half-brothers, did not. But her father was Aunt Rosalind's twin, after all.

Her father went through Aunt Rosalind's things, and asked Millicent to choose some of the watercolors for herself. She brought some to her apartment and stored them for the time being in a drawer, wrapped in brown paper.

Malcolm still came to drive her home from work almost every night, even if she didn't see him otherwise. Once, when Mr. Hopkins sent her home early, Malcolm slipped her mind somehow, and she went on without him. He came and waited for nothing. But he was not angry afterward.

She began meeting him by day again, but then broke a couple of dates, because she felt tired. He took it cheerfully and asked no explanation. She still saw little cigars in his pocket, but she never saw him smoke.

She lunched with him almost daily. Sometimes he took her afterward to his office, while he did some business. She disliked the fights between Malcolm and Yitzy. Yitzy could bellow in anger so deafeningly that she had to stop her ears, and when he did Malcolm forced him to apologize to her.

"Go read a book, ya might learn something," Malcolm said to him.

Malcolm called Yitzy a lefty and Yitzy called Malcolm a reactionary bastid.

Once the dust in Malcolm's office made Millicent sneeze. "Yitz!" Malcolm said. "Run out for kleenex. Ethel, give him a quarter."

Malcolm also sat in Millicent's apartment now, usually if he came for her on her evenings off, and chatted with her roommates. Once he told her afterward that a stock Ella Jane had recommended was too risky. And they kissed good night sometimes, though not always. "I think too much kissing is undignified—if it becomes routine it's cheapened," she said. "I think it should be a spontaneous expression of affection."

She knew that he had his own apartment, presumably a nice one, somewhere in Brookline, but he never suggested that she go there. It was as though, without any need to mention such a thing, he took her virginity for granted.

However he took her once to his mother's apartment in Roxbury. He said he wanted to drop in on his mother because he hadn't seen her in a couple of weeks.

His mother seemed quite old, and kept dropping into Yiddish, of which Millicent understood almost nothing. Malcolm sat back in a chair in the smelly little living room, his hands planted on the armrests and his feet crossed on a hassock. Millicent took an apple from a bowl that the old woman pressed on her.

"Ma," said Malcolm, "talk about education, this happens to be the most educated girl you ever had the pleasure to meet in your life. No exceptions. Latin and Greek, she can read it like English."

"Very nice," the old woman said agreeably, and kissed Millicent on the forehead.

When they had been there exactly fifteen minutes Malcolm slapped the arms of the chair and said it was time to go.

His sister Clara lived around the corner and he took Millicent there also. Clara was big and fortyish, with glasses. A flowered print dress lay on the ribbing of her corset. She grinned at Millicent. She had peculiarly short teeth with a space in the middle. The apartment was hot. A silly, nervous little boy kept hiding behind the drapes, and Clara slapped him. She woke her husband, who worked nights, and he came into the room half awake. He was a huge man, bald and toothless. He said nothing.

"Stay for supper why don't yiz," Clara said to Malcolm and Millicent.

"Naw," said Malcolm. "When I feed the princess, it's nothing but the best."

As they came out to the car a bleached-blonde lady who had apparently chanced by hurried up to Malcolm with a warm greeting.

"Hit the road," Malcolm said to her. "I told ya we're through."

"Who was that?" Millicent asked when they were in the car.

"Nobody," he said.

The next forenoon Millicent received a telephone call from Malcolm's mother. Apparently there had been a dreadful fight, but Mrs. Stack was crying so hard that Millicent couldn't make head or tail of it. If Millicent asked who, the old woman answered yes, and if Millicent asked whether it was Malcolm who had thrown Yitzy down the stairs or whether Yitzy had thrown Malcolm, the weeping became wilder.

It seemed to her, though, that Malcolm must have thrown Yitzy, because Malcolm was the stronger.

She spoke about it to Malcolm at lunch.

"Well, I couldn't take the kid's mouth any more," Malcolm said. "He was getting out of hand. I had to fire him. And the old lady wanted you to patch it up, I guess."

"I'd be happy to patch it up if I can."

"Forget it. I told her she didn't have no business dragging you in it."

"Who'll do your drawings?"

"I got enough drawings. Anyways he's a no-good subversive. The F.B.I.'s got a file on him a mile long."

38

Charles came home on a furlough, and said he expected to go overseas soon. He kept telling his mother he was practically positive it would not be Korea. He said it would probably be somewhere in the Far East, but most likely Taiwan or the Philippines.

When Millicent arrived at the house after Sunday school he flung his arms around her. His yellow hair was shorter than ever, and his eyes even while smiling had the sadness or wistfulness she had always seen in them. Grandma Annie and her husband were there, and Aunt Celeste and Uncle Ira with Jill and Nan. Millicent helped set the table. The house was noisy. During dinner there was some talk of Aunt Rosalind's death and the illness that preceded it, but apart from that the talk was fairly lively. Charles was annoyed with his father for not passing along a stock tip that Caleb Folger had told him months ago. The stock had skyrocketed since and split, though Ed had paid no attention at the time.

After dinner the company moved to the living room, mostly around Charles, but at the first moment at which he was able to speak to Millicent a little apart from the others he put a question to her in a low voice, his face troubled. "Sis," he said, "what happened that time. You know what I mean? About that guy that was trying to make you."

She reddened. He had almost backed her up against the drapes in the bay window, but she pushed away from him. "Let's not talk about that now, for goodness sakes."

She sat between Jill and Grandma Annie on the sofa, and avoided being alone with Charles again. She regretted the indiscretion of having confided anything about that to Charles. She remembered that last conversation with him at her apartment, about all his women, and the idea of giving him an explanation about Leslie seemed morbid and disgusting.

During the next day or two she was in touch with her family by phone. She knew Charles expected to visit her alone sometime. But meanwhile he was busy visiting friends and relatives and polishing the Model T in the barn, so it was easy to put him off. On the first of her nights off he phoned, wanting to come to Boston, but she told him that she and a friend had tickets for the Zürich chamber ensemble. He asked if he could come along, but she said she didn't think there were any tickets left, and that she would see him again on Sunday anyway.

She had thought of introducing Charles to Malcolm at some future time, so that Malcolm might give him some advice on starting a business, but she did not feel in the mood yet to sit between them at a concert. There had never been any occasion to mention Malcolm to her family, and for the moment somehow it seemed simpler not to create one.

Then on Thursday her father phoned. Charles had received a telegram canceling all furloughs in his outfit and ordering him back to his base. The family was going to spend the day together at home, and Millicent could either come there if she wished, or meet them all at South Station when they took Charles there an hour before train time. He had promised to go by train to the base, instead of flying, because Lucinda was upset.

Millicent said she'd meet them at the station.

She spent half the afternoon shopping for a going-away present. She did not know what to get him that he might want or need. He already had a wallet. She thought of a wrist watch with a built-in compass, and looked in two cut-rate drugstores and a large jeweler's, but found none. At last she found a pair of binoculars, ingeniously small and light, with a leather case. It had a beautiful simplicity, with the outer lenses between the eyepieces, and the prisms covered with satiny steel. It was surprisingly powerful. She paid twenty dollars.

Charles seemed quite moved by it when she found the family at six. She saw his thanks in his tender handling of it. Her mother was not crying, but looked as though she had been. Patty, smartly dressed, was also moist-eyed. The whole cavernous station, with its shadowy distances and lighted shops, was ringing with a mechanical music of jingle bells and caroling. They sat in a tearoom that opened onto the concourse. Roland borrowed the binoculars, and gazed at people in a booth at the opposite wall, and then through the windows to the station. Patty asked to try them. Charles said he didn't know the reason for the cancelation. Either his whole wing had been alerted for immediate transfer overseas, or his maintenance crew had been attached to another that had been. They sat for nearly an hour, looking frequently at the clock, and Ed and Charles made most of what small talk there was. At last they rose, Lucinda dabbing her eyes, and found their way through the crowds.

On the long outdoor platform between trains it was cold. The electric bulbs in the narrow shelter were cheerless. The train was already making a noise in its under parts, though it was not ready to move. Millicent noticed it was the same one she had used to take to Chicago, though Charles would get off somewhere between Utica and Syracuse. The cars were tall, and extended on and on up the track.

They stood together below the two doors of adjoining cars. Charles had the binoculars in his overcoat pocket and his visored hat was at a tilt. He carried a canvas overnight satchel that Patty had given him. He wore no gloves and his hands were red.

Lucinda asked Millicent if she would come to Wilmerding Crosswalk with them afterward and spent the night.

"I can't," Millicent said. "I have plans for the evening."

"Do you have a date?" Patty asked.

"I have an appointment with a friend," she said. She felt herself coloring and wished she could keep herself from doing that.

"A male friend or a female friend?" Patty said.

"Leave her alone," her mother told Patty. "You know how she is."

Then they heard a conductor shout and Lucinda clutched Charles. Millicent saw her cry. Yet it was only when she saw Patty kiss him and sob that she felt the sense of a young man's peril in war. Ed kissed him quickly, and Millicent did also. She had seen Charles glance her way, and she did not want to be alone with Roland in not kissing him. Lucinda reached for him again but he pulled from her. "Hey, I've got to get on," he said.

He climbed, and when he turned to wave he was already being borne away.

"Get back!" Lucinda shouted as he leaned out the door.

They walked slowly back, feeling the wind and the dust of the wheels that hammered past them. Ed had an arm about Lucinda. "Well, let's get home," he said. Then he asked Millicent if they could drop her off somewhere.

"No, that's all right," she said.

"Well, I'll take you to your apartment," he said. "Is that all right?"

She said nothing. They walked almost in silence down long blocks to where the car was parked. Then it was a slow ride through traffic. Stores were open for the Christmas rush. Her mother seemed nervous, and seized Millicent by the arm suddenly and kissed her lips as they let her out.

Then the door was shut, and Millicent gave a little wave as the car pulled away.

She pulled open the door of iron and glass. The white lobby looked especially dirty. She climbed, holding the banister.

As she turned to mount the second flight she saw Charles standing at its top, outside her door. For an instant she felt a dizzying confusion. He was fondling the little pigskin case of the binoculars, and his little canvas satchel was on the landing.

"I got off at Back Bay," he said.

"Charles!" she said, her voice strangely high pitched. "Are you out of your mind? We just put you on the train! I left the folks downstairs! Just now."

She had stopped where she stood. He was looking down the stairs at her, not smiling. "I had to talk to ya," he said.

She resumed climbing, somewhat heavily. "You're lucky the folks didn't decide to come up with me," she said.

He gave a slight nod.

"You're just crazy," she said, turning the key in the lock. "What a thing to do. Wasn't that supposed to be the last train you could get?"

"Well, it stopped there, and I just got off, that's all. I wanted to talk to ya. We never talked."

She let him in. "Won't they mark you as a deserter?"

"No. A.W.O.L. maybe, if I don't get a plane."

"But that's serious, isn't it? You seem to take it very lightly."

"No, I don't take it lightly." He slung his coat over the back of the stuffed armchair and sat down low, his feet spread out. They looked large.

"And you realize I'm going out," she told him. "You don't think we're going to sit around here."

"I realize it."

"This is absolutely nutty. I really should be angry. And I am."

"You never answered my question, Sis."

She took off her coat and scarf and put them on the studio couch, as though ignoring him.

"Is this date tonight with that same guy?" he asked. "That was trying to get you in the sack?"

She felt herself tighten with anger. "You're being obnoxious," she said.

"Well, I've been worried."

"You had no call to."

"Well, you should know."

She went to the bathroom to comb her hair and shut the door hard. She knocked a bottle into the sink. Then the cat brushed her leg and startled her. She combed her hair with sharp strokes. That fool, she thought.

When she came out of the bathroom he approached her.

"Are you gonna answer my question?" he said.

She wished she had something to occupy herself with so as to ignore him more easily. She went to the kitchen to get food for the cat.

"Well," he said, "I want to know why you won't answer."

"Because I resent your asking. And I'm expecting company any minute and I don't want you here."

"It is the guy. Isn't it."

"You can imagine what you like." She took the leftover fish from the refrigerator and began cutting it on the drainboard.

"Do you like this guy?"

"Yes, I like this guy."

Charles leaned on the doorjamb and watched her work. He sighed.

"Have you been to bed with him?" he asked quietly.

She worked in silence.

"Fifth amendment?" he asked.

"I chose not to hear you."

"I asked if you've been to bed with him."

"No, I have not. And how many women have you been to bed with since you were up here last, while we're asking questions?"

"Well, if you want to know, I'll tell ya."

"I don't." She put the dish on the floor and the cat leaped to it. She heard Charles sigh again.

"Is he still trying?"

She rose and looked at him. "You're supposed to be on your way to your base," she said. "What are you going to do? Hang around here till he comes?"

"Well, I just want to see what this character looks like. And I'll tell you one thing. If this is the guy that's been trying to make you I'll break his arm as soon as he steps in the door."

"You just do anything violent, Charles Piper Gordon, and I'll call the police."

"Well, I want it understood how I feel about it. If he's got in mind what I think he's got in mind he's answerable to me. Because I'll make a basket case out of him."

"You'll do nothing of the kind. Now please leave."

"I'll do nothing of the kind," he said, mocking her.

" 'Answerable to you,' " she said. "Who do you think you are?"

He tightened his mouth, and looked away unhappily.

"You're not my big brother, you're my little brother," she said, looking up at him. "Just remember that."

He turned, and let himself fall into the armchair. "Sis," he said, "I'll make a deal with you. You want me to get out of here. Can you tell me truthfully it's not the same guy? Because you sounded that time like he almost had you on the verge."

She had walked around to the mantelpiece, and turned and leaned against it.

"Or let me meet him. Let me meet this guy and I'll tell you whether he's a wolf or not. Or if you don't want me to meet him at least promise me he's not going to tumble you in the hay. That's all I ask."

"Nobody tumbles me," she said sourly. "I do my own tumbling. And on clean linen."

"What do you mean by that?"

"I mean I can take care of myself, thank you. I don't need you to supervise my sex life."

"Do you have any sex life?"

She was irritably silent. "Not so far," she said finally. "And don't ever ask me that again."

"Because the next time the answer might be yes?"

"You have some nerve. Because I resent your prying. Mother and Dad never even asked things like that."

She took the perfume from the mantel and opened the stopper. She dabbed it behind her ears.

"Well, all right, Sis. But listen. Whatever kind of perfectly reasonable bull and crap this guy gives you, and however he tries to talk you into it, don't give in. Just don't believe anything he says. Honest, Sis. I know all the arguments backwards and forwards."

"I bet you do."

"When did you start using perfume?"

"I've started using it. It smells good, and if I put a little on I can enjoy the smell. Here. Have a pinch of snuff." She passed the open bottle under his nose.

"That bottle's enormous," he said. "Is that solid perfume? Where'd you get a thing like that?"

"It was a gift."

"From him?"

"Yes." She returned it to the mantel.

"That must have cost about a hundred bucks. Is the guy loaded or something?"

"I have no idea what it cost. I don't think it was any hundred bucks."

"What business is he in?"

"He has several lines."

"That sounds fishy."

"It's not fishy. He's very enterprising."

"Do Mother and Dad know about him?"

"No."

The doorbell buzzed.

"Well, I'm sorry to have to see you off in this fashion," she said. "But it was a very foolish thing you did." She pressed the answering buzzer. "You really better just worry about yourself, Charles. That's my advice."

They waited in uneasy silence. In a moment they heard the rapid tread of feet mounting the stairs. Millicent looked at Charles and he avoided her eyes. She thought his despairing expression both outrageous and absurd.

Then he glanced at her again. "Where are your roommates?" he said.

"Ella Jane's in Chicopee and Natalie's in Canada."

"What's in Canada? Skiing?"

"Yes."

She opened at the knock, and Malcolm stepped over the threshold, smiling and ruddy-faced. His hat was in his hand, but he wore furry ear muffs. A silken print wine-colored scarf was thick but neat about his neck, above the velvet collar of his overcoat.

"Hi," he said. "We got company?" He looked at Charles.

Millicent made the introduction and Charles climbed slowly from the sagging depth of the chair.

"Hi ya," said Malcolm, still smiling, and there was a quick handshake. "It's a pleasure. I've heard a lot about ya." He took off the ear muffs.

"Charles may be going overseas soon, so he stopped in to see me," said Millicent.

"Good luck to ya, chicken," Malcolm said to Charles. He smiled warmly, so that his eyes grew small and his cheeks dimpled.

Charles dropped himself into the chair again, frowning, and the frown brought an awkward silence. Malcolm moved his lips, as if about to speak, and glanced at Millicent, who was standing with her hands together. "Well, I might as well take off my coat a few minutes," he said.

"I just want you to know," Charles said to him, "that if any harm ever comes to my sister, your life isn't worth a plug nickel. I don't care what part of the world I'm in."

"Charles!" said Millicent, reddening. "Apologize!"

"That's all right," Malcolm said. He sat on the studio couch, next to Natalie's stuffed dog, his coat open.

"It's not all right!" said Millicent. She sat on the couch too, about a foot from Malcolm.

"My sister means more to me than anyone in the world," Charles said.

"You got good taste, chicken. She means a lot to me too. I know how you feel."

"Charles has missed his train and he's due at his base," said Millicent. "Do you think we could get him to another train or a bus or something?"

"Why not?" said Malcolm.

"When's the next train?" she asked Charles.

"Tomorrow."

"Where's your base, Charlie?" Malcolm asked.

He sat sullenly a moment without answering. "Griffiss Field," he said. "In upstate New York. Rome, New York."

"Look," said Malcolm, "suppose we run you out to Bedford, and you can probably hitch onto something flying out of there."

"Will that make us late?" Millicent asked Malcolm.

"Yeah, it'll make us late," he said. "So what? If it can't be helped it can't be helped."

"Late for what?" said Charles.

"Don't tell him, Malc. He asks too many questions."

There was a moment of hesitation. "Get on the phone, chicken," Malcolm said. "See if there's any action at Bedford."

Charles almost began to rise but slumped back again. "You know," he said, "I'd rather skip it. I don't want any favors. I'm so late anyway it doesn't matter."

"Look," Malcolm told him, "we said we'd get you there, didn't we? Get on the phone like I said. And if there's no action at Bedford, try Otis. Try Westover. And if they're all dead we'll drive you all the way to Griffiss Field."

"Oh no you won't. You're not taking my sister on any five-hundred-mile jaunt."

"Now look, chicken. Don't get me wrong."

"Charles, get on that phone at once and find out. Or I'll be very angry."

He rose slowly and shuffled to the lavender phone, which he lifted from the floor to the drop-leaf table. Then he dialed.

"I'll pay for the call," said Malcolm.

"I'm paying for it," said Charles.

"I told you to make it, didn't I?" Malcolm said.

"Never mind who pays for it!" said Millicent. "I'll pay for it."

He asked for the number for the Bedford Air Base. There was more waiting. Millicent went over in her mind how she would bawl him out privately for embarrassing her and ruining the evening. She heard him ask for flight operations. Then he spoke to someone, and at last he hung up. He said there was a C-47 from Bedford shortly to Mitchel Field, near New York City, and that there ought to be a good chance of something up to Griffiss from there.

"Okay, all set?" said Malcolm. He stood up. Millicent rose also.

"Do you mind if I talk to my sister privately for a couple of minutes?"

Malcolm looked to Millicent.

She took a breath. "All right," she said. "Do you mind, Malc? We'll meet you at the car. Charles is going overseas, and we've been sort of quarreling, and I don't want to end it on this kind of a note."

"I'll see you downstairs," said Malcolm.

She moved to accompany him to the door, but he went quickly, carrying his hat and ear muffs.

She turned, leaning on the door that had shut behind Malcolm, and looked at Charles furiously. He was standing with hands in his pockets.

"Do you know what you are?" she said. "You're a contemptible little savage. For your information, Malc has two tickets in the seventh-row orchestra for Sing Me A Song Of The Old Country, after which he'll leave me at my door. He's a perfect gentleman, and he's never laid a finger on me. Never once. Or even suggested it. He worships me, for your information. He'd like to marry me."

There was a silence. Then Charles let himself back against the fat arm of the chair and straddled it. "So that's it," he said.

"And he's not the man who was trying to 'make' me, as you so picturesquely put it. That happens to be someone else, that I stopped seeing a long time ago. So all your worries were for nothing. Are you satisfied now?"

A muscle in his jaw seemed to twitch. "Why didn't you say so?"

"Because it wasn't any of your idiotic filthy-minded business! You just better worry about yourself. That's my advice to you."

"Are you considering marrying this guy?"

"I didn't say that."

"What are you wasting your time with a shloomp like that for?"

"He's not a shloomp." She walked nervously into the center of the room again. "He happens to be meticulous about his clothes."

"Yeah? That's about the most non-Ivy-League getup I ever saw in my life. Velvet on the collar. Scarf."

"Well! You're suddenly concerned about campus fashions, for a boy that couldn't finish high school. As it happens I picked out that coat myself."

Charles was shaking his head and gesturing desperately. "The guy doesn't even speak English! How can you go with a guy that talks like that? 'Dese' and 'dose'—"

"He doesn't say 'dese' and 'dose.' "

"Pretty close to it. It sure sounds like 'dese' and 'dose' to me. Unless you split hairs."

"Is your diction so perfect?"

"I don't say 'dese' and 'dose.' 'We sai' we getchih dere, dint we'—'dinhk we'—I can't even do it—"

"Well, he does use a lot of glottal stops." She sat on one of the cane chairs.

"Sis, you don't understand. I'm heartbroken." His voice was pleading and almost tearful. "He looks like a lizard or something."

"A what?"

"A lizard. That's just what he looks like."

"He does not! He happens to be considerate, which is more than I can say for my own brother, unfortunately."

"Sis, I was never so shocked in my life when he walked in here. I can't believe it." He gestured. "The guy's slimy."

"He isn't slimy! He's immaculate!"

"Yeah, he's immaculate all right. An immaculate lizard. I can't stand guys that look like that. He's a phony—can't you see that? He's a draft-dodger type. I can see it in his eyes."

"As it happens, he served four long years in the Army. He was drafted right after Pearl Harbor."

"Well, if I get sent to Korea or some place, I'm gonna send the son of a bitch a poisoned asp."

"Go right ahead," she said. "That would be just the right kind of childishness for you. And I see the Army hasn't improved your language."

"Air Force."

"Malc has never once used uncouth language in my presence, for your information. And he wouldn't allow anyone else to, either."

"It's not half as bad as what I have in mind, that I'd like to call him."

She tightened her lips. "Charles, just don't you make me any madder." She rose. "You're leaving, and I don't know for how long, and it's a terrible way to part. You've walked in here and made a scene, over nothing, and over things that aren't your business."

He came toward her and tried to take her hand, but she pulled it away. She sat on the studio couch.

"Sis—what can I say. He just isn't worthy of ya." He sat beside her, sideways, and tried again to take her hand but she avoided him.

"I never said he was."

"Well, I promise ya I'll never accept him as a brother-in-law."

"It's not up to you to accept him as a brother-in-law or not."

"Sis—I beg ya. Please, please, please. Don't marry him."

"As it happens I don't intend to marry him. I don't like him well enough. But if I did I wouldn't ask you."

"What the hell do you go with him for? What do you keep defending him for?"

"I enjoy his company. I admire him as a person. And I don't mind the way he talks. I think it's rather quaint, as a matter of fact."

They looked at each other.

"And I think we better go," she added, "or you'll miss that plane too."

They rose. She went to the closet and he helped her with her coat.

"Kiss me," he said. "Okay?"

She kissed him quickly.

"Please take that gloomy look off your face," she said. "It's just rude."

She preceded him down the stairs.

"Malc's being very decent to you. He paid a lot of money for those tickets and you've messed up the whole evening."

Malcolm was in the car and the motor was running. He leaned and swung the door open.

"Charles wants to apologize and ask your forgiveness," Millicent said. "It was all a misunderstanding."

"Forget it," said Malcolm. He reached and gave Charles a quick handshake. His smile was only a brief jerk of the corners of his mouth, as though he knew that Charles would not return it.

They tossed Charles's canvas satchel into the back seat and started off, Millicent low and small between them.

"And we haven't even had dinner yet," she said. "I bet we miss the whole first act."

Traffic was heavy and it took them a long time to get out of the city. Malcolm made nearly all of what talk there was. After a while he suggested that Charles keep in touch with him from overseas, with a view to setting up an import business. He told of a refugee who got the American franchise for an Italian sewing-machine needle and became a millionaire.

"All you need is eyes in your head. When you see a good thing let me know, and we'll study it. Something we got that they need, or something they got that there's a market for over here."

" 'Or sumpm,' " Charles mocked him.

"You just got to train yourself to think that way, that's all. You got the brains. I'll tell ya, kid, you send me your address, and keep looking, everything you touch and pick up, and we'll find something. Nothing's easier than doing what you want, once you decide you want it, you know? You got to want it. Especially if you go to Germany—Germany's a gold mine. So's Italy. Japan. Any place where there's been an expansion of manufacture—they're bound to have something new, something different. You follow me? You still with me?"

"I follow you," said Charles. "I'm not stupid."

"I didn't mean you was stupid. But they're looking with open arms. You know how many new patents come out in a year? And everything wants to crack this market. You're from the U.S.A., you got a basis for talking business. You got to pick the right item, that's all."

"Why didn't you keep your own eyes open when you were overseas?"

"Chicken, when I was overseas there was a war on. They wasn't making nothing. I don't say the opportunities wasn't there, but I was too young, you know? I didn't have nobody to take me in hand."

His constant talk began to irritate Millicent. It seemed like a nervous chatter. She wished this trip would end.

He gave many examples—successful imports of which he had heard, and hypothetical ones that occurred to him. They traveled up long avenues, assailed by constantly moving lights, but after the town of Lexington it became almost rural. The motor gave Millicent a headache. She watched the clock glowing greenish in the darkness of the car.

At last the headlights shone on a sentry house in the middle of the road. There was a guard with a heavy side arm. Charles retrieved his satchel and ran forward. They saw him waiting while the guard stepped half inside to telephone. It seemed to take a long time. Then Charles waved once. He turned and hurried. The overcoat was clumsy about his legs.

"Let's stay until his plane goes," Millicent said.

They remained sitting in the car. Buildings closed off their view of the field, but they could see the revolving beam of the control tower.

"Well, I guess the kid didn't like me too much," Malcolm said.

Millicent said nothing.

"Well, he'll change," said Malcolm. "He's still wet behind the ears."

They waited. She expected to see a plane rise like a black shadow with winking lights. It was cold. She huddled in her coat, watching. In a peculiar and unsatisfying way she felt her brother's love for her. It seemed irrational to have quarreled. And it seemed strange to be watching for a brother of her own flesh to be whisked up into the heavens, and grow smaller and smaller until he disappeared in the sky.

She still felt irritated with Malcolm. She had not liked his manner toward

Charles, even when he smiled, and the way he had tried to enlist Charles as a business associate. It was patronizing, as though he were going to take him over. Men just love bossing people around, she thought. One's as bad as the other. They just love running other people's lives. It makes them feel superior, apparently.

"Suppose a plane goes up," said Malcolm. "How do we know if it's his or not?"

She said nothing.

He took the theater tickets from an inside pocket. This time he tore up the tickets more slowly than the other time, and he did it with a resigned scowl. He opened the window automatically, dropping the pieces out.

"You shouldn't have done that," she said. "We might have caught the last act."

"Why do things by halves? I'll get tickets for another night."

"Even so, you shouldn't litter the ground."

They heard the sputtering that meant the experimental exercising of propellers, but it was a while longer before anything else happened. She heard Malcolm's breathing. They sat without speaking. A roar moved across the field and a plane rose and banked. She lost sight of it almost at once. It seemed to have gone directly over them.

"Well, do you figure he's on that?" Malcolm said. He started the car. "Well, since we come out in the jungle here, what about some grub? Ever been to the Wayside Inn?"

"You know what I'd really like, if you'd do me a favor, Malc? Just take me home and let me alone. I just want to be let alone."

"Well, sure, sure."

"I feel dizzy or something," she said.

"You all right?"

"I'm all right. I just don't want to have to talk to anybody."

They rode a while without speaking.

"How come the kid missed the train?" Malcolm asked.

"We put him on it at South Station and he walked off at Back Bay."

"Just like that? Is he nuts, or mixed up or something?"

"A lot of people are mixed up."

"You know what I think? I think the kid's a little spoiled, that's what I think. I mean it's selfish. We was all set for a big night, you know?"

"Getting a serviceman to his base is more important than the theater. For all we know he's going to Korea. The whole United Nations is involved." Her voice was tired and serious.

"Sure, you're right again, princess, you did what you had to. Am I complaining? I meant on the kid's part—I didn't mean I was blaming you."

" 'I dim mean.' The word is 'didn't,' for goodness sake. Don't you ever listen to yourself?"

"Well, I'm sorry. I been doing a little better lately, haven't I?"

"You haven't been doing a bit better. You don't even try."

"I thought I was doing better. Maybe not much. A little better."

"And why, I would like to know, did you have to parade all your worst diction in front of my brother? It was just as if you were doing it on purpose—you certainly didn't make the least effort. And the poor boy was upset enough as it is, and you just wouldn't stop talking. On and on. I thought I'd scream."

"What did the kid say about me when you was upstairs?"

"None of your business."

"I know it, but he said something, and it upset ya. You never talked to me like this before."

She didn't answer right away. "He thinks I'm considering marrying you," she said finally.

"Well, it's the truth, I hope."

"No, it's not the truth. I thought I made that clear at the beginning. You're just a little presumptuous. Do you think you run everybody? You've got plans for everybody, haven't you."

Malcolm wet his lips. He didn't look at her but he was watching the road. "Well," he said, "you shouldn't pay too much attention to the kid. He's just a kid, you know? He don't have too much savvy."

"He has lots of savvy."

"I mean you got to live your own life, you know what I mean? Whatever the kid said, put it out of your mind."

"Oh, stop it! You men! I never had so many men telling me what to do."

"Look," he said, "never mind the kid. I'll take care of him. When he comes out of the service I'll set him up in a job. I'll have him eating out of my hand."

"Charles is not a kid, and you will not have him eating out of your hand, and you will not take care of him. He'll take care of himself. He happens to be very talented." She paused and caught her breath. When she spoke again her voice was lower but shakier. "He risked a court-martial tonight because he was concerned about me."

"How do I sound right now?" said Malcolm. "I mean the way I pronounce?"

"Frankly, it grates. It's too ingrained. You haven't got the ear."

"Well, that's just one little thing when you come to gauge a man's character, isn't it?"

"It's not just that. It's a lot of things. I don't like the way you treat Yitzy. That's exactly the kind of thing I mean."

"All right. I got my faults."

She saw the reflection of passing lights against his profile. The muscles of his mouth moved and tightened.

"Look," he said, "I don't want to make a quarrel. To the extent I been wrong, I'm sorry. Believe me, I'm sorry. But I'm asking ya not to close your mind to the possibility that maybe some things can change and some can't, and I offer what I offer—I could still be a guy that you and your brother and everybody else would be proud to have in the family—"

She was shaking her head. "There's nothing to close, Malc. It was never open to such a possibility. I'm sorry, Malc, but you keep forcing me to be blunt. It's not as if I haven't said it before."

"What the hell did you go with me for?"

"If that's your attitude, I refuse to say another word."

"I'm sorry," he said. "I didn't mean that."

"It couldn't matter less."

"I don't know," he said. His voice was agitated. "If that's how you feel, maybe I'm well out of it."

"You were never in it."

"No, I guess I wasn't. Maybe you just been having a good time making a monkey out of me or something. But you must have seen some possibility in me somehow, some way—right? You wasn't just killing time for the laughs. And all I'm saying is, you didn't give it a long enough chance."

"I never said I was going to marry you. I never said I was thinking about it. I don't know where you get such ideas."

"Well," he said nervously, "if you can't stand me, we better find it out now, huh?"

She was resolutely silent.

"What I don't get is," he said, "you say there wasn't ever any doubt, like you knew right away I wasn't even in the running, and if you was fair, you at least should have been a little bit open-minded, and admit maybe there's one chance in a million you could be wrong about a guy, and not just laughing up your sleeve at a guy like he's a chump or something. I been on the up and up with you. My cards was right on the table, that first night. I told you where I stood because I thought at least you was sincere. I didn't figure I was just getting strung along."

"Will you please shut up? Will you? Do me a favor. I asked you to shut up. You make me nervous."

He was quiet only a moment.

"No dame makes a monkey out of me forever," he began again. "I been nice to you for how many weeks? And if I just been making a fool out of myself, it's time I woke up." He gave himself a little shake, like a shiver. "I don't know," he said. "It looks like a beautiful friendship is ended. Everything was fine until tonight."

"Everything wasn't fine. Not like you mean. Now stop thinking that."

At her building he opened the big door of iron and glass and let her in.

He looked at her coldly. His face seemed thin and sharp. "The dough don't bother me," he said. "But my time's valuable, you know?"

She climbed the stairs alone.

She came into the apartment, and wandered there. She had unbuttoned her coat, but it was a while before she remembered to take it off. There was a weirdness in the aloneness. She saw the perfume bottle on the mantelpiece. She sat down, thinking she was tired and had better undress. Suddenly she was intensely hungry and remembered she had had no dinner. But her stomach felt edgy, as though food might bring on nausea. She went to the kitchen and poured a glass of milk, and stood thinking about whether to warm it or not. She remembered when she and Charles were children. It must be in the nature of life that your life gets worse and worse, she thought.

She brought the milk to the drop-leaf table and drank some of it. She wished she had warmed it. The lavender phone was almost at her hand. She picked it up and dialed the number of the Massachusetts General Hospital.

She thought she would hang up without completing the call. She did not reply until the switchboard operator spoke for the second time.

"May I speak to Dr. Hollander, please?" said Millicent. "Dr. Leslie Hollander?" Her voice quaked and seemed completely uncontrollable.

"I think he's gone to bed," the girl said.

"Could you wake him, please?"

She listened to the ringing, wondering what to do. Just as the operator said he wasn't answering his voice cut in.

"Les, it's Millicent," she said. "It's horrible of me to wake you."

"I wasn't asleep," he said.

"Les, could I come over to the hospital there and just talk? I've just got to see a friendly face, or talk to somebody. My brother's gone overseas, and I've been fighting with everybody—I think I'm going insane or something. Could we just sit somewhere?"

"Well, we could go and sit by the snack machines downstairs," he said.

39

Ed stood at his morning prayers, facing the bedroom wall, his eyes meanwhile watching a spider that hung in the air before his face, its legs working, its thread invisible.

Behind him Lucinda lay still asleep.

Then he went to the window and idled there, watching the sunrise. A heavy snow had at last come, two days before, and it lay still clean upon the fields. The reddish sky whitened above the wooded hills that lay beyond the Davey and Hubbard houses, and the sun blazed in a thicket of tree trunks and branches. He could see the movement of its rising. He saw also the rippling of pink light on the snow fields, leaping ahead of itself and spreading on the gray-white, reaching around the long shadows of trees. A deer must have foraged for crab apples quite near the front of the house, because he saw footprints.

The unpaved winding drive that led down to the road curved gracefully, a blue-shadowed gully between waist-high walls sculptured by Mr. Featherstone's plow and topped with chunks. Its narrow bed, at the point where he could see it, was still blue-white and unsoiled, even in the impression of curving tire tracks. As he watched a party of quail came foraging together over the broad field of frozen crust. They came to the plowed trench and walked down into it and out of sight. He waited for the nearer ones to reappear over the nearer bank, and presently they did, quite near the house, and the rest followed, until he counted the same thirteen as before.

Yesterday Lucinda had told him of seeing a large male pheasant out there.

She put suet or crumbs every day or so on a little bird-feeding shelf that had been affixed to the elm tree, and Roland claimed to have identified several of the birds there that he knew from his charts. There had been black-cap chickadees, downy woodpeckers, rusty blackbirds, and slate-colored juncos. The little ones would wait for the big ones to go away. And Lucinda had been getting wrought up every day about a squirrel that kept raiding the shelf. She had told how the birds all screamed at him, with only one jay daring to get close, but even the jay stayed back when the squirrel looked at it.

It seemed to Ed that the children were enjoying the winter holidays. He had seen a sleigh full of teen-agers with Patty among them go by, drawn by an overworked horse. And he had gone to fetch Roland at Squonkamesset Pond, where Roland had gone fishing through the ice without permission. Bobby O'Shaughnessy's mother had tipped Lucinda that the kids might be there. He had found the pond a plain of whiteness, and here and there on it was a small standing figure of a fisherman, man or boy, his clothing a gleam of color on the desert of snow. On the way home they saw little children walking atop the crust of the snow, far over wide fields, and Roland remarked that the little kids could do that, but that he and his friends were too big.

The afternoon classes at the temple had been recessed when the public schools shut down, and Ed hoped he would get a lot done on his own studies during these two weeks. He also meant to construct a flooring in part of the attic that had only crossbeams. He had been feeling somewhat discouraged about the congregation and was glad not to be at the temple so much. During the week of mourning for Rosalind he had tried to get a quorum of ten together every morning and evening, so that the prayers could be said in proper style, but it seemed that the members had cooperated even less with him than they had with other members in similar circumstances. It had meant endless phoning, searching, waits, and broken promises.

As with the usual services all year long, you bothered a man enough and maybe he showed up once or twice to do you a favor—what good was that? Ed had sometimes told himself that it was good, even so—a man may actually come for himself, though he appears to come for you. It was like the question of the teen-agers who came on Sabbath only in time for the snacks. It was good to have them there at all. And apart from that, from time to time the children of men who came reluctantly showed an interest on their own.

He had gone on with his schedule of trying to persuade each family to add some token of religious observance to its home routine, but he had a feeling of getting nowhere. One man had asked angrily and sarcastically if Ed wanted him to say prayers and put on a prayer shawl and phylacteries, and Ed had replied, "Why not? If you're gonna be a Jew you might as well enjoy it." He had meant it seriously. But it was taken as a flippancy. It was spread around, and scandalized people.

During the vacation it was good having Patty about the house more than usual. She spent most of one day making strudel to send to Charles. But he heard her fighting a lot with Lucinda, and she sulked for days because Lucinda would not let her go to the armory to learn horseback riding.

"Do you want to get thrown from a horse and break your neck like Mr. Briggs?" he heard Lucinda shout at her.

"Briggs fell because he was jumping," Patty said. "I told ya I'd only be on a tame horse for beginners, that can't even walk fast. And Polly's even lost three pounds since she started."

She was still sniffling at supper.

"Millicent's favored because she's the oldest," she said, "and Charles is favored because he's the first-born male, and Rollo's favored because he's the youngest, and I'm the one that can't do anything. Anything I want is no. I'm just superfluous around here." She pronounced it superfloous.

"You do more than most girls," her mother said. "You've got the play, and the Rainbow, and the organ job, and cheerleading, and dating, and piano—what do you want?"

"I can't do anything adventurous."

"Adventure is what gets people into trouble," said Lucinda.

"Well, you know what I think? I think I'm a bastard," Patty said. "I don't think I'm really part of this family. I've been suspecting it for years. I don't even look like the other kids."

"You do look like the other kids. And that's lovely language, right in front of Roland."

"Leave me out of it," said Roland.

"Roland knows lots worse kinds of stuff than that," Patty said bitterly. "And anyway I mean it. I think I'm a product of some indiscretion on your part, or Dad's part or something."

"Do you want a good slap across the face?" Lucinda asked, her voice louder and higher pitched.

"Do you want to see your birth certificate?" Ed asked her.

Patty began blubbering but talked through it. "You think Millicent's beautiful, and you think Rollo's a genius, and you think Charles needs all kinds of love because he's a failure, and I'm just who-needs-you." She pushed out her chair and ran from the table sobbing.

Lucinda sat muttering about everyone wanting to get into danger. Millicent had told her she might take a couple of extra days the paper owed her, since the Sunday school was recessed, and go to New Hampshire to learn to ski if she could get a reservation. And Roland played on the ice and delivered papers after dark and in blizzards, and Charles was in the Air Force and Ed was in the firemen. "It's just terrible," she said. "I'm afraid something's going to happen to everybody at once."

He did not get as much done as he had hoped. Though there were no classes, he kept tutoring some of the slower children who were falling behind. He attended a meeting of the Masonic lodge, and Giles Littleton asked him to be second ruffian on the Third Degree team, and that meant coming back for a rehearsal. He also addressed the men's club of the Congregational church, on the invitation of Newton Stillman. He went with Lucinda to give blood a second time to the Air Force. Then Conrad Bernstein and Phil Walker took him to Boston for a session with the architect. The firemen of Wilmerding Crosswalk had a Christmas dance, and he took Lucinda. Roland took him to a fathers-and-sons night of the Boy Scout troop, in the basement of Caleb Folger's church, and he won an onion there in the three-legged race. And there was snow-shoveling to be done about the porch, and paths to be dug.

He decided to remove the telephone in his study, as Patty used it more than he did. The kitchen phone would be sufficient for them.

He conducted a bunch of the teen-agers down to Rhode Island for an all-day conclave of New England temple youth groups, and ran one of the seminars there and chaperoned at the dance. Patty had gone along and she attended one of the other seminars, not his.

At his seminar there he sat on the floor, with a number of boys and girls about him, and enjoyed looking at them and being among them. Somehow, in the discussion, he told them that the dietary discipline was a kind of partial vegetarianism. A girl whose big rounded knee was near him on the floor disputed this, and he stayed on the topic a while. He said that when Moses got the commandments on Mount Sinai, he was told that the people were to be vegetarians. But, according to the Midrash, Moses told God he'd never be able to sell the people on such an idea. They weren't ready for it. They liked meat too much. I'm afraid if I tell them no more meat, Moses said to God, it would cause a revolution, and they'd throw me out. So God backed down and promulgated the kosher laws as a compromise. A compromise that will remind you that even though permitted, it's basically questionable.

Ed saw that he had the kids' attention. His eyes went from one to another. He said the Bible's dietary laws were so arranged that if you became a vegetarian they evaporate. For a vegetarian all restrictions disappear. And the vegetarian is the kosher man par excellence. Basically the principle was that the whole animal kingdom was excluded as food, but as a compromise a certain few species, which could be raised domestically and slaughtered painlessly, were excepted. Notably beef and lamb, which you had to keep anyway, the cattle for milk and the sheep for wool. Also certain fowl, like those which were kept anyhow for eggs. And certain fish were permitted. It was not known for certain in Bible days, he said, just as doctors aren't agreed for certain now, whether people can be their healthiest on a completely meat-free diet. But the moral problem still had to be faced.

Even the excepted animals must be killed by a man trained in painless slaughter. And you must avoid eating their blood, as a reminder of what you're doing. And you must impose on yourself a penalty, each time you eat meat, of being permitted no dairy products for a few hours thereafter. This was quite a penalty, and the knowledge of it steered you away from excessive meat-eating. It encouraged you to devise meatless meals. You found yourself ordering an egg-salad sandwich instead of the corned beef, because if you ate the corned beef you couldn't have an ice-cream soda all afternoon. After all, dairy products too were a gift of the animal kingdom, and it taught you something to have them withheld when you had eaten flesh.

The eyes of all the kids were upon him. He looked at one of the prettiest girls, and then at a plainer one. He said the dietary discipline was a symbol of man's confusion before a God who creates evil, a God who makes his creatures to devour one another. That was why Isaiah said God creates evil, and that was why Isaiah spoke of the lion and the lamb.

The dietary discipline symbolized also the incompleteness of man's evolution —just as our bodies aren't yet fully adapted to walking erect, so perhaps are we not yet adapted to doing without meat, though our moral sense had already begun to tell us it was wrong.

There wasn't one of us, he told them, that doesn't feel he would improve on God, given the chance. There wasn't one of us who wouldn't have preferred to create a world without evil, injustice, suffering. It's not the way we would want it, he said, that the world should be such a horrifying mystery, and that we, our species, should be assigned the slow labor of cleaning it up. But that's how it is.

The main thing was reverence for life. You had to breed out of yourself the spirit of the huntsman. The Biblical word for nonkosher meant basically an animal taken in the pain and the terror of the chase. The huntsman learned in time to kill for sport, and to polish and love his weapon, and was less likely to grow into a man of nonviolence. In the same way you shouldn't eat a carnivore, because to eat a wolf, or a boar, which in turn eats other animals—it was already too much the jungle. Reverence for life, if you were serious about it, was an attitude worth hammering at and ingraining, worth making part of your basic nature, with every possible approach, day by day and over the centuries. Thou shalt not kill was not enough. A religion that simply taught men not to kill each other would not be sufficient to teach them not to kill each other. The whole way of daily living, how you prayed, how you ate, should inculcate reverence for life. And should bring the spirit of nonviolence into our natures. And in four thousand years, he said, we've managed to become a relatively unmurderous people. To hear of a man of this tradition, especially one who kept these disciplines, being arrested for murder—it was pretty rare.

Ed looked at a bosomy girl in a big sweater, who sat on the floor before him between two boys, her feet to one side. He told her it was also good for calorie control. If you ate a steak, then you could not at that meal put cream in your coffee. Every meal omitted either butterfat or animal fat, one or the other. And he'd read that doctors were starting to talk now about saturated fats. The dietary discipline steered you toward more use of fish and vegetable oils. And restriction didn't make for sameness, it could make for variety—when you omitted butter you might try peanut butter, apple butter, prune butter. Still looking at the bosomy girl, he told her she'd have a husband someday, and that she'd want him to live a long time. And the best way to keep his ticker in good shape was not to pile butterfat on animal fat, and to see that once a week he got the slowdown of the Sabbath. Keep ye My statutes, that ye may live.

He looked around the group. He was sitting now with his knees up, and his hands resting over them. If you don't accept the dietary discipline, he said, then you believed that all the living things about us were fair game to be eaten. Did you want that to be your stand? Accepting a denial of that was already a first long step in the direction of saintliness.

After the seminar broke up he had little to do, except listen to the singing and watch the dancing, but it was nearly one in the morning when he set out for home. One of the Wilmerding Crosswalk girls had lost her coat, and searchings and inquiries at lost-and-found had not turned it up. Ed even arranged for a notice in a bulletin that would reach whoever had taken the wrong coat, but he knew he would have a hassle with the girl's parents anyhow. It irritated him that a girl so young should wear such expensive beaver. He had her ride in his own car, instead of one of the others, because the boys were already talking of keeping her warm.

In a few days he found that there was a rumor in the congregation that he had really gone off his nut and was insisting now that everybody become a vegetarian.

At his Friday evening sermon he tried to explain himself to the congregation, but he felt he was not getting through very well. He was tired, and thought he might be coming down with a cold.

On Saturday morning he devoted his sermon to it again, because the people present were somewhat different. By now he was sneezing a lot, and kept wiping his nose and excusing himself. He even interrupted himself in the midst of his sermon to say God bless you to someone in the congregation who sneezed. He tried to explain evolution, and man's nearness to the animal kingdom. By way of illustration he said that a man and a raccoon were much more closely kindred to one another than either was to a horse. But he didn't feel the sermon went over well, and afterward it turned out that Mr. Brill thought raccoons were colored people.

He had walked halfway home when it began to sleet. It splashed icily on his face and neck, driven by a wind. Lucinda had not come to the service, though she had been the night before. She felt it did the most good for her to be seen on Friday night, when the biggest crowd came, but even then she rode instead of walking with Ed, because she looked best in heels.

Directly after lunch he got into bed, with a bottle of Canadian blended whisky and a volume of the Talmud, a tractate of the order Women. He wanted to find something to add to the answer he had given Millicent.

Lucinda had put on a wool dress, thinking that Ed might let someone drive him home because of the weather, but now she came up to the bedroom and lifted off the dress. He saw her hang it in the closet. He took the bottle and glass from the night table and poured some whisky. Lucinda stepped into a house dress that had buttons most of the way down the front, and pulled it up about her shoulders.

"Don't you take any water with that?" she asked.

He shook his head, and took a gulp. "I like it to taste like whisky," he said.

40

Millicent rode beside Leslie on the rigid upholstered seat and looked out the train window. She saw a frozen river, spotted white and gray. Sometimes the passing fields were divided by little stone walls. Even through the dust and soot of the unwashed glass she could see delicate hues in the nearly colorless landscape.

She could hear the coal-burning locomotive. It would take four hours to get where they were going. But when uneasiness crossed her mind about having come with him, she reminded herself that he had agreed it would be upon her terms. She had raised that condition at once, as soon as he had suggested that she come along, and she had been taken aback by his ready assent.

He had been going to go anyway, alone, and had had the weekend long planned, and had borrowed the things he would need. He was quite right to think of himself once in a while, and not just of his mother and brother all the time.

And it had been good of him to let her tag along like this. It was just what she needed, some change of scene and new activity.

She was of course paying her own way. And it was agreed that she would spend her time in a beginner's class and not hamper Leslie in his skiing.

She glanced at him, but he was staring past her at the scenery. He was in ski clothes, like herself, though his were baggier. She had bought the black stretchy pants in Boston and borrowed the flannel shirt from Ella Jane, and wore as many as possible of her things on the train, so as not to have a lot of luggage. It had surprised her that Ella Jane owned some ski clothes.

And she found she liked the costume, sweater, parka and all. It seemed practical, and unlike ordinary clothing it did not unnecessarily emphasize a distinction between the sexes.

She felt an adventurous exhilaration when Leslie at last helped her down at a small brick railroad station. The icicles were shining. The town turned out to be not a pretty little village such as she had imagined but a nondescript one with a straight main street. But she did not mind that, and Leslie said he had chosen it because the ski area was near enough to walk and they would not need a car.

They went together up the icy sidewalk of a side street, between fences and piled snow, and stopped briefly at an old white inn, where Millicent verified her reservation. She went upstairs and left her valise on the brass bed.

She found Leslie waiting for her on the long veranda, and she let him take her gloved hand while they walked up and down more streets toward the mountain. Sometimes the dug pathways were narrow and slippery. There were many cars, often with sloshing chains, and people coming and going.

At last, beyond a parking lot, she saw a vast dazzling slope on which skiers shot across this way and that, crouching and almost leaping over hillocks and crossing one another's paths. Tiny open cars crept up and down a track, carrying skiers far up the mountain, and other people clasped a contraption of poles and ropes and were hauled uphill on skis. She heard the machinery, and saw a child fall in a cloud of snow. The mountain was fringed with pine. The parka she had bought was black, though of a texture quite different from her pants, but she saw now that many people wore the gaudiest colors. Leslie, carrying skis and poles on his shoulder, had several sweaters on, and the outermost, white and coarse with a few decorative stripes, had worn thin at the elbows. A red knit cap with a stripe about its edge rose to a small tower above his head, like a little boy's, and he had on his glasses. His clothes had a touch of homeliness and poverty, and of being not quite right, that somehow pleased her very much.

The hood of her parka was tight about her face, and on her cheeks she felt already the pleasantness of sun and cold. Leslie talked as little as he had on the train.

At the foot of the mountain was a complex of chalets, and Leslie took her into a dark shop beneath them, where busy men fitted her to boots and ankle guards and skis and poles, and gave her a rental contract to sign. The room seemed crowded with mothers and fathers and children all walking in slush.

When Millicent came out the sunshine was blinding, and the eaves all about her were dripping with thaw. But her breath made steam before her. There were more people walking about than on a city beach in summer, she thought. A tall angular rouged woman in a big shaggy cap was shouting at a child named Wendy.

Leslie showed Millicent how to fasten and unfasten the skis and to slide along a bit on the hard, bumpy snow near the buildings, one foot at a time. Then after a sandwich he installed her for the afternoon in her class, and went off without her to ski on the mountain.

Millicent's class started away single file. They trudged slowly on skis, through snowy glades where forest cut off her view of the mountain. There were snow tufts on pine-needle clusters. A squirrel ran up a pine tree, shaking down some snow that showered like a smoky waterfall. Millicent followed the ski tracks of a short elderly woman. They passed a brook. Its irregular shore line was a rounded puff of white that hid all details. In the middle of the winding black wet she saw rounded white islands like cotton balls. On her cheeks there was a nippy cold. Once a gust blew down a cloud of blinding powder from the pines.

At a secluded hill, surrounded by woods, the instructor lined them up. There were about fifteen pupils, none near Millicent's age except for a married couple, but some much older, and children of various sizes. One man said he was seventy. The instructor was a middle-aged man in a pompon and a sheepskin. He spoke the odd accent of the north, with short vowels where she expected long ones and long where she expected short. The lesson dealt with sliding downhill and braking to a halt by forming the skis into a plow. He did not like the way Millicent thrust herself out, and had various slang words for backside, without quite being offensive. She thought of telling him that she had given blood to the Air Force recently and did not have all her strength back. But she decided against it. She worked hard, but climbing back up the hill after each slide was very tiring. After the first few times down she grew worse, and nervous, until she always fell when she passed the instructor.

When the class was over she waited for Les at the bottom of the mountain. The sun was gone. The skiers on the big slope were few now, but seemed expert. They lowered themselves, turned suddenly, almost sprang, and she heard the smack and the scrape of their skis. She tried to brush the whiteness from her hips, so Leslie would not know she had fallen so much. But it clung to the fabric. She did not see him until he was beside her in his red knit hat, smiling, moist and sunburned, breathing the same agreeable exhaustion that she felt throughout her body.

They walked up the long road toward the town and the inns, stepping often into ruts of frozen slush to make way for carloads of departing skiers. He carried her skis and poles as well as his, and it was a bundle of lumber on his shoulder. She was full of what seemed a cleansing tiredness. It seemed quite natural to lean on him as they walked. Dusk came, giving the snow a peculiar iridescence.

He left the skis and poles on the porch. There was hot cocoa and tea at the inn, but then a long wait until suppertime, so they went to the big living room, which was dowdy but warm, with a low ceiling and a blazing fireplace. There were parts of family groups, and teen-agers in Scandinavian sweaters sat on tables reading magazines, and three ruddy girls of about thirteen or fourteen sat singing on the floor. A Christmas tree was blinking in the corner. Millicent squeezed into a place on the sofa, smelling the fire and feeling its intense radiance, glad she had come here and convinced she must learn to ski properly. Les was on the carpet, and she did not mind that he lowered her socks and massaged the soreness of her ankles, even in the presence of strangers.

He does that very gently, she thought.

But she was barely able to remain awake through supper. After dessert she excused herself and went to her room. Leslie was to sleep in the attic dormitory.

She enjoyed the weight and feel of the quilts. The mattress seemed billowy, and she sank in it. She heard the yells and the feet of kids, from below, from the ceiling, in the hallway and on the stairs. She wondered how Les could possibly sleep in a dormitory with two dozen men and boys.

When she woke she had slept for twelve hours. She looked from the window, and snow was falling before the pines in the yard, and before the houses of the town. All the light seemed gray-green. She felt ambitious.

For breakfast she and Les were assigned to a table with a half-dozen men and women, all in thick sweaters with various zigzag designs, and the talk was almost entirely of skiing. She asked Les if the dormitory had been noisy, and he said that when you're tired enough you sleep.

When she accompanied him to the slope she carried her own skis and poles. Then she enrolled in the same class as before.

Some of the other people were the same and some were new, but she was a veteran now and the instructor knew her by name. Snowflakes were on his face and he kept wiping his nose on his glove and sniffling. The fresh powdery snow made it impossible to go very fast, and this gave her confidence.

The session ended at lunchtime, and she met Les amid the stomping and warmth of the cafeteria. People were pushing, and she saw melted snow running in the creases of blue parkas and pink ones. The lacings of her boots were clogged with it. The instructor had said she could go on to the next higher class in the afternoon, but Leslie offered to show the mountain top instead.

"I don't want to keep you from skiing," she said.

"You won't."

The outdoors was good after the steaminess of the cafeteria. She rode one of the tiny open cable cars up its little viaduct in the woods, beneath the branches, directly behind the one that carried Les. Her rented skis and poles leaned beside her.

Her face felt as if a cool mist lay on it. Snowflakes that had settled on her own eyelashes were even visible to her cloudily. The snowfall came in a steady sprinkle. Clumps of trees a distance off had various shades of dimness, according to how far away they were. When she looked back the parking lot and the base headquarters were already small, far below, as though seen from an airplane, but chalky behind the snowflaky turmoil.

When she looked below again, the whole clump of chalets had disappeared behind the depth of veiling.

She was hauled steeply into rocky places, and yet she saw people skiing, not on a slope now but in strange pathways through the forest.

Leslie shouted and leaped from the carriage ahead. She seized her skis and poles and he put out a hand to help her jump to the ground. There was a cabin here, and people about, and a great spinning wheel on a tower hauled other skiers in swinging chairs from another side of the mountain. Even though the air was opaque at any distance she had the sense of a summit. It was windier here. Before her no two snowflakes were moving the same way. Some coasted sideways in arcs, as if concerned with dodging one another and circling one another, and as many appeared to travel upward as down. If she looked closely she could see each flake wandering and changing direction constantly, with no particular eagerness to reach the ground. Yet if she turned and looked behind her they were in fact going down, but with a strange illusion of two directions at once, some to the right and some to the left, so that in their crossing they seemed to fall with a flickering, like an old movie. And down the steepness she dimly saw square yellow tractors on treads, that beat the snow to make it easier to ski on.

Leslie fastened his skis and told her she could wait for him in the cabin if she got cold. He started away slowly, with a push of his poles, and then he swooped down a bank. She marveled at the way he turned sharply. Then he did it again, further down, the red of his cap visible a while through the swirl of flakes. But soon she could see him no more.

The cabin turned out to be a snack shop. It was warmed by fireplaces, but the air was smoky and oppressive. She went out several times to see if Leslie had returned, and at last she saw him jump from one of the moving chairs. He lifted a projecting little mask of clear plastic from his eyeglasses. He was ruddy, and his face and hat and clothing were covered with droplets. He looked joyful. She sensed his exhilaration. How beautiful he is, she thought. He asked if she minded waiting while he skied down again. She said she didn't. He told her she could take the cable car down the mountain again if she got bored. "If it's not snowing tomorrow maybe you can come up here before train time and see the view," he said.

Several times he skied away, and returned on the chair lift. Millicent wandered about, looking at the skiers, and watching each time for Leslie's return. Sometimes she went into the cabin to warm herself, and once she treated Leslie to hot chocolate there. She got to know how long it took him to ski down and come up again.

How little recreation he gets, she mused, and how hard he works at it. All year long the smell of antiseptics, the smell of death, and now, for two brief days, how he enjoys this cleansing air! How he exults in it, with what vigor. She felt as if she could weep for him. How complex were his labors, how simple his wants.

"Are you still here?" he asked her the fifth time he came off the lift. Then he said he knew of an easy trail on which she could hike with him around the mountain, back to the lodge.

"No, I don't want to break up your afternoon," she said.

But he insisted he had had enough, and at last she got her skis and poles from where she had leaned them against the cabin and walked after him. The soft snow was higher than her boots, but the pants seemed watertight and the boots clasped them firmly. He picked his way, and she followed. He did not go in the direction he had skied, but along the edge of the woods. When they were some distance down the hill he found a winding swath cut through the forest, like a snow-filled roadway, and made her put on her skis.

Then she followed him into the forest, gliding one ski forward and then the other. She felt no wind here. The trail had hardly any slope at all. But her skis moved beneath the powdery surface and she could not see them.

She felt she was a nuisance, and that she had in fact cut short his afternoon. She looked back at their pristine tracks. They were totally alone here. She could scarcely hear the hauling machinery any more, and the snow fell with an audible hush. In the underbrush it clotted in each twiggy fork like an endless fabric of cotton balls. She saw branches of a tall pine laden like a willow. The snow clung differently on each species of tree and bush, delicate high ridges on some, and on some like intact separate flakes bristling as if on a magnet, and on others like a white coral. Everywhere there were whites and grays, an infinite world of angular twigs. Brambles were whitened like patterns of frost. In the forest a bird repeated a rattly whistle. The trial twisted, rose, fell, always with a curve ahead that beckoned.

She was panting. Then she fell, where the snow banked up toward some bushes. The skis held her feet in an awkward position. Leslie had heard her, and he unfastened his skis and ran back. She tried meanwhile to struggle up, but fell again. He unfastened her skis.

She was looking at him, breathing through her mouth. "I must be stupid," she said.

He kissed her. She responded to the kiss, closing her eyes. Then she looked at him again.

"Can you get up?" he said.

"I could, but I wish I didn't have to," she said.

He kissed her again and she lay back into the snow with the kiss, taking him with her. His leathery mitten slid on the silky black parka, under the bulk of her arm and around her body. It was a long kiss, with pauses for breath. I don't know, I can't help it, she said to herself. I shouldn't do this. Some of his weight was against her and she heard snow crush when he moved. His face was warm, despite the wetness she felt between her cheek and his. The kiss stopped, but they scarcely moved. She saw his eye, and the frame of his glasses, and the flakes alighting on his hair.

"Will we be buried in the snow?" she asked.

"I don't think so."

"Will somebody come, and see us kissing and everything?"

"I don't think so."

"They could."

"Well, this is the novice trail, and nobody'll use it today. It's not good for anything in soft powder."

"They might."

"Ya, they might."

But she lay as though she didn't care. With a mittened hand she reached for his cap, where it had fallen in the snow, and put it lightly on his head. He rubbed noses with her and looked at her lazily. He took off his glasses and placed them in the snow. She still heard the snow fall. On the tree trunks each scale and blister of bark was laced in white.

"It's really awfully good of you to let me come along on your trip," she said.

He smiled slightly. He touched his tongue to the tip of her nose.

"You've been awfully good to me," she said. "Always agreeing to everything. And I've never been very understanding of you."

He lay beside her, his mitten playing upon her chest. For a while they said nothing. Snow was falling in her face. Sometimes his mitten made creases in the parka and sometimes it smoothed it.

"There are seven layers between your hand and me," she said.

"Seven?"

"Well, there's your mitten, and the woolen glove inside that, that's two right there. And then there's my parka, and then my sweater, and my shirt, and long underwear."

He seemed to repeat silently with his lips. "That's only six," he said.

"Well, my bra."

"And then you."

His thumb moved.

"I guess you can't feel very much through all that," she said.

He said nothing. She saw a snowflake fall on his lip.

"Remember how we used to neck and everything?" she asked.

"Of course."

The wrinkled leather mitten moved to her pants. She let her legs move, and his mitten felt the tough seams. If I tell him to stop that he'll stop that, she thought.

"I just have three layers of pants," she said.

"Is that all?"

His mitten went to her hip, and seemed to fondle the button and the waistband extension. She wondered if he were going to undo the button and open her zipper. Then he would see her red knit, she thought. And she would be down to two layers. I'll just lie still, she told herself, and see what he does.

She responded to a kiss meanwhile. There was no sound but the steadily falling snow. He's keeping the snow off me, she said to herself. She seemed to recall having heard, perhaps long ago in school, that snow kept animals warm. He must know what's feasible in snow. Eskimos must neck in igloos and not get pneumonia.

What a convenience it would be, she reflected, to have the other point of view, and attach no stigma to it, and be able always to let him do whatever he wished, without scene or argument. Then she would come to know for herself, at first hand, not just by hearsay and theory and words, precisely what it was—this desire for her she had heard of so much. She would be witness to the shape and course and feel of what he wanted, and discover the exact particulars of what her flesh became for him.

She wondered if he were all aroused, inside those clothes. It crossed her mind that possibly he knew of an abandoned hut in the forest nearby, and that in a moment he meant to take her there. She had neither the skill nor the equipment for contraception. There would be only her undefended skin and membranes, waiting with nervous expectancy, relying upon his delicacy.

He caressed the taut black fabric, but he did not unfasten the button or touch the zipper. She began to talk of her ski pants, where she had bought them, and what size they were.

He propped himself on his arm and looked down at her face. "Well," he said, "we better be on our way. Before we freeze. What do you think?"

"Good idea, I guess," she said, starting to rise with him on an elbow.

He picked up his wet eyeglasses and got to his feet, so that pressed snow fell from the creases of his clothes. He slapped at himself once or twice to make more fall, and then reached and pulled her up.

As soon as she stood she embraced him, before he had dried his glasses or put them on. He held her, and she leaned into him with all her weight.

"Okay," he said. He slapped her behind. "Do you think you can manage on skis, or would you rather walk it?"

She said she supposed she'd better walk, and he said skis weren't easy in this fluff. He began to gather the skis and poles.

"I can carry my own," she said. He gave them to her and she jockeyed them to her shoulder. He helped to get them balanced. She noticed that it had turned somewhat darker and colder.

She walked in his wake, sometimes hurrying to catch up, and straightening her poles when they threatened to tilt. The panting seemed to clean her lungs. She was not sure whether this trail really would lead to the base lodge and the road to their inn, as he had said, or whether he was taking her somewhere else. In the layers of underwear that walked with her she felt the heat of her exercised body.

The trail did in fact come out quite innocently on the main open slope, near its bottom. The daylight was fading, and as she walked she saw the cable cars halt for the night.

The warmth of the inn was particularly agreeable after the darkening road, with its ruts of frozen slush. There were some new people at their table, but she could not enter much into the conversation the way Les did. But she listened. Someone told her to keep her weight on the downhill ski, and Leslie said that was right. The dining room was pleasantly noisy. A child at another table was having a birthday; a waitress brought a cake and there was singing.

After supper they went again to the crowded living room. There was one place by the sofa's end, facing the fire, and he told her to take it. He said he thought he'd read a while and go up to the dormitory early. He said she'd better turn in early too, if she wanted to ski a little before the train.

There was a rack of magazines by the sofa, and she sat looking at picture spreads of world events. But she was somehow a little nervous and could not concentrate. Her limbs were tired. In an adjoining room, through an open door, children pounded a piano and played ping-pong. She saw Les study the worn titles in the bookcase. Then she saw him sitting on the arm of a chair, chatting with some gray-haired man. They were saying something about how the speed of the snow would be faster tomorrow, and ideal the day after.

She wondered if Les had understood the craziness of her state of mind during the afternoon. The more she thought of it the more possible it seemed that he had, and the more it embarrassed her. After all, she had thrown herself at him in a way quite unlike herself. As though to tease him deliberately and wantonly, after their solemn agreement that the trip was on her terms. She would go over and apologize to him now for her conduct on that snow trail, if he were not busy talking to that old man. It must have been some intoxicating effect of the mountain air.

It occurred to her that he was staying away from her and talking to that man on purpose to prevent her from apologizing. He did not want to embarrass her further. His intent was to let the matter drop, and he had the poise to behave as though nothing had happened. Just as in the forest he had had the decency and the good sense to protect her from herself.

She stared at the fire. A log popped. She extended her legs, in their black pants, and rubbed the toe of one red sock against the sole of the other.

What a dependable person he was. She was childish and emotional, and when she created foolish embarrassments he knew how to smooth them over.

In a while he came by the sofa and tousled her hair. "Well, I've had it," he said. "I'm dead."

"Good night," she answered. "I think I'll be turning in too, soon."

Then she watched him saunter out to the hall and she heard the heavy tread of his ski boots on the stairs.

She rose listlessly and looked at the book titles. Then she stared absently at the tinselly little tree. The blink and flash of its lights were jarring. She thumbed a few pages in another magazine.

She went slowly up the stairs, thinking she would shower before bed. But the shower room was occupied, so she went to bed without it. She undressed and buttoned her pajamas in darkness. She could still hear the muffled sound of children playing below. The brass of her bed reflected the moonlight, and she saw that the snowing had stopped.

The sheeting in the soft quilts and down was cold at first, but her body warmed it. She did not fall asleep as quickly as last night. She began to doze but woke again.

There was only one morning left before her train to Boston, and she wondered if she should spend it in the next higher ski class, or riding up to the mountaintop to see the view.

She wondered how long it would take her to learn to ski passably well. She wished she could have a whole week here.

The latch of her door clicked. The door opened a few inches. She did not stir. The light of the hallway was behind him, so that he was in shadow, but she could see it was Les, and when he turned to close the door she saw he was not wearing his glasses.

When the door was shut he moved quickly and came into bed beside her, under the quilts. The bed was narrow and his hip and his shoulder pressed by her side, so she moved a little to make room. His foot brushed down past hers. The springs of the bed squeaked a little and became still. Maybe he won't really do anything to me, she said to herself. Anyway it was good to have his company. They were on their backs, side by side, and neither had spoken yet.

"Hi," he said finally.

"Hi," she answered.

He found her hand, and held it gently, under the quilts and under the top sheet. She moved her toes against the sheet and looked at the dark ceiling.

The hand that held hers rested lightly against the thigh of her pajamas.

If I just let him, he'll do it. I don't have to do anything. While I mind my own business, not asking, not interfering, it will happen.

She could give her arms and legs orders, like the border guards of a small nation, to move aside like the Danes, in polite unresistance, while the Germans pour through with inevitability. And her heart would be like the townspeople, frightened, anticipating, curious, awaiting the conqueror's will, his cruelty or his mercy, or the change he would bring to her life.

Leslie dropped her hand. He seemed to stir and roll, as though taking off his bathrobe while he lay. Then he was still, not touching her.

Will he make love by degrees, or pounce?

Maybe he meant only to lie here through the night, and let her decide another time. That would be the kindest thing of all. To sleep, just letting it be calm and good to have him here, not getting too aroused. She did not want to have to argue. She had no more arguments left, and he undoubtedly still had some.

There was a loud muffled boom that seemed immediately outside. "What was that?" she said with a start.

"It sounded like a bunch of snow fell off the roof."

Her breath came back. He turned to her, and his hand came across her breast and arm and shoulder. She returned the embrace and found that he was naked. He had taken off not only his bathrobe but his pajamas too. Her sudden uneasiness was like alarm, and the impulse of her hands was to draw away. But after her first recoil she reached again, quickly, to be certain, and felt the hairs on his buttocks.

She lay back, not touching him. But he kissed her, and she slowly and lightly embraced the bareness of his back, high up. Her mouth was dry and she felt her heart pounding. Even in the continuing kiss she swallowed. Already her feelings were different from what she had expected. That's the excitement of surrender, in the not knowing, she thought. As long as you had been defending you had some control, and to some extent you knew the next moment. But now each next instant, each next happening, was his. That's what makes it now strange, alien country, she thought, in a way it can't be for a boy. His control is your suspense.

Unhurriedly he undid the buttons of her pajama top. She thought of asking about contraceptives. But she didn't. It was inconceivable that his prudence could not be trusted in a matter like that. He pushed the pajama top aside and his hand played and molded, with lifting, shaping strokes, as on occasions in the past. His lips clamped wetly and sucked and drew. And when he paused at that, his fingers had pulled the drawstring at her waist.

"Why do men find breasts so fascinating?" she asked him, and her voice sounded strange to her in its weak breathlessness.

"They just do."

When he shoved the pajamas down her legs he left in place the woolly underdrawers she wore beneath. She had forgotten that she had kept those on. She had never worn underwear under her pajamas before, and it seemed now a vulgar and low-class way of keeping warm. She hoped Les didn't think she did that all winter long. They were ugly things too, thick and ill-fitting, of a heavy weave.

But he didn't seem to mind. He put a hand inside them from the bottom, stretching the ribbing of a leg band, and his tickling fingers staked out claims in those regions. He took his hand out again. She wondered if he had done that to see if she had still something else on beneath, or if it had been only play.

Then he grasped her in a firmer embrace than before, pulling her to him. There was a completeness in his hands upon her back. It made her want to press next to him and remain. He made not separate caresses but motions that flowed into one another. His face came against hers, shutting out the moonlight. She lay fascinated by touch, following his tracing. She could still hear the noise of people up and about on the floor below, and children on the stairs.

"You cold?" Les asked.

"No."

He stroked the woolly underdrawers and his fingertips scratched her through it. She moved her feet to push the pajamas from her ankles. Meanwhile the underdrawers upon her behind moved with his hand and with his fingers. It was as if they had their own way of responding to him. She realized now that the coarse furry woolen slid around on her more freely than a thinner material would have. It always clung to his hand instead of to her skin, and followed his caresses about. Those pants are in love with his hand, she thought. Always the cloth stuck to the palm of his hand and not to her. He lowered them, first in one place and then in another, and at last swept them from her.

She sensed his excitement in many ways. Her skin could feel his whole body, gentle in one place, threatening in another. She gave a shiver, but she moved to accommodate his hand.

You're crazy, Millicent Audrey, she thought to herself. Why are you doing this?

"Is it possible for it to be pleasurable the first time?" she asked him.

"Sure."

"I'm sort of scared."

"Scared?"

"Afraid."

"A lot afraid? Or a little bit afraid?" He massaged all the folds of her flesh, as though he owned her.

"I don't know. A little bit, I guess."

The caress of his finger had a quality almost like vibration.

"Well," he said, "try to enjoy being afraid."

She returned his embrace, but he kept extricating a hand from the embrace to massage her more. For some moments they didn't speak, but she heard herself breathing through parted lips and heard his breathing too. She moved only to welcome his fingers.

"Les—" she said.

"What."

"God must have an awful dirty mind, to have created sex."

She felt him press.

"Oh dear," she said, catching her breath. She made a slight convulsive motion.

"Be still," he said.

She was still. She felt the push, slowly.

"Does it hurt?" he said.

"No. I don't think so."

He was still, and then he stirred, and was still again, and stirred some more. He began to move with more regularity. They watched each other's eyes. His hands moved about her shoulders smoothly.

"How did I get here?" she murmured.

"Shut up," he said softly.

His head came down beside her ear, and she no longer saw his face. He held her tight. She felt the small tremble of flesh hugged in flesh, and then the fervor of his slippery goading, the way his body seemed to believe in itself. He seemed to ebb, and then swell and advance, slowly but strong. Then he would sway and lighten again, and undulate. It became a soothing that craved more and more soothing. She tried to answer his rhythms, but he moved her knees, and she found herself merged with him even more and sinking further in the sheets and the downiness. He had been right that it could be pleasurable the first time.

He lifted his face, and she liked the way he smiled down. He was propped in such a way that he was not heavy. He slowed, until he moved with only the tiniest of occasional shocks, and yet his tone and exultation seemed to remain. He played a very long time, sometimes slowly and sometimes rapidly. Once he told her that if she liked she could rock, like a little boat at a mooring. She did try, and told him she could not. But he didn't seem to mind, and kept making sensations, until their intensity was such that she hugged and shook with him, as though with a paralyzing strength, crushing her cheek and jaw against his. It affected her heartbeat. The quilts slipped away, but joy seemed to pursue joy with such heady concentration that interrupting it was unthinkable. His writhing became quick syncopated convulsions, like a seizure. The breath rushing up and down his throat was loud like a gale.

Then in a moment he lay beside her, as though he had fallen, his eyes shut, his windy mouth at her ear. He seemed far more exhausted than any of the motions seemed to account for.

"Are you all right?" she asked.

He opened his eyes. He was breathing more softly, his mouth closed now. His face looked like a little boy's, she thought. She cuddled tenderly near him, and embraced his sweatiness. He caressed her spiritlessly. It took a long time for his breath to come back. The moon no longer shone at the window, having risen too high, or behind clouds, but her eyes were fairly accustomed to the darkness.

She drew the quilts up over Leslie and herself, and lay near him. She caressed his hands, and his body. She found that hair grew around his navel.

After a while he said he had better get back to the attic, because the innkeeper would begin to suspect where he was. It had not occurred to her that he would have to leave. He said the innkeeper was a blue-nosed young snoop, who prided himself on the family atmosphere.

He sat up and found his pajamas. She watched him stand and put them on. She remained bare under the quilts. He put on the bathrobe and fastened it, and then retrieved her crumpled wooly underdrawers from the bedclothes.

"Can I keep these, for a memento?" he asked.

He was holding them up, bunched in his hand.

"Wouldn't you rather I washed them first?"

"Nope. Just as they are." His hand pressed the crushed cloth to his nose and mouth, and she didn't know if he kissed it or inhaled. Above it his eyes closed briefly and smiled. Then he stuffed it into the pocket of his bathrobe.

He unlatched the door, and stood a long time with it open a crack, while he watched for a chance to leave unseen. By the light of the hall she could see the familiar dull blue-green of the drawers hanging from his pocket, and the colors of the quilting she had drawn to her face. Then suddenly he slipped out, shutting the door behind him and leaving her in darkness.

41

The rubbings and stimulations, while they went on, had been as delightful as she had anticipated, quite up to expectations, both in his preparatory love-making and at last in their union itself, and she could have wished for it to continue and continue. The resting afterward was agreeable too, but after he left she began to have moments of uneasiness that kept recurring.

Making the bed again and putting on her pajamas and going to the bathroom were vaguely a letdown, something like the debris and sweepings of a party. It crossed her mind, lying there, that if Les were in a private room, instead of that unpartitioned attic full of boys' bunks, she would go to his bed now, and slip under the blankets beside him, so that he might talk to her, or hold her hand.

In the morning it was Les who woke her. The day was bright, and he came to her in ski clothes and kissed her in her brown pajamas. There had been no one in the corridor, he said, so he had slipped into her room. "Well, you better slip right out again," she said. "You'll get caught." He replied that it was a decent hour. They could walk out of the room both dressed, to go down to breakfast, and it would appear as though he had called for her. But she refused. She would not let him watch her dress, and made him go to wait downstairs. She put his hands off her pajamas and even pushed him somewhat to help him out the door. "I still have some modesty left," she said. "You have to break me in more gradually."

At their breakfast table for a while she felt quite left out of all the ski talk, though Les entered into it with the other people as though he were scarcely with her. But when the pancakes came, and he smiled and poured syrup on hers, she feared he was too attentive and that the others would notice.

She was thinking during breakfast that she would go up the mountain and see how the view was on such a clear day. She hoped Les would accompany her, but she did not like to ask him, and when it appeared that he was planning to go off and ski by himself she lost heart and went to the class instead.

Once in the class, however, the cold and sunshine and exercise revived her spirits. The gleaming snow, fresh and deep, was as though the world had been made clean.

But later, in the dingy little railroad station with Les, she found herself wondering what he was thinking. There was somehow a lack of conversation. I was someone he didn't have to bring to New Hampshire, but now I'm someone he has to take back to Boston, she thought.

She bought a lot of newspapers and news magazines.

The train was three-quarters empty. She had the window seat again. She began to read, feeling ill at ease, and expecting long silences. But Les spoke to her, quietly, amid the click of the rails. He said that if you got interested in skiing you watched the weather and the reports of conditions day by day, even when you couldn't get away, and you were happy when it snowed. The winter ended too soon. And your changed attitude toward the winter changed your view of the entire year—instead of that dreary low point you saw four seasons full of various joys, and the summer's shortness no longer saddened you. Even if he became a rich doctor he would take his winter vacations in the north, where winter was not just the absence of summer.

He found her hand, and held her thumb. She watched the passing scenery with him, a dull-red barn, and then a black-and-white forest rising up a hill.

He remarked that his friends the Mahadys, the couple who had given the spaghetti supper she had been unable to go to, would be away for the next few months, and that he would have the use of their apartment. Mahady was going to teach a semester in Buffalo.

Millicent began to color, and withdrew her hand.

"Now Les," she said, "just a minute. We've just got to have a talk."

"What do you mean?"

"I don't want you to have an apartment. I think you're assuming much too much, and it's just a little highhanded of you."

"Now, wait a minute," he said, and she heard the smile in his voice. "This deal was arranged long before last night. It's got nothing to do with you."

She reddened darker. "I'm sorry," she apologized. "I just meant—" She became silent.

She felt gauche.

He explained the terms of the sublet. The rent was very cheap. Many interns had places of their own, for their nights not on call, in which they could entertain or just get away from the hospital atmosphere, and it would give him a chance to live in dignity for a few months. He felt it was such a bargain that he'd have been a fool not to take it. Of course his mother had fussed when he wrote her of it, but he had written back that it would give her a place to stay when she visited, so that there would be some saving. He said he was getting tired of the way he lived. In June he'd go into the Army for two years, and before he had any enjoyment out of life his youth would be gone. He had almost not taken the ski weekend because of the apartment, but then had decided to do both.

She felt more foolish than ever. She said she supposed he had done right to take the apartment, under the circumstances. She asked where it was. He mentioned the street, down the hind part of Beacon Hill, toward the West End, where it began to be slummy. It was handy to the hospital.

He took her hand, and she began to feel confused again. She stared at the soiled woven straw of the empty seat before them, uncertain how to say what she wished. She sighed.

"Les," she began finally, "about last night—"

She paused. She felt him waiting for the rest of the sentence. She took her hand from him, on the excuse of scratching her other hand. She pushed a lock of hair in place.

"What about last night?" he said.

"Well, I don't want you to start getting any ideas. I mean, that we're going to have an affair, or anything like that. I mean, I'm not your mistress, just because I happened to get carried away—one lapse. I haven't changed my views just because of a weakness one time—"

"I don't see it as a weakness. I think you rose to the situation magnificently. With courage. I mean it. I'm proud of you, baby."

"Don't call me baby."

"I'm sorry."

She reopened one of the magazines on her lap and closed it.

"Another thing," she said. "I'd like to know how you just happened to have those devices along. Especially since the trip was supposed to be on my terms." Her voice quavered.

She didn't look at him, but she could almost hear the tone of a shrug in his voice. "I just did," he said. "I don't know."

She tried to read, but the motion of the train made it uncomfortable. She did not know what attitude she wanted to display toward him—aloofness or something else. He asked for the loan of a magazine, and then she felt that her forgetting to offer him one had betrayed her nervousness.

The ride was long. After a while he made neutral conversation, which she welcomed, first about items that he read, and then about a patient at the hospital.

"Les," she said after a time. "You really can't afford an apartment, I don't care how cheap. I agree with your mother. You only get twenty-five a month."

"Well, I only pay half."

"Half?"

"I'll give him the rest when I'm in the Army. And I've got a little dough socked away my mother doesn't know about. I give blood every two months. A paid donor. Twenty-five a pint. It helps, believe me."

"Is that good for you? Every two months?"

"The body replaces it. I've done it for years."

At North Station he offered to have supper with her at one of the counters off the concourse, but she took her valise from him, saying she wanted to get to her apartment as soon as possible and get out of her ski clothes. She went home by subway.

Her roommates greeted her warmly. She drew a bath.

"Well, did you lose it in the mountains?" Ella Jane asked afterward, her voice soft and slightly musical, while Millicent stood in her bathrobe warming a pot of soup. Ella Jane was in a robe too, and her good leg and her bad one were over the arm of the stuffed chair. Millicent decided not to answer. She kept stirring the soup. But both her roommates kept watching her and waiting for the answer, so that she reddened.

"If I did I wouldn't tell you," she said, with some sourness, not looking from the soup.

"Well, in case you did," said Ella Jane in the same gentle voice, "congratulations."

Natalie, wearing slacks and straddling one of the small chairs backwards, did not take her eyes from Millicent. She seemed to twinkle with amusement.

"Don't feel badly," Ella Jane added. "There's nothing you'll be needing it for."

Millicent felt like slamming the kitchen door to shut off their view of her. But she knew it would make them laugh. She poured the soup into a bowl and brought it to the drop-leaf table.

"Anyway how was skiing?" said Natalie.

"Fine," she said.

In the morning her mother phoned to ask if she had gotten back safely without any skiing accidents, and also if she were planning to come home for her days off. Millicent said she wasn't planning on it.

At work her mind kept wandering. She wanted to understand more clearly what the possibilities were regarding the future of her friendship with Les. She felt she would like their New Hampshire episode to be something intimate and remembered, but put aside and not repeated. But she had a feeling that such a course would lead to the same old dismal bickering. She wondered if he now had a proprietary feeling. It even occurred to her to dodge the unacceptable alternatives by breaking off with him at once. But then breaking off seemed the stupidest course of all. It was not only stupid in itself, but it made the New Hampshire trip stupid in retrospect.

The next day was one of her days off. Les phoned, saying that he was going to move in that evening, and asked if she would like to come over and help. She refused, making the excuse that Ella Jane and Natalie were expecting a girl friend from Chicopee and she wanted to help entertain.

"They don't need you, do they?" he said.

"Well, I ought to be here," she told him. "I'll come and see your place sometime after you're settled."

She spent the afternoon shopping for a housewarming gift. At last she chose a small barometer, trimmed with brass and polished wood, in the same store where she had bought the binoculars for Charles.

The shopping gave her an eagerness to see his apartment, and improved her mood.

When the day was turning dark and cold she returned to her own apartment, carrying Leslie's barometer gift-wrapped. A flurry of tiny snowflakes blew in the night air.

The girl from Chicopee had already arrived, and was unpacking her things in the middle of the floor and talking in a plaintive voice. Millicent was introduced, and then she put her package on the mantelpiece and unbuttoned her coat. The girl was short and dark-haired and somewhat plump, and her name was Barbie Chisholm.

The girl squeezed her things into drawers and closets where Natalie and Ella Jane made room, and Millicent pressed things down and made room for her also.

The four had supper together, with the leaves of the table spread out. Barbie sounded depressed, but she was talkative, and it was interesting to have someone new around with new problems.

"You should be analyzed," Ella Jane told her.

"I know it, but I can't afford it," said Barbie.

Apparently she had known Natalie since earliest childhood, and she and Natalie talked a lot about people they knew in common. Barbie had some hard-luck stories about jobs. She had taken a course for airline hostesses but had not been placed. She had tried New York for a few weeks but had found it horribly lonesome, and had run out of money. She thought now she would study to be a dental assistant. She felt terribly in the way, and promised she would leave as soon as she had a job and was on her feet.

"You won't be in the way," Millicent assured her. "Please don't think that. It's awfully hard to get started. Everybody has a hard time. Especially if you're a woman."

"Well, you tell me if I get in the way."

"You're not in the way," Millicent said. "Not as far as I'm concerned."

During the evening Barbie was greatly impressed on learning that Millicent worked for a newspaper. "Really?" she squealed. Millicent explained that she was only a copy boy, but Barbie was still impressed, and confided to Millicent that she wrote poetry sometimes. They remained talking until one in the morning, though Ella Jane had gone to bed earlier. Barbie fetched some of her poems for Millicent to read. "Do you think you could get it printed?" she asked. "They use poems on the editorial page."

"Gee—I don't know—" Millicent said, studying a typewritten page.

"It can't hurt to try," said Barbie. "You could show it to them."

After a while they removed the goggle-eyed stuffed dog and Natalie helped take the long cushion off the studio couch, and make it up with bedding for Barbie to sleep on. Again Barbie became self-effacing, and did not want to deprive Millicent of her cushion, and offered to sleep on a blanket spread on the bare rug, but Millicent insisted.

Barbie fell asleep quickly. Her breathing was very heavy. But Millicent lay awake on the cushionless couch, and when she dozed it was not for long. She could feel every spring, and in one place she could feel a slat. It occurred to her that while Barbie stayed here she might use Leslie's place during his nights on call. When he was on call he presumably had to sleep at the hospital, even though he had an apartment. And his apartment must be vacant on those nights, while it was so crowded here. She lay calculating when he was on call and when he was not.

Barbie went out job-hunting in the morning and Millicent lent her two dollars. Millicent left a message with the hospital switchboard for Les, and when he phoned back in late afternoon she explained her idea. It was agreed that she would meet him in midevening in the hospital cafeteria to pick up the key.

When she explained the plan to the girls and began to pack her valise, Barbie became upset about the studio-couch cushion and offered to go to the Y.W.C.A. But there was explaining and re-explaining, and at last Millicent snapped the valise shut and gave instructions about feeding the cat and put on her coat and her overshoes.

"Behave yourself," Ella Jane said with a little smile.

"I told you he's not there," Millicent answered severely, but coloring somewhat. "If you don't believe me you can come and see for yourself."

"Oh, I believe you," said Ella Jane.

In the hospital cafeteria Leslie's eyes were bloodshot. He seemed for moments on end to forget to make conversation, as though preoccupied. He said he had performed four operations during the day, including one that was far more delicate than any he had been allowed to attempt before. And he had done one without any other surgeon present. He told her to keep the keys as he had another set. He said she could have his apartment every night if she liked, while Barbie was on her hands, because he could sleep at the hospital. But she said no, only when he was on call—he was entitled to enjoy having his own apartment for the first time in his life and she couldn't turn him out.

Toward ten o'clock some female voice, harsh on the speaker system, paged him. Millicent thanked him again and set out with her valise. She felt it was still early enough to be safe to walk. She climbed up a very steep street in a dirty neighborhood. Small groceries, closed for the night, were cut into basements. The tenements were of brick and old, tight together. But she could look down to a view of the hospital's loftiness and lighted windows. She found a narrow entry, the step of which went into the slanting sidewalk like a wedge. A rusted bank of mailboxes was set into the wall. Her key fitted the inner door, and then she carried her valise four flights up a stair well, past stenches of old cooking. Except at the bottom level the bulbs were missing and she guided herself with a hand on the wooden rail. It was dizzying, near the top, to look down over the rail to the dimly lit tile far at the bottom. While she felt for the keyhole of the corner door a skylight blinked with some red glow from the outdoors.

When the door creaked open she set down the valise and found the wall switch. The brightness was cheering after the stairs, even though the room was quite unpretentious. A big convertible sofa near her had been unfolded to make a wide bed, and its sheets and blankets were still mussed from Leslie's having slept in them. Along one wall the Mahadys had made a bookcase by resting unpainted boards upon bricks. There was a table with an enamel top, and a couple of wooden chairs repainted a pale blue. A big oval rug of coarse yarn was partly under the extended sofa bed. The wall toward the street slanted a little, except for two dormers cut into it, each with a tall window that came nearly to the floor. They had gauze curtains and old green shades, but they needed drapes, she thought. Mrs. Mahady did not seem to have been much of a decorator. The opposite wall had a recess with metal wall cabinets high up, and a sink, gray washtubs, a greasy stove, a stained refrigerator with its motor running, and a wooden counter over drawers. She saw from the dirty cup and saucer that Les had made himself coffee. A black phone sat on the counter, but Les had told her it was disconnected. The room was the entire apartment, except for the bath. The small closet contained an ironing board and a stepladder. There was no closet space for clothes, only a makeshift wardrobe standing in the room, with a flowered curtain. There were no lamps either, only the bulb that made shadows in the unevenness and cracks of the low ceiling. The bathroom was not bad. It was pleasant to see Leslie's things about, the toothbrush and shaving articles. She went back to the valise for the toothbrush and comb she planned to keep here and placed the toothbrush next to Leslie's.

She put the barometer, still in its gift wrapping, on the counter where it would surprise Leslie tomorrow night. She looked in the drawers and the cabinets to decide where she would store the pajamas she meant to keep here. There were folded linens and towels, and shirts and socks and underwear of Leslie's. But some were empty.

She looked at the Mahadys' books, and read in two of the nonmedical ones, sprawled on the bed. It was agreeable to be here.

She made the bed, but without fresh linens, and when the electric clock said one she retired. The wideness of the bed seemed luxuriant. She had never slept in a double bed before. It seemed a remarkable Providence that had provided this apartment, just when Barbie Chisholm had crowded her own.

She slept long, and even after her first awakening she lay dozing. She heard a truck shift gears on the steepness of the hill.

At last, when she was ready to leave, she remade the bed with new linens for Leslie and took the ones she had slept on down to a laundry in the neighborhood. She bought groceries and returned to stock the refrigerator with them. She swept the floor, with a broom and dustpan she found in the bathroom, and left a note for Leslie that smoked fish and cheese had been put away for his Saturday's breakfast. Then she departed.

At the city room later she got a phone call, and took it at Maud's desk. It was Natalie.

"Are you going to sleep at Les's again tonight?" Natalie asked her.

"No. He's not on call tonight. Only when he's on call."

"Oh. Well, listen. I have a date. So if you're home before I am, would you share my bed with Barbie, like a good kid?"

"All right," Millicent said drearily.

"I mean so I can have the living room, okay? And if I'm home first and he's gone before you get there I'll go in with Barbie."

"All right."

"You're sweet."

When she got home Natalie and her young man had not arrived. Ella Jane had gone to bed, and Barbie was sitting naked on the closed toilet cover, massaging herself with olive oil from a can she had found in the kitchen.

"What's that?" said Millicent.

"Olive oil. The best thing for skin."

"Well you better hurry up, before Natalie brings her boy friend up here."

Barbie showered, and got into Natalie's bed beside Millicent. It seemed very narrow, and Millicent clung to the edge. She thought Barbie still had an odor of olive oil, despite the shower. Barbie fell asleep, and the bed became still narrower, because Barbie tossed and thrust legs out. In anger she tried to return Barbie's crowding, but Barbie didn't waken. The tossing continued, and Barbie muttered unintelligibly. "Hey," Millicent said to her. It had no effect.

Barbie kept moving to a diagonal position across the mattress, so that Millicent felt in danger of being pushed to the floor. She sat up. At last she stole the blankets and pillow entirely from Barbie, and wrapped herself up on the floor. But it was far harder than she expected, and hurt her bones. She rose up and woke Barbie, who promised to stay on her own side. They remade the bed. Barbie fell asleep again. Millicent lay on her stomach, clutching the bed frame, and tried to doze. She determined to tell Natalie the dating arrangement could not be used again while there were four in the apartment.

The next day she took her alarm clock to the city room with her, so she could take it along to Leslie's and be waked up in time for Sunday school. As soon as Mr. Hopkins sent her home she found a taxi and went to Leslie's.

She climbed the dark stairs again, holding the ticking clock in her hand, let herself in, and clicked on the light. Leslie turned in the unfolded sofa bed and blinked at her.

"Oh," she said. "Aren't you on call?"

"What?"

She seemed to have waked him. She was flustered.

"Come in," he said. "Sit down." He remained in bed.

She sat in one of the blue chairs without unbuttoning her coat.

"Aren't you on call every other night?"

"Not on my weekends," he said.

"Oh." She hadn't thought of that.

"How could I be on call when I'm off the next day?"

"That's right." She put a hand to her forehead. "I'm stupid. And I woke you up."

"That's all right."

"I'm sorry," she said. "Gee, I don't know, I'm really awfully sorry." She rose and opened the door, putting out the light.

"Hey!" He sprang to her in pajamas and blocked the door with his arm. "Where are you going? You're here. Stay."

"Les, I have my own place. I've got no right waking you up."

"I'm awake now. What's the difference?" He pushed the door shut with his arm. "Is the girl still staying with you, whatsaname?"

"Yes."

"How is it?"

"We manage."

"You don't really want to go back to that mob of girls, do you? How are you gonna get there at this hour?"

"A taxi. The same way I got here."

"On this street? You'll never find one. You'll walk all the way down the hill. And you might not find any there either."

"I'll manage."

"You're staying." He put a hand to her shoulder to turn her from the door but she resisted.

"No, I don't want to stay. Really, Les. It's not the idea."

"Listen," he said. "I'll get out if you want. I'll go back to the hospital. But if you leave I'm leaving too. So you might as well stay."

She was confused.

"Les, I made a mistake, I thought you were on call. Now please go back to bed."

"And let you walk around the streets alone at one in the morning? You'll freeze to death. How cold is it out?"

She didn't answer.

"Is it cold?" he said.

"Yes."

"Take off your coat," he said more gently.

She sat in the chair again but didn't take off her coat. He took the clock from her hand and put it on the counter, winding it.

"Thank you for the barometer," he said.

"Did you like it?" She saw that he had mounted it on the wall, over the sofa back.

"Yes. Very much. Also the fish."

"Oh. That's nothing."

He sat on the bed. "Well," he said, "I'll go back to the hospital if I have to to make you stay."

"No," she said after a moment, "you don't have to." She was not quite looking at him and she was not smiling. She unbuttoned her coat slowly, sitting in the chair. He got back under the covers, far on the further side, and lay with his back to her.

She drew off her boots and placed them by the door. She hung her coat behind the curtain of the wardrobe. Then she clicked on the bathroom light, leaving the bathroom door slightly ajar, and crossed the room again to turn out the main light. By the glow from the bathroom door she fetched her pajamas from the drawer. Leslie still lay on his side, not facing her. She took her pajamas to the bathroom and shut him in darkness.

Before coming out she turned the bathroom light out also. She felt the yarn of the rug under her feet. She got into bed. He lay in the same position, not moving, his back to her. She lay still and straight, her arms crossed upon her bosom, waiting for him. She stared at the pale images of the windows that spread upon the ceiling. Irregularities of the glass put shadows in them.

He came nestling, and in his touch she felt both restraint and urgency. She lay limp while he moved her arms away and opened her pajamas. His hand both warmed and chilled, as if he created the goose flesh he smoothed. She marched her feet to be rid of her pajamas. He half lifted her and rolled with her, hugging her to all the hairiness of his chest and stomach, and she hugged too, feeling the bones inside him. He grew gentle, and his fingers raked her lightly. It was surprising the way they could be so tickling everywhere, even on quite innocent and ordinary parts of her. I'm clothed in your hands, she thought of saying. I'm not wearing anything but you. But she didn't say it.

"Les," she said.

He neither paused nor answered.

"You fill up my skin," she said. "Your fingers are magic."

His lips kissed her lightly.

"This must be what the clay feels like," she added, "when God shapes a person."

More and more he rubbed her roundnesses and creases, the smooth, soft, pliable belly and the converging furriness. His embrace wallowed.

She tried to match his moods. He would grow still for long periods, as though resting in her flesh, and would then grow agitated, so that she arched up into his squirming ballet.

"That's good," he said. "Do your share, don't let it just happen to you."

Again he would grow still, but his continuing clutch and an occasional fitful stirring deep within her told her he was not calm. Many times her heart raced wildly. It all took a very long time.

At last his exhaustion came. They lay a while holding hands. In the scant gray glow from the windows she could see his closed eyes, and the sweat on his forehead. After some minutes he spoke, and told her a patient had died under his knife that morning.

She didn't know what she could say in sympathy. She remained silent, holding his hand. After a while he asked if she could come here every night, at least while the extra girl was at her place.

"No, I don't think so, Les. That wouldn't be good. Sex every night."

"It wouldn't be every night. It couldn't. For one thing I'm on call every other night. Except my weekends."

"No," she said. "If you don't mind I'll skip it. It's one thing when things happen spontaneously, or by accident. But deliberately spending the night is something else. And anyway I don't want to keep coming in and waking you up like tonight."

"You could come in quietly and probably never wake me."

"No. I'd get here late and you have to be on duty before seven."

"The bed's wide. It's made for two."

She made no answer. But in a moment she began to talk of all the things she planned to do in the apartment day by day. She wanted to clean the stove and refrigerator, wax the floor, and scrub the green from the bathtub and the sink, and wash the bath mat, which was caked with dust. She would put up drapes, and get a bedspread to match. The tile of the bathroom floor was filthy. And on her evenings off she would come here and cook him a good dinner.

"I'd rather have sex than a dinner," he said.

"The dinner's for your health."

"So's sex," he said. "Emotional health affects the whole organism."

He extended an arm toward her. It was thin, and in the darkened room quite pale, but shaped by its muscles and veins. She lay on her side, cradled in his arm, and let her fingers enjoy the warmth of his sunken belly. She traced his ribs.

His caresses grew intimate again, and she was surprised to find that his eager tautness had already renewed itself. There was contagion and warmth in his excitement.

This time it did not take as long. He even swung her above him, but his fierce probing still rose like thumps. She felt a soreness, but then it was drowned in an intoxication that surpassed the other time. "Oh dear," she gasped.

They lay apart. She flung a hand to him. He took it. With her other hand she pulled up the blanket and spread it over them.

"I suppose it's like a new toy," she said. "We'll tire of it."

He kept breathing.

"I have to get up in the morning and teach Sunday school," she said.

He just lay and breathed.

"I better make sure I set the alarm," she said. She got out of bed without putting anything on, and pattered across to the counter.

The room had turned cold. She squinted closely at the clock in the darkness, turning it toward the windows. It was in fact set, from a previous time, but it needed winding. When she finished she hurried to the bed and snuggled next to Leslie's warmth.

But she was chilly even so, whenever her body did not touch him, and before she slept she had to put on pajamas.

She was awakened in the early daylight not by the alarm but by the clang of steam in the radiator. She lay a while listening to it. Leslie still slept. Then she rose, shut off the alarm clock, that it might not disturb Les later, and gathered up her clothes, and took a bath, trying to run the water slowly behind the closed door so as not to wake him.

But afterward, when she stood combing her hair at the spotted bathroom mirror, he appeared behind her, in his rumpled yellow pajamas. He embraced the pieces of underwear she had put on, clutching and lifting in his fond way, and the skin between. She kept combing. He kissed her neck and her ear, his nose and mouth losing themselves in her hair. She turned her head aside, still combing as best she could. His fingers went to the elastic ends that met at her backbone.

"Don't unhook my bra," she said.

"I'll be your bra."

She turned, collaborating in his embrace, and rested her face against his jaw and shoulder. His pressing warm hands chased each other over her flesh, making cozy friction. She leaned into him. For a while he kneaded her buttocks like dough, pants and all. The pants became squashed like a rope about her thighs and he squeezed her harder, as if they both would occupy one and the same space. It was like a motionless fury inside him.

"Again?" she asked.

"I have to," he said huskily. "I'll explode."

She ran with him, leaving the two pieces of underwear in a trail from the bathroom, and flung herself with him onto the wrinkled sheets.

"It's my fault too," she said to him. "I don't even try to stop you, do I."

She saw it all this time. They had no blankets or sheets upon them. The radiator was hissing, by fits and starts. Leslie paused, without extricating himself from her, to remove his pajamas. She helped him get rid of them.

She had time to look at the electric clock on the wall and calculate how much time she had to catch her train. She saw that the frost on the windows was yellow now in the sun. She tried cautiously to knead his buttocks, as he had done to her, but he was hairy and sweaty.

"Is it fun to be a beautiful woman?" he asked afterward when they lay resting. He was fingering her belly idly.

She laughed. It was an average, conversational kind of laugh, but she felt it to be utterly spontaneous and pleasant.

"You have the sweetest little figure I ever saw," he said. "Even in my dreams.

It's full of life, somehow." He was propped on an elbow, smiling at her. "You have no idea how cute you are with nothing on."

She did not mind that he sat on the bed and watched her dress.

"Come back tonight," he said. "After work."

"Well, I don't know, Les. I'd rather wait until tomorrow, when you're on call. You know how it is. We get excited, and we don't exercise any restraint at all."

"Tonight there'll be restraint. You've got nothing to worry about. I haven't got any sperm left."

She had straightened her skirt and sweater and taken her coat from the chair. She buttoned it without smiling.

"Come on," he said.

"I'm not promising. I'll think about it."

He crouched naked on the floor and helped her with her boots.

She was at North Station barely in time for the train. It was only when she had boarded it that she realized she was hungry and had had no breakfast.

She taught Sunday school, and rode from the temple to the house with her father and Roland. During dinner her mother asked about the place where she had skied, and the inn, and whether she had met any interesting people there. Millicent replied in a general way, about the various age groups and types of people.

She left for Boston early, and changed clothes at her own apartment and fed Theodore before going to the city room.

After work she took a cab to Leslie's again. It had begun to snow.

She saw a crack of light under his door, and she found him reading in bed. From a photograph on the page she knew it was a medical text.

"You're supposed to be asleep," she said.

She undressed in the bathroom. When she came out in pajamas he folded his glasses. He put the book on the floor and the glasses on top of it. She turned out the light.

"Now tonight we're going to exercise restraint," she said as she got into bed. "You stay on your side and I'll stay on my side. We've had enough love-making to last us a while."

She curled up on her side, away from him.

"No good-night kiss?" he said in the darkness.

"It's not necessary," she said. But she changed her mind and gave him a quick kiss, and then curled away again. "Now go to sleep," she said.

She closed her eyes, and tried to relax her face, and her hands, and her arms. He changed position. She heard it, and felt it in the springs.

"Let's don't exercise restraint," he said.

"Now listen," she said, without changing position. "You promised."

"Did I?"

"Yes. And I'm holding you to your promise, Leslie Hollander."

"When did I promise that?"

She felt his hand upon her behind, which was firm because of the way her legs were drawn up.

"Les," she said without turning, "did it ever occur to you that you're old enough to control your passions?" She caught his hand by the wrist and removed it from her. "Don't be such a roué. It's time to go to sleep."

He rolled away from her, and she knew it again by the feel of the mattress and sound of the sheets.

"You know when you'll be master of your passions?" he asked, as though addressing the ceiling. "When your passions serve your pleasure."

"Now really, Les," she said more gently. "Let's not discuss it any more."

"I mean it," he said. "That's when you'll really be the master of your passions—when you make them serve your pleasure. Not while you're afraid to go near them."

"Les, you have to get your sleep. You have responsibilities. You have to be on the wards in a few hours. With people's lives in your hands."

She was sorry she had said that. It would remind him of his patient who died.

They were silent.

She heard distant fire engines.

Occasionally he stirred.

She heard him sigh. "I could fall asleep a lot more readily if we had some sex first," he said. "I'm just lying here wanting you."

"I thought you didn't have any sperm left."

"Well, I wouldn't have thought so. But apparently I'm tapping unknown reserves."

"Just try to relax. Think about something peaceful, like flowers in a field."

"I can't."

"Well, you make an honest effort to fall asleep. I don't think you've made an effort. At least really try first. And then if you can't, you let me know."

42

The Sabbath morning attendance was so bad that Ed decided to skip the sermon. He had had to delay the start of the service while someone went out to find another man, and he felt that the few who did come were entitled to have it over with as soon as possible. No women had shown up, except Patty, and she had to prepare the after-service snacks at the seminar table in the library all by herself. While the service was still on he heard her bust something back there, a glass or a plate.

Afterward, when the small group repaired to the refreshment table and Ed poured the wine and said the blessing, squat little Mr. Brill began to bait and heckle him, saying again that there was nobody upstairs and nothing there. "Tell me, rabbi," he said in his thick raspy accent, "what's the purpose, that He makes a boy that a boy should have a foreskin, that it's supposed to be cut off from there? He doesn't want it, He says cut it off, so what does He make it in the first place?" He shrugged, staring about at everyone, to give force to his question. "Or a baby should suffer pain in teething. Why? An infant, to suffer already, for nothing. You say a God, everything is a purpose, a plan, a design. So what's the purpose, a baby's teeth should hurt him. His hair don't hurt him. His fingernails don't hurt him. But his teeth should hurt him, he should cry. For why?"

"Well, evolution isn't finished yet," Ed told him.

"Evolution isn't finished yet," Brill repeated. "You think there's justice in the world?"

"We're not given to know these things," white-haired Mr. Resnick said to Brill.

"No, we're not given to know," Brill said. "You know why we're not given to know? Because it would make such a scandal if it came out. Sure. That's why He keeps it covered up."

"Go on, you're crazy," Resnick said to him.

"No, I'm not crazy. I looked into it."

"You're here," Resnick said. "You're in a shul. In your heart you believe in God. Or you wouldn't come here."

"Nah. I don't believe in God. I wouldn't give Him the satisfaction. When I look in the newspaper I couldn't believe in a God. It would get me too aggravated."

Resnick glanced at Ed with resignation. "Never mind us," he said to Ed. "Go after the children."

Ed was already putting on his overcoat and helping Patty with hers.

"So why do you come here?" Resnick said to Brill.

"I'm a retired man—where should I go?" said Brill. "It's cold. I sit in the house, already I'm in the way."

Ed and Patty descended the icy steps carefully and went down the shoveled walk, between embankments of old snow. Brill tagged along with them.

"That's right, tell it to the children, there's a God in heaven," said Brill.

On Muckanaug Street they turned toward Murphy Square. Ed was wearing his new fur cap, which he had gotten at Rogers Peet, and which he had heard a couple of the ladies in the congregation did not like on him. Patty had a long dangling scarf that alternated white and green.

"I'll tell you something—God gives me a pain in the ass," Brill said in his phlegmy voice.

"All right, He gives me a pain in the ass too," Ed said, even though Patty was along. "He gave Job a pain in the ass. He gave Jonah a pain in the ass. Who are you, somebody special?"

"All right, it's no joke," said Brill.

"All right, it's no joke," said Ed.

"It's no joke," Brill said again. "It's no joke all right. I can see why the goyim wanted a younger man, some New Blood already. Because if God had to run for re-election He couldn't get elected. The Jewish vote He lost already."

At the next corner Brill turned off to go toward his son's house. "Take care of yourself," Ed said to him. He crossed the street and continued with Patty across the common. A path beaten in the snow had grown dirty and hard. When the path narrowed they walked single file, Patty first.

"Mr. Brill has a point, though," Patty said. "I mean, how can anybody say definitely there's a God? Maybe there is just nothing."

"Well, when I look around me, I don't see nothing," said Ed. "I see all kinds of things."

Around the Civil War monument the snow was beaten down more, but then their path narrowed again under the bare trees.

"I tried atheism in my youth, like everybody else," he said, "but it was too light for me. Atheism is a paragraph, and you've said it. Religion is volumes. I'm still studying."

At lunch Patty told Lucinda what Mr. Brill had said, and Lucinda said she agreed with Mr. Brill. She too wished that evolution would hurry up and get finished, and that we'd get to the time when people would learn not to make wars.

Ed went upstairs and lay down for a Sabbath nap.

He felt depressed. His project of visiting and consulting with each family had lately grown more and more discouraging. It felt like a queer thing to be doing. Going about trying to get people to do things they didn't want to, and trying to devise all sorts of compromises to get a housewife or a householder to attempt this or that bit of observance. As though they were to do it for him, as a favor. It not only made him uncomfortable, but he felt he was making everyone else uncomfortable.

But could he just let everything slide, without a fight? The clergy was a humiliating occupation.

All they want of you is that you should be a recorder of births, marriages, and deaths. They don't want you to care about scripture, and they don't want you to care about physics and sociology, ancient and modern history, universes and communities. People are provincial, he thought. Their own time and place are the only context they see, and God's all right—He should come once a year like Santa Claus.

He recalled the gloomy feel of doubts he had had in his beginning years, when he had wondered if it were only a matter of trying to get people to play games, of pretending it's some other century. He shouldn't have come here. To be a missionary took a strength he suspected he didn't have.

Bill Prince had been laid up for the past ten days with bronchitis and laryngitis, so that Ed had been teaching twice as many classes. He had thought that Bill's absence would be a good chance to get more laymen of the congregation to lead parts of the service. He said that any man who enjoyed singing in the bathtub could enjoy leading prayers. It would make the service democratic and put life into it. But none could, or would, except the same ones who had done it sometimes before—Mr. Resnick, and Mr. Munk, and Resnick's son-in-law Wisebard. Ed liked Wisebard, who handled the prayer book with fluency and informality. Wisebard would ham it up somewhat, and kid around, and imitate the mannerisms of the older generation as a kind of gag, but Ed didn't mind that. A man ought to have that kind of easy relationship with his religion.

But this morning, when communal worship had nearly come to a halt for lack of interest, he had felt ready to quit and look for another job.

Yesterday he had had an argument with an intense young matron who had refused to send her children to Sunday school. She told him organized religion was for the birds. He had asked her to regard it then simply as a cultural thing, but she had said no—she wasn't going to have her children taught there was a Benevolence taking care of a world full of death camps and nuclear bombs.

At least she wasn't provincial—you had to give her that, Ed thought. He had sat in her living room, trying to argue patiently, until everything seemed to hinge on his point that despite pain, suffering, death, injustice, it was still good that the world had been created. What good there was in the world justified the world's having come into existence. He said that the saddest music still arose out of an ultimate joy in life. And surely she believed that on balance, despite all its defects, it was still better for this world to have come into being than not. She would not, on balance, want it never to have been. So it was quibbling to deny that creation was basically good, or that it could be seen as ultimately beneficent.

But she met him head on. She said it was not good on balance, and that it was pure Pollyanna to say it was good that the world had been created. Hiroshima, Nagasaki, cold war, hot war, Hitler and neo-Hitlers, and there were whole areas of the globe where every child was born into disease, where the average life expectancy was eleven years. Whole tribes in the Andes were literally starving, and rioting between religious communities had killed millions in India. Either he didn't know history or he was blind to the world about him. He lost the argument.

Arguing with women. What a futile thing the clergy had become, if this was now his job.

It occurred to him now, lying in his bedroom, that that same young woman was very busy on a Ban The Bomb committee. So if she really didn't believe it was good that the world had been created, why then was she so anxious to avert its destruction? Why had she borne three children? People talk like atheists, and don't notice that they act like believers. Even while half the people argue that creation had no purpose, all mankind searches for its task.

People condemn God, he thought, and condemn the world, because the world is imperfect. And yet what they're sore at God about, is that they want that God shouldn't condemn the world for its imperfections.

He thought of Brill again. He knew what Brill was so depressed about lately. Brill's favorite niece, whom he loved dearly, was hospitalized with cancer and had had both breasts removed. Ed had known the girl during their childhoods in Dorchester, and had taken her to dances, though he had lost track of her after her marriage and his, and had not even known until Brill spoke of her this past week that she had any connection to Brill.

He gave up trying to nap, and went down to the barn to make sure the dog had been fed.

In the evening Patty had a sweet-sixteen party, even though she wasn't quite sixteen yet. Ed had not been much involved in its preparation, except to borrow some folding chairs and roll up the new rug, which he stored for the time being first in his study and then in Roland's room because Lucinda said the party might overflow into the study. He even offered to be out for the evening, but Patty said she'd just as soon he was in the house, because at Denise Saint-Onge's birthday party some of the boys had tried to spank Denise.

When it was nearly time for guests to arrive, however, Lucinda ran out of mayonnaise and sent him to Sparkstown for some and also for extra bread and soda. There was some snow in the air. He saw some old cars lined up out front when he returned, and saw kids through the lighted windows of the porch and of the projecting bay to the side, and heard girls singing.

"You ain't a lazybones,
You jest a crazybones,
A-dancin' in the stockroom,
A-dancin' down the hall—"

He brought the groceries to the kitchen, and Lucinda told him Patty had asked for a fire. He fetched logs and kindling. The living room was quite full of boys and girls, so that when he knelt at the fireplace many scarcely seemed to notice him. The record player was atop the piano, making music, and here and there girls were singing with it, and some couples were dancing. Two boys joined him and helped him build the fire. He did not know them. But they were soft-spoken and he was impressed by their manners.

When the fire blazed up there was a great shout of young voices, and even some applause.

Ed started out through the French doors, but it occurred to him that the crowd was large enough so that he could remain and watch a few minutes without cramping their style. He turned, but remained near the door as though he might leave any moment. It was nice to watch the kids dance, and see the graceful footsteps of the girls. Patty pleased him, and so did many others. It was curious, he thought, how his congregation could send him into despair, and then how the sight of young girls could revive him. Just to watch was enjoyment. Faces, and petticoat edges.

"I didn't used to date,
I didn't used to rate,
Then bingo-bongo stabbed me through the heart—
I didn't used to coo,
I didn't used to woo,
Then bingo-bongo stabbed me through the heart—
Sta-a-ab me,
Gra-a-ab me—
Hocus pocus bracada-a-ab me—"

The words could not be more frightful, and yet the sound of the young female voices harmonizing together was a delight to the ear. It seemed to him that many of the girls sang to avoid the embarrassment of having to make conversation with boys. Some even sang while they danced.

"Wa-a-ake me,
Ta-a-ake me
All the way to love—"

He slipped out, but came back again. A boy who introduced himself as Robert Houlihan stood with him a while and made some conversation. They talked about the undefeated basketball team. It had beaten Pepperell, Billerica, Squonkamesset Vocational, and Furnaceville Regional. The boy also told him that the town field which people still called the old Pigs Gusset Indian Reservation was going to be flooded for hockey.

"The teacher caught you stealin'
And my Ma will hit the ceilin'
But your smile is so appealin'
That there ain't no use concealin'
That you give me such a feelin'
And I'm ma-a-ad for you—
You're ba-a-d for me—"

Ed left. It wasn't fitting to hang around so much. He got some books from the study and went up to the bedroom. Music and laughter came through the floor and through the heating register, and occasionally there were feet on the stairs. He heard the piano for a while. Later he went down and to the back of the house for another log. Roland was in the kitchen in his pajamas, sampling refreshments.

There was an inch of snow already on the ground, and snow in the bark of the log when Ed brought it in. He wiped his feet, and took the log to the fireplace. Sometimes the girls sang even when no recording was playing. One had only to begin and others would join.

"He's a juvenile delinquent
And I know he's got a knife.
He snitched it off his nanny
For to carve a slice of life.
And we'll go to jail together
'Cause I'm bound to be his wife—"

He saw Patty dancing with a boy named Wernick, whose parents belonged to the temple.

At midnight the snowfall had become heavier, and after consulting with Lucinda he told the boys they had better go and get their cars out before the driving got bad.

The party seemed to have been a success anyhow. Patty was still glowing as she helped clean up. Ed offered to put the rug down, but Lucinda said she would have to vacuum first.

It was quite late when they got into bed. Ed made a pass at Lucinda but she rebuffed him, saying she was tired. He rolled to his own side of the bed and let her alone.

Live joyfully with the wife whom thou lovest, for that is thy portion, for all thy labor under the sun.

He thought about Brill's niece. When a girl you used to feel up in high school has had her breasts removed, you know you're middle-aged.

Then his thoughts went sadly to his twin sister Rosalind, already in her grave. He would rather have lost his brother Franklin or his brother Maxwell than Rosalind.

"Ed," Lucinda said in the darkness.

"What."

"Do you pray for Charles in your prayers, when you say all those prayers?"

"No."

"Why not?"

"Well, I don't feel a prayer is that kind of thing. It's devotional. It's not like a mail-order proposition. Charles is on my mind all the time."

"I'm the atheist in this shebang," she said, "and I'm the only one that's praying for Charles." She drew a long sigh. "I don't know what you're wasting all those prayers on, if you're not even mentioning him."

"Okay, I'll work him in."

He heard her move in the sheets, as though she could not find the right position in which to settle for sleep. Far off he could hear a snowplow, somewhere down on Massapeequit Road, working in the night.

When Lucinda spoke again her voice was different. It was low, and sounded timid. "The Chinese torture prisoners," she said. "Did you know that?"

"Where did you hear that?"

"In the paper."

"Well," he said, "no Air Force mechanic ever got taken prisoner."

"And what about napalm—the liquid fire they fight with now?"

"We have the napalm. The Chinese don't have it."

Her small sigh was audible against the sheet. "I hope not."

She was quiet only a little while.

"Do you think they could be out flying in this?" she said.

"At night? In snow?"

"Don't they have to train in all kinds of conditions?"

"He's ground crew anyway. He's a mechanic."

Her breathing was deep and irregular. "But don't the mechanics have to take the broken planes up and test them? To see why they don't fly right?"

"No."

"Are you sure?"

"Positive. And anyway how do you know it's snowing at Griffiss Field, just because it's snowing here?"

"It must snow there sometime."

"Well, that's true. But right now, at this hour, he's safe in bed. In a nice warm barracks."

They listened to the snowplow.

"If you want to worry," Ed said, "worry that he does his job right. So no other boy is hurt because of his mistake."

"You're callous."

"Why? What's callous about that?"

But he put an arm about her to comfort her, and she hunched near him. He played slowly with her hair. The wind was gusty at times and he could feel it sway the house a little. He heard Lucinda swallow saliva.

She seemed to be falling asleep, and he lay listening to the wind. He could hear a mouse in the wall. Charles was still at Griffiss Field, but the outfit was alerted and there were to be no more passes. Charles had written that after his discharge, or maybe after more schooling, he might look for some good part of the country in which to set up an air-taxi service. There would be discharged ex-pilots looking for someone to employ them, and he would do the maintenance. You made money by having people work for you. Maybe he would continue his schooling at night.

The family would scatter, Ed thought, like every family. It was too bad.

Families dissolve. Now you were alive, now there was a family, a brief thing.

His parents had had cousins whom they used to visit, and on whom they used to pay condolence calls, but the children of the cousins did not know one another's names now, and had forgotten their common ancestor. He had heard much of his grandfather's father—his sense of the past didn't come from nowhere. And he was one of the great-grandchildren, glad to be one, yet he did not even know all the rest of the great-grandchildren. He did not know in what regions they lived, who they were, or even what their religions were.

How scattered Lucinda's family was. The three sisters—Lucinda, Celeste, Gwendolyn—were still close, but the only brother had gone to the Canal Zone and thence to El Paso, where he had a wife called Pegeen. Grandma Annie's sister was in Chicago, one of her brothers had removed years ago to Hollywood with connections that never panned out, and the other two brothers had gone to the penitentiary together and one had died there. Lucinda's uncles had been fences for scrap-metal thieves. The sons and daughters of the jailbirds had turned out to be among the most respectable members of the family, as it happened, but Lucinda scarcely knew them. His own family was on the whole better than Lucinda's, he thought, though every bit as scattered. It had no jailbirds, so far as he knew, and he had had an uncle in the Massachusetts legislature for years. Only one of his cousins had been in a mental institution, to three of Lucinda's. Some cousin of his mother's, one of a family of nine, was supposed to have become a prostitute in Montreal, but a second cousin on his father's side was a brigadier general in the Pentagon, and a more distant cousin through his father's mother was said to have invented the basic chemical process which underlay all the new synthetic fibers. Rosalind had years ago talked to the old folks and worked out the relationship. So what. He didn't know those people.

Your mother's relatives, your father's relatives. You have relatives who are not relatives of one another, and your relatives have other relatives who are no relation to you. And each relative has a different set of in-laws, with whole other connections. Its multiplication embraces the world. You make the acquaintance of still other relatives at funerals, in houses of mourning, so every time you lose one you gain some. You're born endowed with introductions, with an army. Who can keep track of relatives?

You're born in one family—you die in another. In old age a man has a family that never knew the family he remembers. You can't go through life with those you loved in your youth.

He saw how it was with his grandfather. A very old man—one day a daughter tells him of the death in an old-age home of his last sister, an old childless sister, whom he had still used to write to—and he cries.

Man's preoccupation is permanence, Ed thought, to defeat death, but God's concern is evolution. Its flux and waste. You come into the world loved—you go out of it less so. Maybe He thinks if He can keep us in ferment long enough we may produce something of excellence. Man is conservative, God is radical.

It was too bad, he thought, that Rosalind had never done a portrait of their grandfather. She had done their grandmother, at the round oak dining table, and Ed's own children. That same dining table that he and his sister had used to run around and be chased off of. The priceless, unappreciated antiques that had been in that house. Only Rosalind had had the wit to save a few knickknacks, and Maxwell's wife probably now had those. Someday you're the last to remember certain people fondly. Grandchildren will wonder who those yellowed snapshots were. Gone, like the little girl's hair, and the sunsets of Abbottsford.

He heard the clock downstairs chime three, and fell off to sleep.

Roland's arising woke him before it was fully light. Lucinda sat up too. "That kid's not going out in this weather," she said. She called Roland.

He didn't answer, but they still heard noises. Ed went down, followed by Lucinda, and they found Roland in the kitchen, buttoned up for the storm and pulling on his boots. Snow was flying past the windows in the half daylight. Lucinda told Roland angrily he was crazy and that nobody expected him to deliver papers in a blizzard like that, and Lucinda and Roland got into an argument, the boy pleading, while Ed watched silently. Lucinda said no other boys would be out, and Roland said they would. He said he had no business having a route if he didn't show up. Lucinda said she would phone his boss and tell him a thing or two, but Roland burst almost into tears, pulling her from the kitchen wall phone and begging her not to. Ed felt for him. It seemed plain that as Roland saw it his reliability, his integrity was at stake.

"Look," Ed said to him, "it's not the United States mail, after all. Why don't you phone your customers and explain to them you couldn't make it? You'll bring them later."

"Yes," said Lucinda.

"No!" said Roland. He looked desperate and his eyes were moist.

"Well, all right, look," Ed said to Lucinda, "I'll go with him, okay? To see that he doesn't get lost in the snow, and we'll get done faster. I'll help him."

"In the car?" said Lucinda.

"On foot. How would I get the car out?"

She seemed confused by this betrayal, but Roland looked relieved. She put out her hands in a gesture of exasperation. "You're crazy too," she said.

Ed went upstairs and dressed quickly. He came down and got into his outer things without having said his prayers.

The wind was fierce. They made their way to the barn in snow that reached in places to Ed's knees, though for a stretch between the house and barn it had been blown away clear to the ground. Roland got the sled with sides, that had been loaned him for the Sunday papers. The dog was lying on a rag pile and Roland put a blanket over him. It seemed to Ed that the dog smelled.

They hauled the empty sled in deep soft snow, but could not see their curved driveway or even guess exactly where it was. Each step was a kind of plunge, and quickly made Ed warm and breathless. He had not realized it was quite this bad. Sometimes the high ground under the snow disappeared and his foot sank lower than he expected. Great cold galaxies of dry snow dust went spinning and rollicking over the undulating field.

At Massapeequit Road they climbed over the high ridge left by the plow. Ed dragged the sled up and let it down. Snow beat in their faces, collecting in every groove of their hats and scarves, and they could not look into the wind. They walked backwards up the middle of the road. He wondered if Millicent's train would be late, and in the next instant he realized Sunday school would have to be called off in such a storm anyhow. Ed saw the snow lying on the planes of the house roof, its porch and the attic gable and the lower roof of the kitchen, and on the roof of the barn. The scrub woods behind were filling and transformed. The snow did not seem just to lie along twigs and branches—the whole woods seemed to have been turned over and immersed in it. There was nothing there that was not some shade of white. As they retreated the woods grew dimmer behind the turmoil of flakes, but he saw the whiteness swept from the nearer plane of barn roof by a gust, leaving it black except for strewn ripples. Then all the snow dust still on it turned around like a wheel, billowing up, and was gone. He could almost see the air currents as flakes poured up over the ridge of roof.

As they approached Murphy Square the storm grew worse, until they could scarcely see two houses away. The air seemed exploding, and the roaring of wind rose and softened and heightened again. The world was in a cloud of paleness that purged it of people and of color, and made familiar corners hard to recognize. The white had no brightness, but the grays were made alive by the busy thick air.

They found Roland's papers tied with ropes, half buried against the locked door of Yerxa's Pharmacy. Roland had a knife and they loaded the sled, their red wet faces breathing hard, and they did not speak. Ed had begun to expect and hope that the bundle of papers would not have been brought, but apparently the main roads had been kept plowed. They tucked the papers under a piece of canvas.

Their load followed them easily on the slippery street, and the wind was at their backs for a while. The route lay among the hills beyond Caleb Folger's end of the Square, where the town rose among new houses before the long slope down again toward Wilmerding Mills. They stopped frequently, both of them making deliveries and Roland giving instructions as to what paper went to what house. Ed labored. Roland still got into mischief, he thought, and this past week had blown his trumpet loud into a girl's ear at the orchestra rehearsal, so that her ear rang all the next day and her parents complained, but basically he was serious-minded, a marvelous child. Despite all his interests his schoolwork had not suffered. He was possibly even more of a student than Millicent had been.

They went up a side street that was still unplowed. The sled sank on its runners, not riding on the snow like an Eskimo sledge, and spilled over. They righted it, and straightened the papers, but at the first tug the sled spilled over on the other side. They fixed it again, and Ed resolved to keep it straight by pulling the rope higher on whichever side sagged. But it spilled again.

"You walk behind it and steady it," Ed said, "and I'll pull."

They tried that, but before they got started a paper blew apart, its sections tumbling in the air, and the open comic section plastered itself high against the side of a house, growing wet. Roland said it was a good thing it was a Post, as he could call that copy his own. The wind was worse here, perhaps because the street was more exposed. The gale roared over snow dunes, lifting and spinning powderlike flames of white. Clouds of fine white dust blew smokily down from trees and roofs, strands of it pulling apart and spreading in the air like primordial gases photographed by an astronomer. The houses were set further back here and did not have porches. Roland said the papers would have to be tucked into storm doors, if they were unlocked. "If it were daily papers I'd teach you how to fold them," Roland said, "but the Sunday ones can't be folded." Ed pulled the sled, Roland pushed.

"Let's rest a minute," Ed said.

Roland nodded, his lips parted. They stood unsheltered in the storm. Ed noticed that a little distance behind them their deep wake had already begun to fill and smooth again. Roland pointed with his mitten to a certain brick house and said they would not deliver there until later, as they would pass this way again on the way back, and he wanted that house to be the last on the street to get its paper. And in summer he always threw the paper there in such a way as to belly in the screen door and ruin it. Because the guy there was a louse.

"What do you want to be when you grow up?" Ed asked him.

"I still haven't decided," Roland said.

"How about President of the United States?"

" 'That's a joke, son,' " said Roland.

"Well, who knows?" said Ed. "It's possible."

"How much does the President get?"

"It's a hundred thousand a year, I think."

"How much is that a week?"

"Well, fifty weeks into a hundred—figure it out. It's about two thousand a week, I guess."

"Does he have to pay the Cabinet out of that?"

"No."

"Well, there's things I'd rather be. Come on, we have to get going."

He directed Ed with a certain paper to a certain house and told him to look for money under the mat there.

Ed struggled. There were drifts in the front yard, with curves of mathematical beauty, and the wind that had made them came upon him from the side. The stairs that led up to the door were completely enclosed in a simple bulge of white, with no hint of each separate step, and it was hard to find his footing when he climbed. But he saw drifts molded about the corners of the house and garage in wonderful height and depth—near the rain pipe it had scooped down to the pebbles of the ground. Powder scudded over surfaces.

The storm door was locked. He rolled and squeezed the bulky paper into a square of the latticework that extended from the doorway. Three feet of snow had blown against the door, and he burrowed down into it for the mat, as Roland had told him. Down deep the snow was packed and slippery, and he had to take a glove off and scrape with his fingers before he could lift a corner of the rubber. He picked up the coin.

He heard the steady loud motor of a plow, and turned to hurry back and pull the sled out of its way. He fell down the covered steps, making an avalanche. Then he hurried on, trying to find his old footprints. Roland got to the sled as he did, and they pulled it aside together.

They saw the burning yellow headlights coming up the curve, but the rest of the plow was a dim shadow in the blind gray-white. Then it became loud and visible. Chunks of the mountain it threw up came tumbling down at them and the sled was pushed to a tilt against their knees, but did not spill. They stood a moment looking at the wide shiny path the plow made as it roared up the hill.

"What would you rather be," said Ed. "An explorer? Zoologist?"

"Zoologist, maybe."

"What about a rabbi?" said Ed.

"Nope."

Roland gave Ed a paper and pointed to the next house.

Ed started through the snow with it. It occurred to him only belatedly, when he saw the garage set far back, that a subsurface depression of driveway might lie down an embankment hidden by the flat blown waves of snow before him. You could not judge depth by the surface. When he did think of it he was already sinking. He tried to step lightly and struggle up, but it gave way beneath him until he was stuck, immobilized up to his waist.

43

On her day off Millicent washed her own socks and underwear and Leslie's in the washtubs of his apartment. She draped them to dry on the long heavy radiator in the main room and on the tall narrow one in the bathroom. Then she scrubbed all the woodwork. To reach the cabinets and over the doors she stood on a chair. She was winded when she finished, but she went on to other tasks. She had bought a preparation that was supposed to rub the green stains from the bathtub, but it didn't work very well.

She swept the bathroom floor, and poked hard with the broom behind the radiator where chips of dried paint had fallen. The floor needed a scrubbing. But her arms were tired. It was past midafternoon. She put an old coat over her jeans, and gathered up some shirts of Leslie's and the soiled bed linens, and took a walk to the Chinese laundry.

But she still didn't feel ready to go back and scrub the bathroom. So instead she took a walk to her own apartment, to see if she had any mail. She had not been there for a couple of days.

There was snow in the city, piled at the curbs, and the ponds in the Common and the Public Garden were frozen. Barbie Chisholm had found a job, as a saleslady in a dress shop, but she had not found an apartment yet, so they had worked out an arrangement. Barbie was to pay Millicent's share of the rent, in Millicent's behalf, while Barbie stayed there and Millicent stayed at Les's. But it was understood that the apartment was still one-third Millicent's and that she could come back whenever she wished. And Barbie was still looking meanwhile for a place of her own.

It could amount to quite a saving for Millicent in the meantime. And it seemed entirely fair.

She found the mailbox empty. So she decided to climb the stairs and warm herself a while, to justify her having walked all the way over here.

She found Ella Jane at home, sitting in a bathrobe and drinking coffee. "What's the matter?" Millicent asked.

"I seem to have intestinal flu," said Ella Jane. "I haven't been to work for two days. And it's lucky you dropped in—your mother's coming over. She's in town."

"My goodness! Why?"

"She's shopping. She called. And she asked me how I liked her noodle pudding. Don't worry—I said we loved it. I covered for you."

"Oh, good. Thanks. I took it to Les's."

"I figured."

"I wish she wouldn't come in to town unannounced like that," Millicent said. "Without sending a postcard or anything."

In a little while Lucinda came. She said Millicent had a nerve, leaving her roommate all alone when she was sick and feverish. Ella Jane could fall, God forbid, and damage her leg, and it had been a very inconsiderate and thoughtless thing for Millicent to do.

Millicent said she had had to do an errand at the laundry.

Her mother sat chattering, about Ella Jane's symptoms and what she had eaten, and whether she could make her some rice soup, but Ella Jane kept refusing and saying she was on the mend. Millicent wondered if her mother would get out soon. She wanted to be home when Leslie got there from the hospital. Then it struck her as odd that she thought of Les's place as home now. It was starting to become dark, but Millicent didn't put the light on.

All at once she wondered, with a flutter of panic, what she could say if her mother should miss the cat. She had taken the cat to Leslie's, and had explained to Leslie that she thought the girls didn't always feed him when she wasn't there.

Lucinda talked of her shopping, of the crowds, of the mud puddles. Ella Jane began to rise, saying "let's have some light," and Millicent switched it on. She tried to think of some excuse about the cat, in case her mother should notice. She could think of none. Also her little clock was gone from the mantelpiece. She found herself unable to concentrate on what her mother was saying, and she answered absently when spoken to. At last her mother rose, saying she had to catch her train, and gathered her bundles and left.

"You're as white as a sheet," Ella Jane said to Millicent when the door had shut.

"Wouldn't you be?"

"I was wishing there was some way I could get in touch with you or signal you over there."

"There isn't," said Millicent. "The phone's disconnected. Les can't afford a phone. If it happens again we'll just have to make excuses."

She waited long enough to be sure her mother must be down the block and out of sight. Then she set out for Leslie's. It had grown dark. As she walked she felt calmer. Actually her mother did not drop in like that more than once in a month or so. She did not phone often betweentimes either, as it was a toll call and there was rarely anything that could not wait until Millicent came for Sunday school. And with a little effort she could keep herself informed of her mother's intentions. As a matter of fact her mother often did send a postcard ahead.

And there was nothing wrong with being out anyway. It had been absurd to panic like that. It occurred to her now that if necessary she could have said that the cat was exercising on the roof or out back in the alley. But it would be a good idea to bring her clock back. Les had one anyhow.

When she got back to Leslie's she drank some warm milk, and then began scrubbing the tile floor of the bathroom, on her hands and knees. He arrived while she was in the midst of it.

"Hi," she said, not looking about or rising and not interrupting the scrubbing. "This floor was a sight. I just had to do something about it."

"Hi." He watched her scrub.

He poked his toe at the seam of her jeans.

"Don't be juvenile," she said without stopping.

He told her they were going to go to a movie with some of his colleagues. An English thriller. One of the group was to call for them in a car.

"Okay," she said.

"It's about time you met some of my friends."

"Okay."

He said he would lie down for a nap meanwhile. She heard him unfold the bed from the convertible sofa.

In a few minutes she finished the floor, and went out of the bathroom. She saw him lying on the bed naked. His eyes were shut, but they opened when he heard her steps. She put the pail and soap and brush in the cabinet under the sink.

"Come and keep me company," he said.

"I thought you wanted a nap."

"I do. Come and sit here until I fall asleep."

She sat on the edge of the bed. He smiled at her.

"I'm bushed," he said.

With a finger she closed his eyelids. He opened them again.

"If you're gonna sleep," she said, "how come you're getting all sexed up and ready?"

"I'm not. It does that all by itself."

"I saw you like that sleeping once. Sunday when you slept late. You were lying there all sexed up in your sleep. Really, it was grotesque. In your pajamas."

"It's possible."

"What were you dreaming?"

"Who knows."

"It's amazing the way it knows to get ready when I'm near. It's like the door in the supermarket that opens when you get near it."

She played with the rough brown hair that ran up his body and spread itself in whorls on his chest. Then she stopped.

"You told me to be like a little boat at a mooring," she said, "but you're like a submarine with a periscope."

She enclosed some fingers about his flesh, gingerly. His skin seemed stretched like the strings of a violin. His breathing deepened.

"It's just like one of these toy clowns that won't lie down," she said. "It's so persistent."

"Your fingers are magic too," he said.

"Are they?"

"You've got the light touch."

She brought her eyes near to study the mysterious response, until she knew they must be very crossed.

"Is it sensitive way under here too?" she asked.

He made no answer.

"Is it?" she repeated.

"Sweetheart—I'm speechless."

"You'd think caressing and gentleness would soothe it, wouldn't you. But it doesn't. It makes it rear and bristle."

"I'll never make love to you if you're so nice to me," he said. "You'll make me lazy. You have to be coy, you know—leave something for me to do."

"I'm sorry," she apologized. "But you said you were tired."

"You'll spoil me."

" 'Lullaby—' " she sang. "Do you like me to do this to you?"

"You're a darling."

"I'll play it like a harp string," she said.

"Play it like a flute."

"What?"

"Like a flute."

"That's disgusting."

"Don't say that. What's disgusting about it?"

She took a breath, and bent and dribbled a kiss along the variety of his textures. She renewed the moisture of her lips and did it again. Her hair hung on her forehead and about her face.

"There," she said.

"More."

"No. I don't want to. I'll do it the normal way if you want."

"Take off your clothes."

She unbuttoned her shirt, pulling the tails of it from her jeans. He turned and reached under the pillow meanwhile.

When she was nude he was still lying there. "You don't really want to," she said to him. "You're too tired."

She got onto the sheet on all fours, and crept playfully on hands and knees. She planted her hands on the pillow, on either side of his head, and kissed his lips.

Then she put a knee across him, to the other side.

"I'm a wolf," she said, "and you're Romulus and Remus."

She bent her elbows and moved down to sweep his face. His hugging lips slid over her skin with drenching swallowing kisses that pulled at her softness like a plumber's helper.

In a while she straightened her arms again and looked down at his face. They smiled at each other.

She began to sit back on him, but he held her hips and guided her slowly. He wriggled a little and they adjusted themselves carefully, with many hesitations. At last she sat up. Her knees were on either side of him, fleshed out by the squatting.

She leaned, lifted herself a bit and settled again, testing the feeling. She found that while he lay still she could give herself as much or as little stimulation as she wished.

She took his hands. She held his hands lightly in the air. She made a little riding motion. " 'Ride a cock hoss, to Banbury Cross,' " she said.

He laughed.

" 'Ride a cock hoss, to Banbury Cross,' " she said again. She rode rapidly, and then slowly, and then just rocking. They still held hands lightly. "Ride a cock hoss to cranberry sauce."

She excited herself, and let herself cool, and excited herself again. All at once Les went into his throes, breathing helplessly. She watched him.

The cat jumped to her shoulder. She gave a cry and half struck at it, as though to grasp her shoulder, and the cat leaped to the floor.

"Oh!" she explained to Les. "He gave me such a start! He scared me half to death." She turned to look down at her shoulder, and rubbed the white scratch marks. "Claws and everything."

She looked at Les again. They separated themselves, and sat side by side on the edge of the bed.

"We're rotten," she said.

"No."

She ran a step over to the chair where he had hung his clothes, took the pipe from his jacket, and sat herself down beside him on the edge of the bed again, pretending to smoke his pipe. She puffed, though it had no spark. He tried to take it from her but she snatched it back and restored it to her mouth.

"Sleep with a man," she said, "and the next thing I know I'm smoking."

He tickled her foot with his toe.

"See?" she said, holding the pipe. "It just goes to show. Sex leads relentlessly down the road to tobacco."

He took up the weight of her breast, and she felt his cool fingers circling.

"What time are we supposed to meet your friends?"

"Eight."

She looked at the electric clock.

"We should take a bath, actually," she said.

"You want to take a bath together?"

"I didn't mean together necessarily."

"Why not? We'll get slippery together. I'll wash you and you'll wash me."

They stayed sitting there.

"We don't smell the same," she said, "do you know it? There are two different smells."

"Don't you like it?"

"Oh, I didn't mean I didn't like it. It's kind of gamy, actually. You're more gamy. I'm more sicky sweet."

"Come on," he said, and hit her knee.

She followed him to the bathroom, leaving the pipe on the table. He turned on the taps of the tub, and she sat on the edge of it to regulate the temperature. He dropped the contraceptive in the toilet.

"What size do you wear?" she asked.

"What?"

"Those things."

"What do you mean?"

"When you buy those things don't you have to tell your size?"

"No."

"You mean they're like stretch socks?"

"No, they're not like stretch socks." He seemed to laugh at her.

"Well, what?" she said. "Tell me. They're just one size? You mean all men are standard?"

"I don't know."

"Could I get pregnant from washing together in the tub now?"

"No."

"Well, you wash a little first. I don't want them swimming at me in the tub."

She watched him turn a faucet at the sink.

"You smell like rotten meat," she said, "and I smell like rotten fruit, that's what I meant."

The tub was deepening and the pouring was noisy. She got into it and lay back in its warmth, trying to keep a little to one side to make room for him.

"You have knobby knees," she said.

"That's all right. You're beautiful enough for both of us. We don't both have to be beautiful."

He shut off the water into the tub and the noise stopped. He stepped in, and her body squeaked wetly as he got down beside her. The water rose and rocked. The tub was small and sloping, and its bottom was quite rounded, so though they tried to lie giving one another room they tended to press together and were tilted toward one another.

She leaned in his arm and his other hand played on her wetness. The light glistened on all her curves. She moved her feet and the water stirred with little splashes. She laughed.

"What are you laughing at?" he said.

"I'm just smiling out loud."

"See? It's good for your soul."

"You smell like electricity," she said.

"What does electricity smell like?"

"Lightning."

Their feet and the water kept moving. The ripples heaved in all directions at once—seemingly simple yet infinitely complex when looked at. One of her breasts lay on his chest.

"Teach me how to make naughtiness beautiful," she said.

"Are you a willing pupil?"

"Yes."

"You don't mind any more, about taking the brunt of the sexual revolution?"

"No. It's a nice brunt."

His hand dug between them for some water and he poured it on her chest. His fingers traced upon her. "I can see blue veins under your skin," he said.

"Blue veins dimly seen?"

"Blue veins dimly seen," he repeated. His fingers moved along her lovingly. Her eye followed his hand. In the upper frontiers of her thigh, where it spread to her belly and hip, she saw more veins.

"It makes me feel naked, my blue veins dimly seen."

"You feel very naked to me," he said.

"Let's play doctor. Is it a perfectly normal belly, doctor?"

"No, let's just play. It's simpler."

His hand moved, and she tried to straighten.

Matted hair rose and fell with the water. He swept a wave on the landscape of her front.

"Do you ever wish I were a blonde?" she said.

"No," he said softly. "No. You're just fine. You've enriched my life, sweetheart." He lounged in the water, eyes half closed.

"You've enriched mine, too," she said. Her feet kept the water moving. "I'm still not sure if the reasons for living this way are good, though. It's just that the reasons for not doing it had been there so long that I voted them out of office."

She looked up at his eyes, and then down at his body.

"Are you gonna get excited again now?" she said.

"I don't know. I might."

"Don't you know it isn't nice to point? Anyway we better get ready, if we're gonna meet those friends of yours. We don't have to fool around here." She reached across him to grasp the edge of the tub and pull herself, but she slid and fell on him. At last she climbed out and seized one of the towels.

He followed her, dripping, and they wiped themselves. They had not touched soap.

"Will we catch our death of cold," she asked, "going out right after a bath?"

"Not necessarily."

When she began to dress he became playful. He made the elastic of her underpants snap against her, and snatched away pieces of clothing for which she reached. He pushed her down onto the bed and wrestled with her.

"Hey, this is silly," she said. "I put things on, and you take 'em off again, and I get bathed, and you get me sweaty again—"

She tried to pitch him from the bed. They fell together slowly to the floor in a dragging fold of the blanket.

"Come on," she said, climbing out of the tangle. "We have to be sensible." She tossed him his underwear.

They dressed, and he watched her.

"Why don't you get some sexier underwear sometime?" he said.

"Why?" she said. "You mean like lace, and frilly garters?"

"Well, garters, and see-through stuff—there's all kinds of things. Pants cut way high—"

"I hate those things." She kept on dressing.

"Why?" he protested. "Your stuff is so plain."

"Because I may be your mistress, but I'm not your plaything. You put frills and decorations on little children, and on 'women' you know—'women' in the sense of something a man owns. And the more you put on the more the person is not a person but an object, to be loved as a thing."

"No," he said.

"I'd feel ridiculous," she said. "It's not even dignified." She rose and went to the wardrobe. She pushed aside the curtain and found a dress.

"And why white all the time?" he said. "You always wear that plain white stuff. There are sexy colors, you know. Like pink or something."

"Why don't you accommodate to me, and find something sexy in white?"

"White's so bland. When you're in underwear you should look underwearish, that's what I'm trying to say. Otherwise it's a lost opportunity."

"I'd think you'd be interested in me, instead of my underwear. I mean, it's what's in the underwear that makes it sexy, isn't it?"

"Well, I suppose. But clothes do have some erotic value, you know—all these things contribute. Why don't you explore the possibility? It enhances things. Even a body as perfect as yours."

"No. It embarrasses me."

He put on his jacket and knelt to tie his shoes. She got her coat.

"Gee, we forgot all about supper," she said suddenly. "We'll be starving."

"Well, there's not time now. We'll have to eat later, I guess."

They went down the stairs. She wished Leslie could afford a new overcoat. His sheepskin looked as if he had had it since his teens.

They waited in the little doorway of their building. The roadway and curb were steep. She looked up at him and he smiled. He still looked as if he needed a haircut, but that she didn't mind.

In a moment the car came by for them. They made seven passengers in all, and Millicent sat on Leslie's lap. In the confusion and excitement of introductions she caught none of the names. The doctor who was driving had a little blonde wife hunched down in black stringy furs next to him, and another doctor, who had no girl with him, was squeezed next to the wife on the other side, with his arm draped around. There was a dating couple in back with Les and Millicent. The talk was at once lively and warm, though she found no way at first to enter into it.

The theater was not downtown but a few miles in another direction. In a while the doctor who sat in front asked Millicent what her work was, and when she told him he said it must be interesting. She answered that it wasn't, not by comparison with his.

"It ought to be, I would think," he said. "Or it could be."

"Well, that's it," she said. "It could be. I should get busy."

The other man in back had a pointed face and straight black hair and big teeth, and made quips and jokes a lot, particularly when they got into the movie. To some extent they all did, and the pointed-faced one was especially witty at the expense of a travel short and the previews, so that Millicent thought they must sound like a group of college students.

When the film was over someone suggested going somewhere for drinks, but Les suggested that they all come to his place for scrambled eggs instead. She was glad he did. They piled into the car, the other girl offering to lap-sit this time, but Millicent ended on Leslie's lap as before. The other girl was skinny and long-legged and talkative, but the little blonde wife was pregnant and retiring and silent.

All at once Millicent had the mortifying thought that the bed was still unmade. They had rushed out without folding it into the convertible sofa again. She wondered how she could remind Les, or head them off. There was no way to. To speak of it, to announce in advance that she knew the condition of the bed, would disclose their relationship even more dramatically.

She thought of nothing but the unmade bed the rest of the way home and up the stairs. As soon as Leslie turned the key she burst over to the bed and scurried about it, straightening the blankets, and at last lifted and folded it into the sofa. She grabbed the pieces of soiled clothing that lay about and flung them into the bathroom hamper. She hung new towels. She wanted only to get this embarrassing exhibition over with as quickly as possible. Yet she noticed, somewhat to her surprise, that the company paid not the least attention, as though it were all quite natural, and continued to chatter unperturbed among themselves.

"There aren't enough chairs—I'm afraid we'll have to do it buffet style," Millicent said, her voice shaking.

She rushed about busily at the stove and refrigerator and counter, using all the eggs, and while the eggs were cooking she started a salad. She put in some of Mrs. Mahady's spices from the upper cabinet. The cat was curled asleep near the floor cabinets, with slanting tight eyes, and she was careful to step around him. Conversation and merriment continued behind her, and the long-legged thin girl was being gay and laughing loudly. Someone asked Millicent for an ashtray. There were none, but she supplied a saucer. Since there were only the two chairs and sofa one of the men had sat on the boards that formed the makeshift bookshelves.

"I'm afraid we don't have coffee," Millicent said quavering. "There's ovaltine—it's better anyway. Oh, there's not enough milk for it, to go around. Would anybody like some ginger ale?"

The pointed-faced doctor, whom everyone called Fritz, took a pot from the sink to help her with the ovaltine.

"You can't use that—you have to wash it first," she said. She took it from him and began to wash it. "Do you want to make everyone sick?"

Several of the company laughed, as though Millicent had scored a point, and the pointed-faced doctor shrugged and smiled and flinched.

"Well, you ought to know better," she said. "You could see there was old dried milk on there."

"Don't you know a washed pot never boils?" he said.

There was laughter again, the thin girl especially shrill.

"Please, I hope you're not one of those people with a propensity for puns," Millicent said. "I find jokes of that kind very upsetting."

"Upsetting?"

"I can't just laugh at will, when I'm not amused," she said. "And it upsets me to be expected to."

"Okay."

There was some more laughter, somewhat milder, though Millicent had not meant to be amusing. She put the eggs and salad and bread and butter and dishes on the table.

The party continued, the group seeming quite congenial, though Millicent busied herself as hostess, feeling tense, and did not enter in much. The small blonde wife complimented her food and then they all did. The doctor who had driven the car, a big, square-faced hulking man, sat on a board and read one of Dr. Mahady's medical journals. Les and Fritz and the one who had asked Millicent about her work talked about developments at the hospital and about doctors on the hospital staff, and in the course of it Fritz imitated the mannerisms of the people he talked about, so that the skinny girl particularly kept laughing. At one point they happened to speak of a surgical operation in which Les had been involved, and which the others seemed very much impressed by. The man who had asked Millicent about her work asked her now if she appreciated what a brilliant surgeon Les was. She began to answer, but the man asked if she had heard about the new way of correcting a slipped disc. "Only two men in the world can do it," he said, "and Dr. Leslie H. Hollander is one of them."

"Leslie D. Hollander," Les corrected him.

"Is that true?" Millicent asked, wide-eyed. "You never told me that."

"I've only done it once," said Les.

"Well, tell me."

"I'll explain it sometime, if you're interested."

"I'm very interested."

But the conversation went on to other matters, and Fritz came upon the corrugated carton full of Malcolm Stack's party hats, which sat on the floor next to the wardrobe. Millicent had brought it here because the girls' closets especially after Barbie's arrival were hopelessly crowded.

"What's this?" Fritz asked, picking up a hat in each hand.

"Oh, I used to have a friend in that business," she told him.

Fritz tried on a pointed little hat, pulling its elastic under his chin. He put a little top hat with a feather on the skinny girl. Meanwhile the conversation and laughter continued. The doctor who had been reading showed the others an article by a certain Dr. Demarest.

It was past midnight when someone suggested leaving, and the company pulled down the overcoats that had been thrown up over the top of the wardrobe. The departure was with smiles and handshakes and Millicent found herself telling one person after another to come again. At last the door was shut. She looked about the room, at party hats and at emptied and half-emptied plates of food. Leslie seized her in an embrace, strongly and hotly, leaving her breathless a moment, and stood clutching her to his chest and cheek.

"You keep happening to me," she said.

His lips moved on her face. Then he looked down at her, not smiling.

"You don't need lacy underwear," he said. "You have lacy-underwear eyes."

Her skirts made way for his stroking embrace.

"Shall I take your clothes off from the top," he said, "or from the bottom?"

"Rub them off," she murmured.

"You're nice to hold tight," he said by her ear. "You're so nice to hold."

"Is it really me that makes all that electricity in you?"

"Let's sleep in the nude tonight," he said.

"Okay."

He went to the sofa and opened the bed. She stepped from her underpants, which he had made fall out of her other clothing, and ran to brush her teeth and prepare for bed.

She came out of the bathroom nude. The apartment had already grown chilly. Leslie was in trousers and undershirt, sitting in one of the painted chairs and reading the Demarest article in the medical journal, with his back to her.

She put her hands over his eyeglasses. "Boo," she said.

When she took her hands from his glasses he went on reading. "Just let me finish this," he said. "I just want to see something here."

"Look," she said. "I'm ill-clad. One-third of a nation."

He kept reading.

She got under the blankets.

"Beddie-bye, anyone?" she said.

He closed the journal, finished undressing, put out the light, and got into bed. He folded his glasses and lowered them to the floor. Then he embraced her.

He warmed her gleefully. She returned his hug.

"You were very sweet tonight," he said. "I was proud of you."

"Proud of me?"

"You look so cute the way you prepare a salad. So busy tearing the leaves off the lettuce. You look as if you learned it at your mother's knee."

"I guess I did."

He hugged her harder, with a little tug.

"I should have coffee, I suppose, for people who want it," she said.

He didn't say anything.

"Are you very tired?" she asked.

"I'm all right."

"I'm going to hold you by the handle," she said, "so you can't roll away from me. So you have to face me."

His face was so near she could feel the gentle breath from his nostrils.

"I just want to hold it some more," she said. "Because it's mine, just as much as if I were a boy, only it's on you."

"Take it easy."

"I won't hurt it," she said. "Don't forget it's mine too. Yes. I have one, just as much as if I were a boy, and here it is, on you. It's ours. We share it." She nestled, and stretched next to him. "We have a half interest in each other's flesh. My breasts are your breasts. Do you like having breasts?"

He said nothing, but she knew from the quality of his breath that he had smiled or chuckled inwardly.

"I love how it grows," she said. "It comes reaching. Oh, it's mad. It's just mad. It's hot. Does it feel hot to you?"

His hand played with her ear.

"Do you think I insulted what's-his-name, Fritz, about his pun?" she asked.

"No, that was all right."

"He thinks I have no sense of humor."

"You do have a sense of humor," Les said. "I've been noticing it lately. I didn't used to think you did. You used to seem so serious and blue-nosed all the time."

"I do have," she said, "when it's appropriate. I just don't believe in making jokes all the time."

Again his arms tightened about her. His hands moved. She liked his touch.

"You have sensational skin," he said. "Gee, you feel good."

"You're so nice and warm," she answered. "Hatch me."

For a moment his lips made a vacuum on her cheek. They embraced each other's buttocks. The whole expanse of his front and hairy chest pressed her.

"I like having no pajamas," she said. "So we can get more next to each other. It's so sleepy-warm." She had found she could make her voice very small and soft. "I'm very next to you. Let's get nexter, and nexter, and nexter."

They really seemed to do so. The hard muscles of his stomach pressed her.

"I love you," she said in the same small voice as before. "Let's get all sweaty and stinky together. Let's be Siamese twins some more."

"Stop talking," he said in a husky whisper.

He rejoiceth as a strong man about to run a race, she thought. It was good to enclose that nervous fullness. She listened to the soft agitation of his nostrils. He made himself heavy, and light, and heavy, and light again. She coasted with him in an easy mutuality. The grip of his arms was gentle, yet she knew they would tighten if she tried to remove them.

A sleepy, dizzying tingling came even into the sides of her head.

Their oily slippage prolonged itself marvelously. Her body seemed to become full of wildly spinning engines. Yet he was not finished. The exultation continued. If she thought it had died it would begin again. He rested his chest upon her and his chin in the crook of her neck, and his hands lifted her buttocks until her legs danced. Even when she felt too worn to assist him he surprised her with quickenings that made her gasp.

Acceleration transfixed her. She responded in great twitches and tightenings, again and again, until exhaustion came on her like a flood.

Her heart was racing. His face had descended beside her. He seemed utterly spent. She listened to the slow rush of wind, back and forth, in and out of his lips. Then his lips closed. His eyes were closed too. The cycle of his exhaustion and endless renewing, she thought.

She looked at his face, in the bit of light that came from the street. The shades were only up an inch. She could see the breathing of his stomach. Sometimes in his sleep he looked angelic, but now he looked only tired. She kissed him.

He half opened his eyes.

"And so tired, too," she said. "I'll be the death of you. You mustn't make it so delicious, Les. I'll get too depraved."

"Like riding on a dolphin," he murmured.

"Can you believe that's what babies come from? I can. I really can. You're just like a maple tree dropping seeds."

"You're as watery and velvety as the womb," he said.

"Am I? That's nice."

"You're as soft and syrupy as ice cream."

"Do you like me enough to make me pregnant someday?"

"Do you want to be pregnant?"

"You're a fountain of life-giving seed."

They lay quietly.

"Do you feel sad after we do it?" she asked.

"Sad?"

"I've read that men do. That they feel sad and empty and drained."

"Well, I don't know. Maybe a little. Depends."

"What do you think about when we do it?" she asked.

"What do you think about?" he asked her.

"Well," she said, "sometimes I think about doing it, like a panorama of all different couples, and sometimes I think about other positions, and sometimes I think about a baby, and sometimes I think about you, your face, how you look at different times, reading, and thinking, and saving that man's life."

"What man's life?"

"Monday. You told me they brought in this emergency case, and you massaged his heart, and restored him to his family. His wife and children."

"Well, that's all in a day's work. Lifeguards at the beach save lives every day."

"Tell me about that operation. I mean that new operation, that only you can do."

"Now?"

"I mean when there's time."

She wondered if he were going to fall asleep.

"I feel wide awake somehow," she said.

But she turned away, intending to sleep.

"It's cold," she said. "I wish they wouldn't shut off the radiators at night. That's the coldest time."

He said nothing.

"I'm going to put on my pajamas if you don't mind," she said.

"Go ahead."

She rose in the dark and got pajamas from a drawer beneath the counter. She brought Leslie his pajamas also. Then she put on socks and her bathrobe. "Do you want your socks and bathrobe too?" she asked.

"No."

She huddled under the coverlets. "I love you," she said. "I used to think that would be very hard to say. I didn't see how I could ever say that. But now it comes very naturally."

Their backs were to one another, but she pushed back her feet until the soles of her socks touched his leg.

"Do you love me?" she asked.

There was a beginning of a little snore, as if he had been dropping off to sleep.

"You do love me," she said softly. "You're too fine not to love me."

She worked her toes against his leg.

"We hardly ever get to see each other, do you know it?" she mused. "Just these few hours of sleeping, when you're not on call. You're up and out at six-thirty in the morning, and by the time you get back I'm at work, and when I get back it's past midnight and time to get some sleep again. And the one morning when you can sleep late and be around in the day I have that stupid old Sunday school. Just whichever of my nights off you don't happen to be on call—that's all we get to relax and be together, or go anywhere, or be with people. One evening. That's all."

He didn't answer.

"It's awful cold," she said. "It feels like zero in this place."

"Want me to stuff the windows with newspapers?"

"No. I don't want you to go away."

"Put my bathrobe on too if you want," he said. "Wear two if you're cold."

She got out of bed and found his bathrobe. "Don't you need it?" she asked.

"I'm okay," he said.

She put the bathrobe on over her own. "I'll be warm now," she said. "As soon as I warm up inside all the insulation. Everything's freezing when you first put it on."

She got under the blankets again. This time she lay on her back. He still lay curled away from her.

"Les," she said, "what would you suppose the chances are that you and I will end up married to each other someday?"

"Probably a good chance."

"You do? Would you say better than a fifty-fifty chance?"

"Sure. I'd say so," he said. "Why?"

"Nothing. Just speculating."

"Well, you never know, of course. But it's obviously possible, if you're reckoning possibilities. Why not?"

"If you were gonna get married right now, would you marry me? Of all the people you know now?"

"If I were gonna get married right now? Sure. Obviously. You're good enough to marry."

"Have you ever met any you liked better?"

"No. I don't think so, actually."

"What about as well?"

"No, you're probably about the best I've met so far," he said.

"I'm keeping you awake," she said. "Aren't I."

"I'm not too sleepy either," he answered. He turned, and lay on his back.

"Do you know the Song of Songs?" Millicent said. "When I was little my father used to read the Song of Songs to the family every Sabbath, but my mother made him cut it out, because we found the translation and it was too sexy."

"What kind of a nut was your father?"

"No, very pious people are supposed to do that. Really. The Song of Songs is the only book in the whole Bible that's assigned in the prayer book for weekly reading."

"I don't get it."

"It's supposed to be read in the synagogue," she said. "You know, just like they have a hymn that calls the Sabbath a bride and all that, and they're supposed to read that thing about a good woman is worth more than rubies, so they'll appreciate their wives, but if they didn't read it in the synagogue my father would read it at home, and that night the father and mother are especially supposed to make love, and married women are supposed to make themselves especially sexy on the Sabbath."

"I never heard of it."

"No, that's true," she said. "That's the orthodox way, and my father tries to be as orthodox as they let him."

"You're pulling my leg."

"I'm not. Honest."

"How long does it take to read the Song of Songs?"

"Well, my father would kind of sing it. About ten minutes, I guess. He especially liked to do it if we had company. Maybe because my mother bothered him less if there was company there. Or maybe because he wanted to set an example, I don't know. And sometimes the kids would start their baths meanwhile."

"Did he have a good voice?"

"No, he can't carry a tune. He's like me."

Les rolled to his side again, with his back toward her.

"Is everybody's father a nut?" she asked him. "Was your father a nut?"

"No, he wasn't a nut, exactly."

"Why are there two sexes?" she said. "I mean, what if there were five sexes, and five different kinds of people had to get together to make a baby."

"Much too complicated," said Les. "I wouldn't like it."

"I mean, think how it would be," she said. "Five people would have to be congenial and get along together, and when you finally get four together they'd all have to agree on who to get for the fifth, in order to make a marriage. And then the one they agreed on might say, 'I'll join if you get rid of so-and-so—I like the people you have for the first, second and fourth sex, if you get a nicer number-three sex.' And if one died, the others couldn't do anything until they got somebody else of that particular sex. And think of all the genders of pronouns."

"I'm glad you aren't God, if that's the way your mind works. That's all I've got to say."

"And five different kinds of clothes and underwear."

"Go to sleep."

"You poor man," she said. "You have to be working in a few hours, and I'm talking and talking. I won't say another word. I promise."

She resolved to keep the promise.

He did not move or speak. She lay awake a while even after she was sure he was asleep. I shouldn't have kept him awake so long, she thought. She recalled the evening, and his colleagues. It must have been so obvious to them that she was living with Les, and yet it didn't faze anybody.

The problem now, she thought, was to prevent sex from becoming disproportionate, or overemphasized, lest their friendship become based on it. But, she told herself, some disproportion was probably inevitable in the beginning, until they get used to it.

Day by day lately she had been growing more and more aware that there was not an inch of her flesh that could not be aphrodisiac in his eyes. If she pulled a foot to herself to trim its nails, she was aware of the widening of her thigh, straining the legband on which she sat, and its effect on Les. She knew she was sexy in clothing and sexy bare, that clothing itself suggested nakedness. The flow of a hem, however modest, or the crinkle of a blouse suggested to a man the woman beneath.

Whenever she assumed he had grown used to the sight of her body, there would be new evidence of his enjoyment in seeing her undress. In her underwear he would come and embrace her and feel her. He had even said to her that the mind's eye forgets and gradually gets out of focus, and that having her around all the time—this continual renewal of loveliness in front of him—he just couldn't tell her how great it was. He had said he didn't know life could be so great.

And she liked the way his face looked when he looked at her in the nude, and the way his face looked when he touched her. Something in his excitement was contagious.

Saturday, when she had slept all morning, he had come home at one in the afternoon and found her doing calisthenics in her pajama top, and he had watched her without a trace of reserve. He had walked about, and even sat on the floor behind her for a better view. She had told him it was silly, but his interest seemed unflagging, especially when she touched her toes. She kept exercising, and took his bold gaze for granted. He would look at the rising of the cloth, or he would pass near and touch the round skin as she bent, and once he opened a hand before her so that a breast came down into it, spreading as it struck. "Stop," she had said. But it had not interfered with the exercise. It had seemed a friendly restatement of the relationship between them.

It must be strange, Millicent thought lying here now, to be a man, and want to assault someone who's across a room. Just because she's female. And just because she's there.

Even on Leslie's nights on call, she enjoyed sleeping here on this wide bed. She liked the buoyancy of the pillow, the hard flat breadth of the mattress. And she was pleased that he shared with her even in his absence.

A snore began to bubble in his throat.

She slept.

One of the alarm clocks woke her. Leslie usually set both, his and hers, for about ten past six, so that the second might wake him if the first did not. He leaped from the bed and shut off the clocks. Sometimes she slept through without hearing, but she did not like to, as she wanted to make sure he had a good breakfast. She heard him washing, and there was a line of light at the bottom of the bathroom door. She rose and put on the light in the room. Outdoors, around the edges of the shades, it looked pitch black. She began to boil water for oatmeal, and opened a can of frozen juice.

He came from the bathroom. "Go back to sleep," he said.

"I'll go back to sleep when you've had your breakfast," she told him. "You don't sleep, and you give blood—you at least have to eat."

She cleared away the company's dirty dishes that had sat all night on the enamel table. She sponged off the table quickly. He began to dress, but when he was in underpants she put juice on the table, and he sat and drank it.

She undid the two bathrobes to begin her exercises, and dropped them with her pajama bottoms to the big oval rug, stepping forth in her white socks and unbuttoned top. It was cold, but she knew the exercises would warm her, and that the radiators would begin to steam in half an hour. She saw he was watching, so she chose the angle that seemed least obscene. She began exercising her arms.

"Get dressed if you've finished your juice," she said. "Don't watch me. You've seen all this before."

But he sat there, not with his eyeglasses but watching nonetheless, and smiling. She counted, and tried to pay no attention to him.

She went to the stove and stirred the cereal.

"As a doctor you ought to appreciate that I take my calisthenics seriously," she said.

"Oh, I do."

She poured him a bowl of cereal.

"Aren't you having any?" he said.

"I'll have mine after my calisthenics. You can't exercise after a meal."

She went through the whole gamut of her exercises. He ate, looking on meanwhile. She counted with her lips, breathing more deeply as her muscles strained. She touched the toes of her socks thirty times without bending her knees, and rotated from the waist, this way and that.

When she lay on the oval rug to swing her legs he left the table and walked slowly about her, shamelessly looking down. Their eyes met briefly and she looked at the ceiling again, counting. She pushed the cloth shut on her bosom. She raised her hips, with her forearms as props, and bicycled.

At last she rose to her feet again, and counted squats. Past the twentieth it grew more and more difficult, but she wanted to do thirty. He stood facing her and did them with her. He watched her face as they went up and down together. In one of their squats she heard his tight briefs rip, but he kept on. When she had done thirty she stopped. He did a few more and stopped. She was still standing face to face with him, panting. He spread the pajama top from her shoulders. She let the sleeves tumble down her arms and it fell to the floor.

"Hi," she said to him.

His warm hands moved from her ribs to the spread of her hips.

"You tore your pants," she said.

His hands moved on her slightly.

"Take them off, and I'll see if I can fix them," she said.

He took off his underpants and handed them to her.

"That's easy," she said, studying them. "It's just a seam."

She went to the drawer where needles and threads were kept. She wetted an end and threaded the needle. She sat on the edge of the bed and he sat beside her, both of them naked. He picked up his eyeglasses, and watched her fingers sew.

44

Charles rang the bell and saw that a fourth name, B. Chisholm, had been added to the three on the mailbox. He peered through the decorative holes in the metal.

When the door buzzed he went upstairs. His uniform was rumpled and the Air Force overcoat hung unbuttoned.

A short, plump girl in skirt and blouse, with long dark hair, opened the door an inch. "Who are you?" she said.

"Charles," he said. "Millicent's brother."

"Millicent's not here."

"Well let me in. I been hitchhiking all night."

She opened the door wider and he entered. He looked about, squinted and yawned. He was beginning to need a shave.

"She's out already?" he asked. He looked at Barbie. "Are you B. Chisholm?"

"I'm Barbie Chisholm," she said.

"What are you doing here?"

"I live here."

"Where do you sleep?"

"Right there." She indicated the studio couch with its mussed linen and blankets.

"And where does my sister sleep?"

"I can't give you any information."

He yawned again, and sat down heavily on the bedclothes.

"Get off my bed please," Barbie said.

"I'm not contaminating it," said Charles. "What do you mean, you can't give me any information?"

Barbie reddened a little. "I have to get out of here and go to work in a couple of minutes," she said. She returned to her coffee at the drop-leaf table.

"Did she get up early to do errands or something?" Charles asked. "Did she give you any idea if she's coming back before she goes to work at least? Is she coming back? Or gone for the day, or what?"

"She didn't tell me."

"Or did she go home yesterday? Are her days off different or something?"

"Look, don't ask me," Barbie said.

He watched her sip coffee. He took a little ribboned package from his pocket and fingered it.

"Are you staying here temporary or permanent?" he asked.

"Depends."

"Will you tell me where my sister is, please?"

"I don't know."

"What's the mystery?"

"I didn't say there was a mystery."

"Why did you say you couldn't give me any information?"

"I meant I didn't know."

"First you said she didn't say where she was going, and then you won't tell me if she slept here last night. And do you know I'm aywol so I could see her? I'll be court-martialed for it when I get back. So don't be so secretive. She could be murdered for all I know."

"She isn't murdered."

He walked across the room, returning the package to his overcoat, and opened the closet door.

"You won't find her in the closet," said Barbie.

He felt the clothes. "Whose are these?" he said.

"Mine. Leave it alone. Quit snooping."

He dropped his hand. "Do Natalie and Ella Jane still have the bedrooms?" he asked.

"Who do you think you are? Sherlock Holmes?"

"Well, do you mean she moved out or what? She still gets mail here, doesn't she? She never sent any change of address. There was a thing for her in the box, some political thing."

"You have some nerve, prying in the mailbox."

"You're a real friendly type, do you know it?" he said.

"Same to you," said Barbie. "How do I know you're really her brother anyway."

He stared at Barbie, looking very tired. Then he looked downward, with a grimace. He left.

45

Millicent worked at improving the one-room apartment. She cleaned the stove and refrigerator. She took Mrs. Mahady's curtains to the cleaners, and bought a new drape for the front of the wardrobe. She bought oilcloth, which she cut to fit all the cabinet shelves, so they could be more easily kept clean, and made progress on the bathroom rust with some new powders from the hardware. She even bought light bulbs to replace the dead ones in the stair well, since the landlady apparently had no intention of doing anything about it. She wished she could do something about the stains in the bathroom mirror, but apparently there was no help for it short of resilvering.

She washed Leslie's socks and underwear along with her own in the washtubs. It was absurd that men didn't learn these elementary ways of taking care of themselves.

She also bought him some warmer pajamas. Les had been right in those arguments they used to have, she said to herself. Being a woman was better than just being a person, and the only way to be a woman was in relation to a man.

Meanwhile in the city room Bob Lyons told her that Aptaker, the wire-service reporter who worked at the State House, was real gone on her.

"I couldn't care less," she said. "Anyway I don't believe in office romances."

"He's not exactly in the office," said Lyons.

"I don't care," she said. "It's the same principle."

A few mornings later, as she lay in bed alone, after one of Leslie's nights on call, she discovered some scary lumps under her flesh, a pair of them, one on each side, and the thought lodged in her that in a few months she would be dead of cancer. She paced about distractedly, testing the lumps again and again, and did not dress or have breakfast for a long time. They did not show, and she had to press to feel them. What an irony that would be, for her life to come to an end now, so stupidly. She got as far as a telephone booth in a cigar store in the neighborhood, but stopped short of calling Les. She did not like to interrupt him at the hospital. And anyway she would certainly live through the day.

At night she showed him what she had discovered, and he said it was a simple mastitis of no importance, and that the lumps would dissolve of themselves. She was relieved, but wanted to know if he was positive, so he said he could arrange for a complete check-up at a cancer clinic. He said that by calling it an emergency he could get her in without the usual wait.

She had an all-day appointment on her day off. She wore a sheet, and it was a complete going over, in one room after another, with one doctor or technician after another. The proctological part, with a tube inserted by a nurse, was so painful that at last she wept, lying there prone on the table and appealing to the nurse like a child.

She went to Wilmerding Crosswalk on Sunday without yet knowing the results of the tests.

As she finished teaching her class a young man with thinning hair entered to call for his niece, and followed Millicent through the corridor and entrance when she went to wait for Ed.

"Can I give you a lift home?" the young man asked Millicent, walking beside her and pulling his niece by the hand.

"Thank you, no," Millicent said.

"We could have a Sunday-school lesson," he said.

"I only teach children," she said curtly.

She reached the steps outside and stood in her coat, waiting for her father. There was a sunny cool freshness in the air, and old snow by the walks. The young man remained beside her, his hand on the child's shoulder.

"Aw, come on," he said to Millicent. "You're the cutest Sunday-school teacher I ever saw."

"Good day," she said without looking at him.

"Did I say something wrong?"

"Good day," she said again.

He hesitated a moment, and then led his niece down to one of the cars. Conceited fool, she thought.

In a moment her father came, with Roland, and she rode home with them. She learned from them that Charles had at last gone overseas, and was in Japan.

Her mother too talked of nothing but Charles half through dinner. "Every time I pick up a newspaper I die," said Lucinda. "Now they're talking that they're going to make tactical atom bombs, little ones, to throw at people." At last she asked whether Ella Jane was better. Millicent said she was. Lucinda said to let her know whenever Ella Jane got sick, and that she would go to Boston herself to look after her during hours when Millicent or Natalie or Barbie could not be there. "That poor girl can't even get around," she said.

She also mentioned that Mrs. Herzlinger had said her nephew, Freddy Winkler, who was an assistant professor at M.I.T., was doing some special research about what happens to metals when they get very cold, and that it might be a good news item for Millicent to put in her paper.

Then when Millicent set out for Boston her mother gave her a jar of chicken broth and a cheese-and-macaroni pudding for her roommates, and some scraps for the cat. "Isn't it awfully crowded with four girls?" her mother asked.

"We manage," said Millicent.

Monday morning she phoned the cancer clinic for the results of her tests, and was told she was in perfect health. Her impulse was to phone Les and tell him of the good news, as well as of the correctness of his diagnosis. But again she did not want to chance interrupting in the midst of his work, so instead she took a walk to the hospital and left a note for him, sealed in a envelope, at the information desk.

Then she telephoned Mrs. Herzlinger's nephew at the Massachusetts Institute of Technology and made an appointment to interview him. She was glad to have at last found something she could write about and submit to Mr. Killian.

That night in bed she told Leslie of her plans for the M.I.T. interview, and it occurred to her that she might also write an article about the new disc-operation technique that only Leslie and one other doctor knew how to do. She wondered why she had not thought of that before. It suddenly seemed true what Mr. Killian had said—that material was all around her if she developed a reporter's eyes.

Les promised that he would explain the operation to her on her day off.

In the afternoon of her first day off she went by subway to M.I.T.

She found Fred Winkler in a tiny cluttered office. He lounged in his chair with a limpness that seemed almost double-jointed, and had an agreeable smile that opened first on one side of his mouth and then spread. He rose, more than average height, with a lock of black hair drooping across his forehead, and helped her with a chair, and then sat back. She rested her note pad on a corner of his desk.

He had very intelligent eyes, and complete ease of manner, sometimes even to the point of languidness, and smiled at her often, but she found his scientific explanations hard to follow. She wrote things down as best she could, and when she asked questions, or when he seemed to guess that she wasn't following, he tried to use very simple terms. His face was wide at the top, narrow at the bottom, and she judged his age as twenty-eight or twenty-nine. Sometimes he took her little pad from her and drew arrows and diagrams on it, but much of the time he played idly with little animals made of pipe cleaners, that were strewn here and there on his desk.

He spoke of extremely low temperatures, more than three hundred degrees below zero, so cold that they were as though heat did not exist, and he said that under such conditions familiar metals and gases develop peculiar properties, and behave in strange ways. He said he was collaborating with a physical chemist, and that they were developing a theory about how molecules move.

Then he took her down long corridors to a laboratory full of small strange noises, tanks, and coiled tubes.

At last she thanked him. He wished her luck with her story, but said he doubted that many readers could find his researches interesting.

He walked with her in corridors to show her the way back to the entrance.

"Would you let me know if you hear of any other material for features?" she asked. "Among your colleagues?"

"Well, I'm sure there are some," he said. "I'll keep my ears open."

Their feet echoed together in the corridor.

"There's a guy that calculates algebraically the formulas of the curves of women's figures, just for the hell of it," he told her. "You might make some newspaper copy out of that. Are you interested in that?"

"No," she said, coloring a little. "I don't think it's funny. And I don't work for the Daily Record."

They parted. She did not return the way she had come, but strolled over the long, low avenue bridge that spanned the river at its widest. She looked down at the broad field of gray ice. When she looked back at the Institute dome it had already turned from white to pink in the sunset.

She got to Leslie's just as he got back from the hospital. He fed the cat for her while she prepared supper. She told him of the interview, and about the low temperatures, and he seemed to understand it better than she did.

After supper he helped her clean the apartment. She liked the awkward way he squatted with a dustpan when she swept, and the curve of his back when he twisted in his undershirt, reaching to put up the curtains that had come back from the cleaner's. It occurred to her that any termination of this friendship other than marriage would be an unhappy one. It was not simply between friends—a special dependence had been established. She liked the concentration on his face when he repaired a faucet.

In the evening they sat at the table, and he tried to explain the disc operation, the old way and the new way, while she took more notes. He sketched out bones and tissues on the enamel of the table top, and pulled up his undershirt.

When they went to bed she felt she had done a marvelous day's work. It seemed that she had never been happier. She felt free.

She looked forward to writing the two articles, and to handing them in to Mr. Killian. Her career would begin, at last. And journalism was the best way to come into contact with men and with women, because you met them at their work, and their work was what they talked about. And in a sense shop talk was the best talk, the truest conversation, because it dealt with what people were really doing, with what they were giving their lives to.

It was infinitely better than socializing, the mating-market kind of thing, in which everyone put up a front and the talk was never genuine.

She couldn't very well socialize with many men anyway, while sleeping with one. This was the way to know men, through their work. It was not sex-conscious. And if she and Les should end up deciding to marry each other, the whole stupid chore of socializing would not only have been a horrible bore but unnecessary anyhow.

The next morning, as soon as Leslie had left for the hospital, she began work on the Winkler article, writing in longhand on sheets torn from her note pad. She began it many times, throwing it away as she became dissatisfied. But she finished it and began on the Leslie article. She stopped only for a sandwich in midafternoon. The articles were both quite short, but it took her all day to do them. Leslie was on call at the hospital that night so she spent the evening polishing her sentences.

On Friday she went to work ahead of time and copied her articles on a city-room typewriter. She expected Mr. Killian to be quite surprised and pleased with her. However he did not smile or lavish praise on her as she had thought he would.

"Good," he said, taking the sheets from her and putting them aside.

Then she thought he would call her to his desk when he had read them, and would perhaps make criticisms. She felt anxious excitement while she worked. But he did not call her to his desk, and at length he went home.

Late in the evening, however, Mr. Hopkins gave her her pieces to take upstairs to Mr. Valentino, and she saw that Mr. Killian had marked one of them for Sunday and one for Monday. Sunday's paper was always fat, and Monday's was usually short of news. She saw he had made scarcely any corrections or changes.

The next evening, while still at work, she found the Winkler article already in print. It was strange, seeing those words that she herself had written. And on Sunday, when she looked it up for her family in Wilmerding Crosswalk, they were excited and awed, even Patty and Roland. She told them she had also interviewed a surgeon and that there would be another article tomorrow, about a new way to operate on slipped discs. Her mother wanted extra copies for the aunts, and especially to send to Charles. Her mother had saved each little paragraph that Mr. Killian or Mr. Hopkins had ever let Millicent copy out from a press release, except when Millicent had not bothered to point them out, but this article about the metals at low temperatures sounded quite professional and learned. When she reread it after her parents' praise it seemed even better than before.

She made love with Leslie that night. There was rain and sleet that they could hear on the windows, so that the apartment and the blankets and Leslie's arms gave her a special sheltered feeling. He kept wetting her with kisses, bathing her with kisses.

They embraced a long time. "You're my clothes," she murmured. "You're all I've got on." He kissed her throat. Their noses fenced. His hands moved on her skin like brushes. His hairy stomach ebbed and rose in time with his breathing.

They rolled together slowly, like a double star, or as if they had been in a barrel.

Afterward, when they had put their pajamas on, they lay reminiscing, and calculated how long they had known each other.

Somehow he mentioned that it had been lucky, her calling him again just when he was acquiring the Mahadys' apartment, because he had been about to move into it with a nurse. On the day they were supposed to move in, he was in New Hampshire instead with Millicent.

Millicent was flustered by the unabashed way he mentioned it, as if in passing.

She found her voice. "What was her name?"

"Francine."

"What was she like?"

"Nothing special." There was some uneasiness in his voice now and she knew her shock had communicated itself to him.

But she couldn't decide how she wanted to feel.

"Sort of a flattish face, if you know what I mean," he added. "Kind of coarse—what you call coarse-boned actually."

"Bright?"

"No."

"Something must have attracted you."

"It was strictly sex, nothing else," he said.

"It doesn't sound very sexy."

"Well, I don't know. It was something about her hips, the way she looks in a uniform. Sort of horsy, or skittish in the hips—I don't know."

She knew he regretted the conversation, but it did not make her feel any better.

"The whole thing was all at a time when you and I weren't even seeing each other, after all," he said. "It all came to an end when you and I got together."

"I know it," she said. "Is she still at the hospital?"

"She's there. But we don't even say hello, hardly. She knows I've got another girl."

"I'm not 'another girl.' "

He reached for her hand under the blankets but she withdrew it.

"I don't want to be 'another girl.' "

"It's just a phrase. I didn't mean anything. You're being silly."

"Women are just mistresses to you, aren't they."

"Aw, for Christ sake. I'll never understand these crazy emotions women have. I shouldn't have told you about it, I guess."

"Why did you?"

"I don't know, I just did. We were talking. I thought we were good enough friends by now not to have secrets. I didn't know you were jealous."

"I'm not jealous. But I'm monogamous."

"Now, look. Honestly. Was I unfaithful to you? When I was going with her

I thought we were through. You wouldn't even see me. Remember? You said, 'I think we better not see each other.' "

"It certainly didn't take you very long to find somebody else."

"Why should it?"

"And you certainly treated Francine pretty shabbily. Ditching her overnight because I called you up. She was probably in love with you."

"It's possible," he said.

"You could at least have had a decent period of mourning," said Millicent. "It seems to me I've read that a man that's really mature thinks of a girl's emotions, and he protects her from being hurt by him."

"Oh, come on. If I always had that in mind I'd never get off the ground. I'd still be a virgin."

"Well, that's pretty irresponsible," she said. "An unhappy parting is a very real possibility in such things."

"Look, you can't go bothering your head about unhappy partings, or you'd never make a friend. You have to live in the present sometimes. You have to let yourself love life. Not just worry about the dark side."

"You still shouldn't have encouraged a girl you knew you didn't care for."

"You're not being reasonable," he said.

"I'm not?"

"My getting together with Francine when I did was the most natural thing in the world. I'm a guy that works pretty damn hard—I've been knocking myself out to make myself a useful member of society. I never had any childhood and you can say I never had any youth—just school, and jobs and struggling for scholarships—I never even had summers."

"You're only twenty-six and your youth isn't over yet."

"A pretty frustrated twenty-six."

"I'd say 'frustrated' is hardly the word at this point."

"Well, it was just coincidental that you and Francine happened about the same time. You know the saying—when it rains it pours. I don't know—maybe I just reached a certain stage of development where I automatically had more confidence or something. And if you really have some feeling for me you ought to be glad."

"Of what?"

"That the dam broke, and I started living a little."

"Is it just for you? Do you think your pleasures are all I care about? I'm not your mother."

He patted her hip. She neither responded to the caress nor fought it.

"You felt good," she said, "didn't you. Going straight from her bed to mine. You didn't feel any shame, or promiscuousness."

"Not especially," he said. "I didn't. It's perfectly normal for a guy to feel attracted to various women. I haven't had so much. A guy my age should have had fifteen different girls by now."

"That isn't the way you used to tell it."

"Yes it is. I've never been anything but honest with you."

"Why don't you sleep around all over the lot, then?"

"You always said you'd like to have a lot of men friends," he said.

"I didn't mean to sleep with."

She pushed his hand off.

"Why don't you make love to somebody at the hospital?" she said.

"When I'm at the hospital I'm up to my neck in work."

"What about nights there, when you're on call? You do get a few hours to sleep there."

"And when I do I'm too bushed to do anything but sleep."

"You could bring a girl here some evening when I'm working."

"Don't worry about it."

"Why don't you, if it's so normal?"

"I just wouldn't, that's all. Because you'd be hurt. You can't compare the thing with Francine to my relationship with you."

"Why?"

"Because you're entirely different," he said.

She stopped discussing it. He said nothing more either. But she hardly slept.

She fretted miserably all the next day, trying to understand his attitude. She wondered if in fact he was tempted at times by nurses or student nurses. She wondered if women were permitted to visit the interns' dormitory quarters. In any case, a hospital was full of beds.

Before going to work she strolled to the girls' apartment to see whether she had any mail. There was a letter from Charles. She opened it without going upstairs.

Dear Sis,

Here I am in Japan. I tried to see you one more time, so I went AWOL and hitch hiked to Boston and back, only you weren't there. I just wanted to tell you not to get involved with that guy. I met that new girl whathisname that is staying at your apt. When I got back they gave me a summary court martial and a week in the stockade. I wasn't even gone 24 hours but they were tough because we were alerted. I am lucky they called it AWOL because I could have been shot for desertion because the outfit was ready to move. Anyway I never served the week because they sprung me when we moved. Don't tell the folks that I have a court martial on my record. You keep my secret and I'll keep yours. I also lost my stripes but don't tell them that because I figure I can get them back in a couple of months. They would think I can't succeed at anything because they were proud of me for the first time when I got those stripes.

Sis, I know you are living with somebody or I have a pretty good idea of it. Maybe it is the lizard and maybe it isn't but it is somebody. I didn't see any stuff around that looks like yours and you haven't even got a bed there and everything is a big secret, only your name on the box is all. She kept talking funny like she can't give me any information. Sis, if it isn't true that you are shacking up with some son of a bitch write to me and tell me it isn't true so I don't have to get sick about it.

She had hardly the strength to read any further. She squashed it into her pocket. It was queer that Barbie had not told her of Charles's visit. Barbie was either malicious or stupid. But, she thought next, it wouldn't have made any difference anyway.

A few minutes after she got to the city room Mr. Hopkins called her over to the copy desk. "Wait till Dexter gets his hands on you," he said. He raised his green eyeshade an inch, and told her it was lucky for her that Mr. Killian had gone home early, because Mr. Killian was furious, ready to wring her neck. Her stomach sank with fright and mystification. Mr. Hopkins's tone was quiet, and not unfriendly, but he said Dexter was just wild.

Mr. Hopkins asked what she had been trying to pull with that medical story. A big surgeon at the Massachusetts General had telephoned that morning, angry because a surgical technique he had developed had been ascribed to some young intern. He had found out that the intern was Millicent's boy friend and assumed it was some publicity trick, and Mr. Killian had thought so also.

She began explaining, becoming tearful, but Mr. Hopkins misunderstood her explanation and seemed to think she meant that Leslie had duped her. She could not make Mr. Hopkins understand, but he remained sympathetic and told her she had better leave Dexter a long note explaining in full. He said Dexter had been threatening to fire her, and that he wouldn't be surprised if the surgeon fired her boy friend. Apparently he was mad enough to.

She went about her work weeping.

"Sneezy, you look like you had a bad night last night," Danny McBride said as she tore copy from the teletype machines, but this time instead of slapping her behind he poked his thumb in a disgusting manner, making her jump.

"I'll report you if you do that again," she told him with tears in her eyes.

When she did her errands to Heustis Garvey and to the State House she skipped her supper so as to have time to phone Leslie. He would be off his regular duty around supper time but at the hospital on call through the night.

The switchboard lady thought he had just gone to the cafeteria. At last she spoke to him. He had not been fired, but he said he had had to do a lot of explaining and had been warned to leave press relations to the hospital's publicity officer. She had written that Dr. Hollander described the new technique, and never even mentioned the doctor who developed it. She had not thought of it at the time, but it did seem stupid and misleading now.

A short time after her return to the city room Mr. Hopkins told her there was a call for her, and she took it on Maud Dickinson's phone, since Maud was not there.

"Hi, this is Fred Winkler," the voice said.

"Oh. Hello."

"That was a nice story, in Sunday's paper."

"Oh. Thank you."

"Very nice indeed. You got everything all wrong, but that's okay."

"I did?" Her voice began to break. "What facts were wrong?"

"Well, just about all of them, I should say. I didn't make those pipe-cleaner animals—my kid cousin did. And the scientific stuff you had completely backwards—I guess you missed the point."

"Oh my God."

"Don't worry," he said. "No harm done."

She thought she would faint. "I'm just sorry," she said. "I'm just no good, I guess. I don't know what to say."

"Forget it. I said there's no harm done."

"Are you sure there's no harm done?"

"I'm sure. Listen, can we get together socially?"

"Socially?"

"How about some country dining?"

"I couldn't, really. It would be awkward. I mean I'm rather busy. My time's taken up."

He hesitated a moment.

"You mean you're engaged—involved—something like that?" he asked bluntly.

"Well, something like that." She was surprised to find herself admitting such a thing to a stranger. She wondered what had gotten into her.

"Okay."

"But please don't mention anything like that to the Herzlingers or anybody," she said hastily, "if you talk to them."

"Don't worry," he said. "I wouldn't dream of it."

She hung up, shaken.

Louie Alpert, the big pear-shaped man with a drooping mustache, slapped her on the behind. "Come on, get to work," he said.

She looked at him indignantly, and hurried to Mr. Hopkins. "Mr. Hopkins, would you please speak to Mr. Alpert," she said as she got there, her voice quaking terribly. "Some of the men in this office just have no moral sense."

Mr. Hopkins put his head back so he could see from under his eyeshade.

"What's the matter, Louie?" he said.

"What?" said Alpert. He was going flat-footedly toward his own desk.

"What's the trouble?" said Hopkins.

"Nothing. I gave her a pat on the rear end and she wants to make a Federal case."

"Well, she's right," said Hopkins. "Keep your hands to yourself."

Millicent resumed her work, tense and rattled. The evening seemed very long. She tried to compose mentally the note of contrition and apology she would leave on Mr. Killian's desk. She dreaded to think what Mr. Killian would say if he knew that the M.I.T. story was all wrong too. She wondered how she could have gotten both those stories all wrong. After all she had an I.Q. of a hundred and fifty one, which was well up in the genius category.

Also Charles's letter kept coming to her mind. She wished she could run away, or become ill. She was glad that Leslie was on call tonight, and that she would not have to see him or talk to him or sleep with him.

46

Leslie bought a motor scooter, in partnership with the intern called Fritz. He told her of it one midnight when she returned from work, and told her to get into something warm, like ski clothes, so she could have a ride at once. The extravagance of it amazed Millicent. It seemed completely out of character, as though he had lost his mind.

He explained to her that his share of the installments would amount to less than ten dollars a month.

"Even so," she said. "You haven't got it. The apartment costs you."

"One pint of blood takes care of the scooter until spring."

"That's awful. I'm going to start paying toward the rent if you're going to do that."

"You're already paying for the food."

"That's all right. You take more than half your meals at the hospital anyway. And I can afford it. Barbie's paying my rent."

"You don't have to," he said.

She followed him down the narrow wooden flights in the stair well, wearing ski pants and parka. He had on his sheepskin jacket.

The gray scooter was parked at a slant, the front wheel turned toward the curb. She saw that a green doctor's cross had been affixed. She swung a leg over somewhat sullenly and mounted the rear seat.

"Are you sure you know how to drive this thing?" she asked as the motor started.

It moved at first bumpily downhill on the cobbles, but when they got to the broad main street the ride was rapid and smooth. The buildings of the city were darkened and there was scarcely any traffic. The scooter's motor dominated the air. It was as though the empty nighttime city belonged to them.

There was a late-February balminess but the wind had a coolness on her face and made her squint. Leslie's sheepskin was bulky before her. There was a curving windshield mounted on the handebars and he wrote no goggles.

"I would have arranged with my brother for you to use his old car if I'd known you wanted a vehicle so badly," she told him.

He didn't answer, but told her to lean and put her leg out on the curves. She was surprised that she could hear him so clearly despite the motor and the wind, though he didn't turn his head. He went faster, and she felt an exhilaration and joy.

They sped up open avenues, stopping for occasional street lights, slowing for turns, swerving to pass a lone car.

After nearly an hour they returned and parked again on the cobbles.

"I find speed very relaxing," he said as he dismounted.

"Even so, it's a very foolish and unnecessary toy," she said. "You don't need it. And your mother would have a fit if she knew, and she'd be right."

"Well, I'll tell her about it," he said. Millicent followed him on the stairs. "I'll present it to her as an economy," he continued. "I'll tell her it'll save money when I make a trip down to Connecticut, and that I'll get most of it back when I sell it. What the hell. I need some recreation. My life has been school and work, school and work, and I'm losing my youth. For the first time in my life I've got an apartment, with a woman in it, and I'm living a little. And I want that thing on wheels while I can. I never enjoyed college, I never enjoyed anything. I always worked too hard. And I'll be in the Army in four months."

"She'll wonder where you get the money," Millicent said. "She doesn't know you give blood."

"She knows. She found out."

They came into the apartment and she began getting out of her ski clothes.

"My biggest regret is that I didn't start living this way sooner. I should have started younger. I should have started living with girls about seven years ago."

"I wish you wouldn't say that."

"Well it's true. When you consider how little of this I've had, and what a tiny, minuscule fraction of my time is spent in pleasure—these articles about the younger generation just amaze ya."

"Even so, I wish you wouldn't talk about these regrets about affairs you didn't have, and girls you didn't sleep with. It makes you sound sad. What does it matter? You're happy now."

"The first time I got laid I was older than you are now," he said. "Do you realize that? I started later than you. It was a girl in Baltimore." He spoke slowly.

"Please, honestly, Les. I'd rather not hear about it. And I'm just as glad you weren't sleeping around all those years."

She went to the bathroom mirror to comb her hair. It had blown into quite a tangle. Leslie said nothing more. She used the comb and brush together.

He slapped her on the shining round underpants.

"What's that for?" she said. But she did not look about or take her eyes from the mirror. She kept combing.

"You're cute."

"Mrs. Grasser thinks we're married," she said.

"The landlady?"

"When I take the garbage down she calls me Mrs. Hollander."

She found fresh pajamas in the drawer and he prepared the bed meanwhile. He was under the blankets before she was. When she got in beside him his hands came to her at once.

"I'm gonna peel you like a banana," he said.

He undid her pajamas, and lifted her arms and legs from them, and tossed the pajamas from the bed.

"Want to try a new way?" he said.

"No, I like the old way," she answered. "Old ways are best."

Their nearness seemed to intensify. His fingering traced lightly how concavities flowed into convexities, all over the mathematics and artistry of her body, until she seemed everywhere lined with nerves. He wet her with his lips and drew the soft flesh upward.

She was wrapped in his embrace. The taut, unhurried fullness would rub juicily, or grow still, while seeming to pulsate.

She clutched. "Grab me as you would an opportunity," he said.

Afterward she lay awake a long while, even when his bubbly snoring had begun. Her skin felt the linen and the wool. Her hands lay on her stomach and were moved by its breathing.

She heard her belly rumble.

Leslie's snoring sounded like Patty's, she thought. He could have been angry with her about the newspaper story, but he had not been. He had understood.

It was only a few days since the trouble with her newspaper articles, and while she did not feel back in Mr. Killian's good graces the worst of it seemed to have blown over. Mr. Killian had not fired her, and the abject note she had left on his desk, outlining her faults and promising never to repeat them, had apparently headed off a bawling out. And he had never found out about the errors in the Winkler story. At least there was no sign of it.

Leslie had been taken to task at the hospital, but he told her his standing had not seriously been damaged.

She saw the motor scooter by daylight when she went down the next day.

She was very tired in the office, from insufficient sleep, and it aggravated her sneezing. Late at night there was little for her to do, and she wished she could be sent home early. But Mr. Hopkins was off, and the man who took his place never dismissed her ahead of time. Even the teletype machines that brought the wire-service news could not keep her busy and for long periods did not clack. Louie Alpert played solitaire.

Millicent sat at an unused desk at the back of the room, sneezing occasionally and holding a handkerchief to her nose, and doodling on paper. She wrote a series of names to see how they would look.

Leslie D. Hollander, M.D.
Leslie D. Hollander, B.A., M.D.
Millicent G. Hollander, B.A., M.A.
Millicent Hollander
Mrs. Leslie Hollander
Mrs. Leslie David Hollander
Millicent Gordon Hollander
Millicent Audrey Hollander
Dr. and Mrs. Leslie D. Hollander

She thought about what Leslie must have been like as a little boy. Then she thought about how much he had accomplished since they had known each other. She had done nothing of any account, except those two stories finally, which were no good. And she did not know where she would get another one, or whether Mr. Killian was in a mood these days to print it if she did. But Leslie's work and his learning went on full blast, whether he had a love affair or not. Neither sadness nor happiness could distract him. How strong he was.

At last she was allowed to leave, and took a cab. She usually did at night, when she could find one, as the way to Leslie's was not as easy by subway as the way to the girls' had been, and from the subway one still had to walk a long way up a steep hill through narrow streets.

When she stopped by the girls' for her mail the next day there was another letter from Charles.

Dear Sis,

I sent you a couple of things from Tokyo including a Chinese Communist bayonet I bought off a guy. Incidently it was used. Some day I will tell you the story. Also I sent a watch I bought you at Griffiss in the PX.

You are the only one that hasn't written me. I am worried as to what the answer is. I don't know if I figured it right and you are trying to get back on the straight and narrow first and then write, or you are too ashamed to write. I did some investigating on my own and wrote and asked the folks if you still have the same apt. with Ella Jane and Nattalie and they said yes. So apparently they don't know you moved out, like I suspected they didn't, or this other slob wouldn't have made such a big deal mystery out of it when I asked her.

So make a clean breast of it so at least I'll know. I am still your brother and you should confide in me. You are the only fly in the ointment. Outside of you I have no complaints. I told a friend of mine about this terrific sister I have, beautiful, smart like nothing he ever saw, and then I felt like a shmuck. I love you Sis. You are life and death to me. You are more to me than Mother is.

This is crazy country. It is terrificly beautiful some times, especially coming into it by plane.

Please answer my question. I give you the benefit of the doubt but the way it looks it stinks. Especially if you don't answer I have to draw my own conclusions. I remember all these talks we had and I wish we could have them now, especially when there is something to talk about. There is lots to think about here. You should see how the people live. Sis, write me something spiritual. I appoint you my chaplain. When we flew over here we flew up right into this gorgeous omenous cloud bank, and you could look up and swear God must be right on the other side of it, that is how it made you feel. It was real stormy. You know how a real awful low storm cloud looks. And then you come thru and there is nothing, only blue sky, and you are over a big flat layer of white clouds that just looks like a mattress or something, and the sky is just empty and completely different. I would like to know what you think about bombing across the Yalu.

Affectionately,
your loving brother,
Charles

P.S. The son of a bitch is my mortal enemy whoever he is. I would like to break his jaw. If I were back there I would chuck you right out of his little love nest and drag you home. I want to see if you deny it. You say you don't like to discuss some things but I wasn't born yesterday and I know what is going on. I think about it all the time. At least tell me it isn't the lizard.

She began to stuff it away unfinished, telling herself it didn't deserve to be read. But then she read on.

> Think how you would feel if you caught Mother in the sack with some guy or how would you feel if you found out Dad was sleeping around. It would be just like a knife in your heart. I know it would be just like a knife in my heart. Well that is exactly how I feel when I think about my sister taking her pants down. I feel like we are a no good family.

She walked to the city room, highly agitated. On the way she tore up the letter into a sidewalk trash barrel, but as an afterthought retrieved the corner of the envelope bearing his address.

At work her thoughts kept returning to Charles in a distraught way, as her mind kept thinking of angry replies. Toward midnight she had time to beat out an answer to him on plain copy paper, at a typewriter that wrote with crooked letters.

> Dear Charles,
>
> Don't you ever write to me in that fashion again. You are very misguided, and you have a filthy mind. I do not have to issue denials to the likes of you.
>
> No doubt you have been visiting all the geisha houses in Tokyo. You are perfectly horrible. I wish you would look after your own spiritual improvement.
>
> Your loving sister,
> Millicent

She blacked over errors with no regard for neatness. Then she took one of the newspaper's envelopes and an air-mail stamp from Mr. Killian's drawer, and put her letter in the outgoing mail.

In bed she told Leslie about Charles's letters.

"Poor Charles," Leslie said.

Yes, she thought, poor, benighted Charles.

By the following afternoon she was still feeling some agitation, but it had grown more diffuse. She hung around in the girls' apartment for a while, just in case her mother should happen to phone, and also just to have spent time there. No one phoned.

At work she tried to recall what phrase Les had used when he told her his affair with Francine was somehow in a different category. But she could not remember it. She was positive he could not have said anything nasty, like tramp.

But even if he did not use such words, what was it that made one affair different from another? Was there some rule of thumb, or was it in the spiritual attitude? Spiritual attitude on whose part?

There ought to be some clear-cut definition. Everyone knew exactly what an alcoholic was, for instance.

When she had a chance, late in the evening, she tried to find an answer in the city room's big Merriam-Webster.

However tramp was not listed, in that sense, so she looked up whore. But to pin down what it said she had then to look up harlot. She chased the meaning through the dictionary, avoiding terms that referred to prostitution. Harlot meant a loose woman. And loose turned out simply to mean unchaste.

She looked up alcoholic. It said someone addicted to excessive use of alcohol. That was beautifully clear. You had to be addicted, and it had to be excessive, or else it didn't count.

Someone shouted to her and she had to take some copy upstairs. But when she came down she picked up the Roget's Thesaurus from Mr. Killian's desk and looked in that also.

It was sickening. Strumpet, wench, fallen woman, trollop, woman of easy virtue, hussy, drab, jade, minx, slut, harridan, trull, wanton, tart, broad, chippy, floozy, pushover, woman of the world, courtesan, hot pants, sex pot, a bit of all right, bag, baggage, piece of tail—she slammed the boot shut, reddening. Everything derogatory. She wondered how to look up decent, wholesome, friendly love affairs.

47

She turned her head to the sheet, near where his knee knelt beside her, and then looked up again at his sleepy eyes. His panting began to subside.

"I spit it out," she told him.

"Why?"

"I'm sorry," she apologized. "I had to."

"Oh, you're chicken," he murmured. "You should have swallowed it."

"I couldn't help it."

"You missed the best part. Weren't you curious what it tastes like?"

"I got enough of a taste."

His knees were on the sheet, and he still straddled her neck and shoulders. He was smiling down at her. "What did it taste like?" he asked her.

"Salty, sort of."

He stroked and smoothed the hair about her forehead and her ear.

"Are you insulted because I spit it out?" she asked.

"No."

"It's the texture that's awful, really. Maybe if it were cooked."

He moved his knee across, and crouched restfully next to where she lay.

"Why does it taste salty?" she asked.

"I don't know. Maybe because life came out of the sea." He kept looking at her and smiling. "Anyhow, thank you."

"You're welcome."

"I'll do the same for you now."

"No." She drew her knees together and up. "Thanks just the same, but no thank you."

"Why not?" he said. "You're entitled to the same treatment."

"No, but I'd rather you didn't, actually. I know you mean it affectionately, but it would make me feel like a spittoon."

She pushed herself up.

"Anyway I want some grapefruit juice," she added. "I sort of need it after that." She got out of bed and tugged at the sheet. "And I'll have to change the sheet now," she said. "Get off."

He got off the bed and helped her pull the bedclothes.

"How does it feel to be a sex object?" he asked her.

She said nothing, but her hand offered him a caress, with a squeeze and a pull.

Then she gathered up the sheet and carried it to the bathroom hamper.

"You'll be late," she said. "All this fooling around."

She got breakfast started, and while it cooked she put on clothes. She saw him shaving.

She looked at the clock. Now that he rode to the hospital instead of walking he had an extra fifteen minutes in the mornings. The motor scooter was a convenience in that respect.

When he had gone she finished making the bed. She hung up his pajamas. She remembered that she had meant to tell him that if he would cut his toenails more often she wouldn't have to darn the same socks over and over.

She felt too keyed up for a morning nap, though her night's sleep had been scarcely more than three hours. She went out for a stroll.

The trees on the Common were still bare, and the squirrels she saw looked thin, but the snow lay wet and heavy, as though spring were no longer far off.

She walked past the uptown shops. In a window she saw a bra and panty set of the erotic sort that she knew Leslie wanted her to have. It was displayed on a chromium rack. The yellow color had drawn her eyes. It was briefly cut, the pants of a bright silky stuff that would fall to her skin in clinging wrinkles, and with lace. She imagined herself in it. Then she saw another made completely of lace, in white, close-fitting and transparent, scalloped and with curlycued designs. She swallowed. It looked quite expensive, too. She walked away from the window.

In time she returned to the one-room apartment when she had walked enough, and settled in bed for a nap. It occurred to her that if her name were Millicent Gordon Hollander she would have the same initials as the Massachusetts General Hospital. She shut her eyes to the light in the shaded room, and tried to stop thinking and sleep. Naps had grown important, since their hours of nighttime sleep were so short.

She knew that Leslie often caught caps here in the evening though he always arose in time to call for her on his motor scooter. On any night when he was not on call he would be there waiting when she finished work, to save her the trouble of hunting for a cab. The city-room men all knew who he was by now, and sometimes he came up and waited at one of the desks. Mr. Hopkins was very nice about trying to let her go as soon as possible after Leslie appeared.

She would ask Leslie if he had fed the cat, and he always had.

Usually they would go directly to the apartment, without taking a spin about the city, but then she would prepare a snack and they would play for an hour. She had learned how to saunter past him, her hand brushing him, and a little shake that she gave her shoulders would vibrate in her breasts. He would clutch her. Once she told him she was glad she had pants on, because her pants held his hands more tightly to her skin.

Even if she left the city room early it might be one a.m. before they rolled into bed together.

Sometimes the raw friction of their love-making would grow ravenous, so that perspiration seared, and she would tell him they were like two trees climbing each other. She had learned how to make her body pinch him in spasms. And sometimes, when that high-strung joy had struggled free of them, it was as though it had never been, and she wished they had detained it yet another moment. Even in the flooding relief she regretted sometimes the loss of tension, and was sorry the teasing pressure had escaped. We lie like punctured balloons, she thought.

In their fondling he told her she had nice ribs, and she remarked that she ought to have shaved under her arms. "Why should you?" he said. Once she asked him if he would like her better if she weren't cross-eyed.

"You're not very cross-eyed," he said. "If you even are."

"Do you think I'm cross-eyed?"

"It's hard to tell," he said. "Sometimes it seems so. It depends on the angle. It's queer."

They would talk seriously also. He talked to her about his work more than formerly, sometimes for a long time in the darkness.

The presents Charles had written of arrived, almost all at the same time—the little chromium wrist watch from the PX and the grisly looking Chinese bayonet—and also one he had not written about, a carving in ivory of a smiling old man who sat carving still something else. They came to the girls' apartment, and she opened them there. The ivory figure was about six inches high, and beautifully detailed.

The delicacy of the carving, and the taste he had shown in choosing it, particularly touched her, and she wrote him warmly. But her letter crossed in the mail with another of his, which upset her again. He said they should write to each other more often. He begged her, please, please, please, to give up this guy who was just a wolf so she could respect herself in the future. He urged her that it was still not too late. She sent an answer at once.

> I'll write to you more often when you learn to mind your own business and not discuss certain things. You might have the decency and the intelligence and

the consideration to write me letters I can show the folks. They're starting to ask if I hear from you. Can I show them a letter like that?

You are generous in some ways, but there are more important kinds of generosity.

She showed the presents to her parents when they came to Boston to give blood to the Air Force again. Ella Jane had phoned her at the city room to tell her of the postcard from her mother, so when they arrived she was ready for them at the girls' apartment. She had brought the presents there and also the cat. She went with her parents to give blood, and then they went to the apartment once more. Lucinda talked of letters that Charles had written home, and Ed spoke of having been to the town meeting. Lucinda noticed a rip in the curtain and asked if the cat had done it. She said the place looked terrible. "Don't you girls ever clean it? I know it's hard, being so crowded, and you go to business every day, but you could all pitch in a little. I think it was nice of you to take Barbie in, but you can't let things go like that. I'd like to come in here with a maid some afternoon."

Lucinda also told Millicent that Aunt Gwendolyn had mentioned that she could never reach her. She had tried a number of times to get her on the phone.

"Well, I've been out a lot," Millicent said shakily. She waved away her father's cigarette smoke. "I have errands and things. And I'm going to try and look for stories more. I can't just hang around indoors all the time."

"I know it," her mother said apologetically. "I didn't mean you should have been here."

"As a matter of fact," Millicent said, "if you tell her to call about eleven, when I get up, she'll usually get me." She resolved as she said it to come here every morning about that time, to pick up her mail and wait a while by the phone just in case.

That night in bed she told Leslie she hated having to lie. She said she kept having close calls. And she disliked having to tell her mother how the girls had liked noodle puddings that she had in fact shared with Les. One of these days her mother would suspect something fishy, and catch her off guard with the wrong question, and she would put her foot in it.

"Don't worry about it," Les said. "Modern mothers usually don't ask questions, even if they do suspect."

"My mother isn't all that modern," said Millicent.

She did stop in at the girls' apartment Friday and Saturday, but there were no calls.

On Sunday she prepared a breakfast of the smoked fish and cheeses that Leslie liked. She bathed, saying she didn't want to teach Sunday school smelling of fish and sperm. He soaped her back, but when he grew playful she told him there wasn't time to be silly.

He took her to North Station on the scooter. She rode sidesaddle in the flared blue coat.

"If you think Sunday-school teachers don't get laid you're naïve," he said.

"I don't think any such thing, and I'm not naïve."

It was almost springlike, and she went to the house with her father after Sunday school on foot, as he had not brought the car. Roland had gone ahead on his bike.

Alongside Massapeequit Road a cottontail rabbit dashed from them amid the leafless bushes, and Ed remarked to Millicent that they should appreciate living in a time when such animals still exist. He said wild creatures already existed only on man's sufferance, and that it was good that in a town like Wilmerding there were still patches and corners, overlooked by man, where a rabbit or a woodchuck or a muskrat could make a living. In time to come, probably, there would be none.

She asked him about the town meeting. She was wishing she had known of it and had arranged to go, since she would have been eligible to speak and vote. Ed told her there had been several hundred people, and that they had voted on seventy-five appropriations, the largest of which was for the schools. They had met in the high-school gymnasium, though when the town was smaller they had used to meet in the Unitarian church.

She pressed him for more details of what the meeting had been like. She had never been to one. He said the moderator had been a man named Gidding Thompson who wore two pairs of spectacles. There had been much angry questioning and recrimination because the hook and ladder that had been voted on and purchased the year before could not make the sharp turn down at the covered bridge, without a lot of backing and maneuvering and delay. There had also been debate about the sidewalk snowplow, which had been horse-drawn, and run by a man named Di Giacomo, but the horse had died, and the meeting turned down an appropriation for a new horse, voting instead to investigate the possibility of using the little bulldozer from the dump. Girls from the high school had sold refreshments at the meeting for some fund.

Millicent determined to attend any such meeting in the future. If she had been there, and had turned out to have an opinion on something, it would have been good practice to ask for the floor. She supposed she could begin to become known that way to local voters, even without having been elected to anything and even without connections as yet. It was high time she began to get the feel of political strife, even if she had to begin on that level. She felt there was real danger that she would be a nobody all her life.

At the house she was given letters to read that Charles had written to the family. She was struck by how different in tone and content they were from the ones he sent to her. He told how the mechanics worked eighteen hours a day and sometimes slept on the wings of their planes.

He told also how planes flew missions from Japan right into northern Korea, and how they would first hear the returning planes in the night and then begin to count them. And he wrote in detail of a wounded infantryman, just out of the hospital, with whom he had drunk beer in Tokyo. The infantryman had told him the infantry was the softest job in the Army. If there was an advance, the first regiment got wiped out, but otherwise things just settled down, and for ten weeks at a time you just sat. You could get a corporal's stripes by volunteering for a Browning Automatic Rifle, but if you did you got a Purple Heart the first night, because a B.A.R. lit up the sky like a machine gun and they could pick you off. A little old Garand was a lot healthier.

Millicent felt somewhat jealous that he did not write so newsily to her. The part about the infantryman had upset her mother. Even though he was not in Korea, it bothered Lucinda that he met and associated with boys who had been there. He wrote also that he was sending Patty a kimono.

Ed had written Charles a letter, not yet mailed, and he showed it to Millicent in the study and asked if she wanted to add anything.

> We gave blood again Thursday. We called for Millicent at her apartment and she joined us. Here's hoping you never need it.
>
> Patty just sent you some more of her special brownies again. I understand Aunt Celeste also put some sort of package in the mail this week.
>
> We are all very impressed by your letters, especially by the way you write that you hold the lives of many men in your hands, and by the way you realize the importance of accuracy and conscientiousness in your repair and maintenance work. I know that you also understand what is at stake in the whole national effort. As I said before, any job you do is either God's work or a boondoggle. Either you're God's agent or you're doing nothing.
>
> A-1 mechanics are probably even scarcer than good pilots.
>
> I am not sure if I agree with your views on MacArthur. But you gave me some food for thought and I will answer more fully in my next letter.
>
> I hope you don't forget the tallis and tefillin and prayer book I put in your stuff. Pray when you are healthy. When you are sick or things go bad you will feel too rotten to pray.
>
> It occurred to me lately that you can think of religion as like a mountainous country, bordering poetry on the west and bordering science on the east, and you can get lost in it, or lose your way in it. It's what keeps science and poetry apart, because it lies between them. Its peaks and clouds seem full of color where they rise from the watered hills on the west, but treacherous and dark and high on the east, where lightning beats on sheer cliff, and fogs fill ravines. You must pick your way through tribes of madmen hunting in the eastern slopes, and tribes of pixies in the western. The middle part is unknown. It's too steep.

She read the letter through. Then she added the word love under her father's signature, and her own name.

On Monday night Les told her he had had word from his mother that she would visit him on the weekend. His aunt from Glens Falls was going down to New Britain to look after his brother and mind the store. Millicent would have to vacate the apartment so that his mother could have the use of it, and Les would sleep at the hospital.

"How long will she stay?" Millicent asked.

"Just the two days. She gets some special half-price weekend deal on the bus if she sits up all night."

He reminded her that she would have to take all her clothes back to the girls' place, and remove all evidence that she was living with him. She said it was a lot of lugging and carting for just two days. He said he would help her.

It made her uneasy. But she realized that of course it was necessary.

Wednesday evening they had a little argument over whether the big corrugated carton full of Malcolm's paper hats had to be taken back to her own apartment. He said that the fewer things there were for his mother to ask questions about the simpler his life would be. But at last he agreed that he could say it belonged to the Mahadys.

She asked whether she could have him and his mother to dinner at her own apartment on Sunday or Saturday. She said her roommates could share dinner with them too and it would not look too suspicious. But he was disinclined.

"You know how mothers are," he said. "I don't want to start giving her ideas."

She asked if she would meet his mother at all, and he said he supposed that could be arranged.

"If you're not afraid to tell her you've got a motorcycle I don't see why you're afraid to tell her you have a girl friend," she said.

"Listen, I said you'd meet her, okay?"

"I'm a lot cheaper than that motorcycle. As a matter of fact if you consider the food and the laundry you're making a profit."

"What do you want? Do you want me to tell her I'm sleeping with ya?"

Day by day she brought clothing back to the girls' place. It was more than she had bargained for. Barbie's things had expanded into every cranny. The girls helped make space in drawers and closets that were already full, but it was next to impossible. Some things she left piled on Natalie's dresser, and Natalie assured her that for the few days involved she could manage.

She wanted to give Leslie's place a thorough cleaning, to have it spic and span for his mother's arrival, but he told her his mother would suspect something if it was too neat.

Early Friday morning, before he went to the hospital, he insisted they make a search for any forgotten evidence that she or the cat had been there. He went through the cupboards and cabinets.

"It's like a search for leaven," she said.

"I just want to make sure you didn't drop a bobby pin in the bathroom or anything."

"I don't use bobby pins."

"Well, anything. You don't know my mother. She has an eagle eye."

"And what's so terrible if she does find out?"

"Nothing's so terrible. But it's just reasonable to look around and pick up these things."

When the search seemed complete she sat at the table in her bathrobe, holding the cat, and watched Leslie put on his sheepskin.

"How about you meeting my folks," she said. "How about coming to Wilmerding Crosswalk for Passover?"

He buttoned the coat without answering.

"Will you?" she said.

"Well, we can talk about it. There's time, isn't there?"

"What if the landlady talks to your mother about me?"

"Oh, she won't."

"Well, you better tell her. Tell her your wife and your mother don't get along, or something."

After he had gone she made the bed. She did not make it as neat as usual, but tried to leave it a little sloppy, as she thought a man would do it. She made sure there were no contraceptives under the pillow. She thought of how Leslie would always place them there and then carefully fold his eyeglasses. She liked those precise ways he had. And she thought about the time she had been obliged to make this bed in full view of his friends, and how glad she had been that no contraceptives had been there then.

48

It felt strange, Friday night, to be back among all those girls. No one had a date, and Natalie and Barbie had done laundering, and clothing was hung everywhere. The long cushion was removed from the studio couch, and she made it up with bedding for sleeping on the floor.

Barbie irritated her. She had not liked the way Barbie shoved Theodore with her foot from a pile of soiled clothing. And she was not surprised on Saturday when Ella Jane confided to her that she would be glad when Barbie got a place of her own. Barbie played the radio too much, and was quite untidy, and did things like leaving the cream out to spoil, and expected Natalie to get her dates.

But Barbie was not looking for an apartment very hard. There was some possibility of Natalie's moving to share a place with two of the girls she taught with, and Barbie had said that if Natalie did so she would like to stay here.

Leslie phoned Millicent at the city room, quite late at night, and said she could have lunch with him and his mother in the hospital cafeteria Sunday if she liked. They would have had breakfast late, and would wait for lunch until about two, to give her time to get back from Wilmerding Crosswalk.

So after Sunday school she did not go to the house, but told her father she was meeting some friends for lunch in Boston.

On the train ride she began to feel some uneasiness about meeting Mrs. Hollander. For either Les or herself to introduce the other to a parent meant that their friendship had somehow to be defined. And it had no definition.

She was at the cafeteria ahead of them. There were basement walls painted a gentle green, and shiny tables. There was a mild smell, she could not tell whether a combined one of foods in which no one item could be distinguished, or of antiseptic. In a little while Les came, towering over his mother. She was a tiny woman, not at all as Millicent had pictured her, and quite worried-looking. She drew off a glove and gave Millicent a moist hand, but didn't smile.

They pushed their trays along the rails. Mrs. Hollander remarked that the prices were quite expensive. This judgment surprised Millicent. But she supposed Mrs. Hollander must mean expensive for a hospital cafeteria.

Millicent took a salad and Leslie and his mother took hot plates. There was no table completely free, so they had to share one with a hunched, middle-aged man who was already there, breaking bread into pea soup. They took off their coats, and Leslie began to take them to the coat rack, but his mother pulled him back by the arm.

"Just put them down here on the chair and then we don't have to watch them," she said. She pulled an empty chair and it grated on the floor.

"No one'll steal them here," Les told her. He went off to the coat rack.

"He needs a haircut," Mrs. Hollander said to Millicent. They sat and waited for him. Mrs. Hollander kept looking at Millicent. She was older than Millicent's mother by perhaps ten years, though without a trace of gray in her permanent. But she had small, nervous eyes, and the lines of an anxious, almost frightened expression seemed deep in her face. Her lips were tight, and her face was rouged and powdered. The surrounding noise of clattering trays and utensils seemed bothersome.

"Did you have a good trip up?" Millicent asked her.

"Oh, it was horrible," Mrs. Hollander said. "They have some nerve." She began to tell of it, while she ate, and Leslie returned meanwhile and drew in his chair. The bus had taken all the bumpiest roads and gone a roundabout route by way of Providence and New Bedford, stopping in scores of cities and towns. In New Bedford the layover was three hours, in the middle of the night, during which the driver disappeared, and she had remained in the bus all alone. From there to Boston there was one other passenger, a man sleeping in the back, and there had been no heat.

"Couldn't you get a better bus?" Millicent asked.

"Anything to save a buck," said Les.

"So am I to be blamed for that?" his mother asked him.

Leslie ate without answering. The hunched man with pea soup ignored them, breathing loudly and wiping his mouth often with a paper napkin.

"At least I'll get a ride home with someone," Mrs. Hollander told Millicent.

"Who?" said Millicent, not quite understanding.

"A lady I know. Mrs. Mintz. And I want you to try to cash in that ticket stub," she said to Leslie.

"Are we back on that again?" he said irritably. "You can't cash it. It says right on it—no refunds. It's a special excursion between certain hours and it doesn't even amount to a regular one-way fare. The whole thing's only four bucks."

"You could try," said his mother.

"And waste time, and make a fool of myself. You'd have to do it in Hartford anyway."

"It still seems to me I'm entitled to two dollars back," said Mrs. Hollander. "If I ride back with Mrs. Mintz I've only used half of it."

"Well, you're wrong."

"I'll go there myself if you won't."

"Go ahead." Millicent noticed that his voice, usually so soft, hesitant even, was quite different when he spoke to his mother.

His mother put a hand to her lips and asked Leslie to get her a glass of water. He pushed his chair back noisily and went for it.

The stranger at their table ate as though hearing nothing.

"I brought those two boys up all alone since my husband died," Mrs. Hollander said to Millicent, "and a lot of thanks I get for it."

"Are you enjoying your visit?" Millicent asked.

"Well, he's my oldest, and if I didn't come to see him I'd never see him, I suppose. I'm lucky if I get a letter out of him once in two weeks."

"I know he thinks of you," said Millicent. "He speaks of you quite often."

"Do you see him often?" Mrs. Hollander asked.

Millicent took a mouthful of food, and swallowed it. "Well, he's very busy," she said. "And so am I. We both have our work."

"Leslie told me what you do—I forget."

"I'm a newspaperwoman."

"Oh that's right."

They ate in silence a moment.

"The Mass General takes only the very best, you know," Mrs. Hollander told her. "Just a very few from each of the top schools."

"Is that so? I more or less suspected that," said Millicent.

"Oh yes. It's the outstanding hospital in the country."

Leslie came back with the water and resumed eating. His mother drank some.

"Leslie was Phi Beta Kappa in his third year, you know," Mrs. Hollander said.

"Millicent's also Phi Bete," Leslie said.

"In her third year?" said Mrs. Hollander. "They don't take very many then, you know. Only the very top."

"I was a greasy grind," said Leslie.

"Oh yes," his mother answered him sourly. "I suppose they take just anybody in Phi Beta Kappa."

She took a small bite.

"He was salutatorian in high school," she said to Millicent. "Did you know that?"

"No. I didn't know that."

The man finished his pea soup and rose, buttoning an old coat.

"And he ranked in the first five in medical school," said Mrs. Hollander.

"And he was a transfer student, which put him at a disadvantage. He went to Johns Hopkins first."

"There was no disadvantage," said Les.

"He contradicts everything I say. In my day children didn't contradict their elders." She took another bite and wiped her mouth with a paper napkin. "Do you contradict your mother?" she asked Millicent.

"Sometimes."

"But everything she says?"

"Listen, there was no disadvantage," said Leslie. "What do you want from me?"

They ate a while without speaking. A skinny woman came by collecting plates on a wagon and making noise. Then, with everyone nearly finished, Millicent said she had to leave for work.

"Do you have to work on Sunday?" Mrs. Hollander asked.

"Yes. I'm off Wednesday and Thursday."

As they rose Mrs. Hollander drew a neatly flattened green paper bag out of her purse, opened it, and dropped Millicent's uneaten rolls inside.

"Mother, will you stop that?" Leslie said.

They went toward the coat rack. Mrs. Hollander went by a vacant table on which a pair of soft uneaten rolls still lay on a tray, beside dirty plates and a crumpled napkin, and gathered those rolls into her bag also. Millicent saw her glance at other tables as if looking for more.

"Mother, don't be so cheap," said Leslie. His voice was low, but he sounded furious.

"Oh, so I'm cheap. I scrimp and do without, to put a boy through school, and that's what I get."

"Yes, you are cheap," he said. "How cheap can you get?"

"Did you hear that?" Mrs. Hollander said to Millicent. "What do you think of a boy that calls his mother cheap? I bet you don't talk to your parents like that."

Leslie was red-faced. Millicent felt for him, but avoided looking at him so as not to magnify his embarrassment. Mrs. Hollander buttoned her coat. It had a woolly surface, kinky and tightly curled.

"What do you think those rolls are worth?" Leslie said to his mother as they started out into the hallways. "All of two cents?"

"That's all right. Every penny counts. And I don't believe in waste. Every penny I spent on myself I always felt was out of the mouths of my children," she told Millicent, walking beside her. Leslie was behind them. "But I suppose it's wrong to expect gratitude from a child."

They passed through the lobby.

"My Jackie has no gratitude either," she told Millicent. "The younger one gets it from the older one. Their mother's just a doormat, to wipe their feet on, that's all. As soon as they're both through school and on their feet I'll commit suicide and I'll be out of their way."

"Mother, for Christ sake. I'm embarrassed."

"That right. Be ashamed of your mother."

He held the door. They went onto the steps and into the sunshine. Millicent stole a glance at Les but he was not looking at her.

"Talking of being cheap," his mother said, "I wish you'd get a new coat. That sheepskin's too frayed and it makes a very poor impression for a doctor."

"I can't afford it. When my mother steals garbage I can't afford it."

"You can afford it much better than you can afford that silly motorcycle." She started into the street alone, crossing against the traffic lights.

She was somewhat bowlegged, Millicent noticed. Leslie hesitated a moment, and then hurried into the traffic after his mother, raising a hand and dodging a car. Millicent let them go, without having said good-bye, and walked to the city room.

Monday morning she rose when the other girls did. She waited for Leslie's phone call. He had told her he would phone when his mother had finally left, so she could move her things back at once.

At ten she had not heard, and wondered if Mrs. Hollander had delayed her departure or missed her ride with Mrs. Mintz, or whether Les was simply too busy at the hospital to telephone. She busied herself gathering together the articles she meant to take back to Leslie's. It would require more than one trip. She would not trust Charles's ivory to a valise, and the cat would have to be carried.

The door buzzer sounded. She pressed the button that would release the downstairs door and went to the landing to see who it was. She heard footsteps on the flight below.

Then at the bend in the stairs her father appeared. He had never dropped in on her like this before, though she knew he sometimes had errands in Boston. It's lucky I'm home, she thought.

"Hi," she said.

"Hi." His voice was heavy and he did not look up at her.

When he got to the landing he went into the apartment, looking almost a little absent-minded. His coat hung open. He sat back heavily in the fat worn chair with broken springs. She thought he looked very tired and drawn.

"Sit down, Millicent Audrey."

She sat in one of the rickety chairs by the drop-leaf table. There was a gloom in his manner that frightened her. It crossed her mind that somehow he knew about herself and Les, but then she told herself it was not possible.

He looked at her, and then rested his closed eyes on his fingers, rubbing them a little. His hat lay on the back of his head.

"Millicent," he said, not very loud, and almost in a monotone, "get ready for a shock." He seemed to draw a breath and let it out again. His eyes were still hidden. "Charles was in an accident, in a helicopter. He's dead." He became still.

Millicent drew a breath. It seemed to her that it was not real, and yet she knew it was real.

He took his hand from his eyes. He looked at her almost in a dazed way. "I'll take you home," he said. "We want you home for a few days."

She swallowed. It surprised her that she didn't cry. Her father's eyes turned to the wall before him. They looked glazed.

"I'm numb," he said. "Six boys, in a helicopter. A mechanical failure. They were being taken from one base to another, or something. I don't know. It's being investigated. I tried to get a phone call through. I can't get through yet."

"How's Mother?"

"She's had a sedative. The kids are with her. Celeste's there, and Grandma Annie's there."

His eyes moved to her.

"Are you all right?" he said.

"I'm all right," she said weakly. She still wondered that she hadn't cried.

He looked at the wall again. She saw his eyes wander to Natalie's crucifix above the table.

"What do these girls eat for breakfast?" he said. "Ham and eggs?"

"Just coffee, usually."

His eyes lowered somewhat, and looked at nothing. "I'll phone your office," he said. "You give me the number. I'll tell them you won't be in."

"I can call."

But neither of them moved.

"You got some schnapps?" he asked.

"The girls may have some." She pushed herself up. She went to the delicate old cabinet that stood at the end of the room, and opened one of the doors of inlaid wood.

49

She poured whisky into a shot glass. It seemed to her that her father's hand shook when she gave it to him.

She got her coat from the crowded closet, trying to keep the items pressed against it from falling down. She saw her half-packed valise lying open on the studio couch, with clothing about it, in her father's view, and yet he seemed not to have noticed it at all. Following him down the stairs she felt at last the warming gush of tears, and was glad that she did. She had begun to fear that she wouldn't.

She wept in the car also, slouched down and using a handkerchief. Her father put his hand on hers now and then while he drove. It seemed to her that he drove with reckless abandon, so that she thought they might have an accident. But she said nothing. Several times her father seemed about to speak, but he didn't.

As she entered the house her mother seized her, clutching her to her and sobbing, and Patty and Roland and Aunt Celeste and her grandmother crowded around, as though she herself had come back from death. Her own crying began again. She knew it was real, and it weakened her as she stood in her mother's arms. They led her to the sofa, and she could not stop or control her sobbing. But she was glad somehow that they saw it. Patty was blubbering and the others were crying too, especially Aunt Celeste. Everyone's weeping seemed to affect everyone else.

At length her mother was persuaded to go upstairs to lie down, and Celeste and Grandma Annie went with her. Millicent went to the kitchen and made cocoa. She felt as though she needed the comfort of food, yet her stomach was too nervous for anything more solid. Patty sat with her red-eyed while she drank it, saying nothing.

Afterward she heard her mother crying again, and went up to sit with her and the others. Her mother cried not hysterically or loudly, but in an endless, quiet, forlorn way, as though she were worn out and had no strength for resistance. When her mother dozed off Millicent went downstairs.

The framed portrait of Charles was on top of the piano, beside the picture of the four children, and now a candle flame was up there also, its wick burning in a tumbler of wax.

Millicent helped Aunt Celeste prepare some lunch. The phone was tied up, as Ed was trying to place a call to Japan to find out more about what had happened, and he also phoned Washington. In late afternoon, when Lucinda had come down to the kitchen to have tea, he told them all he had arranged for the body to be flown home for burial. He said he thought it would take about two days. He seemed to speak with some difficulty, and Millicent saw that his eyes were moist. Roland asked him if the box would be flown with a flag draped over it.

"Yes," said Ed. "A flag on it. So no other freight will be put on top."

"That's good," said Lucinda. Her voice was hoarse and heavy, and dragging, and she sat hunched over her tea. "I want the best for him." She remained calm a while and then the forlorn, weak, helpless crying began again. It was horrible to watch. Celeste put an arm about her. It made Patty cry also.

"This is what's meant by 'in pain shalt thou bring forth children,' " Ed said. "You know that? Not the childbearing. This is what it means." He was looking mainly at Millicent, his face contorted.

"Well, I've got to get out on my paper route," Roland said.

"For years you worry about a kid's schooling," Ed said. "And about getting him ready for manhood. He flunks in school, and you think that's a disaster. All your love for a child is tied up with pain."

Lucinda had eaten little all day, and ate almost no supper, though they urged her to. Afterward Millicent and Patty sat with Ed in the living room, and Patty was tearful about a fight she had had with Charles shortly before his enlistment, in which she had told him she hated him. They assured her that Charles must have known she didn't really, because she had sent so many brownies since, but Patty seemed not satisfied.

Millicent felt now that she ought to have taken him into her confidence more. She should have had him meet Les, or at least told him more about Les, so that he would have realized how fine a person Les was. Then he would have understood, and would not have worried so. It was as though she and Charles had been on the verge of a great understanding, a great closeness. But instead there had even been a kind of teasing in her anger—she had teased him and plagued him, the way she had kept him in the dark. She felt she had given him no warmth at all.

"You know what I believe?" Patty said tearfully. "I believe that in just about a month from now Russia's going to come in, and the bombs will start to fly, and they'll bomb Boston and New York and every place, and we'll all die a horrible lingering death, the whole world, all lying around all scorched and burned, so that what happened to Charles was a great mercy. That's what I believe. He died just in time. God spared him."

Later she spoke of a kimono that Charles had sent her, that the mails had not brought yet, and she said that when it came she would wear it every day.

Ed called Roland, and then asked the three children to join him in evening prayers in the study. He gave them prayer books, and prayed in a whisper, facing toward the east, occasionally louder to give them a clue as to what paragraph he had arrived at.

"How can you love a God that allows wars?" Patty said when he closed the book.

"So if I embraced atheism," he said, turning to her, "would that give me answers? Atheism I don't need. Because a religion that doesn't give answers, I have already. Do you think I know why things happen? Why things are how they are? There's only one thing I know, and that is, that whatever God's doing, He isn't cheap. That's all. Look, Patty." He put a hand on her. "This isn't the world we'd choose, if we had a choice. There isn't one of us, that if we were God, that we'd set up the universe the way God did. Not one of us. And if anybody said he would, you'd think there was something wrong with him. But so I can stand to live, I try to trust that there's a level on which things make sense. And I try to live as if things made sense. Because we're boxed in, whether we like it or not. Even in death we can't get out of this universe."

They all went to bed early. Millicent slept on the spare iron cot in Patty's room, as she had used to. The bed in Charles's room was vacant, but somehow it seemed sacrilegious to suggest using it. She had a fit of weeping as she lay in her blankets. Thinking of how she had wept earlier in the day seemed to set off a repetition, until her face was drenched in the darkness.

She could remember correcting his infant speech. He had been littler than she, and then bigger. She could remember all sorts of unimportant events, not in a saintly way, but as though he were still alive, and it seemed a profanation.

She remembered a time when they had gotten silly together and had not been able to stop laughing. And she remembered a time when he was sent to bed without supper. But he had been in the wrong.

She slept, but awoke in the middle of the night. She felt she had dreamed of Charles. The candle in the living room downstairs even sent some trace of its glow to the upstairs hallway—she knew it was that by its occasional flicker. It must shine enough through the French doors for some of its light even to rise up the stairs, she thought.

She was too nervous to lie there. She put on a bathrobe and went down. Her father was sitting in the tall rocker by the bay window, also wearing a bathrobe, and holding a glass of whisky.

"Couldn't sleep?" he asked her.

"I woke up," she told him. She sat near him. There was no light except the wick burning in its tumbler. "Isn't it unusual to light the candle before the funeral?" she asked.

"Well, Patty lighted it," said Ed. "She didn't know. So leave it. We'll light another one."

He stared vacantly and tiredly at the opposite wall. For a time he didn't say anything, and the silence grew long.

"Well," he said at last, "a life—it's everything." He looked at her, as if for confirmation. Then his gaze drifted away and became vacant again. "And in the end," he said, "if we're really living, we're all cut down before our time. Life's too short to let you complete anything. But at eighteen, it's a terrible time. At that age his life is all input." He gestured slightly and shook his head hopelessly. "Millicent, it's awful to outlive a child. To remember back years before he was born, and to have seen both ends of his life, and know how short the whole thing was. He's dead. Such potentialities—what was he given them for? And there were other boys too. Beginnings, that evaporate without purpose. Tell me, what use was the seed he carried? This death, it didn't just kill him—it killed off a whole line of descendants, all the sons and daughters that might have sprung from him. It makes a man a random thing, doesn't it? Like a seed that falls on a stone. And we're like a broken set, the rest of us, you know that? We'll never be whole again. And no joy will ever be whole again."

His words disturbed her. Some of them coincided with her own feelings. It seemed to her too like a permanent brokenness.

Her father took a sip of whisky. I'd rather he'd drink whisky than smoke cigarettes, anyway, she thought. It's cleaner.

"Of course I've got parents in their graves, grandparents," he said. "You live with the dead. But the dead should be behind you, not surrounding you. And Rosalind, only three months ago."

He took another swallow.

"That was a blow too," he said. "She was the person nearest of kin in my own generation. Certain things only we knew. Things about our parents, our brothers. You know what I mean? Nobody else can ever fill that role for me. Some deaths only grieve you, and some deaths change your world. Even though

I didn't see her often, as long as she was alive, I knew my childhood world still lived. I could talk about it—I wasn't alone. And when she was gone, I was a middle-aged man—I live with the dead now. That's what a middle-aged man is. He can work, and he can fight for his family, like he did before, but his world is peopled with memories of people that are dead. Even your own children don't replace the people who went before. And your parents, grandparents, are still different. None replaces another. You know what science should bend itself to, and what the taxpayers' billions should be spent on? A search for a way to resurrect the dead. That I'd be in favor of. Let's study a way to bring back the dead, so wrongs can be repaired. Reconstitute a boy from the grave—that's worth a few hundred billion, a crash program. I've seen so much death. Funerals. And they talk about dying philosophically. But even an old man dreads his time. And the speed with which he sees his remaining little boiling away, just like steam. If he loves anything. You live so fast, and you do so little. And just recently I buried a man thirty-nine years old in this congregation. Just croaked at his desk, and his children found him on the floor. A girl twelve, a boy ten. A Ph.D. in mathematics. And what's the use of stuffing in all that learning, a Harvard Ph.D., if you're gonna be dead at thirty-nine? He hardly got time to use what he learned, and his brain is dead and empty again. And I read somewhere, in the paper today, a young girl with leukemia, Charles's age. And we forget death, really, we stop believing in death for years and months at a time, so long as it hasn't recently struck near, so long as it doesn't strike the few people who really matter."

His eyes looked sunken and his face was drawn. She had not seen him cry, but Patty had told her he had cried very much in the morning. Apparently he tried not to in front of the rest of the family.

"I can't sleep," he said resignedly. "I sleep two hours, or three, and I dream about him and I wake up." He gave his head a little shake. "Did I will this child into the world? Some night eighteen years ago I decided to make your mother pregnant. But could I will that he be a boy, or that you be a girl? Or your temperament and your whole nature, or your size and your looks? Could I will this particular child? We desired a child, that's all. I can remember him newborn. How a baby's littleness reaches out to you. It fills you with tenderness. And you don't stop and think then, that this child is someday going to have his day in the funeral parlor too, that it's the surest thing in the world. That it's the one certain thing about him, actually. All you see is life."

He blew out a long, despairing sigh, and sat quietly. After a while he patted Millicent's hand.

"Why don't you go to bed," he said.

She went upstairs. The next day her mother seemed to her drier-eyed and more controlled, so she left the house for a while and telephoned Leslie from Yerxa's Pharmacy. It turned out that he had phoned the city room and knew what had happened.

He offered to visit her family as a friend of hers, during the condolence week. She said he didn't have to.

"What can I say?" his voice said in the receiver. "I wish I could say something more comforting. It just has to be accepted, Millicent. You have to go on living."

The words moved her. It struck her how full of truth and meaning these old phrases became, now that they applied to her. The more commonplace, she thought, the more when it applies to you it suddenly contains revelation, all the truth in the world. She thanked him for what he had said. Then Leslie remarked that going off to war was one male privilege she didn't have to envy.

She asked if he would pick up the cat from the girls' apartment when he had a chance, and remember to keep it fed.

She was grateful for his having taken time to speak to her, especially as he was at the hospital, and the minutes must have been stolen from his work and his patients.

Her mother still seemed quiet when Millicent got back, but also rather nervous, and in some ways her behavior was strange. One moment she said they must move and sell the house, that she could not stay here a bit longer. But a few minutes later she said Charles's room upstairs must always be preserved exactly as it was.

When Ed said his prayers it irritated Lucinda, as though such attention to routine implied that he wasn't thinking about Charles.

"You've lost a child!" she shouted at him.

"I know I've lost a child," he said.

"Ask your damn God if He was ever a mother," she muttered.

Tragedy hasn't brought them closer, Millicent thought. She thought about the antique car out in the barn. She wondered if that would be kept always just as it was, also.

Lucinda began to speculate on how Charles had suffered at the end, and Ed assured her that from what he had learned it must have been sudden, and that he had not been burned. But Lucinda said he must have been frightened, when that machine began to fall.

"Why did you always tell me not to worry?" she said to him. "If I'd worried more I'd have realized how dangerous it was."

In the afternoon Ed received word when the body would arrive. He said his brother Franklin would make the arrangements with the funeral parlor and arrange for the body's being picked up. Millicent wandered about the house, and also outdoors. It was the first day of spring. A whole flock of birds had all perched in one crab-apple tree, and Roland had said they were grosbeaks migrating to Canada. Her father had said it was the wrong time to die. It was mainly little recollections that brought tears to her eyes again and again. She kept thinking of how she had directed him in the construction of a dam at Abbottsford.

She came in by the kitchen door, and found her mother telling her father she would never forgive him for letting Charles enlist.

"If he'd been in school he would have been deferred," Lucinda said. "He got the interest in motors from you, and he got the impulsiveness and the recklessness from you, too. I know about him crawling around in Moon's Garage. Why didn't you make him study? Every time it's Saturday he couldn't study because it's the Sabbath. And you backed him up."

"Well, a man's entitled to a Sabbath," said Ed.

It was decided during supper that Patty would have to give up her part in the De Molay play. The understudy would have to take over.

In the evening Lucinda seemed to grow very mild and very tired. She sat on the sofa squinting, and looking old. "They lose him for you," she mused, not very loud. "You send him to the Air Force, and he's out of your sight, and they lose him. Just like a screwdriver or something, that they left out in the rain. They lose him like a glove, so carelessly. They don't care. They can get another mother's boy."

Late the next day they were told they could view Charles at the funeral parlor any time from about midnight on. It seemed to Millicent that the body had come very fast. Lucinda wanted to be there at the earliest time, and sit at the funeral parlor through the night until the funeral. Ed didn't want to leave her there alone, and there was some argument, but finally it was decided that the whole family would go.

"Who'll do my route in the morning?" said Roland.

"Call Bobby O'Shaughnessy," said Ed. "Or call your boss, and tell him the circumstances, and maybe he'll do it himself. If he can't I'll drive you back special at five in the morning and help you deliver it, okay?"

At the funeral parlor Lucinda broke down again, and when she went near the casket Ed and Patty had to support her. It seemed to Millicent that Charles looked strange in death. The profile, with cropped hair and closed eyes, was still his, but his features had somehow taken on a different cast. It was hard to recognize them with that inertness. The undertakers had done a good job, but she could see traces of bruises and cuts. She had heard he had been thrown clear of the craft, and died of concussion and multiple fractures. He rested on satiny quilting, a prayer shawl draped on his Air Force uniform. She remembered a summer when she had nearly drowned at a beach, though none of her family knew of it even now. An alert lifeguard had caught her in the nick of time. And she had thought then in the water, before she saw the lifeguard, of how her family would react to her death.

Lucinda wanted some of Charles's hair, and Ed said he would arrange for the undertakers to cut some. Then Lucinda fell to her knees, hugging Roland to her. "I just have one son now," she sobbed.

"Leave the poor kid alone," said Ed.

50

Lucinda was persuaded after an hour or two that it was better not to sit all night at the funeral parlor, and they went home.

But in the morning they returned, well ahead of the funeral hour, and stayed in a room set aside until everyone was fairly composed. Then they filed into the main chapel, where the casket was, and sat in the front pew that had been reserved for them. Millicent knew she must be as red-eyed as the others. Roland was not red-eyed, but he looked grave and solemn. When she looked about there were very many people. She saw among them relatives she knew, and some old friends of her parents, and others she did not recognize. She had been saying to herself that her mother must not be allowed to become hysterical, but in a while she became aware that all five of them were weeping in a quiet, controlled way. She was between Roland and her father and held hands with both.

A man she did not know gave a eulogy. She had somehow supposed her father would do it and would lead the service, but she realized now it made sense for him to have engaged someone else. He was a dark-jowled man and grayer than her father, though perhaps no older, and he seemed really moved by the tragedy of so young a man's death and by the family's grief. He mentioned the full name, Charles Piper Gordon, and spoke of Charles's bravery, of his ambition, of his inventiveness, of his devotion to his family. It was all true. He recalled many incidents that he must have been told by her father or by someone in the family—he even knew that at the age of twelve Charles had taught himself to move a car back and forth on the driveway. He mentioned also, at one point, that if it were not for such young men, who were willing to go into the service and risk everything, we would all be slaves.

In the limousine that followed the hearse none of the family spoke much, except that Patty remarked on what a big crowd had come. Millicent looked back too, and saw that the cars with headlights burning in the daylight stretched back in a very long line on the highway. It seemed strange to her that the weather should have turned out so bright and full of promise. And some hours before, on entering the funeral chapel, she had noticed a rolled newspaper in someone's coat, and it had struck her that even while a life ends, headlines proclaim new international events and new developments the dead would have liked to follow up.

It was the warmest day of the year so far, and as she walked on the cemetery paths she thought of how the trees would bud soon and insect life would begin again in the ground, and how her brother would lie here through all the variety of changing seasons. Among all this population of monuments that stretched around on the little hills and valleys. He would be here among all these old people who had died.

She recognized the family plot when they got to it, and the familiar headstones in it. The crowd gathered about solemnly. There was a new oblong hole next to a pile of fresh dirt. Her mother had broken down once more, with that crushed, destroyed kind of crying, and her father and Celeste were supporting her. Patty leaned with Aunt Gwendolyn and they were all close together. Another service was being read. Every death of someone near you brought you nearer to your own death, she thought.

It seemed as though her mother would keep up that desolate sobbing forever. It was not even a protesting kind of sobbing, but a sobbing that seemed to understand that everything was forever ruined.

Happiness involved a blacking out of some things, she thought, a forgetting. There was something fraudulent in it.

> *Glorified and sanctified be the great Name throughout the world which He has created according to His will—*

She followed the prayer. According to His will. She knew that phrase occurred elsewhere, in other prayers too. Her father had told her once it was a backhanded phrase, a kind of veiled protest, with an undertone of bafflement. It almost seemed to mean, God, I trust it makes sense to You. Because it doesn't to me.

> *May He hurry up and establish His dominion while we're still alive—*

Her father had told her it was a trick, placing this prayer here—to make you affirm order in the world when there least appears to be any. It was a prayer to be said when you had the greatest urge to blasphemy. Because our blasphemy only leaves us all the more aware of how helpless we are. God doesn't cringe before it. She said the responses.

> *Worshipped, praised, glorified, exalted, extolled, honored, adored, lauded, beyond any capacity of word or hymn—*

She heard Patty's broken voice, and her mother struggling to say the words one at a time as her father repeated them slowly, guiding her.

> *Let us have peace—*

She poured water over her fingers, after her father, from a copper pitcher that one of the natty undertaker's men offered, putting her hands out ahead of Roland. She saw that her mother also did so, distractedly, when Patty urged her. Peace, shalom, really meant completeness, her father had told her once. And now there could never be completeness. Her mother walked down the path unsupported, though her resigned, defeated kind of crying went on. She looked ghastly.

They did not go back in the undertaker's limousine, as the funeral parlor would have been out of the way. She saw her mother and Roland get into Uncle Ira's car, and someone directed her into Uncle Maxwell's. She rode in the back seat, her father between her and Patty. Uncle Maxwell began to smoke a cigar as they rode. It bothered her and she lowered a window. Aunt Tessie remarked that she thought the eulogy had been very lovely.

"It's his first day in the grave," Patty said. "He's been there twenty minutes. And tomorrow I'll think, he's been in the grave a whole day now. And it'll be two days. And a week. And someday I'll think, it's a whole year already, and then five years, and I'll be shocked at how long it is."

Ed patted her knee. Uncle Maxwell seemed to be avoiding the city, and taking them instead around it, directly to Wilmerding Crosswalk. He drove fast. For a time no one spoke. When Millicent looked at her father he looked very tired. It occurred to her that either of her parents would rather have lost the other, rather than any of the children.

He seemed lost in his thoughts. Once or twice she thought he was about to speak, but then he seemed to change his mind. At last she saw him squeeze Patty's hand more tightly, still looking at no one.

"You see what I mean, Patty?" he said slowly, as though apropos of some thought of his own, or of some remark of a previous day. "This is the universe we have to live with. This is your life, and this is your death. You can't get out. All roads only take you back to the same question mark, and you start making religion afresh."

He pressed Patty's hand again and Millicent's also, staring vaguely at the upholstery before him. She heard his breathing.

"God has us over a barrel," he said.

Most of the relatives came to the house, so that it was full of uncles and aunts and cousins. Some had brought foods that could be prepared easily, and Gwendolyn and Celeste set to work at once with efficiency, laying out plates on the dining-room table and seeing that everyone ate, though not all at the same time. They washed the dishes also. Millicent saw that as her mother discovered each person a new flood of tears came, and her mother would babble about something that particular relative had done for Charles in the past—a toy sailboat from an uncle, or that he and Steve had gone double-dating together. Millicent heard Uncle Maxwell say to someone that it had cost a fortune to fly the body halfway round the world. He said it was Lucinda that had insisted on it, though in the past she had always used to say she didn't believe in funerals. But she had said not a word this time about no service, or no burial, or giving the body to science. It irritated Millicent to hear a hypocrite like Uncle Maxwell talk meanly of her mother that way. "She didn't even let him lie in Japan," Maxwell was saying. "She had to bring him home, save a lock of his hair. Whether she still doesn't want a funeral for herself when she goes, I don't know," Maxwell said. "Maybe she's got different standards for herself and the kids."

She also heard him say her mother had fainted when they first got the news and that Ed feared she had gone into shock.

And she heard Patty telling people that Charles was sending her a kimono.

The next day the condolence callers began, especially in the afternoon and evening. Relatives came again, and members of the congregation, especially prominent ones and officers of it, and some other townspeople, and old friends of her parents' and distant cousins that Millicent scarcely knew. She heard the same sorrowful greetings expressed over and over. "What can I say, Ed?" And she was struck again that such words no longer seemed banal. The fact of death and the fact of temporariness had lost their triteness. Many of the women, even those not related, arrived with tears in their eyes and embraced Lucinda, and Millicent saw Polly Cook and Denise Saint-Onge and some other girls sitting with Patty, some of them quite wet-eyed. There were endless gifts of food. People kept bringing more.

Men and women who had not seen each other for a while visited together in all of the downstairs rooms, and Millicent heard introductions being made. There were conversations everywhere, on a variety of topics. Jill told Millicent she had met a Hindu at a dance and was thinking of marrying him.

The atmosphere was sedate, but not gloomy, and Millicent found it pleasant to talk to people. There was some talk of Charles, but she was also asked about her job, and a man told her some interesting things about politics. In late evening, when all the company had gone, and her aunts were busy washing dishes, it occurred to Millicent that she was glad of the condolence-week system. The house would have been awful without all those people about, and she was glad there would be more of them tomorrow. She had even come to like some relatives she hadn't much cared for before.

Ed came into the kitchen, and said he had had word that Charles had named Millicent as the sole beneficiary of his G.I. insurance. Ten thousand dollars. She reddened.

"I couldn't take it," she said. She was sitting at the table. "I don't want it."

"Well, it's yours," said Ed. He sat down.

She knew that all the others, even the aunts, felt the oddness of Charles's doing such a thing. Her voice had been faint. She could say nothing more. It seemed to make her feel his presence. She rested her face on her open hands, covering her eyes, breathing through her mouth.

No one spoke, until her father did again. "It was a surprise to me," he said to everyone present. "I just assumed he named you," he said to Lucinda, "or maybe all the children. Maybe he thought Millicent would be an old maid and she'd need it for her old age."

She continued the quiet breathing. She wished Roland and Patty would stop looking at her.

"Well, whatever his reason was, it shows he thought about it anyway," said Aunt Celeste. "Most boys would just leave it to their mother like everybody else does without a thought."

"That's what I was thinking," said Ed. He looked pensive. "I guess we never really knew him."

"I knew him very well," Lucinda said sourly.

51

Millicent stayed in Wilmerding Crosswalk five days in all, including her days off, from the time Ed had brought her there, but then she felt she had to return to her job. The condolence week and the daily arrival of visitors continued without her. Ed's stomach was nervous and he ate little, though there was always food about. He stayed in the living room, sitting with callers, and usually in the evening enough men came, relatives and men of the congregation, so that prayers could be said in traditional form. He felt as though life was a shambles. He slept lightly, and once he dreamed that the report of Charles's death had been a mistake. He mentioned to one of the visitors how all through the children's lives he had worried from time to time, about the many dangers that could befall a kid—a small boy drowned or hit by a car or falling fifty feet from rafters in some forbidden exploration, a little girl kidnapped by a lunatic, a son blinded by a friend's rifle. Yet the fears never seemed real, because they didn't happen—like your fear before a child's birth that he might be a mongoloid. And now it had happened.

He told how Charles when little would come out with amazing bits of knowledge and information, that he had never dreamed the child had heard or remembered.

He hardly went out, except to the barn to bring the dog its dinner. Who could have guessed that that old sick dog, half blind for the last couple of years, would outlive Charles?

Caleb Folger gave a lecture to a joint meeting of the sisterhood and brotherhood of Temple Beth El, but Ed did not go, and Caleb was introduced instead by Amethyst, as president of the sisterhood.

But when the condolence week was over Ed returned to work, even though it seemed to him that every few minutes Charles came to mind. After a week you don't cry much, he said to himself. And it was forbidden to grieve longer than seven days. He was glad he had not relapsed into excessive smoking.

Most of the grass was still brown, and the trees had no leaves yet, but the crocuses had been up, and there were birds in the mornings and swamp noises at night. The phoebes were building a net again in the porch eaves. He kept busy, with his classes and his tutoring, and made visits to the Concord Reformatory and the Sparkstown Hospital, and traveled to three different towns where he lectured to small audiences of women on how to set a Passover table.

He gave the Weekly Wilmerdingian a message to be published among the Easter messages. He answered two fire calls, one caused by a short circuit in the Eng Hop Hand Laundry and the other by a greasy smoke duct in Bingle's German & Yankee Cookery. At the house he got the screens and cleaned the cellar dust from them, and began to remove the storm windows. It seemed also that he kept hearing of deaths of teen-agers and children. Whenever he picked up a newspaper his eye caught something like that.

Charles's effects came, in a big cardboard box. They were placed up in his room. The mails also brought his Purple Heart medal, and a little square banner with a red border and a golden star. The Gold Star was hung in the living-room window.

Lucinda seemed spiritless and aged to Ed, particularly if the weather was good. On an especially fine day, when the sun was bright, she would remark, "Poor Charles. My poor son." She chased away some children who went into the barn to play in the Model T.

She often let the housework and the cooking go now, and even the shopping. She said she disliked to go out because whenever she did she saw boys who resembled Charles. But Patty took over to a large extent. Ed was struck by how efficient Patty was. It seemed as though Patty had a good effect on Lucinda also. Seeing Patty start the laundry or prepare a meal often would make Lucinda bestir herself. Lucinda's sisters visited often, meanwhile, and were of help.

Then one afternoon Patty went horseback riding with Polly Cook, without having asked permission, but she mentioned it at the end of supper, after Roland had left the table. Lucinda was at once furious with her. "Do you want to get killed?" Lucinda shouted across the table at her. "Don't you ever sneak off like that again! Don't you know it's dangerous? People get thrown from horses!"

"You don't get thrown if you pay attention to instruction and if you have a gentle horse," Patty said.

Ed was repeating the Grace After Meals very quietly, as though not listening.

"A horse can get frightened!" Lucinda said to Patty. "Or you can get kicked! Or bitten!"

"Okay, so I didn't get hurt, did I?" Patty said.

"It doesn't make any difference! Even the gentlest horse in the world can stumble. And you never know about a horse. There was a case of a horse that ran wild and carried a girl for miles and miles."

"When? A hundred years ago? It seems to me it's a lot safer than cars."

"I'm not crazy about cars either for young kids. There's altogether too many cars in this town."

"I can't stop living," Patty said.

"Nobody's asking you to stop living."

"You're withdrawing from life," Patty told her. "Just like Daddy said."

"I'm not withdrawing from life," said Lucinda. "I'm just withdrawing from any more deaths in the family."

"Do you realize they put babies on that horse?" Patty said.

"You never mind what I realize."

"I can hardly wait to grow up and get out of here."

"Patty—" Ed cut in. He waited until she looked at him. "Do what your mother says for now. All right? And in a few weeks we'll talk about it. Maybe we'll all go around and meet the horse, and see what we think."

No one spoke. Ed rose from the table and put a hand on Patty's shoulder.

"Why don't you pour your mother another cup of tea?" he said.

Lucinda was angry with Ed afterward for having taken Patty's part, but he said he had not taken her part and that he hoped she would forget about horses. He said he couldn't afford the boots and riding breeches and other expenses.

"I just wish they'd all stay away from anything dangerous for a while," Lucinda said finally. "Just in case anything happens. I couldn't stand another one so soon."

He went to his study, and looked at the text from the Prophets for the Sabbath before Passover and some commentaries upon it, in order to prepare the sermon.

> *—and on that day will I turn the eyes of the children toward the parents, and the eyes of the parents toward the children.*

Lucinda had argued at first that it wasn't proper to make the usual Passover celebration so soon after Charles's death, and that none of the relatives expected them to, but Ed had said it was proper and necessary.

"Oh, sure, the show must go on," she said bitterly.

He said he thought Patty could prepare the meal if she didn't feel up to it. But later on, she remembered that Millicent had spoken of inviting a young man for Passover. She brightened somewhat, and told Ed that Millicent had said the boy was from out of town and had no place to go on Passover. She said they really ought to invite him. She telephoned Millicent to find out whether the boy could definitely come, and reached her at last at the city room.

Lucinda's sisters and mother and Ed's brothers and their families were invited for the first night, as usual. Some of them were planning to go to relatives on the other side of their families for the second night, as they usually did, but this year the feeling among them was that none should bother Lucinda for two nights in a row in any case. So the plan, as it finally worked out, was to have no guests on the second night except Millicent's friend, who was an intern and could not come the first night because he would be on call.

Lucinda did the preparation as usual, with the assistance of Patty, and Celeste, who arrived early in the day. Millicent said she could not get the first night off, after taking off so much time for the funeral. Lucinda said she had thought of setting a place for Charles, just as though he were there, but that she was not sure now if she should. Ed and Celeste advised her not to.

Ed had come home at five o'clock, and began at once to put extra leaves in the table and to lengthen it still further by placing card tables against it, so that it extended through the arch into the living room and it took two cloths to cover it. Patty and Jill laid it out, with slim books by each napkin, and little wine cups, some of silver and some of glass, and the two crystal decanters with deep-red wine. At the end of the table, where he would sit later, the herbs and bone and cracked egg sat high on a square of cloth that covered the layers of unleaven. His grandfather's wine cup with filigree had been put there, and beside his chair there was another chair with a pillow on it, so that later on while partaking of unleaven he could recline a few moments as at an ancient banquet.

The relatives were prompt, and they were subdued, even the children. Ed did not bother to make comments or explanations in the service, so it went rather quickly. At the end he gave the cue for one of the songs, but he found himself feeling half-hearted in it, and he let it go at that. The ladies all insisted that Lucinda do none of the cleaning up, and even so the evening ended early.

Ed and Lucinda sat silently in the kitchen.

"I keep asking," she said finally, "was his life really necessary for the defense of the country? Did it do anything? The risks he had to take?"

"Well—he worked—men—it adds up. All their contributions add up. His work went into missions, and the missions—" He trailed off.

"But it adds up such a little," she said, and for a moment they were silent again. "I guess," she said after a while, "to make the whole world free, I'd give up Charles. But how many square miles did Charles save for freedom, if you divide it, or if you take just his missions—just the planes he fixed? I wish I knew. I keep thinking he was sold too cheap."

"Well, we can't think like that. It doesn't do any good. It's rotten, and we can't justify it, but—I don't know."

The next day Lucinda cleaned the house again, though Ed said she shouldn't.

"I can't let her bring a boy home to a dirty house," she said.

"Why didn't you start a few days ahead, instead of all this rush?"

"I did, but things always get dirty again. Come on, help me move this. I can't do it alone."

Roland came back from his paper route and Lucinda went up to change. She came down after a long time, looking quite striking for the first time in many weeks, Ed thought—her hair swept and combed, and a touch of paint and of costume jewelry.

There was a noise like a motorcycle, and instead of diminishing down the road it seemed to swerve into the yard toward the barn, louder than ever, and Ed saw its solitary light pass a window. The motor slowed its puttering and then coughed silent. In a moment there were footsteps on the porch steps, and Lucinda opened half the double door to Millicent and the tall young man behind her. Millicent was red and wind-blown, hatless but with scarves about her neck, and she wore mittens despite the mild weather. Her eyes were bloodshot.

"Was that a motorcycle?" Lucinda asked.

"A scooter," said Millicent.

"You said driving—I thought a car," Lucinda said.

Millicent introduced Leslie. Ed came forward. He saw Patty gazing with awed approval as she took the man's hand, and Roland leaning around the door to look toward the scooter.

"Close the door," Ed said to Roland.

"Excuse me—if I knew you were on a thing like that I'd have had heart failure," said Lucinda.

"I know it," said Millicent.

"All the way from Boston," Lucinda said.

"It's perfectly safe," said Leslie.

"What did you do, ride sidesaddle?" Patty asked.

"Dr. Hollander—please—I know you meant well," Lucinda said, "but try to remember that girls have mothers."

"Oh, Mother, stop," said Millicent. "Dr. Hollander has a mother too. And we got here safe and sound."

They were moving into the living room. Patty took Millicent's coat and Leslie's sheepskin.

There were a few silences amid the small talk, but the guest explained where he was from and where he was interning, and that he liked it there. He sat leaning back on the sofa, legs crossed and hands clasping a knee. He seemed boyish and without pretense, Ed thought, even somewhat shy. But then he thought it was perhaps only the effect of being looked at by the whole family.

"Well, maybe we should get started, in view of the hour," Ed said.

"Was I very late?" Leslie asked.

"No, no, I just thought we might as well begin," said Ed.

In the dining room Leslie put on the skullcap Ed gave him, and pulled out a chair for Millicent. Roland sat at Ed's left, and Patty after Roland, opposite the guest, and Lucinda at the end. The wall lamps made a soft and yellow light.

The guest filled the wineglasses of both sisters, and then Lucinda's and the rest. Ed raised his silver cup and led the benediction.

When they had drunk he asked Dr. Hollander if he had had any Hebrew training.

"Well, I had some Sunday school," Leslie told him, "but my mother took me out. You were supposed to pay twenty-five cents a week, and we couldn't really afford it, and she had her pride, I guess."

Ed made sure everyone had the right page, and began. In a while he noticed that Patty was staring at Dr. Hollander, and when it was time for her to get the basin and the pitcher for the handwashing he had to remind her.

Roland helped Patty carry the basin and pitcher and hand towels. Ed saw Millicent's and Dr. Hollander's eyes meet, and heard Millicent giggle when a little water splashed between them.

"Does your family celebrate Passover at home?" Ed asked Dr. Hollander.

"Well, not really. When I was a kid we used to go up to my grandfather's in Glens Falls."

"Well, maybe we can make it seem like your grandfather's," Ed said. Then he looked at Roland. "Is there anything you want to ask?" he said.

"No," said Roland.

"The Four Questions, stupid," said Patty.

"Patty—" said Lucinda.

"I'm sorry," said Patty.

Roland recited his part of the ritual confidently, in a stylized singsong. Ed saw Dr. Hollander watching Roland with a little smile, perhaps approving, or perhaps impressed.

When Roland finished Ed began the response. He paused occasionally to clarify the text, or to let the wineglasses be refilled, or for the eating of herbs as the text directed. He related the Passover to other rites in the year's pattern, and talked of the interconnection of freedom and law and responsibility, directing most of his remarks to Dr. Hollander, who nodded attentively. But in the midst of the spilling out of drops of wine to count the plagues Lucinda began to wipe her eyes and sniffle. Suddenly she pushed back her chair and hurried from the room—not toward the kitchen but toward the hallway and the stairs. Ed stopped in the reading and Dr. Hollander stared after her.

"Shall I go with Mother?" Patty asked.

"No," Ed said. "Let her alone. I think she'll be all right." He glanced at Dr. Hollander. "We've had a tragedy recently," he explained.

"I know. I'm sorry."

Ed resumed the reading, without looking at anyone. At first he read with some faltering, listening for Lucinda. He wanted to sound normal, but also to get through the service quickly. He heard the others turn a page, approximately together.

After a while he paused, and said he had meant to explain before that the spilling of wine was in memory of the boys in Pharaoh's army who had drowned in the Red Sea. He said it applied to the North Koreans and Chinese also, and that your joy in victory should be tempered by the realization that your enemies are also God's children.

"Is that what upset Mrs. Gordon?" Les asked.

"No. I think it was just in general. She's used to having the family together."

He asked Patty to go upstairs and see if Mother was all right. He continued, and a page later Patty came down.

"She's all right," Patty said. "She's coming right down."

Ed proceeded with the reading. They ate the bitters.

Lucinda came back just before it was time to serve the dinner. She was smiling, though the evidence of having wept was still in her eyes and voice. "I'm sorry," she apologized to Dr. Hollander. "You'll have to excuse me. I'm afraid we're not a very gay household. We've had a terrible loss recently."

"I know, I heard," he said solemnly, and rose to help her with her chair. "I'm very sorry."

Lucinda sat, pulling her chair in as he got there.

"I should have expressed my sympathy before," Dr. Hollander said.

"Are you ready for dinner?" Lucinda asked Ed.

He nodded.

Lucinda and Patty went to the kitchen. Millicent said she had better help, and followed them. For a moment Ed faced the guest without conversation. He felt awkward.

The eggs were brought, and the soup, and Lucinda made conversation with Dr. Hollander. It seemed to Ed that Dr. Hollander spoke easily and was not so shy any more, though he wrinkled his forehead often, and had a mannerism of lowering his head and looking up from under his brow, especially during the chicken soup while he talked to Lucinda. He was a little freckled, and brown hair lay across his head haphazardly combed. His voice was soft and sometimes he had a trace of a smile. He told about his hours and about his work.

The chicken was brought, and the conversation was about Leslie's childhood and how he had decided to become a doctor. Ed listened without saying much. He noticed the way Millicent gazed up at her friend. It gave him a mixture of feelings. It was good that she had suitors. Leslie seemed impressive. He hoped that if this boy were going to be the serious one and the permanent one, he would also turn out to be someone congenial, who could be close.

Then, as he watched Leslie holding forth to the family, and Millicent beside him hanging on his words, he began to have an uneasy feeling. It was strange. Somehow they were not like a couple engaged or courting—Leslie hardly looked at her, as though he were completely sure of her. It was as if he could afford to ignore her. As though she would go to bed with him at the crook of his finger. The boy's composure was almost smug.

The idea was like a rending of Ed's own flesh, as though he himself were raped. He made himself push it aside. Why worry about such a thing, when you cannot know, and it may not be true anyhow? Maybe, he told himself, it was just a father's natural reaction to the realization that his daughter is ready for marriage. To be taken as a mistress was not in Millicent's nature, after all. And it was not the action of a girl who asks her father what the Bible and its commentaries say about sex.

Lucinda told Leslie that if he liked the chicken she'd give him some more in a paper bag to take home.

There was a dessert of fruit, and then tea and honey cake. Ed resumed the service, but he did not take long with it. When it was done Roland asked if he could go out and look at the motor scooter.

"No, not by yourself," said Ed.

"Can I help with the dishes?" Leslie asked Lucinda.

"No, that's all right," she said. "We'll do it later. I've got two girls to help me."

"Well, if you want to start it now, Roland and I will go out and look over the scooter with Dr. Hollander," Ed said to Lucinda.

"All right," Lucinda said. She told Roland to put on a coat.

Ed and Leslie put on no coats. The porch light was still on, and the sky was starlit. The air had a chilliness. Roland straddled the scooter and studied its controls.

"Shall I give him a ride?" Leslie said to Ed.

"No, I'd rather you didn't," said Ed.

They stood idly on the porch steps, looking at Roland. Leslie was taller than Ed.

"What are your religious views?" Ed asked.

"Well, I'd have to think about that," Leslie said pleasantly. "I'm more concerned with medicine than theology these days."

"Do you get to read contemporary philosophy at all?" Ed asked him. "Existentialism, and this and that?"

"Well, not really. They keep us pretty busy."

Ed's hands were in his pockets. "To my way of thinking," he said, "what a lot of these moderns are trying to say is already said better in Deuteronomy. Moses quotes God as saying, 'I offer you this day good and evil—choose.' Good and evil come from the same source. Flowers and cancer come from the same molecules, and the same science applies throughout. And still man chooses. It says, 'I offer you good and evil, life and death—see that you choose life.' In the midst of an urge to goodness man still chooses, and spreads good or evil on the earth. God makes a recommendation, but He offers good and evil, and man takes it from there. That's a fact of life, I think, whether you're religious or not."

Leslie made no answer, but he seemed to listen thoughtfully, standing by the column at the top of the porch steps.

"And in Isaiah," said Ed, "you have 'I am the Lord, creator of good and evil.' There's no devil. No dualism. We don't have a devil in the Bible. Except in the Job story, where he's only some kibitzer in the heavenly court. The evil done to Job is done by God."

He saw Leslie nod a little and look somewhat downward, as though pondering this idea.

"What about the serpent in the Garden of Eden?" said Leslie. "Isn't that the devil? Or the principle of evil, or something?"

"No," said Ed. "What does it have God saying to the serpent? 'From now on you'll have no feet, and crawl on your belly, and eat dust'? Does that make sense, to be said to the devil—that he should have no feet? There's no devil in the story. And eating the fruit wasn't a sin, as a matter of fact. Before there was knowledge of good and evil how could there be sin?"

"What's the serpent then?" said Leslie.

Roland looked up at them.

"The serpent, the snake," said Ed, "—it means the degradation of the rest of the animal kingdom that occurred as a result of man's achieving awareness. The story uses a snake because the snake is a degraded animal."

"The animal kingdom is degraded?" Leslie asked.

"As one of the consequences of the emergence of man, yes. My son here puts tadpoles in a jar. Come on, let's go in. It's cold."

Roland climbed off the scooter. They went in. Ed and Leslie went to the living-room sofa. Roland did not follow them to the living room but went perhaps to his own room.

"In the Eden story," Ed said, "as you know, there were these two trees mentioned. And these two trees represent the two things that man lacked in order to become Godlike. That is, that animals lacked, or the pre-man lacked. One was freedom from death. And the other was knowledge, knowledge of good and evil. Awareness that things could be different. And we didn't eat one, but we ate the other. In the story Eve is still talking with animals, and somehow, out of our animal nature, evolving in the midst of our animal activities, we stumbled on awareness, and became human. Eden represents the condition before that. Eden is like the pre-human state. An animal may have pain, but animals aren't aware that things could be different. An animal who suffers probably thinks it's necessary, or at least he doesn't know it's unnecessary—it's just there. And when an animal has enough pain it dies, but it doesn't have the added pain of seeing it as unnecessary and evil and rotten and unjustifiable. To know the futility, the waste, the unnecessity—to know that it's not part of a higher good—this is to know evil."

Millicent had appeared while he was talking, from the far door of the dining room, and she came toward them through the dining room and the arch.

"Hi," she said.

Leslie rose for her, but she sat on the piano bench, and Leslie sat down on the sofa again.

"Eden is without evil," Ed continued, "but it's not life, Leslie. Can I call you Leslie? At best, Eden is pleasure without responsibility. And that's not life. It's masturbation."

"Oh, Daddy, for goodness sakes," Millicent said with irritation.

Ed saw Leslie color a little at the ears.

"The awareness that things could be different leads to unhappiness, and it also leads to work," Ed said. "And so to the end of Eden. But even so, we see knowledge as an instrument of good. We're told that an ignorant man can't be just. And you need scientific knowledge to improve the conditions of life, don't you?"

"What is it exactly," Leslie asked, "—'tree of knowledge?' Or 'tree of knowledge of good and evil?' "

"Both," said Ed. "We need all the knowledge we can get—moral and scientific. Everything bears on everything else. You try to have knowledge of what we should do, without having knowledge, and you're like a superstitious old woman. But you look for knowledge without knowledge of what we should do, and you've got a laboratory at Auschwitz."

"You're glad man was kicked out of Eden then?" Leslie said.

"Well, would you rather be a man or an oyster?" said Ed. "But we pay a price. Man labors. Man works. He's aware of leisure, and he's aware that the earth could be improved. Take a gorilla, or a sea gull—it may forage for food all day long, but it doesn't see it as work."

"Horses work," said Leslie.

"Yes, horses work," said Ed. "Horses labor. But they didn't used to. That's man's degradation of the other species. Symbolically they've all had to crawl on their bellies and eat dust."

"Well, even before that," said Leslie. "Lions ate antelopes. Maybe they ate wild horses too. And animals eat one another. In the sea, the air. I don't know how Eden-like that was."

"That was different," said Ed. "They had a fair chance. And since there was nothing higher you couldn't say it was degraded. Anyway, consider a fish. Or a starfish, or a real low animal. You're already talking about mammals, that are closer to the human state. But even so, Leslie. Wild animals, untouched by man may know moments of pain, and terror, in their natural condition, but on the whole a wild animal functions and passes most of its days in a state of health and well-being. I think it's safe to say that man is the only truly unhappy creature."

"That may be true," said Leslie.

There was a pause, as if they were all contemplating this.

"And even if the world had been made differently," Ed said, "so that it was immune to pain, and evil, and injustice, I suppose you could say that God would still know that there could have been worlds with pain and injustice. Even if there had been no evil, and everything was right, God would still know it could have been otherwise. So that to know evil is to be like God."

"Well, you can't justify evil," said Leslie. "I can't see evil as necessary to some higher good or anything."

"Of course it's not necessary," said Ed. "If it were it wouldn't be evil. If man, by his ingenuity, can derive some piece of good out of an evil, as by taking a lesson from it, well, good for him—but the evil itself, like the death of a child at Belsen, it stays rotten. Nothing will ever justify it. That's why it's evil."

"Well," said Leslie, "I'd prefer a world without evil. Creativeness, and so on, but not evil."

"Yes," said Millicent.

"I can agree with you," said Ed. "Better not to be like God, better to have evil blacked out of the world, better not to know this whole possibility. Better that life should be a party where everything goes right. I agree, I agree."

Patty and Lucinda came from the kitchen, through the dining room as Millicent had.

"You agree to what," Patty said.

"We were discussing religion," said Ed.

"I might have known," said Patty.

Leslie had risen again. Patty sat in the middle of the sofa, between Leslie's place and Ed, and Lucinda sat in the tall rocker.

"I believe that it's still early in the whole evolutionary process," Ed said. "I think the spreading of justice is part of it. Knowledge grows, and religion grows. In the twenty-first century, or the twenty-fifth century, medicine will be better, and cars safer, and the planets will be nearer, and also our interpretations of Torah will be profounder. New insights. Scholarship is cumulative. And in five hundred years there'll have been that many more generations of scholars putting their heads together, that many more archaeologists, discoveries that throw light on things. New exegesis. Better translations. More commentary.

New conditions. So much more to study. I'd like to be around in five hundred years. I'd like to see the next chapter. And I'd like to see more of how history goes. Why do you think I work toward it? 'The task is great, and the workmen are laggard.' "

"There may not be a twenty-first century," said Leslie. "A nuclear war could break out on the Fourth of July and civilization could be ended by Christmas. Man could even be extinct."

"That's right," said Patty.

"No," said Ed. "It won't happen that way. I don't believe it. Half of humanity, maybe. Or two-thirds. But civilization will never have to start from scratch again. That's what we call God's promise to Noah. That possibility we've put behind us. We have what it takes to avert that, at least."

"Well, I hope so," said Leslie.

"You know," said Ed, "what men do is also God's action. If you're just, then God is just. God will be godly when men are godly. And today mankind is going through a period of anger at God, furious anger at God, and disbelief, for what He permits. For man's failure to be godly we're furious at the God who made us, and permits us. You see, we're still animals, and we're just beginning to evolve into something more, and in that first awareness of a better possibility we react with angry resentment, that God started us so low in the scale. Someday we'll come around to the view that God is just not to be comprehended. We ask, how do you explain the rottenness? But how do you explain the goodness? How do you explain that the rottenness isn't rottener? How do you explain that you're alive, and in good health? You can't. You can't explain the good and you can't explain the evil."

There was another little pause. Then Leslie said that he had a long ride ahead of him, and that he had to be up at six-thirty.

"So early?" said Lucinda.

"He's on duty before seven," said Millicent.

"We could put you up on a cot, if you'd like to stay over," Lucinda said.

"No, I'd better go."

He rose, and looked about as though for his sheepskin. Patty fetched it from the study, and Lucinda went to get the chicken she had promised.

They went with him to the door. He stuffed the bagful of chicken into one of the old jacket's huge pockets. He shook hands with Ed, and thanked them. Lucinda gave him her hand. "I hope we'll see more of you," she said.

They went out with him onto the porch.

"Drive carefully on that thing," Lucinda said.

He turned once more at the top of the porch stairs, and smiled at everyone. "Well—" he said. He looked at Millicent.

"You can kiss her," said Ed. "She's kosher for Passover."

"Daddy, I'll thank you not to make such jokes," she said. "It's very embarrassing."

Leslie gave them a last nod, with one foot down a step, and went to the scooter.

He made it sputter, and then roar. He waved, and it turned and started off. They watched its forward glow and the tail light go down the curving dirt drive and then disappear down the road.

They turned to go in. "A very intelligent young man," said Ed.

"Yes, he is," said Millicent.

"Dreamy," said Patty.

"I thought he was very nice," Lucinda said.

52

Millicent remained in Wilmerding Crosswalk overnight, on the iron cot in Patty's room.

When she next slept at Leslie's he was at the hospital on call, so she did not see him until the night following. Then they lay awake talking. He said he had liked her father. That pleased her. She told him that her father was a man of broad interests, who knew much about motors, and who liked to read about American Colonial history and about zoology and evolution. She said she even remembered he had once been much interested in cameras and photography.

Millicent was pleased too that Les had been willing to meet her family.

And he had been comforting to her about Charles. They had lain in bed, and he had told her all about how upset he had been in his childhood when his father had died. It occurred to her that a doctor's whole aim was to help people stave off death, to extend life as long as possible.

On the Sunday after Passover, when Sunday school was over and she had returned to the house for dinner, Patty asked her at the table how her boyfriend was.

She resented the designation, and she also resented Patty's familiarity.

"Dr. Hollander is in perfectly good health, as far as I know," she answered coolly.

"Do you like him?" said Patty.

"Please! He's a friend. Don't get any ideas," said Millicent.

"You don't start ringing wedding bells every time a girl brings a boy home for Passover," Ed told Patty. "Next year she might bring a different guy."

"That's right," said Lucinda. "And it was very thoughtful to invite him. He's far from home and he didn't have any place to go."

"You ought to get a different job," Patty said. "You can't get any romancing in, working nights and weekends on that crazy job. You're going to work when he gets through."

"Millicent doesn't go in for romancing," said Lucinda. "You ought to know that by now."

"I know it," said Patty. "They discuss the higher things."

"Will you stop?" said Millicent. "Everyone? Or must I leave the room?"

"We'll stop," said Lucinda.

"I'm beginning to think I shouldn't have invited him."

"No, it was very nice," Lucinda told her, "and you just invite anybody you want, any time."

During the week she practiced ironing Leslie's shirts, on Mrs. Mahady's ironing board. He had been complaining about the way the Chinese place starched them, and she saw no reason why she could not learn to do this, especially since the Chinese place was expensive.

The following Sunday she had a quite normal dinner at Wilmerding Crosswalk and none of them asked anything about Leslie. The early flowers had begun to come up, in yellow and white and purple, and she had a pleasant time inspecting the garden with her mother after dinner. The city room that evening happened to be unusually serene, with very few stories, and she sat chatting with Maud, who told her all about how she had gotten started in the newspaper business years ago. Mr. Hopkins sent her home early. Leslie was at the hospital, and she had a long untroubled sleep alone in the wide bed.

Late the next afternoon her mother telephoned her at the city room, saying she was at Millicent's apartment. She said she had come in to shop, and had stayed late, and Natalie had let her into the apartment, and she wondered what time Millicent took her supper hour, so they could eat together.

"Well, they usually send me out at five-thirty," Millicent said. "But I couldn't go up there. I only get thirty minutes to eat, and then I have errands."

"I'll meet you," her mother said.

"It's really not worth it," said Millicent. "It's out of your way and it's inconvenient."

"No, that's all right, I'll meet you," Lucinda insisted.

Millicent told her where the spa was. Then she ended the conversation and returned to work. It seemed to her that her mother was being stupid. It would have made much better sense to get the early train home.

Toward five-thirty Mr. Killian beckoned with a toss of his head, and stood up, with a foot on a pulled-out drawer, and gave her a press release. He had a reporter's assignment for her. She was to have her supper, and then make her usual call on Heustis Garvey at Police Headquarters, but skip her usual trips to the State House and City Hall. If Garvey had nothing urgent, she was to go directly to the Copley-Plaza Hotel, where the registrar of motor vehicles was speaking at a convention. But if Garvey had something urgent, she was to bring it to the city room by taxi, and then go at once by taxi to the Copley-Plaza and cover the registrar.

It was the first time she had been sent to cover a speaker really all on her own, without a copy of a prepared text. She put the press release in her shoulder-strap bag and started out to the elevator. She would have to listen carefully and jot down only the most important things. It was not like interviewing an

M.I.T. instructor who sat in his office and explained, and who waited for you to get it down.

She went up the street to meet her mother. The spa was large, with a long marble soda fountain, and the walls were of mirrors and dark mahogany. The place was so deep that it extended through the block to another front on another street. Lucinda was in a corner booth, with a cup of coffee, and her tired eyes greeted Millicent pleasurelessly.

Millicent slipped into her booth, opposite her. "What's the matter?" she said. Then she noticed that instead of bundles and shopping bags her mother had a valise on the seat beside her.

"Oh, nothing," her mother said, and took a sip of coffee. She put down the coffee and looked at Millicent steadily. "Tell me the truth," she said. "Look me in the eye."

"What?"

"Are you living with a man?"

Millicent stared at her mother in bewilderment. She felt a warming in her own face and saw a slight but perceptible hardening of her mother's, but she could say nothing. The strength seemed to go out of her.

"I think I know now why it's been so impossible to find you at home," her mother said. "We got a letter from Charles. He wrote it before, I mean. And he said he asked you and you didn't deny it. He looked for you just before he went overseas and it was just a phony address. You don't even live there at all."

Millicent felt her eyes moisten. She saw that her mother's eyes were wet also, and a tearfulness had come into her mother's voice. She could not on such brief notice devise a reply or even decide what kind of reply. But her confused silence humiliated her too.

"Well, aren't you going to say anything?" Lucinda said.

Millicent still didn't say anything.

"Do you want to see the letter?" her mother said.

"No."

"Patty found it," her mother said. "He wrote it to Dad, but Dad hasn't seen it." Lucinda's voice began to break and she found a handkerchief. She dabbed her eyes nervously and wiped her nose. "Oh, poor Charles," she said.

A middle-aged waitress clad in pink came with her pad and looked at them. Millicent also was trying not to break down.

"Egg salad on toast," she managed. It was what she always ordered.

"The same," said Lucinda.

"Coffee?" the waitress asked.

"Milk," said Millicent.

"Coffee," said Lucinda.

The waitress left.

"Well," Lucinda said, still tearfully, "is it true? It's true, isn't it. Do you deny it?"

Millicent glanced to see if people noticed they were making a scene, but her mother had kept her voice low.

"I think it's pretty rotten of Charles," Millicent answered, quavering.

"You can speak decently of a boy that's in his grave. Poor Charles. He loved you. He was so worried. It's Dr. Hollander, isn't it. I'm really amazed that you could bring him home to meet us, as cool as a cucumber. I'm just amazed. Well, aren't you going to answer? Is it true or isn't it?"

She tried to avoid her mother's eyes but couldn't. "What do you want me to say?"

For a moment her mother's face didn't move. It seemed lined. "How often are you there?" her mother asked. "At his place. Every night?"

"Just about."

"And how long has it been going on?"

"Since about January, I guess."

"January? You mean when I saw you at your apartment different times—when we came to give blood that time—you hadn't even slept there that night?"

"No."

"And what's your old apartment for? Just a phony address, for appearance's sake?"

"No, it's not phony. It's still mine. I have things there, and I sleep there sometimes. And I'm there practically every day, almost. Mother, I'm a grown woman." Her voice was quaking terribly but she could not steady it. "I'm entitled to live as I please. And not have people prying."

"I'm not people! I'm your mother! And you just listen to me, Millicent. The party's over. You're coming home with me. I've got a valise for your things, and what we can't take now we'll pick up later. But I'm putting an end to this before it's too late."

"I can't go home. I have to work. I'm working. Don't you know that? I have errands to do, and I have to go to the Copley-Plaza."

"What's at the Copley-Plaza?"

"The registrar. The registrar of motor vehicles. It's a reporting assignment."

"Oh. Well I'll wait."

"Mother, please! I work until midnight."

"That's all right. I'll wait until midnight. We'll find some excuse. Your father doesn't have to know."

"Mother, no. I'm not going home."

"And where are you going to sleep tonight? At that man's place again?"

"I don't know where. You shouldn't be asking. There are some things you don't ask."

"Oh, that's it. Very sophisticated, aren't you. Very modern. Well how would you like me to have to tell your father? Do you want him to see that letter?"

"Mother—"

"I know, you want to spare him," her mother said. "And so do I. But if I can't do anything with you he has to know."

"It would be pretty rotten," Millicent said, feeling almost ready to cry.

"Oh, now we're all rotten," her mother said, her voice choking up also. "I'm rotten, and poor Charles. It seems to me you're the one that's rotten. I wouldn't even use the word for what you are! I'm too much of a lady to tell you what you are. And I'll tell you one thing, if you don't come home now you'll never be welcome again."

The waitress appeared with their sandwiches. It was clear that she must have heard, but she remained poker-faced. They were silent while the waitress set the plates and cups in order.

When the waitress left Lucinda began weeping quietly but openly, wiping her eyes and nose with a little embroidered handkerchief. Millicent felt herself crying also. "It's just too bad that poor Charles had to die knowing what his sister was," Lucinda said.

"Mother, will you stop it?" I've got to control myself, she thought. I have to keep my head. "Mother, you're destroying something beautiful."

"Beautiful she calls it. You don't know what's beautiful."

"I haven't done anything I'm ashamed of."

"And what do you mean by that? That you haven't done anything to be ashamed of, or you're just not ashamed of it? Very sophisticated, aren't you. Oh, I know, it's very de rigueur in the highest intellectual circles. It's just too bad you can't send a daughter off to college without—without—that's what you learned at Chicago I suppose. And I don't think those girls are a good influence on you, either. Those roommates. Do they do things like that?"

"I don't know. It's none of my business. And it's not yours, either."

"Oh no. It's none of my business where my daughter sleeps. Or who with. Maybe I should go and do the same thing."

"Mother, you're getting hysterical. I can't explain it. You just have to trust me and don't worry about me and don't make assumptions."

"Oh, now it's an assumption, is it?"

"I'm not a child."

"You're my child. And you think you know it all. You think you're in love, don't you. You can't give him up, no matter what happens, can you. He just has to look at you and you melt."

"I don't melt."

"Well if it isn't that I'd hate to think what it is, then. Do you think you're gonna get him to marry you that way? It's just stupid. You think you know everything but you've got rocks in your head, that's all. A boy wants to marry a girl or he's sleeping with her contemptuously, that's all. Having a good time with you. I never let your father touch me like that, before we were married. He respected me. Your doctor friend hasn't said a single word about marriage I bet."

"We haven't decided anything. He has his career. And I have mine."

"I knew it." Her mother's eyes filled again.

Millicent had eaten nothing and neither had her mother. She took a bite of the sandwich, but she had no appetite.

She wiped her mouth. "I have to go," she said, rising. "I can't talk any more. I'm supposed to go to Police Headquarters."

Her mother appeared to be in despair, staring feebly at nothing with wet eyes. "Watch out on the crossings," she said.

Millicent left her mother sitting there with the valise and did not look back, though she was relieved to notice that the booth that had been at her back was empty. She hurried along the street. It was impossible to think. She coughed and gagged, and her stomach felt as though it could scarcely retain the one mouthful she had eaten. She tried to calm herself, but found herself impatiently crossing in front of moving cars despite her mother's warning.

She got to Police Headquarters without an awareness of what streets she had traversed, and hurried through the zigzags of the corridor.

She pushed the door open and found Mr. Garvey lying on the floor. He was on his back, spread out, with eyes shut, and apparently unconscious. He was alone. A dark wet blotch appeared in his pants while she watched. It spread, and at last began to make a puddle. The sight of him stunned her.

She cleared her throat. "Mr. Garvey?" she said timidly.

The phone on his desk began ringing. There was a little bubbly sound down in his throat, but he didn't stir.

"Mr. Garvey," she said again. She gave his hand a little nudge with her foot, but nothing happened.

She wondered if she should answer the phone. She knew how he felt about things like that. He might wake up and accuse her of stealing his job.

The phone kept ringing. She had a vision of the other reporters out on some important story and Mr. Garvey being scooped. She stepped across his extended leg and picked up the telephone.

"Hello?" she said into the phone, looking down at Mr. Garvey.

"Hello, Heustis?" said the rough voice in her ear.

She cleared her throat again. "Could I take the message, please? Mr. Garvey just stepped out for a minute."

"Tell him to call Sergeant Corcoran," the voice said, and the phone was hung up.

She stood wondering what to do. Her coat hung on her unbuttoned. The body on the floor was silent, without even the bubbly sound. But the puddle was bigger. She picked up the directory and began to look for the police department, but then remembered that one of the desk phones was a direct line to the police. She decided quickly which it must be, and picked it up. She stared absently at the calendar with the bare-bosomed moron.

"Headquarters," a man's voice said in the phone.

"Sergeant Corcoran, please," said Millicent, her voice shaking.

"Sergeant who?"

She repeated it.

"Nobody by that name here," the man said, and hung up.

She clicked the phone again at once. She heard the ringing a long time, and then the same man answered.

"Please, I must locate Sergeant Corcoran," she said. "It's very important. Or maybe it was Cochrane. I'm not sure."

"Is he in detectives?"

"Yes, he might be," said Millicent.

"I'll give you detectives." For a little while there was a noise of equipment. Then a brisk voice said, "Lieutenant McLellan."

Her whole body was shivering. "Lieutenant, I'm calling for Mr. Garvey, one of the reporters in the press room—you know? Mr. Garvey isn't feeling well, and could I take the news? If it's important?"

"I ain't got no news."

"I think Sergeant Corcoran has some news. Could I speak to Sergeant Corcoran please?"

"Corcoran ain't here."

"Well," she said, "I'm here at the press room helping Mr. Garvey, and if Sergeant Corcoran has a press release—"

"He wouldn't have no press release."

"Can you tell me how to find him, please?"

"No, I wouldn't know how to find him."

She wondered what she could say next. "All right," she said finally. "Thank you."

"Okay."

She hung up. Oh dear, she thought. It occurred to her that if she waited Sergeant Corcoran might call back. She wished she had had the foresight to keep him on the phone the other time. She looked at Mr. Garvey. What a horrible condition, she thought. She wondered if she should try very hard to wake him, or if it would only embarrass him too much.

It occurred to her to ask the old policeman in the lobby alcove if anything was happening. She went to the lobby. The old man sat behind his counter, half in a doze. The lobby was dim. The elevator man leaned by an open elevator and watched her. She went to the old man. She cleared her throat and gave the counter some nervous little slaps to get his attention.

"I'm Millicent Gordon from the press room," she told him in her quaking little voice. "Mr. Garvey sent me to inquire if there's any news."

"About what?" the old officer said. But he did not seem hostile.

"About anything."

"No, I don't know of anything," he said.

"Have the other reporters been here?"

"Not tonight. I haven't seen anybody."

"Do you know a Sergeant Corcoran? Or Cochrane? Does he work in this building?"

She looked at the elevator man too. Both men shook their heads a little with mystification.

"Who gives the news?" she asked. "Where do I go to get the news?"

"What news?"

"Any news."

"The press room," the old policeman answered. "Any reporters back there?"

"I just came from there."

"Well, I don't know. You better ask in the morning."

She sighed. "All right," she said. She hurried back toward the press room.

She was growing frantic. If she phoned the city room and reported that Mr. Garvey were dead drunk he would lose his job, and at his age he might never find another. But if she did not, and the paper were scooped on a big story, he might be fired in any case, and the paper would be hurt besides, owing to her negligence. She made a little whimpering noise. She could not help it.

She found Mr. Garvey exactly as she had left him. It occurred to her that he might not be drunk, but terribly sick. She had heard stories of unconscious men who were thought to be drunk and were then found dead of a heart attack. But if she called an ambulance and he were not sick, it would create a scandal for which she would never be forgiven. There was a tingling in her head and stomach. She thought of phoning Leslie at the hospital and asking him how to tell if Mr. Garvey were seriously ill. He did not even look alive now. She remembered Leslie was not at the hospital. He was not on call tonight, and would be at his apartment, where there was no phone.

It occurred to her to have the old policeman and the elevator man look at Mr. Garvey and see if they thought he was ill. But they might put him in a cell to sober up.

She wished she knew whether that Sergeant Corcoran had had a story or not. It also occurred to her that Sergeant Corcoran might have been leaking special information to Mr. Garvey against regulations, and now she had given it away. She had heard that Mr. Garvey had personal arrangements like that.

She thought of phoning the city room and saying that she herself had taken deathly ill and had gone home, and would not be able to cover the registrar, and then remaining to cover the press room for Mr. Garvey, and perhaps fetch him some smelling salts from the drugstore. If a story came in, she would phone it directly to Maud, who could be trusted. And Maud could tell the copy desk that Mr. Garvey had phoned her directly instead of informing the desk, because it was so urgent.

But no, that was no good.

It wouldn't work anyway. What if Mr. Hopkins phoned the press room to ask for Mr. Garvey and Millicent answered?

She stepped over Mr. Garvey's outstretched arm and picked up the telephone. She dialed her own apartment.

She heard Ella Jane's voice answer.

"Ella Jane?" said Millicent.

"Hi," said Ella Jane. "Natalie said your mother was here."

"I know about it. Listen, I need a big favor right away from you or Natalie."

"Natalie's gone out. I guess it'll have to be me."

"There's a man's whole life and career at stake," Millicent said.

"What?"

Millicent begged Ella Jane to get into a taxi and come and cover the press room. She explained about Mr. Garvey, and what confidence Mr. Killian had in him, and how if anyone phoned she could say she was Mr. Garvey's niece, or was delivering sandwiches, and take the message.

"Are you out of your mind?" said Ella Jane. "I don't know anything about newspaper work."

"There's nothing to know. You just take messages. I'll keep phoning you. It'll be an adventure for you. And I want your opinion whether he's sick or not. Please, Ella Jane. You can't just let a man die. He's got nobody. This job is all he has. It's everything he's built up for sixty years."

Ella Jane sighed. "You're nuts," she said.

"Oh, Ella Jane! Please! You must. It's an act of mercy. I can't just abandon him like that."

"Well, I can't go right away."

"You have to. As soon as you can then. It's very near. Honest, you can be here in a couple of minutes. You'll save his job for him and you'll save his life. You'll be glad all your life."

"Oh, all right."

Millicent explained where it was. "Just ask the man at the front desk where the press room is," she said. "You can even say you're a new copy boy. Honestly, really, you're sweet. I could kiss you. I didn't know what to do."

Then she went out, relieved that she had solved the problem of Mr. Garvey, and hurried nervously in the streets to the Copley-Plaza. It was only a few blocks, but she went some distance the wrong way, as if she were thinking of the Statler. She retraced her steps.

When she got to the Copley-Plaza she was breathless. She looked for a phone booth. She wanted to call the press room and find out if Ella Jane had gotten there yet. The apartment too was not many blocks, and if Ella Jane had found a cab immediately it would not take long. She thought also of the calendars on the walls and it embarrassed her a little to have Ella Jane see those.

The hotel lobby gleamed in a tasteful, subdued way, with columns and long counters and little illuminated signs. There seemed to be many wings to it. From her phone booth she could see a meeting already in session through a double doorway that opened onto a kind of mezzanine at the top of a carpeted staircase. She hoped the registrar hadn't been introduced yet.

Ella Jane answered the telephone. "Millicent?" the voice said.

"Oh, good! You're there. Did you just get there?"

"Yes, I just got here. What is this? My God! And this pig? The place is spooky."

"Oh, you're a real friend," Millicent said. "Honestly, I'm so grateful. And I'll call you back as soon as I get a minute. My meeting's already started. Okay?"

"Okay," Ella Jane said gloomily.

Millicent hung up the telephone and started toward the carpeted staircase, but then she had an afterthought and went back to the phone. She called Ella Jane again.

"Listen," she said, when Ella Jane answered, "see if he's breathing, will you? And see if you think he needs a doctor. I wouldn't want to call a doctor if he doesn't really need it, because it might get back."

"Oh, he's breathing—he's muttering, so he must be breathing—"

"What's he saying?"

"Oh, something about cutting people up. What's the difference? And listen, sweetie pie, I'm gonna get a cabdriver to drag this guy into a cab and dump him on his doorstep. Or I'll get the guys out front to do it. And then I'm going."

"You can't do that!"

"Oh can't I."

"He's the dean of the New England press corps."

"The what?"

"The dean of the New England press corps."

"You're dreaming. You're kidding."

"No. I'm not kidding."

"Well, now just a minute. This dump is giving me the creeps. And if you think I'm gonna baby-sit this stinkpot you've got another think coming."

"How would you know where to send him?"

"He's got a wallet, probably, with an address in it. The driver'll find it."

"How do you know the driver won't just rob him and throw him in the canal?"

"Sweetie, you're a worrier, do you know that? Just don't bother your pretty little head."

"But Headquarters will be unstaffed. Unmanned."

"Well, that's too too bad. It just is. It's not your problem, and it's not mine. Millicent honey, you're cute, and you're sweet, but you just have to get a grip on yourself. I mean, what are we? The Sweet Sisters of Charity? Now I've done you one favor tonight and that's enough. So good-bye and good night." The receiver clicked shut.

Millicent looked at the phone. She sighed.

She hurried to the meeting. When she had climbed the carpeted staircase she was panting. A stoutish lady was sitting on a chair just inside the doorway, apart from the other people, and looked up startled.

Millicent flipped the press card out of her sock. "Press," she said.

"Oh, that's nice," the lady said, rising. She led the way toward the front.

"Have I missed much?" Millicent asked her.

"No, he's just begun," the lady said.

The speaker was a thin gentleman with gray hair curling over his ears. The lady whispered to another lady who sat at the same table behind which the speaker stood, and Millicent was shown to a chair at that same table also. It embarrassed her to have been put in such a place of honor right beside the speaker, and facing the audience. There were about seventy-five or a hundred people, more women than men. She rummaged in her shoulder-strap bag and found note paper, but she had lost her pencil. Oh dear, she thought.

"Excuse me," she whispered to the lady at the table beside her. "I don't have a pencil."

She felt foolish. The lady nodded. It occurred to Millicent that the lady might be the president of the organization. But the lady left the table and in a moment brought Millicent a gold fountain pen. Millicent had been trying to listen meanwhile, though every few seconds she realized she was not. She remembered that she had been supposed to call the city room from the press room before coming here, and tell whether Mr. Garvey had anything urgent or not. She wondered if they were still waiting for her call, and whether her forgetting it had by now caused them to call the press room. She did not see what she could do about it now.

The speaker began to hold her attention. He was quite an old man, but he spoke with conviction. He told how wild horses in the West were shot at from planes by dog-food packers. They did not even kill the horses outright, but tried only to cripple them, in order to keep the meat alive and fresh. Wounded beasts lay suffering from pain and thirst for days on end, under the prairie sun, the colts starving beside their mothers, until the men had time to come back for them. Then the wounded horses were hauled carelessly onto trucks, or dragged for distances over rough ground in such a way that the skin was ripped from living flesh. The lands were public and the horses had no protection. A bill in Congress was stuck in committee, and unless it was passed the wild mustangs of the public lands would be extinct within two years.

She took notes furiously. The elderly speaker piled horror onto horror. The cruelty sickened her. She determined to get every detail onto her note pad, and to do her best to get the outrage publicized. She considered that the world must be full of such wantonness that never comes to light. But for the accident of her being sent here, she would never have heard of this one. The old man said a favorite trick was not to shoot the horse at all, but lasso it from the plane in a certain way and drag the horse until its legs broke. It was cheaper than bullets. Millicent had to put a hand to her head. He said the dog-food packers were in competition to kill off the remaining horses before their competitors did. And these were the last of the wild mustangs of the prairies, the descendants of escaped Spanish horses, the horses ridden bareback by the Sioux.

When he had finished and people gathered about to shake his hand Millicent asked him in a shaky voice what the chances were of getting the bill out of committee. She addressed him as sir, and one of the ladies told him that Millicent was from the press. He smiled and spoke to her. She told him she would certainly do everything she could to help, and then she left for the telephone booth.

She told Mr. Hopkins it was a story that deserved a lot of space. He told her to hold on, and then he was silent, while typewriter and city-room noises filtered through the receiver. At length he switched the connection to Louie Alpert's phone. Millicent told Mr. Alpert about the horses, interrupting herself often to let him take notes on his typewriter. But he said almost nothing and she could not tell if what she said moved him. She wanted to urge him to write it effectively, but his bored, cold, businesslike way made her timid. She could visualize him, with big nose and drooping mustache, the way he hunched over his belly and pecked at the machine. When she had told it all he clicked the phone and transferred the call again to Mr. Hopkins.

Mr. Hopkins was a little surprised that the speech was over so early. But she assured him that it was.

"Okay, come in," Mr. Hopkins said.

She found the subway. She stood on the platform, thinking of the dog-food people with indignation. The whole nation had to be aroused about this. It occurred to her that at last this was true journalism—not just reporting a little story to advance herself in her job, but an involvement with urgent facts, that had to be brought to the people.

She felt it was the first story she had ever had that really and truly mattered.

When she got back to the city room Mr. Hopkins sent her down to the street to chalk some bulletins on the blackboards. She had a sneezing fit while she stood there writing. A breeze played with her skirts.

She returned upstairs and resumed her duties. She wondered about Mr. Garvey. There was no indication that anyone suspected anything, or that any scandal about his absence had been discovered while she was at the Copley-Plaza. But there was no way she could ask, without giving him away.

And apparently no one had noticed her own failure to telephone from the press room before going to the Copley-Plaza.

Maud was not there. The city room was in fact fairly empty. She wished there were someone around she could talk to. She could hear the great presses rolling overhead and feel them shake the building. She remembered that she had eaten no supper. Yet she hardly felt like eating anything. She remembered that Charles had left her his insurance. She had never endorsed the check and had not even wanted to look at it, and did not know what her father had done with it. It made no sense. Nothing was right in the world.

Mr. Hopkins sent her home an hour and a half before she was due to finish. He said there was little doing, and that she looked under the weather.

She was glad to leave. If Mr. Garvey were found out at the last minute she would rather not be there.

She took another taxi, even though her money was running low. She was not sure if she were going to sleep with Leslie, or if she were only going there to tell him that she couldn't.

She rode up the dark hill in narrow streets. Despite the many times her parents had been unable to locate her, she was sure they never would have suspected, if Charles had not betrayed her.

And she could not now remember how Charles had managed to worm that confidence out of her.

She found Leslie already in bed. She clicked on the light without thinking, and it woke him. She apologized. Then she sat down hard on the bed near him, coat and shoulder-strap bag and all.

"Oh God, Les," she said. "I've had such a night. You wouldn't believe it."

"What happened?"

"Everything. Just everything. I think I'll go out of my mind."

"No you won't."

"Well, it's nice of you to say that." She began to undress, starting with the shoulder-strap bag and coat, and as she dropped each piece of clothing to the floor she told him with emotion of the experiences of the evening. "And that's not all," she said several times, and went on. She spoke of Charles seeming to come back from the dead to hurt her, and her mother empty of any understanding. And then Mr. Garvey, and those poor horses she could not get from her mind. She left her clothes in a heap, not bothering to hang anything. She did not even put on pajamas, but clicked out the wall switch and got into bed. She snuggled close.

"It'll all blow over," said Leslie. "It'll all look better in the morning."

"How can people be so cruel to dumb beasts? I mean, after all, horses are human too, you know. I don't mean human—you know what I mean."

"I know what you mean."

"They love their children just as we do. Les, I just have to cry, or have sex, or something."

He held her close, and patted her buttocks.

"I was looking at Mr. Garvey lying there," she said, "such a mess, old and sick, and his pants wet, and now here's you, and how can one man be so ugly and another so beautiful, and where's God's justice? The world's such a mess. I wish God would just throw the world away and start over."

"Maybe He will," said Les.

"It's just horrible, horrible, horrible. Can people in this country be so unfeeling? They must hear them whinnying—how can they stand it? It's like what my father said. You remember what my father said, about man degrading the other species?"

"Yes."

"My father always taught me never to inflict cruelty on animals," she said. "He'd open a window and throw a bug out rather than kill it. I couldn't even stomp on a beetle. Could you?"

"No." He tried to comfort her by stroking her.

"My mother said an awful thing. She said you sleep with me contemptuously."

"Well, it's a reflection of attitudes when she was young, I guess."

"You don't sleep with me contemptuously, do you?"

"No."

"She's narrow."

"Well, you can't talk across generations about such things," he said. "Those things are private within each generation."

"I know it," she said. "But my mother doesn't know it."

"Well, she'll learn the hard way."

She felt that her body had excited him. His pajama bottoms seemed to have disappeared. She kept close.

"And Charles," she said. "Such a gruesome thing to do. It's just as if that awful letter came crawling out of the grave. I never heard of anything so ghoulish."

"He couldn't help that part," said Les. "He didn't know he'd be dead when they got the letter."

"Well he should have thought of it. I don't know. I loved him alive, but I think I hate him dead. They're all filthy-minded. They're trying to destroy a beautiful relationship. And I'm mad at him for hurting my parents, that's what."

She received his flesh, slowly, and moved her hips, as though breathing with her loins.

"Les, don't ever leave me."

She hugged him, wanting to merge, and the embrace deepened. He made it last a very long time, as though savoring her. She responded with her swallowing throbs, but he went coolly on. His lips wet her, he shaped her breasts, and he rolled, carrying her. He resumed the probing and delaying. At last, as though in a finale, he joined in her frenzy.

"That was nice," she said when it was done. "Thank you."

She clung to the remains of his embrace, until he moved away to sleep. She knew he was very tired. She lay a while in the darkness.

"Les—" she said.

He said nothing.

She rolled and pressed against him.

"Oh God, Les. When you're not holding me I'm all alone."

"You're all keyed up."

"Let's be one."

"We did."

"Let's do it again. I want to be one with you. I'm too scared to be just me."

"I'm tired," he said. "You know how many hours I got last night? Exactly zero."

"I know, Les, but I'm a nervous wreck. You don't know what a night I've had. Just hold me."

"I can't sleep if I hold you."

"Then do it to me just once more, and then I can sleep and I'll let you sleep."

"No."

"Please."

"Shut up, will ya? You woke me up when you walked in here and now I have to get some sleep." He moved from her.

"Oh, Les. I never say no to you."

He didn't answer.

"If you were a girl," she said, "and I were a boy, I wouldn't refuse you."

"Thanks."

"Oh, you're a bum," she said. "You're the only male in this bed and you should regard it as a public trust."

She reached her hand over and caressed and cajoled him.

"Now what?" he said. "Cut that out."

"No. I'm gonna tickle you until you want to."

He removed her hand gently but she put it back and resumed the cajoling. "Leave me alone," he said.

"I can play with it all I want," she told him, "because everything we have belongs to each other. Come on, now."

"You little bitch."

"Rise and shine. There, see? You're starting to want me." She changed her position. "Diddle de dum, diddle de dum, dum de dum. I'm gonna be obscene. Let's be obscene, Les. There, do you like that? I'm using all ten fingers."

"I know."

He came to her, breathing heavily, and she made way for him. She pulled at his shoulders and back, wanting to sink upwards even closer. His style was different now from the other time.

"There, aren't you glad now?" she murmured. "I told you you'd be glad."

She felt the pressure of his weight. Then he became not quite still, an occasional stir asserting his presence, and he made his weight light upon her. She knew he was not resting but prolonging the tautness. Her hands felt the stiffening of his backbone, and pressed the shoulder blades that moved just under the skin.

"Let's make it very long," she said. "And never end."

He kissed her throat and put his face in the pillow, his cheek against hers.

"Can we stay like this all night?" she asked.

"I doubt it."

"Let's."

"Not possible."

She let her feet float up in the darkness.

"Les—"

"What."

"Do you love me?"

"Yup."

She pointed a toe ballerinalike toward a corner of the ceiling, but could scarcely see it, shadowy in the black air. The city had grown silent and she heard a clock strike once somewhere. She wondered if it were eleven-thirty.

They played slowly, and slower still, as if to reduce the sense of touch to its subtlest delicacies. He brought her to feverish excitement even so, until the teasing endlessness was intolerable. When she gave in to convulsions he remained like stone, and when she lay shuddering he began again.

She squeezed and he seemed to swell. Even when they stayed utterly still it was like a stillness on a tightrope. Again he waited out her convulsiveness.

"Les, Les," she said. "You're marvelous."

He was not so still any more, and they pushed with their feet to a fresh place on the wrinkled sheet. When he ended, it was not with a grand passion but a kind of falling to pieces. He kissed her good night and rolled away. She lay with her hands resting on the hollow of her belly. She arose, and felt her way to the bathroom in the dark, and returned to bed.

"I feel better," she said. "I'm glad we did that."

He didn't answer.

"Les—"

She waited and then repeated his name softly.

"What," he said sleepily.

"Do you think I'm a nymphomaniac?"

"No."

She was quiet, until his breathing started to deepen again. "Let's have an orgy," she said.

"We can't have an orgy," he said. "It takes three to make an orgy."

"Oh. Well then let's don't have an orgy. I don't want to share you with anyone."

He had not moved since he had rolled from her. He lay with his back to her.

"Let's have a revel," she said. "Can two have a revel?"

"What?"

"A romp. Two can have a romp."

"Go to sleep, will ya? I've got to be up in the morning. Be a good girl."

She closed her eyes, and tried to imitate his regular breathing. She opened her eyes.

"Les—" she said. "Hey."

"What."

"Let's do it again."

"What?"

"I do need it one more time. I'm not satisfied yet."

"No," he said, without moving.

"Yes."

"Look, dopey, I haven't got any more."

"Yes you have. You told me you have untapped reserves. A whole private hoard. Just like the emergency tank in a Volkswagen."

"I'm not a Volkswagen."

"You're a sperm whale. You're my itsy-bitsy sperm whale."

"Shut up, will ya? I don't want to be dead on my feet again tomorrow. There's too much at stake. And don't try that trick again." He pushed her hand away. "You'll kill the goose that laid the golden egg."

"Aw." She withdrew her hand and sighed. She lay on her back, her hands folded on her stomach. "I wish it could keep sneezing and sneezing. Like my nose."

They were silent. She sighed again.

"Okay, I'll be good," she said. "I'm not gonna bother you any more. I'm gonna go seepy seep."

"Just go uppy shut. Geh shlofen. Do you know what that means?"

"Yes."

They were silent once more.

"You know what's gonna happen tomorrow?" she began again. "Patients are gonna die, and it's my fault. Patients are gonna die because I kept you awake, and you're gonna make mistakes."

She waited for him to reply. He didn't.

She rolled away too, so that they were back to back, several inches apart. She closed her eyes and for a while tried to sleep. She heard tires on the street.

She thought again about the events of the evening.

"Les—" she said.

He gave a startled grunt and half turned toward her.

"Oh, Les, honestly. Were you ever so lonesome on a dark night that you wanted to holler?"

"I was almost asleep," he said. "You woke me up to ask me that?" He rolled back.

She put her face to the sheet and sprawled naked in the linen, her hands spread. She relaxed her jaw. I can't sleep, she thought. Everything's the matter with me. I need sleeping pills.

She wondered how much space her paper would give to the story of the wild horses. She ought to have told Mr. Hopkins that she was the only reporter there—it was a scoop. Mr. Alpert was so phlegmatic and sullen all the time you couldn't tell if you had reached him. She ought to have told Mr. Alpert how very strongly the registrar felt about it. It was unusual after all that he should have devoted his whole speech to that. You'd think he'd talk about cars, or the Massachusetts traffic laws, or something like that.

Suddenly a panicky feeling took hold of her, behind her ears, in her neck, and in her stomach. She tried to remember some indication that the old man was in fact the registrar of motor vehicles, that she had heard him addressed by name. But she could not. And she seemed to remember that the meeting was to have been in the ballroom, and that room had not seemed like a ballroom.

She turned and lay on her back. She could not possibly have made such a mistake. Yet the more she thought of it the clearer it seemed that she had.

She touched Leslie. "Gee," she said. "Les, you have to forgive me. I have to say one more thing. I just had a horrible thought."

"What."

"Do you think I covered the wrong meeting? Those horses? I bet it was the wrong meeting."

Leslie said nothing, though she knew he was fully awake.

"Oh, Les, I'm scared to death," she said. "I just walked in there. I just assumed it was the right room. I didn't think about it or anything. And what if that wasn't the registrar at all?"

"Who would it have been?"

"I don't know."

"Well, are you sure it wasn't? Maybe it wasn't wrong."

She had sat up. "No. I just know it. Oh my God. What'll I do?"

"Well, let's get dressed and go out to a phone booth if you're so worried. Tell them not to print it just yet."

"Maybe we better. Only they'd have gone to press already. Oh Les, they'll murder me. I'll lose my job."

"Well, is it possible they won't notice?" he said. "Maybe they'll never know the difference. Mistakes do go unnoticed."

"It's possible, I suppose. It's my only hope."

He put an arm to her and she lay down against his hairy chest and wept quietly.

But in a little while he said he had to sleep and that she had better sleep too. She lay against the pillow, her face tear-streaked.

53

Leslie slept, but she did not for a long time, and when she did she kept waking fitfully and anxiously. When it was time for Leslie to rise she was already up, though even the cat still lay curled and sleeping in his corner by the cabinets beneath the counter. But she prepared a breakfast of smoked fish and the odor of it woke the cat.

Her eyes ached and she felt exhausted. She had begun to sneeze. It was hard to wake Leslie. When at last he had washed and dressed and shaved he bolted his breakfast and rushed off.

She went to bed again, and slept in daylight for several hours, until the cat woke her in the afternoon by jumping on her neck.

She took a hot bath. She thought she should go to the girls' apartment and see if there was mail, and perhaps phone Ella Jane at Ella Jane's office to find out how much she owed her for the cabs. But she didn't feel like it. If she went to the apartment her mother would probably phone her there, and she did not want another encounter with her mother or with any of her family. Instead she busied herself shopping, and replenished the groceries. She did not see how she could go to Wilmerding Crosswalk next Sunday. But not going would surely make her mother tell her father, and produce an even worse crisis.

She wished Leslie would ask her to run away with him somewhere.

She walked to work, at the last possible moment. Danny McBride came out of the entrance as she arrived, as though on his way to some reporting assignment. "Oh ho!" he said when he saw her, widening his eyes. "Wooh! Wait till Dexter gets his hands on you!"

She went in, to the big elevator cage. McBride's expression had shown some amusement, so she was not sure how much he might be exaggerating Mr. Killian's anger. Even so, the effect was frightening, and she went up to the city room with her heart pounding.

Bob Lyons was typing at his desk, and said hello to her in his usual way when she entered. He did not seem to have heard that anything terrible had happened. The city room was busy as it always was in midafternoon, with the noise of typewriters, wire-service machines, telephones, voices, and sometimes the scrape of a chair. Millicent went at once to the wire-service machines, at the far end of the room. They were spilling their stories to the floor, and she used the ruler she kept there to tear them into sections.

But in a moment Mr. Killian spoke her name sharply, and when she looked he beckoned with his head.

She went the length of the room. Mr. Killian rose, hitching his belt. The phone rang on his desk but he didn't touch it. "Take it," he said to Mr. Hopkins, and Mr. Hopkins pressed a button on another phone.

Mr. Killian put a foot on the pulled-out bottom drawer of his desk. He was glowering and haggard, his hair unkempt.

"All right, where were you hiding?" he said.

She did not immediately get his meaning.

"Your roommate said you were out," he said. "Seven-thirty in the morning, she says you're out. Couldn't be reached. Am I supposed to believe that too?" The muscles of his face became more tightly knotted. He planted a fist on the desk. He lowered his face into hers so suddenly that she was startled. "The registrar had me on the phone at seven, and half an hour later the other guy calls up, and I can't even find you to give him an excuse. Millicent, what's in your skull? Marshmallow? Don't tell me it's brains. I know it couldn't be brains. What is it? What is it, huh? Cotton candy? Is it? Is that what it is? Answer, damn it."

"I don't know."

"And that boob Alpert. I'm not through with him yet either. Never even questions ya. You tell him the registrar's up there raving about horses on the prairies and he sits there taking it down like a dummy. And he says to me, 'she said she was there and she heard the guy say it.' And if I see fit to send you there he's got to assume you're competent. And there he's got me. He's right. It still comes back to me. It's my fault. But the dumb boob still should have checked it. He should have called me out of bed if he had any doubt. I don't know—what a staff I've got." He flung his hands, and tossed his head hopelessly. "I'm the laughingstock of New England now, and sure, I'm to blame. I've got no judgment of human beings, that's all. I'm a damn fool. Heustis Garvey told me after two days down there you were no damn good, you didn't have it. You didn't know a sheet of copy from third base. But no, I knew better. I was gonna make you into something, I saw possibilities, I believed in you. I was gonna be a father to you. I don't know, something blinded me. I used to pride myself in my ability to size people up." She began to sob, though she tried to hold it back. "From now on you're a copy boy and nothing else, understand?" he said. "You'll never do another story as long as I'm in this office. I can't fire you because the Guild would make a grievance. Doing a reporter's work at a copy-boy's wage. So you've got me over a barrel. That's the Guild for you."

"I'll resign if you want," she said through her tears.

"That's right! That's right, quit! Go ahead. Leave me flat, right at edition time! Five editions to go tonight and no copy boy. And a full basket of copy on the desk. Commit suicide, will ya, God damn it! You ought to be put out of your misery. Get out of my sight."

She started confusedly to take copy from the basket to take it upstairs.

"Look at me when I'm talking to you!" he snapped, and she put the copy down. "There could be a triple murder on the floor of the Legislature and the Post Office on fire, and you could be the only one here, and I still wouldn't send you on it. If you were the only one left I wouldn't send you. I couldn't, could I? Could I?"

She couldn't stop sobbing. "No," she admitted.

"No. If I sent you to cover High Mass at the Cathedral you'd cover the barrelmakers' convention. And tell Louie Alpert the sermon was dirty jokes. And that doctor story. And I gave you another chance, like an idiot. Maybe women's troubles was at the bottom of it. Maybe it's the wrong time of the month for you. Or maybe you had a fight with that boy friend of yours. Or maybe you just don't care. Maybe you think the paper's going under anyway."

The phone on his desk rang. He seized it and spoke gruffly to someone. She waited, sniffling and trying to suppress her sobs, uncertain whether she should take the copy upstairs now or whether he wanted to talk to her some more. But he remained on the phone a long time, conversing angrily about another matter.

She took the copy. She saw Louie Alpert give her a black look.

By the time she got to Mr. Valentino she had managed to stop crying, and he was busy at a linotype machine and scarcely looked up. When she came down to the city room she noticed that Mr. Killian was quite busy with other matters, as though he had put her from his mind. She kept at her own duties, and thought meanwhile of the letter of resignation she would write. She would thank him for the confidence he had had in her and the opportunities he had given her, and apologize for having let him down. It was true that she had not turned out to be a newspaperwoman he could depend on. She had no excuse to offer, and she would leave at his convenience, as soon as he had a new copy boy. She tried not to let the people about her notice her tears, which had begun again.

She had her sandwich miserably at the spa. The recollection of the bawling out made her cry anew. Now that her newspaper career was at an end there seemed nothing to do but go to law school, but she had no enthusiasm for it any more. She would have to get some sort of a filing job, like the one she had had with Miss Bancroft, and go to school at night. It seemed long and dismal, not exciting like newspapering.

When she set out for her visit to Mr. Garvey she was wondering how he had fared. She felt she had not handled that situation very well either. She had had no right to let a friend of hers send him home, in the middle of his tour of duty, without telling anyone. His troubles were even worse than hers, she thought. And besides she had gotten Mr. Alpert into trouble, and it must have been far more humiliating for Mr. Alpert than for herself, because Mr. Alpert was a married man with children to support. And yet she had wept more over being bawled out than over hearing that her brother had died. I'm a rotten, self-centered person, she thought.

When she got to the little press room at Police Headquarters she was surprised to find Mr. Garvey looking quite hale and chipper. He was playing cards with Cox and Tilton. He handed her a list of police promotions and police transfers to take back to the city room. "How are ya, Scoop?" he said cheerily, and gave his raspy laugh, a single wheeze down in his throat.

She left red-faced. His laugh had clearly been one of derision. He knew of her downfall. And it was nasty of him to rejoice in it, she thought.

Apparently he had come through the evening unscathed. It was quite plain that no stories had broken in his absence, and that no one had scooped him, and that Mr. Killian and the city-room people had never found out. If she had left him lying there on the floor it would have made no difference at all. For all she could tell he had never even been curious as to how he had gotten home.

When she got to the city room Mr. Killian had gone home. Maud said a comforting word when Millicent passed her desk. She sat by Maud a little later, when she had a chance, but began to blubber again as soon as she spoke. She said she had ruined Mr. Killian's reputation and made him the laughingstock of New England. Maud told her that Dexter's reputation had already been ruined about five hundred times before. She told Millicent not to resign. "It'll all be forgotten in time," she said.

"I don't see how," said Millicent.

But in midevening she told Maud she had decided it would be cowardly to resign. If she resigned now, Mr. Killian would never hire another woman again. Her duty was to remain, and work hard at whatever lowly tasks were given her, until the faith Mr. Killian had at first had in her would at last be vindicated, and until his faith in his own ability to judge people, especially women, was restored again. Even if it took years. Her first move would be to buy some stock in the paper, just to show him that she didn't think the paper was going under.

"Don't buy any stock," Maud told her.

She found the correction of her error when she carried down the first editions from upstairs. It made her realize anew the humiliation she had brought upon the entire paper, its owners, and all her fellow workers. The correction said that the registrar had addressed the Lions convention Monday evening on Better Highways For Better Business, but that a talk given before the Conservation Society by former Representative Hird of Kansas had been erroneously ascribed to the registrar in yesterday's editions.

Maud assured her that she had seen the correction and that she still didn't think Millicent should resign.

About nine o'clock there was a phone call from Ella Jane, who said Mr. Killian had phoned in the morning.

"I know," Millicent said tiredly. "Has my mother phoned?"

"No," said Ella Jane.

Several times in the evening she had wanted to apologize to Mr. Alpert, but whenever she picked up a piece of copy from him he seemed so full of unforgiving anger that she had not the courage to speak. Maud told her that Dexter had phoned Alpert at his home, waking him up, and then had bawled him out again in the office, much worse than he had bawled out Millicent.

"I don't see how it could be worse," Millicent said.

"Oh it was," said Maud. "He told him his I.Q. was the cube root of minus zero. He chewed the hell out of him."

So Millicent determined anew to try to apologize. The next time Louie Alpert handed her a piece of copy, without looking at her, it was near midnight.

"I'm sorry, Mr. Alpert," she told him with tears in her eyes.

"That and ten cents'll take me home," he said sourly, looking at the typewriter. Then he looked up slowly. The mustache hung. The eyes, close at his nose, seemed to hate her. "There's one reason you weren't fired," he said. "One reason. Just one. And that's that Killian's in love with ya."

"What do you mean?" she said, still with tears in her eyes. "He can't fire me because of the Guild."

"That's baloney," said Alpert. "Any incompetent can be fired. It's right in the Guild contract. Incompetence is grounds for dismissal. The guy's got a big crush on you. The whole office knows it."

"I don't believe it!" she said with a catch in her voice. "He's a married man!"

"Go home," Mr. Hopkins said from the copy desk.

"I have a piece of copy to take upstairs," she told him.

She took it up, and when she came down she left.

Leslie was on call. She saw her own wet eyes beyond the stains in the silver of the bathroom mirror. She lay on the wide bed a long time without undressing. She wished he were there.

She wished she could go out to a phone booth and wake her parents, and tell them about this terrible mistake she had made in her reporting assignment. But she couldn't, on account of that awful letter from Charles.

She sat up. She would play with the cat if he were awake, she thought. But he was curled asleep. He was hardly a kitten any more.

Mr. Killian's remark about the wrong time of the month came back to her. She was in fact due, and even a day's delay was quite unprecedented for her. She rose, and got the wallet calendar from her shoulder-strap bag, and studied it. She went to the bathroom, and came back, and got into pajamas.

One day's delay didn't mean anything. It would be stupid to start worrying about a disaster like that. It couldn't have happened anyway. Les was always so methodical and careful about those things.

54

She awoke shortly after five in the morning, even though Leslie was not there. She tried to go to sleep again, but gave up finally.

It was Wednesday, and she was off, and it would be a long day before Leslie came home at suppertime. She frittered it. She was nervous and had a headache. It would have been a good long day in which to find a news item in the city on her own, except that Mr. Killian had made it clear that she was not to aspire to be a reporter any longer. She had no more future there. She wondered whether her decision not to resign had been a wise one, since her job would only keep her in a rut now and keep her from doing anything else.

She was sneezing and her eyes hurt. And the period was still delayed.

It was five in the afternoon when she finally went to the girls' apartment to see whether she had mail. There was none, but Ella Jane told her her father had phoned just a few minutes before.

"What did he want?" said Millicent.

"Well, he asked if you were here, and then he said he wants to come in here tomorrow and see you. He asked me to get the message to you."

"What time? What time's he coming in?"

"One o'clock, If you were here five minutes ago you'd have caught him."

"I'm just as glad I didn't."

"I didn't know how to get a message to you when you're off. I was going to call Les at the hospital and ask him to tell you."

She asked Ella Jane what she owed her for the cabs to the press room and back, and for Mr. Garvey's cab.

"We took his out of his wallet," Ella Jane said.

"Well, how much was yours? Your cabs," said Millicent.

"Oh, that's all right."

"No, I mean to pay you when I get my check."

She did not stay long at the girls' as it was nearly time to meet Les. When she did meet him she insisted that they go out to a movie. She told him how furious Mr. Killian had been, and that her father was going to come to town looking for her tomorrow, and that she was too edgy and nervous to stay in all evening.

She did not enjoy the movie.

Leslie asked her if she would meet her father. "I don't know," she said.

She had pretty much decided she would not meet him. It would be an extremely unpleasant and probably emotional interview, about very personal things that were none of her family's business, and she had no stomach for it. Her father had no right to come bothering her like that.

She thought again of how detestable it had been of Charles to write that letter. It was tearing the family apart. How mixed up he must have been.

In the morning, however, she was in a stew about whether to meet her father or not. He was going to ring the bell at the girls' apartment, and the feeling of hiding from him would be sickening also. Moreover she was not ready to break off permanently with the whole family, or keep on the run from them forever, so a minimum of civility was needed. Even if she found excuses not to teach Sunday school for a while. Anyway she was afraid she could not hide from him very long. He was tough when his mind was made up, and if she persisted in avoiding him he might waylay her at her job, or confront Les at the hospital.

It might be best to be at the girls' place when he looked for her, and have it out with him coolly, and tell him that she was grown up now and that he would just have to accept it. And he would have to, if she kept calm, and stuck to her rights. She wished this embarrassing confrontation could be avoided, but it couldn't. Sooner or later she would have to get it over with. It was one of the burdens of her life. He couldn't drag her away by force, and he couldn't punish her physically.

She went there ahead of time, feeling somewhat frightened. The apartment was not as tidy as it used to be, and she was quite sure it was mostly Barbie's fault. The milk carton had been standing out and open since breakfast again. She cleaned the table and folded its leaves. She made herself some cocoa and toast for lunch, but did not have appetite enough to finish the toast. When the doorbell sounded she was sitting primly. She sprang up and pressed the buzzer.

She heard her father's tread, and stood on the landing to meet him. "Hello," she said unsmiling, as he came up. He smiled a little.

She went in with her back to him and sat on the studio couch, legs crossed, her hands clasped tight about a knee.

"You got my message," he said, and sat in the stuffed chair with broken springs. His hat rested on the back of his head and his tweed topcoat was unbuttoned.

"Yes." Her voice was already shaky.

"Well, I guess you know what it's about."

"Now listen," she began, plunging into some phrases she had prepared. "You can't know what's best for me. So if you have any regard for me—I have a right to my own life. So please—I just want to be respected and let alone."

"When are we gonna see you?" he said. "Are you coming Sunday."

"I don't know. Mother's the one who said I'm not welcome."

"You're always welcome," said Ed. "And I speak for Mother."

"Stop trying to make a nervous wreck out of me. I've got my own problems and I've got to work them out in my own way."

"So can't we talk? Is a father nothing just because you're over twenty-one?"

"Some things are personal and private."

"Don't you know how much each of you children means to us?"

"You're all hysterical. The whole bunch of you."

She was sitting stiffly, trying to be poised, despite the wobble in her voice. She saw the lines in his face. He was being more subdued than she had expected. She thought he was going to try to shame her. When he spoke his tone had dropped.

"Is this all you could do," he said, "with all you've been taught? Some young snotnose has to flatter himself that he's a man of the world, a man with a mistress, and it has to be you?"

"There happen to be different moralities, and I hope you'll decide to be civilized about it. And I don't think a certain letter was so civilized. And I don't think ambushing me is so civilized either."

"Ambush? I didn't lie in wait for you here."

"Well, persecuting me. And I don't think much of Mother getting you involved in something that wasn't anybody's business. And I understand Patty had a hand in it too."

"Well, as far as that goes," he said, "I already suspected it before."

She was startled. "You did?" she asked. "Why?"

"What made me suspect it? The fact that I'm your father made me suspect it."

"Well, I don't believe I've done anything wrong," she said. "And you won't make me believe it's wrong. You and mother didn't make me, after all. I mean not in the sense that God did. And you have to let me live my own life. You've just got to catch up with modern times. You can't live in the age of the Bible forever." She was shivering.

"Look, I'm aware this is an era when fathers have to look the other way while their daughters sleep with their lovers, but I don't know—how shall I say it—on you it doesn't look good. It's not your speed, and it never was. You're not the type. Even when I suspected it I couldn't believe it. Shacking up with a guy."

"I'll decide that. And do you have to use these expressions that vulgarize things?"

"I'm just using the expression. You're doing it. You gonna be seeing this guy again tonight?"

"For your information Les happens to be on call at the hospital tonight, all night long. He might spend half the night doing emergency operations for all we know. Saving human lives." She shivered again. "It's gotten chilly or something," she said. "I'm going to make some warm milk." She rose and went to the little kitchen, leaving the door open. "Would you like some?"

"No, that's all right," he said.

He sat watching while she lighted the gas.

"Tell me honestly," he said. "Are you happy?"

"Are you an advice-to-the-lovelorn expert?"

"Are you happy?" he asked again.

"Are you?" she said.

She had not looked at him, but watched the pot of milk.

"People have needs," she said.

"You need it like a loch in kop. And his needs I don't care about."

"I happen to care."

"When he needs to sleep with my daughter I can stop caring about his needs."

"And I happen to believe in equal rights for women," she said. The shuddering and shaking would not stop. "I don't believe in a double standard."

"Yeah," he said. "Equal rights for women. Next thing you know they'll want equal rights for children."

She gave him a look of disgust.

"Well it's true," he said. "That's how things are going. They'll be giving little girls to little boys for a bar-mitzvah present." He got up, slowly. "Millicent," he said. He seemed to remember finally that he had his hat and coat on. He took them off and put them on the chair. "There's something I want to say to you. I should have said it before only I never really thought it was necessary." He came nearer and stood by the doorjamb. "Listen. I don't know, maybe if you talk to girls you'll hear of cases where a girl got a guy to fall for her by going to bed with him. But if you're smart, Millicent, it's a myth."

"What a mind you have—" she said angrily, without turning, but her throat was tight and she scarcely could find breath.

"I've seen people, I've known people, I've talked to people, and I'd say if that ever worked once, I've heard of a hundred cases where it didn't. Where it didn't work at all. Guys get laid. They don't propose in the morning. But girls romanticize these things. A girl likes a guy, and she starts sleeping with him, and for two years she tries to get him to marry her, while he hems and haws. I've seen this system, and it's a bunch of crap. It's no good. I know, there are girls these days who think the way to get a husband is to move in with a guy like that, on a trial basis. And become necessary to him I suppose, a habit, but to my mind it's stupid. You're at his mercy and it takes you out of circulation. Because after you give in to a guy, he's not a suitor any more. You become the suitor. You don't see a man down on his knees, begging the woman he sleeps with every night to marry him, and the woman saying no. He knows he can marry her at will. Today, tomorrow, chuck her, marry her. The woman living with him is the one that asks for marriage. Don't kid yourself."

"Well you're wrong. I haven't asked Les to marry me. I'm not ready for marriage. And he's not either."

Ed shook his head. "Look," he said, "a girl goes through, say, five affairs, and she marries the fifth guy. Why? Because the fifth guy was willing. You call that freedom? You're out of your mind."

"Girls throw men over too."

"Sure. When it gets through to them that there's no future, then they make a great show of having a choice."

The milk boiled over. She turned off the fire, and tried to cool the milk by pouring it back and forth between a glass and the pot, cooling the glass and the pot alternately under the water tap, but her hands shook as she held them and her motions were confused.

"I don't know," said Ed, "maybe it works for a certain shy type, that's grateful for a woman making it easy. But your friend didn't impress me like that."

"Would you get out of the way, please?"

He stepped aside, though he was not actually in the way. She took the glass to the living room and sat at the drop-leaf table. He turned to face her, though she sat not facing him.

"I don't see what you'd know about it," she said. "Or Mother either."

She took a drink of the milk, holding it with both hands.

"Aren't you cold?" she said. "I'm freezing."

"No." He was still standing at the doorjamb, his hands in his pockets. "What do you think, Millicent?" he said. "You think it's the way to keep him from seeing other women?"

She kept sipping the warm milk. He could not see her face. But he sensed that the question made her angry.

She put the milk down on the table, but still held it with both hands.

"Has it ever occurred to you," she said, still not looking at him, "that maybe a physical relationship helps to create love?" He saw the shiver as she spoke, and heard it in her voice. "Maybe it brings out a closeness," she added, "that was only latent before."

"If that's the case, when are you getting married?"

She remained sitting quietly, with the warm glass. He looked at the delicateness of her ear, of her neck, and the little hairs about it.

"Millicent, I'm not dumb, and I know something about love, I think. And a girl has a right to say no. When a boy says come on—why should we wait—she has a right to refuse. And her refusal doesn't mean 'I don't love you.' It means 'I don't belong to you yet.' You know what advice I'd give a girl? Suppose she has her eye on a man. All right. And say she's even got competition, her rival, some other girl, that he can sleep with. I'd tell her this. You go to him. You say, 'look, my rival goes to bed with you and you don't have to marry her. Me you have to marry. But—marry me and I'll promise to obey. And I'll obey you in bed. Will my rival promise that?' You'll get him. If he likes you. If he likes you best. Because a man wants a woman who'll court him in the long years after marriage, not just before. I guarantee it. And you won't have to sleep with him first, even if your competition did. A guy doesn't marry his second choice rather than his first choice just because she took her pants down faster. Or if he does, then he's so short-sighted he'll never get rich. I promise ya that. He's not a guy that makes his own life. What's the matter—you think you have to sleep with him to prove you have sex organs? He couldn't take your word for it? When I married your mother I took it for granted she had sex organs. She didn't have to sleep with me first to prove it."

"And has it occurred to you that some people might like to find out first if they're compatible or not?"

"Yes," he said, "and Millicent, it's easy to be compatible in bed. What's difficult is to be compatible out of bed. That's my opinion, and my experience, and when you're married that's what you'll find out over the years. And I think the premarital sex, instead of showing whether you're compatible, it does just the opposite. It prevents you from finding out if you really like the person. It can obscure the fact that you've got nothing in common." He moved to the stuffed chair and sat on its arm, so that she would be facing him. "I think that's the worst of it for some of these kids today—the pleasure of getting to know somebody sexually can put a very rosy glow on things, and blind you to things that are going to be of first importance when the knot's tied. It blurs. It obfuscates, so you don't see what a pain in the ass the other person is. When you're all of a sudden married and stuck, that's the time you really need the sex. Because you're stuck, and you need all the rosy glow you can get. That's when you need the new-found pleasure, to tide you over the first couple of years."

She looked at him contemptuously over the glass of milk, which rested on the table with her hands around it.

"And would you give a son the same advice?" she said. "Or is it supposed to be different for a boy?"

"No, I'd tell a boy the same. If a son of mine were mixed up with some broad and he was gonna marry her, that he'd been sleeping with I mean—I'd tell him, all right, she accommodates you now, when she's on the make, but will she be in such a rush to please when the knot's tied, after the deal's clinched? You know, when sex becomes part of courtship, they put their best foot forward there too. I'd tell him, look, man to man, you've had the best of that one already—if you're gonna load yourself up with a family you're entitled to a fresh experience at least. I'm glad of one thing, that your mother and I didn't have to start off with something that was stale before it began."

She glared at him in red-faced fury. "I see now where Charles got his filthy mind. It was inherited. Is that what you married Mother for? Sex? Love means nothing to you, does it."

"Yes," he contradicted her. "Yes. Love does mean something to me. And that's why I'd tell a boy the wisest thing he can do is search widely, for the girl that's even-tempered, and that shares his values, so he can invest in good love and sex for the lifetime that follows marriage. But this affair business gets him into a rut with a girl, maybe a girl that isn't so right, because he doesn't expect it to be permanent, and he neglects the search. He loses months and years, in bed with a girl who happens to be around, when he should be looking intensively for what he really wants. That's what I'd tell a boy. You can search better, and you can see clearer, when you're not hooked on sex."

"And did you tell Charles that?"

"Well, I never went into it with him that much, I guess. But that's what I think."

"And Charles died at eighteen," she said. "Do you happen to know whether he had any sexual experience or not?"

"I don't know."

"Would you want him never to have had any?" she said. "It seems to me sex organs were meant for use."

"Well, nobody expected him to die at eighteen. Sure, they're meant for use. So what? The uterus is meant for use too—that doesn't mean you have to have twenty children, does it? It keeps, Millicent. You can leave it idle years on end. It doesn't get rusty." He shook his head at her, with an expression almost of exasperation, and then he nodded a little. "I know you're worried about women's rights," he said, "but did it ever occur to you that the first time anywhere on the face of the earth that women had any rights in marriage was when the Talmud spelled out that marriage contract two thousand years ago? That contract is about a wife's rights and a husband's obligations, nothing else. And what you've got here with your friend is a marriage, except that you've been done out of all your rights. He can divorce you at will. That's not progress—you've put yourself back to where women were three and four thousand years ago. You're washing his socks for him, probably, and all he has to say is 'phooey, I'm ready for the next one,' and you're divorced. You've got no rights, no claim."

"That's not true," she said, with a new flush in her face and the quaver in her voice becoming prominent again. "Because I can divorce him too."

Ed shook his head. "It's not women who seek divorces," he told her quietly. "That's just a polite convention, but women don't get divorced because they want to."

"That's a pretty broad statement."

"You'll find out. Millicent, once you start going to bed, the man's got the upper hand. That's what the marriage contract tried to counterbalance. You've become the suitor now." He tightened his face, and gestured tiredly. "You're a sucker. Do you understand that? That's what hurts me."

"I don't see it that way."

"Tell me something. Tell me. Are you engaged? Do you consider yourself engaged?"

"I don't suppose so. I haven't thought about it."

"You haven't thought about it."

"What would it matter to you if we were? You still wouldn't approve."

"No, you're darn right I wouldn't. You know what I think of engaged couples? If he can still change his mind, and back out, she's being played for a sucker. And if he's so committed that he can't change his mind, he's on the level, he can't back out, and they're all ready to start sleeping together and it's no secret, then in effect they're already married. It's the same. If he can't get out they're married. And if they're married, why not have the ceremony? Sex deserves a wedding. What's the big deal these days, that the ceremony has to be after? In the old days it was sexier—the party celebrated the night she got it. Not like today—that the party celebrates that they're already an old married couple for a couple of months or a year or something. Millicent, Millicent, please." He gestured with both hands. "With a woman, this affair business is just no good. As soon as she's not too young for it she's already too old for it. If an affair ends badly, if they're wrong for each other, then they shouldn't have done it. I don't think most girls remember their affairs as happy ones. They're all unhappy, because they end unhappy. They're not gonna get married, so they start quarreling. And if the end is good then they should have gotten married sooner, and saved it for the marriage, when it would have been sweetest. Millicent, look. I know it's hard for a woman to give up a guy, when there's hope there, but have the strength to quit. Your family's all upset—you have the excuse now. And then if he wants you and loves you he'll take you in a way that gives you your rights. And if you can't, if you're afraid of losing him, then you're in a bad way. It's what I'm saying. He can end it but you can't. You say you can divorce him too? So prove it. Millicent, listen to me. Quit now. Let him ask you to marry him if he wants you so much. If he doesn't love you what do you need him for? Millicent, if he doesn't feel responsibility for you, you're just like a photograph for him to masturbate over. That's all. You're being had. You're being used. That's what kills me. Sure, the excitement's fine, the moments of excitement. But after the excitement you lie there, and you're empty, and there's a void, an awful void. And it needs to be filled by love. You know, people enjoy orgasm, but it's the same for all. So how can love of an individual be based on it? Obviously it has to be based on a lot of other things—"

"Will you please leave me alone?" she shouted, her voice rising high, and a gesture of her hands knocked over the glass so that what was left in it spilled across the table. She burst into tears. "Daddy! For goodness sakes! Leave me alone!"

"All right." He rose, and picked up his hat and coat. "I have to get back anyway. I have to meet a class."

He buttoned his coat, looking at her. She was sobbing, not looking at him.

"Well, so long," he said. "Can I still figure on you for Sunday school, I hope?"

"I don't know," she said through her sobs.

He went to the door, opened it, and turned to look at her. Her elbows were on the table, a foot was tucked under her, and her face was hidden in her hands while she sniffled quietly.

"Believe me, I wish I could pull you out of here," he said. "I wish I could take you home. I'd spank you if I thought it would do any good."

She looked up at him tearfully. "Oh sure. With my skirts up, I suppose. You'd enjoy that, wouldn't you."

"Well, don't worry about it," he said. "We're forbidden to strike a grown child."

He stood there frowning, watching while she buried her face in her hands again.

"This affair is making you bitchy," he said. "It's hard to believe you're happy in it."

55

By the time he had driven a third of the way home he felt he should have stayed longer, even if it meant missing his class, and even if it meant that the children would come to a locked temple for nothing. When he had had Millicent upset and crying, that had been the time to press his advantage, he thought now. He should have kept insisting until she agreed to come home with him. He felt he had been too mild and reasonable, and he had a panicky feeling now that he had missed his best chance.

His strategy had been to be understanding, so as to incline her to listen, but he was not even certain now that she would grant him a second interview.

He found seven or eight children gathered at the temple for their after-school class.

When he had taught them he drove slowly home. He felt worse than sick. Millicent, this sensitive angel—could it be her fate to be a slave and mistress to the convenience of some punk with other things on his mind? This wise young lad with the medical degree, couldn't he have taken his problems to some other girl? Could that boy know what it was to be a girl's father?

Ed gave a despairing shudder. When your daughter starts going in for this sort of stuff, the bottom falls out. I don't want my girls taken, he thought, until I give them, signed and sealed, with my right to be in the act guaranteed.

To Lucinda he tried to put the best possible face on it. He said he had given Millicent plenty to think about, and would talk to her again when she came for Sunday school, and if that didn't work he'd go to the Massachusetts General Hospital and talk to young Hollander. Lucinda said nothing, but he could see she was not satisfied. In the evening he tried to telephone Millicent at her job, but they told him she was off.

When he heard Lucinda's sighs in the next day or two he hardly knew if they were for Charles or Millicent. He guessed they were mostly for Millicent, even though she still woke nightly with dreams of Charles, and reported seeing boys on the streets who resembled him, and went to the cemetery once or twice a week to put flowers on his grave. She even went surprisingly often to weekday services at the temple and labored unfluently through the kaddish prayer. Patty could do it with facility and usually helped Lucinda with it.

Saturday night he phoned Millicent worriedly at the city room and asked if he could count on her for Sunday school. She told him coolly that he could not, and when he asked to see her again she called him a Victorian and said she would not discuss her private affairs further. She said it was too upsetting. She also told him she was busy and could not tie up the company phone this way.

"I've got a good mind to go down to the hospital then," he said into the phone, "and have a talk with your friend."

"And hit him, I suppose," she answered.

"I didn't say hit him."

"Because if you did," she told him, "he'd give you measure for measure. And that would be just lovely, wouldn't it? Haven't you got anything to do besides try to make me feel dirty? I wish the men in this family would let me alone, that's all. And I don't want you to try to see Les. It won't do you a bit of good, and it'll only embarrass me and you and Les and everybody and I don't want such an encounter. It's quite unnecessary." The voice on the phone wrung him.

"Millicent, I can't leave you there. For God's sake listen to me. It's gonna get worse and I'm scared of it—"

"I can't discuss it—"

"You know," he went on, "when a man discovers that his mistress is a human being, with all kinds of unsexy problems, and that the whole person has to be lived with, it's not Eden any more, and he finds he's married. Except that he's free to get out and start over with somebody else, with all the sexiness of new beginnings, and sex isolated again. That's why men walk out on these things—"

"We're not tired of each other."

"It's not par for the course yet. These things generally run three to six months, that's all. Sometimes eight, nine, maybe. And then you've had it."

"Les is going into the Army in June."

"See? What have you got? You'll find out. Men are of two minds about what they want."

"I'm what *I* want."

"You don't sound it."

"We're two clean-minded people—"

"I know, and it hasn't hurt you. But I guarantee when it starts to hurt it'll hurt you more than it hurts him. You're matched about as equally as a matador and a bull, don't you know that? You're not in control of this setup. So he goes in the Army—" He heard her try to interrupt but he didn't let her. "Millicent, the end of an affair usually results in the beginning of another, and what a series of affairs comes down to is looking for a husband. And there's no evidence that you find a better husband that way than the other way. It's no good for a girl. How can she keep being pursued when she's been caught so often?"

"Dad, I can't talk any longer. You asked if I'm happy—you're certainly not helping to make me happy. I have to find my own way and live my own life, and right now I have to go to work. I have to hang up."

She sounded very agitated. There was nothing he could do but let the conversation end.

He told Lucinda that Millicent wouldn't be home. Lucinda said nothing, and seemed to take it calmly. Ed went to his study and spent the evening working.

A little past ten he heard Lucinda go upstairs and he thought he would go to bed also. But he went to the kitchen first, to see if the back door was bolted, and found Patty and Roland there, sharing a snack of milk and cookies. By the sink there was an uncooked chicken that Lucinda had put out to thaw. The wood of the table was damp as though Lucinda had just wiped it.

"Mother's still crying about Charles," Roland said to Ed.

"She's not crying about Charles, stupid," Patty said.

"Sure she is."

"No she isn't. Not about Charles."

"What about, then?"

"Millicent," she said.

Ed glanced at Patty sharply but did not catch her eye.

"What's the matter with Millicent?" Roland asked.

"Never mind," said Patty. She took another swallow of milk.

"Why's she crying about Millicent?" said Roland.

"Well, we wanted her to live home," Ed explained to Roland, "and there was a big argument about it, and everybody's mad, and she's not coming tomorrow."

"Oh," said Roland. "Is that all. I thought she got raped, or was gonna have a baby or something."

"God forbid!" Patty burst out. "That child! Twelve years old—where does he get such ideas!"

Ed bolted the door, looking at Patty sourly.

"Everything," Lucinda muttered tearfully, when he had gotten into bed next to her. "Everything has to happen. A boy has to go to war and never come back, and a girl has to go wrong. I don't know what I had children for. I'm afraid for the next two already."

"Well, maybe I'll talk to the kid at the hospital," said Ed, "and ask him to have some consideration for her emotions. Get married or let her alone. Maybe I can shame him a little, if he has a conscience."

"I'm just heartsick," said Lucinda. "Did you ask her if they take precautions at least?"

"No. I didn't think I had to ask."

"You should have asked."

"Look, they're not stupid. And the boy's a doctor."

"To you it's just one of those things, isn't it. And if she got pregnant it would be just one of those things."

"Please, don't start that," he told her. "I'm as worried as you are."

"No you're not. You were in favor of letting her have that apartment, and go and live with those girls. I wasn't. You were. You talked me into it. And you were in favor of the enlistment papers for Charles, too, when I was against it. He'd be in school today. He'd be alive." She choked. "So don't tell me a father feels it like a mother."

He patted her hand.

"Oh, don't pat my hand," she said, withdrawing it. "You probably patted Millicent's hand too. You're wishy-washy. A father's supposed to be firm, do you know that? That's the trouble with clergymen—they're afraid to cross anybody. They always want everybody to like them. Especially their own children."

"So how firm could I be? You can be firm, you know, and when a child is a certain age the child is in a position to be even firmer."

"Why didn't you tell her it's a sin—tell her it's against the Bible. You believe in the Bible and all that."

"I tried to tell her what I thought she'd listen to. Look, for all I know the guy took six months to talk her into it. So can I talk her out of it in an hour?"

"I never went in for all the religious chazerei," Lucinda said, "but I still knew that some things were wrong. I never knew of any law that it's all right all of a sudden just because they're over twenty-one. But she can wrap you around her little finger."

He said nothing more, and Lucinda did not either, though for a long time he knew she was not sleeping.

Maybe, he thought, he should have told Millicent point-blank that our Law forbids it, after all, and in the long run nothing in the Law turns out to be stupid. It was forbidden that she should hand herself over to a man who was not committed to be a husband.

He had brought her up as best as he could. You teach her the Law and tradition. But if she chooses to say no to Law and tradition, then what? How do you make her choose?

How do you teach a girl to love God? How can you manage it? There are people who manage it—how do they? What can you do, except train her to love yourself, so your soul can say to her: love me, love my God?

I want that girl to love me, heart and soul, he thought. But I don't think she ever will. To love somebody is to stand before God with him. To stand with him looking into the Unknown.

Maybe you must rely at last on her human need for God, and try to teach her that belief is permitted.

And as for Law, if you don't commit yourself to it, then you will be tyrannized over by the fashions and the times. Some tyranny will move in on you.

Millicent—she had seemed so wise, so sensitive. It was hard to believe that she was only another reacting female. Those eyes were a fraud.

Women were weather vanes. Take Lucinda—if he were to die she would no doubt continue with Sabbath candles and whatnot for a while, out of love of his memory, with more emotion than before, but if she remarried, to a man who wanted no part of it, she could as easily chuck it. To teach a woman, to bring up a woman, to convert a woman, was to write your name on water.

And how do you get the boys to keep their hands off the girls? This new morality makes girls a bunch of sitting ducks. Clay pigeons, that's all. It's not for the convenience of women. But they're too stupid to see it. They think closeness creates love—it does for a woman, so they assume it does for a man.

What was it that God said to Eve? And thy desire shall be toward thy man, and he shall rule over thee. That's not Victorianism. It means that girls tend to fall for the guys they sleep with, which leaves them open for a hell of a pushing around.

Or maybe the trouble was that evolution was still unfinished, still too incomplete. We were still too close to the lower species. In one species after another—salamanders, moose, dogs—the female's instinct is to get pregnant, he thought, but the male's instinct is to make as many females pregnant as he can lay his hands on. And thus a boy, when his juices build up a head of pressure, can go from girl to girl, even enjoy a one-night stand and look for another, while a girl feels left. Surely a God who creates animals to eat one another can create men and women to be at odds.

Just as our stomach muscles were not yet fully adapted to walking erect, so were we not yet fully adapted to our moral knowledge. Some species, lions for instance, have evolved to faithful monogamy, but man not yet.

Still, it seemed to him, society had something to do with it. In a society that makes the girls available, a boy must avail himself in order to feel masculine. The knowledge that men desire her will make a woman feel like a woman, whether she says yes or no. But a man to feel like a man must feel the urge to initiate, and if he does nothing in a society where the girls lie around wide open then his urge may be questioned. When girls cannot be had except in marriage, it's another matter. In such a society his ability to win a wife is what makes a man feel masculine. His ability to be a husband, a father. He's not questioned for not making girls that couldn't be made. Where there are no mistresses, no easy lays, and no brothels, a man's successful wooing still makes him a man, and there had been such societies.

Law was part of evolution. It tried to speed up evolution, to shorten this painful evolving. It had urged young marriages, with relatively flexible divorce, in which the courts functioned as a reconciliation agency. The Talmud had even suggested eighteen as an age for marriage, and twenty for earning a living—in other words a man might marry before his education is complete. He ought to have told Millicent that the Talmud recognized common-law marriage, since she was probably taking the view by now that a ceremony was just artificial nonsense. As the Talmud saw it, the open and admitted sleeping together made the marriage—the ceremony was only a betrothal. In the Talmud's view Millicent and Leslie already had a marriage, except that the Talmud would impose on him all the obligations of a husband.

He wished he had made that clearer to her. And this present-day eroticism, it's just Victorianism turned inside out, that's all, because it's still a covering up of the truth, a phony sex to hide the real sex. Lasciviousness is sex in isolation, isolated from reproduction, and isolated from the fact that you grow old and die and your woman too. It's a sugar-coating for men who can't bear the facts of life.

He thought of Patty. Patty dated more than Millicent ever had. Yet Patty impressed him as having a hard sensibleness, conventional in the old way, and probably tough in defense. He hoped so. Probably she'd marry young. Still, if kids persistently took two hours to get home from the movie in Sparkstown, two hours and three hours, it would lead where it had to lead these days. He had been young.

You couldn't ask. You couldn't talk of the details of love play. You couldn't ask her if the girls she knew let the boys put a hand in their bra. You had to talk in generalities, hours, places. And hope she'd postpone the days of necking, and the days of unbuttoning.

Well, he thought, maybe it couldn't be helped. It was the damn age we live in. Sooner or later Patty's brassiere would be outflanked, and tumble, and become open country, the holy grace of emerging womanhood degraded for the excitement of some idiot pipsqueak. Details of her figure, unknown to me, yet familiar to a punk who cares nothing for her. Then you hope for a defensive action at the waistline for a few years. Holding actions. Rear-guard actions. Delaying tactics.

Being a father of women was like being a woman yourself. Worse. You had no control over bodies that were yours. You were not even there to protest, to say no to the clowns who tramp in to wipe themselves and burn your own beauty to warm themselves.

Ed sighed, and settled to a new position in the sheets.

Where there's no long view, he said to himself, every wavering is mistaken for growth, and today's enlightenment becomes yesterday's foolishness. The Victorians had thought they were enlightened too, because in Washington's day every farmer's daughter had been pregnant.

And meanwhile, all these fashions, these turns of history that men grope in—did it serve some purpose that the world could not have been made right and whole in the beginning, but must suffer instead an evolution moving so erratically, and history at a snail's pace? Why could I not have lived later, when all this is straightened out? Why do my children have to be guinea pigs in God's laboratory?

I'm tired of God's restlessness, Ed thought. God must be restless—if He weren't restless He wouldn't have created the world.

Particles, radiations, stars, suns, galaxies, so busy. And then He had to go and put life in it. And then He had to put mind in it. And still He wants to patschke with it.

What kind of a God is it that even allows Himself to go out of fashion?

What is there that He won't try at least once? How many fashions, empires, detours between here and the End of Days?

Why did He not create a world already just? Why did He give man, that poor shlemiel, the long slow job of putting justice into it?

What could one answer to such a question? No answer. Only that if the mind of God were as simple as believers and nonbelievers alike presume, He'd have built the world out of an Erector set.

And how many other universes has He got running? I'd hate to see them. Even the stars rot. The astronomers have said so. My Charles, how long is the boy in his grave? And while he lies there the war goes on, as if it never needed him in the first place, stalemated, no end in sight.

"Will you stop tossing around?" Lucinda said to him.

He sat up in the darkness, his feet over the edge of the bed, his back to her. "I can't sleep," he said.

"I can't either."

"Maybe I'll go down and make some tea or hot milk. Do you want some?"

"No," she said.

He sat there a while, but then lay down again.

"Aren't you going down?" she asked.

"No, I guess not," he said. "Unless you want something."

"No."

"Did the kids ever go to bed?" There was no light from the hall.

"Yes, I heard them," Lucinda said.

"You know what I think?" he said. "I think we should have another baby. Seriously. While there's still time."

"What?"

"Why not?" he said. "They say a pregnancy is good for a woman psychologically, when she's lost a child. It makes sense to me. Don't you feel that?"

"Well it doesn't make sense to me."

"There's still time," he said, "before the gates close. I don't mean it would replace Charles—it would be a whole new child, naturally. And one more chance that maybe one of the lot will turn out all right."

"Well I couldn't," she said. "I couldn't stand any more children. I couldn't begin to go through all that again."

He didn't answer. It was clear from her tone that there was nothing to do but let it drop.

"I haven't had enough heartache," she said. "I need more."

He lay quietly.

"You're heartless," she said. "You're just heartless. You can bury a child in the ground, and it's 'back to the old drawing board.' That's all. All you can do is give me babies. You can't bring Charles back. You can't even bring Millicent back."

"Listen," he said, "if I could change places with Charles I'd do it. I wish I could."

"I wish you could too. I should have divorced you when the children were small."

"If you want a divorce go see a lawyer," he said. But he was sorry he had answered.

"You're sick in the head," she said. "You must be. It's crazy. The things you come out with. It's sick."

"All right, it was just a suggestion. Forget it."

"I won't forget it. You're sick."

"All right, I'm sick. But why the bitterness. We're in it together."

"Yes, I'm bitter, aren't I. I have no right to be bitter, do I. I don't understand you, do I. Why don't you be a celibate clergy, so I can't bother you. Go and move in with Father Donahue, in the parish house of the Most Precious Blood or whatever they call it. Clergymen aren't fit to be husbands and fathers. It's all just a bunch of religion with you. You probably sat there with Millicent debating the Talmud. You're crazy, do you know that? You're as crazy as she is. You were gonna handle it—you sure handled it. And if this ends up in a disaster I'm gonna divorce you. I'm gonna follow my own judgments hereafter—"

"Listen, why do I have to fight you? Isn't one hysterical woman enough?"

"Is Millicent hysterical?"

"I don't know," he said tiredly.

"Well I'm going in there again myself. And if she doesn't come home I'm telling her she's no daughter of mine."

"You already told her that once. Don't say what you don't mean."

56

Danny McBride kept taunting Millicent about the horse story when she next came to work. "Hey, Sneezy," he said, as soon as he saw her, "what were you trying to do? Sabotage the joint?" She looked the other way and did not answer him.

Mr. Killian was not there, and she was glad not to have to face him again just yet. Later in the evening Maud Dickinson told her Mr. Killian had gone home during the day feeling ill.

She half expected her father might be lurking about the sidewalks in order to meet her on the way to or from work and talk to her again. She watched uneasily when she went down for her errands and again when she left at the end of the evening, but he was not there. On Saturday night, however, he telephoned the city room and upset her with a long conversation.

She told Leslie afterward that her father might try to bother him at the hospital. "Do you think he might come here?" Leslie asked her.

"No," she said. "He doesn't know where this place is."

She was glad Les was there. He had had one night on call since her father had had that awful meeting with her, and two since her mother had told her about the letter, and his nights on call seemed to her now lonelier than ever.

She had also told Les about her delayed period, but he had answered that it was psychological and due to all the recent stress, and that she should not worry about it.

Sunday she hoped they could go out and enjoy the morning together, strolling by the river or riding the motor scooter since she was not going to Wilmerding Crosswalk. It was lovely spring weather. But he slept. Toward noon he opened his eyes and asked what time it was, but at once dropped back to sleep. She waited for him to waken, and played with the cat.

But at two o'clock he was still asleep and she left, meaning to stop by the girls' apartment on the way to work.

When she had entered past the big iron and glass door she found that her name had been removed from her mailbox. There was a new card in the slot, with three names neatly inked.

MCCARTNEY JESPERSEN
CHISHOLM

Barbie must have done that, she thought angrily. In her shoulder-strap bag she found a pencil. She added the name Gordon, squeezing it into the corner. Then she hurried up the stairs.

Natalie was there alone, washing her hair. Natalie admitted that it was Barbie who had put in the new name plate. "We didn't think you'd mind," she added.

"Well I do mind," said Millicent. "She had no right to just go and take my name off, without even asking me. It's still my apartment. That's our arrangement."

At work her mind kept returning to the name plate. What upset her most was that Natalie and Ella Jane had allowed it. She was surprised at them. They ought to have had sense enough to tell Barbie she couldn't do that.

She was still uneasy after work, when she took a cab to Leslie's place, and when she got between the sheets next to him. She asked him if he had fed the cat. He said he had. He lay on his side sleepily, not touching her. He was naked. He had been sleeping that way for a week or two, and had told her he always did in spring and summer. But Millicent wore pajamas.

"Les," she said, "I'm getting pretty worried about my period."

"How many days is it now?"

"It's a week now."

"Well, it still doesn't mean anything."

"Les, I've always been as regular as clockwork."

"You would be."

She fingered the sheet, which lay against her lips. She looked at the pale diagrams that the street lamp threw onto the ceiling.

"Les, I know you think it's psychological, and you think I'm a worrier, and I worried about cancer for nothing, and I worry about atomic war and everything, but sometimes things do happen. And we aren't immune. You can't say that bad things can't happen to us. If I'd worried about my brother you'd have said I was a worrier, and my mother used to worry like crazy, but then he really did get killed. And when I thought I'd covered the wrong meeting you thought

I was worrying for nothing, but then it turned out I really did cover the wrong meeting. Les, you work in a hospital—you see accidents, and horrible diseases, and you see people die—you know the worst really does happen."

"Well, all right," he said. "But I'll tell you when to worry. Okay?"

"But two or three days is one thing. Shouldn't it be straightened out by now?"

"Not necessarily."

"Is it possible that it's not psychological?"

"It's extremely unlikely."

"But is it possible?"

"It's just extremely unlikely," he said again. "You have to look at the whole picture. For one thing I know how careful I've been. And then consider the shocks you've had. First your brother's death, which is a trauma in itself, and then that damn letter all of a sudden, crawling out of the grave so to speak, and your parents' attitude. And your boss down on you besides just now. Maybe your boss is a father figure for you or something. You're full of all these guilts and you want to punish yourself. It's the most natural thing in the world. It would be amazing if you weren't delayed."

"But if it's only psychological, wouldn't the fact that I know it's psychological make it come?"

"It doesn't work that way."

"Les, try to think back. That night when my mother met me and everything, and I made you do it twice. I don't think you put one on."

"If that's what you want to think go ahead and think it."

"Did you put one on?"

"Of course."

"And did you put it on again the second time?"

"Not the same one. What do you think, I use the same one over and over?"

"A new one?"

"Yes. A new one."

"But it's such a habit, Les—maybe you didn't and you just thought you had. You were awfully tired that night. Maybe you just think you remember. That's possible, isn't it?"

"No," he said. "It isn't."

"You're really positive? Nobody's infallible."

"I'm positive. That's one thing I don't forget."

"Maybe it slipped off."

"It didn't slip off."

"They do slip off sometimes, don't they?"

"No. Not just like that."

"Maybe we did it so long that it wore through," she said.

He didn't answer. She sensed his irritation.

"Maybe we should go to the hospital and have a test," she said. "Or you could take along a urine sample, or whatever they do."

"Forget it," he said. "Just wait a few days. You've got nothing to lose. And you'll see that no test was necessary."

"Well, I'd rather have a test. I'll get a drugstore test if you won't give me one."

"Go ahead, if it'll set your mind at rest. But I'm telling ya you don't need it."

He settled in a new position as if he would go to sleep.

"Do you love me?" she asked him.

"What's that got to do with it?"

She tried to make out his face in the darkness.

His eyes were closed. But she kept watching him.

"Les," she said, "what would you do, if you got two different girls pregnant at one time?"

"What kind of a question is that?" He didn't open his eyes.

"I was just wondering. I mean, what would you do?"

"Well, I don't know."

"That's no answer," she said.

"What are you accusing me of. Do you think I've got someone else on the side? At the hospital or something?"

"If you don't love me I don't see why you shouldn't."

"Well I haven't."

"But what would you do?"

"Let me sleep, will ya?"

"Not until you give me an answer."

He lay in silence, his eyes still closed.

"Les, listen," she said. "You're not gonna talk me into an abortion."

She could see his face become pained, even though his eyes didn't open.

"Will you lay off?" he said. "If you were due just then you weren't even fertile."

"Suppose there was a fluke and the egg got stuck somewhere, and it got fertilized."

"Forget it. You're not pregnant."

"But suppose I am."

"Don't worry about it. There's no problem that can't be solved. And chances are you're not."

"I don't care what you say—we can't be sure. Wishful thinking won't make it go away, you know. What if we wait, and it doesn't blow over. What then?"

"We'll see then. We'll cross that bridge when we get to it."

"That's what I mean—you don't say yes and you don't say no. What are we gonna do when we get to that bridge?"

"I haven't thought about it."

"You haven't even thought about it?"

"I don't know, I don't know! Are we gonna be up all night?" He lay on his back now, his eyes open.

"You had plenty of sleep today."

"I needed it. And I don't want to start off tomorrow morning bushed again."

"I just want your assurance that you'll do the right thing."

"The right thing being defined as marrying you?"

"We thought we might get married when you go into the Army anyway."

"We did?"

"Or sometime."

"Well, maybe we are gonna end up married—I don't know—we'll think about it. But I don't want it like this. I don't go for this shotgun stuff. It's not my style. I'd rather marry ya in my own good time, at the proper time, you know what I mean? Like if this blows over, and we start off on a clean slate. I don't want to feel forced. If I marry you I want to feel I married you voluntarily."

"But if I'm pregnant we are forced."

"That's what I don't like about it. It's not how I see myself. We'll get married when we decide to, and we'll get pregnant when we decide to. I don't want my life run by accidents. I plan things. And I'm entitled to a tiny bit of youth and freedom somewhere in my life, for Christ sake. If I have to be an s.o.b. I'll be an s.o.b. for a certain length of time, but I'm not gonna louse my life up just to avoid being an s.o.b. one time. What am I, just a work horse? Other guys have affairs and it's like nothing. A love affair doesn't have to end in marriage, for Christ sake. We don't have to be maneuvered into getting married, you know. Just because we've slept together. Or lived together."

"I know it. I didn't say we did. But there's a question of whether an accident's taken place, and the right thing is that when you father a child you give it a name."

"*You* give it a name," he said. "Call him George."

"That's not funny, Les. Not a bit."

"Or Charles. Name it after your brother."

"It's not something to joke about. You're being in very bad taste."

"What's bad taste about that? Naming a baby after your brother?"

"I'm disappointed in you."

"Sorry I broke your heart."

"I won't say you broke my heart, but you disappointed me. I believed in you."

"Look, first of all you assume you're pregnant. I assume you're not."

"You can't assume I'm not."

"I thought you didn't want to get married for several years," he said. "Remember when you said that?"

"Well, I thought then that it was a tying-down arrangement, but I see now it doesn't have to be. Because if a man and a woman are sort of permanently fond of each other, the way we've been, and the possibility of pregnancy is always there, they're as good as married anyway, so what's the tying down? Married or unmarried, it's the same. So why not have that assurance?"

"Assurance of what?"

There was a brief pause before she answered. "Les," she said, "we're already married."

"No we're not," he told her.

There was another silence.

"What about your newspaper career?" he added. "You'd blow your career just like that?"

"That's not important," she said. "Love is important." She turned, half propped on an elbow and a hand, and looked at him. "Les," she said, "listen. I'm not gonna have an abortion. I don't believe in it. I don't approve of it."

"Are you a Roman Catholic or something?"

"No, I'm not a Roman Catholic or something. I'm just a human being."

"And a typically female one at that."

She suddenly began to weep, and lowered her face onto her hands. "You're a hound," she said.

She wept quietly a few minutes, but he made no move to comfort her.

He rose and walked to the bathroom. He had nothing on. She stopped weeping. She saw him urinate in the lighted bathroom.

He came back into bed. She looked at him wet-eyed.

"Les," she said, "I know you think you don't get your share of fun out of life, but how can you love life when you want to snuff out a life that's here inside my belly."

"That's a fine statement from a girl who used to resent being female."

"Well, abortion would make me more female than ever. To present a man with children when he wants them, or kill my children at his bidding if they don't suit his convenience. Just because I'm a woman it doesn't mean you can manipulate me. I'm not a piece of meat for your friends to go inside of with knives."

"It's just a couple of cells. It's not a person."

"I don't care. It would be a person. How would you like it if somebody had aborted you out of your mother's belly?"

"That has nothing to do with it. Suppose my parents hadn't even gotten laid that particular night, or suppose my parents never met or never married—I wouldn't have been conceived. You don't worry about people that aren't born. If you're gonna worry about unborn souls I'm depriving somebody of life every minute that I'm not having intercourse."

"I think you're a prude, do you know it?" she said. "That's the real prudery, when people don't want to face that babies come from it. Like all that lacy pants that you wanted me to put on. Men ought to see their children actually being born, that's what I think. They ought to see women in childbirth. Then they'd know what it's all about."

"I have seen it. I've delivered them."

"But you don't relate it to your own sex life. Lacy pants. Like these transparent nightgowns they advertise, and the girlie magazines in the drugstores. As if sex were a party, that has nothing to do with life."

"What's so terrible about lace panties?"

"Because it's just like a G-string with tassels and rhinestones—it's a denial of what sex is all about. That's why it's obscene."

"Listen," he said, "lace is an adornment, that's all. Just like when God takes a mess of mammary ducts and shapes it with fat and covers it with skin to look pretty. Do you know what a bunch of gizzards are inside of a beautiful woman? I've cut up a stiff. And I've operated on the living. You cut open the prettiest girl in the world and there's intestines full of excrement. And pretty skin on the outside. Just like your father wants to adorn the cruddiness of the world with religion."

"My father said the female instinct is a desire for children."

"That's what he told you the other day?"

"No. He told it to a group a long time ago."

"Well, it isn't sound," said Leslie. "The sex desire is an instinct to sex. The parental instinct doesn't appear until after the birth of the child."

"My father explained it scientifically."

"Well, he was wrong. He was fantasizing. Clergymen do that—they take a little bit of science, that they don't know the first thing about, and they misinterpret it to suit themselves. But the sex instinct still isn't the mother instinct. Not in itself."

"Can't people improve on their instincts?"

"Not just like that, they can't. What do you think life is—a big Sunday-school lesson? Do you want to take the fun out of sex? It is fun, whatever else it is. And lace panties are fun. And I'm sure your father knows it."

"Well, I don't know. I'm confused."

"Your parents are really on your back," he said. "Aren't they. Especially your father."

"Your mother's on your back."

"I do what I want," he said. "I wasn't afraid to tell my mother about the scooter. Or the apartment."

"Well I have a family," said Millicent. "Do you think I'm just somebody in your life? What I do affects a lot of people beside you."

He didn't answer. She began weeping again, her face in the pillow. She heard him sigh restlessly. He didn't touch her.

"Listen," he said after a while, "maybe I'll marry you, if it seems the best way. I don't want a child of mine to be aborted. But let me think, for Christ sake. Let me get used to the idea slowly. And try to understand. I just said I hope it blows over so I don't have to know all my life that my mate was chosen by a forced marriage, by a dopey situation like this, that's all."

She turned, and sought his hand under the sheet. His fingers were limp and unresponsive in hers, and he still lay on his back.

In a short time his breathing grew heavy. But the tireder she grew the more impossible sleep became.

She was sure she was awake the entire night.

When she got to the city room the next afternoon her eyes ached. "Maggie, you look like you had a bad night last night," Danny McBride said to her.

Mr. Killian was there. It was the first time she had seen him since he had bawled her out and he at once beckoned her to the desk and bawled her out again. He said both organizations were sore, the right one and the wrong one.

Maud told her afterward that he was edgy because there had been complaints to the publisher and Mr. Coddington had had him on the carpet. But Maud said she shouldn't worry about it.

That night Leslie was on call. The loneliness and stillness in his apartment seemed unbearable. She sat a long time on the edge of the mattress, with the light on, staring at the cat, before she could bring herself to prepare for bed.

The following night he was there in bed when she arrived, but they had scarcely any conversation.

"No change?" he said.

"No."

She slipped into bed, and touched his bare shoulder, but there was no love-making. She didn't talk. She felt she owed it to him to let him sleep, after keeping him awake so long the previous time.

The next day she was off, but Leslie was to be on call and would not be home that night. The day and night seemed horribly long.

She had meant to do house cleaning and washing that she had been putting off until today, but now she did not have the spirit to begin. It was rainy. Her life seemed pointless, and her career seemed dead.

Late in the day she began to get some housework done, listlessly. She kept arguing mentally with her father. She was sure that her father did not appreciate how devoted Les was to his work, and how much he deserved a little normal pleasure in his life. She imagined herself telling her father that she had seen a man become happy, and that that was worth something. But she knew her father would say that she could make him happier in marriage.

She looked at the washtubs, under which the cat slept, and remembered her father saying that she probably washed Leslie's socks. He didn't know that she even did Leslie's shirts.

She went shopping in the rain and returned. She regretted the dinginess of the hall and stairway, and what her father would think of it if he saw it. There were cracks in the wall paint, and the bulbs were dim, with two missing again, and bags of garbage stood outside many of the doors.

Toward eleven at night she took her little umbrella and went out again for a walk. Many of the buildings were completely dark. The street lamps were fuzzy in the drizzle and reflected in the irregularities of the empty street. The brick sidewalk went steeply upward, so that doorways jutted into it at angles. She passed a roaring sewer.

It's ten days, she thought. She knew that Leslie's certainty had diminished more than he admitted. She had felt it in the way they lay apart in bed, as though in unspoken agreement to take no risks until the present crisis had blown over. Even in his touch she could sense that she was making him unhappy.

If she did have a child, she thought, she could care for it alone, with the ten thousand dollars of Government insurance that Charles had left her. Leslie certainly couldn't afford it. He had more residencies ahead that paid next to nothing.

She turned a corner, changing the angle of her umbrella, and the hill turned downward.

It must be raining in the cemetery now too, soaking the grass and earth on Charles's grave. Let this darkness and this cold be like a taste of death, she thought. What was it like to be dead?

Far down at the bottom of the hill she had to stop at a crossing. The rain was more than a drizzle now but still fine. It slanted into passing headlights. The traffic light did not work in the usual way at this hour but only blinked, and the wetness of the street kept brightening red here and yellow there and darkening again. She crossed, and as she got to the opposite curb there was a splash of rain that she heard on the umbrella. In her shoes and on her jeans she felt the damp.

She turned toward where the shops were, even though they were darkened.

Perhaps, she thought, she owed it to Leslie not to have the baby, if in fact there was one. Les had been considerate in taking full responsibility for the contraception problem, so that she would not have to become involved with messy internal things. She had taken advantage of his kindness.

No man had ever spared himself less than he. His life was all labor and strain and sacrifice. He had given himself only the months with her, and the motor scooter to take her riding on. But it seemed as though she had brought him only a little joy—instead she would bring him more strain and swamp him when he could least manage it. You couldn't call him irresponsible—he was laden unto death with responsibilities. She had taken none of the responsibility—she had been quite content to lie back and let him be the careful one. She had not considered how frightfully exhausted he always was, or how much longer his hours of work were than hers, or how much fewer his hours for sleep, or even how giving blood so much must strain him, or how much more full of crises his days were.

That's what happened, she thought. One of those times when he had dozed in their embrace it had loosened.

Later on, at a better time, there would be seed enough for all the children they could handle. And he could marry her freely, when it made sense.

She supposed Leslie had connections at the hospital for such things, even though he hadn't said so.

But the thought of it, of the tampering, of the flesh, made her grimace. Who knew what a genius, what a great person she might let be scraped out?

She was passing just then a darkened shop window in which there was a display of children's clothing, and she stopped and looked at it. The outfits were small, and attractive, and they pulled at her. How dependent she was on this man, who would marry her if at all with the greatest reluctance. It wasn't fair. Here he is, making the decisions, and the decisions are my life and his convenience.

She walked on in the rain, feeling cold, but torn with nervousness and knowing it would be useless to go back to that little place and lie in bed. She went block after block. She constructed a fantasy in which her body would right itself in the next hour, ending the whole problem neatly, and she would go back by cab.

At an intersection of avenues there were signs still lighted, and a little pizza joint and a drugstore still open, side by side, with people having coffee in both places. A movie theater across the way had not quite closed. She went into the pizza joint, because it looked livelier. She sneezed.

It was crowded with people younger than herself at little tables. They must be students, she thought. Boston University was nearby. There was a smell of wet coats. She got a cup of hot chocolate and found a small table, leaning the umbrella between her knees. There were groups of boys, groups of girls, and mixed groups, and dating couples. It struck her that she could tell at a glance the state of each love affair. She sipped her chocolate, looking at the gay laughing couples who hadn't been to bed as yet, and then at the somber girls clinging worriedly to their wooden-faced lovers. There was really no difficulty telling those who had slept together from those that hadn't yet.

She left her chocolate unfinished. When she came out, opening her umbrella, she saw the drugstore again. She stopped at the glass door, thinking she would go in and inquire at once about a pregnancy test. She could see a few people at the food counter in damp hats and coats, and shiny racks of thermos bottles and all sorts of articles. She pushed her way in. It was a large place. There was a round, tall rack of paper-bound books, that turned at a push, and she idled at it. There were philosophy and politics, and even a book on prenatal care. She did not touch it.

She saw the pharmacist from a distance, a thin-lipped, sour-looking, fussy little old man. She could not ask him.

57

Ed got Marilyn Prince, the cantor's wife, to teach the youngest Sunday-school kids in Millicent's stead.

Millicent seemed continually on his mind.

But Sunday afternoon he got around to bawling out Patty finally for having opened Charles's letter. He sat on the desk in the study and took Patty to task at length while she sat in the Morris chair. She had in fact not opened the letter at once, but had first kept it secretly a long time. Charles had sent it not to the

R.F.D. box at the foot of the winding dirt driveway, but to Ed in care of the temple, so that the rest of the family might not see it. However the postman brought it on a Saturday, while the service was still in progress, and handed it to Patty, who was preparing refreshments in the big vestibule.

Even so, it had been much delayed, and apparently had traveled at least part way by surface mail, or had been mislaid for a time in a post office. Ed even theorized afterward that Charles might have sealed it but left it unposted, and that someone else had dropped it in the mail posthumously.

It had seemed spooky to Patty, in any case, getting a letter from the deceased, and besides she knew her father would not open it on the Sabbath.

For a while it remained hidden in a drawer in her bedroom. It seemed to her, she said afterward, that her parents ought to be spared the grief of a letter from Charles so soon after his funeral. She had even thought of burying it unopened. She would even have sent it back, except that there was no one to send it to. She changed the hiding place a number of times, and thought of perhaps delivering it to her father in a year's time. When at last she opened it she told herself there was no such thing as privacy in the case of a dead person anyway.

"It had my name on the envelope," Ed told her. "And my name alone. Nobody else should have opened it, let alone read it."

"I'm sorry."

"You shouldn't have read it, and you shouldn't have shown it to Mother. You should have given it to me unopened."

"Mother said I should have shown it to her sooner."

"Well, that's neither here nor there. The point is, it's very wrong to go snooping in a letter not addressed to you, and I want to make sure you know that. It's a sin, as a matter of fact. It's against our religion."

"I didn't know it was a sin."

He told her of an eleventh-century ruling, by the leading rabbis of that time.

Then he asked her what she had to do between now and Yom Kippur if she had sinned against her fellow man.

"Satisfy my fellow man," she said.

"Right. Now, I'll consider that you've satisfied me, if you'll just make yourself forget what was in that letter. I don't mean you can really forget it, but you have to pretend like you forgot it. In your feelings about your sister, and in anything you ever say, to her or to anyone, be like you never saw it. Do that, and we're square. You know nothing about her private life. Understand?"

"Yom Kippur's a long way off," she said.

"That doesn't matter. You start now. I didn't like the way you started hinting around last night, and got Rollo asking questions. It's not his business. And it's not gonna be Polly Cook's business. Or Denise's business. Do you understand?"

"Yes."

He sat looking at her another moment, and then waved her away.

He worked, but it seemed to him that he worked constantly in a state of depression. Someone else had taken over his visits at the Reformatory but he had begun helping out in services for patients at the mental hospital at Danvers, and was trying to get some of them placed in private homes.

In his study one evening he took notes for a sermon on the sacrifice of Isaac. Thoughts of Charles were never long out of his mind, and had given him the idea. It seemed to him that what God had asked of Abraham, governments ask of parents every day. He had used to wonder in the past what he would have done in Abraham's position. He felt he could not have sacrificed a son. It seemed too much for God to ask—yet governments ask it daily. Every day the government asks for our sons, and we flinch, but we say okay.

He did not intend to give the sermon soon but to hold it until that portion of Genesis came up for its prescribed reading.

God asked Abraham, he jotted down, would you give as much for Me as your ancestors gave for the old gods? And would you give as much for God as you would give for American defense? Nothing is more devastating, nothing more powerful to alienate you from God, than the death of a child. Nothing can say more strongly than a child's death that the world is purposeless, senseless. That justice is not in it, that any God who could have made such a world must be unworthy of your allegiance. Of all atrocities, those against children appall you the most. And that's what God asked of Abraham: will you stay with it? Even then? Will you still devote yourself to the idea of a world making sense, even when your eyes are opened to the rottenest? Will you still be one guy standing for law, when you've discovered that the molecules are all mad? And Abraham answered: I'll stay with it even then. And God said: You could see the child die and still assert that this world must make sense. A mind like yours could really believe that murder is forbidden. Therefore He said: Don't kill the child.

Ed looked at what he had written. It was in a loose-leaf notebook, with other notes for sermons. He added a line. Can you take the rottenness that living in a world of infinite possibility will expose you to, and still stand for justice?

He jotted some more.

That's what the story means from Abraham's viewpoint; but what about Isaac? It isn't about dying, as it turns out—he doesn't die—but it's about a willingness to die. If you're a person there are things worth dying for. And if they're worth dying for, then you'll fight for them. Because when you fight you put your life on the line. Isaac would have been out there fighting—he didn't hide in the cellar. As a practical matter there'd be no truth, no freedom, no United States, if there weren't men willing to die for those things. There'd have been no Britain in 1940. Churchill knew he was putting his life on the line when he made that speech. He was like Isaac. And as it turned out, he was spared. Mussolini was strung up instead.

Ed read again what he had put down. Then he went to work on a talk he was to give to the members of Caleb Folger's church, before a joint meeting of their men's club and ladies' auxiliary. Caleb had spoken at the temple one night, during the condolence week as it happened, and it was Ed's job now to return the courtesy.

On the night of his talk Ed went to the church early, but Caleb was already there to greet him, tall and bald, with his vest hanging limp on his leanness. Caleb showed Ed about the building. The interior woodwork had a simple elegance. The pulpit had a little flying staircase that Caleb said dated from the Federal period. He showed Ed the ladder to the steeple, but they did not go up it.

The meeting was held not in the main part of the church but in a low auditorium beneath it, which could be entered either from the church or from a side door direct to the outside. The members of Ed's temple had also been invited, and several were there.

Caleb gave a little introduction, in the course of which he happened to remark that all religions say essentially the same thing, but then Ed began by taking issue with that, and saying they did not all say the same thing.

He talked about forty minutes, saying that his own religion was a continuing tradition that had come into being in order to clean up religion, and that that ought to ring a bell here since Caleb's own church stemmed from the Puritans. He said good religion should meet certain tests—one, it must elevate society as a whole; two, it must never be detrimental to health; and three, it must not insult your intelligence. Otherwise it was a defilement of the Name and would cause the land to vomit out the inhabitants. Religion that insulted the intelligence drew sapheads into the ministry, which made the churches lose influence, so that the breakdown of society accelerated. He said it had happened to the ancient pagans and that the same dynamic still operates. His own religion and that of his forefathers had put a ban on the antirational, in order to create conditions in which belief would be possible. Because when religions pretend to know what we can't know, they not only hamper men in the pursuit of truth but eventually make belief impossible. There was even a tradition, he said, that God Himself studies our commentaries and our debates and decisions and writings, which is a way of saying that religion needs all the creative intelligence we can give it. That was really the sacrifice God wants on His altar.

During the question period a fluttery white-haired lady asked whether love wasn't the sacrifice that God wants on His altar. Ed said yes, that too, and that in the ancient Temple there had been two daily sacrifices.

In time Caleb thanked Ed, and said it had all been very enlightening. Ed went home feeling the evening had gone quite well. But Conrad Bernstein, who had not been there, phoned him the next day to say he had had complaints from several of the Beth El members who had attended, and from others who had heard about it, and that Ed's talk had not sat very well with his own parishioners. For one thing, he ought to have said that all religions did in fact say the same thing.

Conrad went on at length, though Ed felt quite sure that neither Caleb nor Caleb's congregation had been offended.

Conrad said he gathered that more had been said about differences than about similarities. "We're trying to build good relations," said Conrad. "That's the purpose of these meetings. You shouldn't give the impression that your religion is the only brainy one."

"Well, it was Folger's idea to explain the differences," Ed said, "but I guess it isn't a good idea to discuss differences."

"That's right, it isn't," said Conrad. "We all have to live together. Folger talked about his debt to us, and you should have talked about our debt to him, and his crowd. He was being a gentleman, and you weren't. The man went out of his way. He was courteous. And you showed about as much tact as Sheridan marching through Georgia."

"Sherman," Ed told him.

"All right, Sherman. But public-relations-wise, you stunk."

Then a few days later Ed got into more trouble, that seemed to reach the proportions of a scandal. A young man whose parents belonged to the temple decided to marry out of his religion and to drop his religion altogether, and his parents made him go to Ed to discuss it, but Ed did not succeed in changing the boy's mind.

They chatted a couple of hours in Ed's study, but the boy had had scarcely any religious training, and his family's affiliation was of the most inactive and marginal kind, and it was apparent to Ed that the boy's mind was made up.

They talked of one thing and another. The boy remarked that he and his girl were both atheists. Ed replied that an atheist was simply somebody who had swept the puzzle to the floor in impatience. He said the agnostic has left it on the table but refuses to touch it, and the religious man still works at it, even though he can't find a solution.

"Why do you keep working at it if you know you can't solve it?" the boy asked.

"Well," Ed told him, "because I've learned some things, and I hope I'll learn more. When you work at something you get some insights."

But the boy insisted that he and his fiancée were mature, and Ed admitted that in an hour or two he could not impart a sense of tradition that had been absent for a lifetime.

However the boy apparently told his parents that Ed had admitted the boy was right. Several ladies phoned Ed or stopped him angrily on the street and demanded explanations. "And after you did such a wonderful job with the Stokes girl," more than one of them said. "They're heartbroken," some said of the boy's parents. "I'm surprised at you," said others.

Everything began to go wrong. Mr. Dembitz had been leading the morning prayers now and then, but someone told him Ed had said he sounded like a tobacco auctioneer, and he stopped coming around. Actually Ed had been trying to encourage another man also to volunteer, who was too shy because he lacked Mr. Dembitz's fluency, and Ed had simply said that it was not necessary to read like a tobacco auctioneer.

58

Millicent's period began at last, quite normal except for the delay. It had started while she slept, after that long walk in the drizzle and rain. For a moment she was almost stunned with relief. She had all but stopped hoping that she would escape so easily. Her next thought was to go out and phone the good news to Leslie. But then she realized that such a thing was hardly something to tell him at the hospital, where the switchboard girl might be listening in. Even if she confined herself to saying only that there was good news, the meaning might be obvious to eavesdroppers and gossips.

It would be better to tell him when he got home.

Her respect for his medical wisdom and his common sense deepened. He had been right to keep cool.

She went shopping and bought some delicacies that he liked.

He arrived about six-thirty. She flung the door open as soon as she heard him on the stairs, and when he crossed the threshold she embraced him smiling.

"Hi," she said. "Guess what."

She could tell from his answering smile that he knew what.

"When did it happen?" he said.

"This morning."

With a sweep of her arm she showed him the enamel-topped table laid out with appetizers of smoked fish, and the steak ready to be broiled.

"Are you glad you don't have to marry me?" she asked while she cooked the steak.

"I didn't have to anyway," he said.

"We'll go out to a movie after dinner and celebrate," she said.

She stood on the little step stool to look into the oven above the stove, and his hands moved tenderly on her waist and her legs.

"We can't really celebrate, of course," she said, "but we will in a few days. It never takes me long. And I'll spend my next pay check on lacy pants if you want."

"You don't have to do that."

She explained to him why she hadn't phoned him the news. Then she asked him to start his appetizer. When she took the steak out, its edge of fat sizzling, she wafted it under his nose.

"Did you have a good day today?" she asked when she was settled opposite him.

He was eating, and shrugged.

"I shouldn't have asked that," she said. "You work so hard every day. I suppose if you helped somebody on the road to health it's a good day."

He gave a nod.

In the movie he was tired. She hoped he wouldn't fall asleep, but he did.

For the next few days she remained somehow depressed. She had thought the happy end of the crisis would lift her spirits, but it did not really, after the first evening. Leslie was not on call, as his weekend had come, but he was tired and did not talk much. Her father had not bothered him at the hospital after all, and her family had not been in touch with her, and she wondered how the estrangement would be resolved. She thought about Leslie's going into the Army. And she wondered if she should look for another job. But if she looked for another newspaper job now she could hardly expect Mr. Killian to recommend her. It was nearly a year since she had graduated and she was worse off than a year ago. She was older, and had not gained an entree or a foothold in anything. A year ago she at least could have said she had not yet failed at anything.

Sunday he awakened her at daybreak. She felt the sweep of his lips and then returned his smile, knowing from the light and the quiet and from the feel of her body how early it was. He pressed her near. She stretched, and made herself sleepily convex so that her whole front seemed to kiss him. He drew apart the string at her waist and played agreeably with handfuls of her flesh. Her toes pushed her pajamas into a wad.

She harmonized with him, rocking and caressing. Such discomforts as she felt passed quickly as her eagerness rose. She saw his face grow taut and feverish until he seemed no longer himself.

She could not catch his surgings. When it ended she bore his perspiring weight, patting and comforting his stillness. His face lay buried by her ear.

"I'm sorry," he said. "I couldn't help it. I sort of got carried away, I guess."

"That's all right," she said. "I don't want you to hold back."

Their love-making had turned out like that sometimes on other occasions too. When it did it seemed as though she watched his experience with greater vividness from the vantage point of calm, and derived pleasure of a different sort.

They lay side by side. He got up after a while to get rid of the device.

He came back to bed. "There," he said. "You're at the safest possible time, but I still took precautions. So don't tell me I forgot. And don't tell me next month you're pregnant." He sounded grumpy.

"Are you going to say that every time we do it?" she asked.

He rolled over as if he would go to sleep again.

She lay brooding upon his remark. Then she asked if he wanted to sleep some more or if she should make breakfast.

"Okay," he said.

She got up, with nothing on. She cut some bagels on the enamel-topped table and spread them with sweet butter. She put cocoa powder in two glasses and started the milk warming. She got cheese from the refrigerator and squeezed some oranges.

"Les," she said when she poured the cocoa, "do you think I wanted to be pregnant, to get you to marry me? I mean, do you think that's what caused the whole thing?"

"I'd say so."

"Les, that's horrible. You can't think that."

He got out of bed, with no clothes, and sat at the table opposite her. He drank his juice.

"Do you really think that?" she said. "I mean did you think it before I said it?"

"Why not?"

"Well that's just awful. It's not true."

"I don't mean it was conscious," he said.

"I know you don't, and that makes it worse," she answered. "You're so smug about my subconscious and everything. I was worried sick about ruining my life and ruining your life, and you were just thinking the whole time that I was so eager to marry you that I was having psychosomatic symptoms."

"I didn't say you could help it."

"I understand you perfectly well, Leslie Hollander. I was too stupid to face it consciously so I worked up pregnancy symptoms because it's the only thing that would get you to marry me—that's what you think, isn't it."

"Listen, you had your family bearing down on you, and guilt about your brother, and subconsciously I suppose it seemed like an easy solution."

"Well I don't believe it. It wasn't that at all."

"Okay. Have it your way."

She watched him eat silently. He didn't believe her, she thought. He really did think that. It was humiliating.

"Do you know what I think?" she said. Her voice was beginning to shake.

"What."

"I think you're very smug and self-satisfied."

He shrugged. She thought he looked almost bored.

"Do you think that just because a girl goes to bed with you she's madly in love with you and trying to marry you? Really, your conceit is just appalling. You think I'd like nothing better than to trap you into a marriage, don't you. Well it may flatter your ego to think that but it just isn't true. I'm not trying to marry you and I don't want to marry you and I'm not breaking my heart over you."

"Okay," he said easily.

"I have just as much right to sleep with you as you do to sleep with me."

"Sure. I told you that months ago."

"I mean it doesn't mean I have to be in love with you. Really, the conceit men have just sickens me. You're like my father, full of double standard right up to the ears. Men are such frauds."

She bit into a slice of bagel and chewed.

"Don't get hysterical," he said.

"Don't patronize me!" she said angrily. "That's exactly what I mean!"

"Listen, you did offer some arguments in favor of marriage. You can't blame me for thinking it was on your mind."

"That's because I thought I was going to have a baby."

"Oh."

There seemed to be a superior coolness about him and it made her furious.

"You just better apologize," she said.

"For what?"

"For your attitude."

"I'm sorry I hurt your feelings," he said.

"That's not an apology. I want to hear you apologize."

"I'm not gonna get maudlin."

"You think it's all a matter of your convenience, don't you," she said. "You don't even respect me."

"I respect you very much."

"Oh, sure. If you respected me you'd apologize."

"I have nothing to apologize for."

"My father was right, do you know it? You can't be both married and not married."

"Sure, and I'll tell you why he's right!" Leslie said. "Because women can't get anything through their heads. You explain to a woman that you don't have to be married, and she'll fix it so you're married when you're single. That's right. With a woman it's plus ça change plus c'est la même chose. Why is it that if a guy sleeps with a woman she has to move in with him? A guy can't just lay a woman two or three nights a week and be on his own the rest of the time. She'll move in with him every time. Seven nights a week. Even on sexless nights she's got to be there with him. Just so he's hers, you know what I mean? Just so she knows where he is." Millicent opened her mouth indignantly, but Leslie continued. "Explain to a woman you're not married, you don't have to be married—it's meaningless."

"You wanted me to move in!" she said.

"I wanted to sleep with you. You moved in."

"Ooh, you're rotten!" She clenched her fists. "Ooh, what a liar!"

"Think about it," he said. "You don't remember. Women never remember. It's amazing the way a woman's mind rewrites history. They remember things the way they want. There's just no concept of facts or of truth, where their emotions are concerned."

She stiffened up. "It's always men that try to get women to live with them! Always!"

He shook his head. "That's not true. Men want love, sex, affairs, mating—call it what you want. It's women that turn it into living together."

"Ooh, you stink, Les! You really do!" She pushed back the chair and stood up facing him. He looked up from his chair, a little startled. Her belly and navel seemed to breathe. She opened her mouth, but with her jaw taut, and shuddered, though she didn't sob. "If you think I'm the one that moved in with you I'm moving right out again!" She dragged the step stool into position to get her valises. "This arrangement has just about run its course."

"Don't get sore," he said.

She was already reaching for her valises on top of the upper cabinets. " 'Don't get sore!' " she repeated indignantly without turning. "You think you can do anything you want to me and say anything you want to me."

The valises were quite high. She jumped a few times, but only touched them. The jumping shook and wobbled her flesh in a feminine way, and she felt ridiculous. She knew he was watching her. She caught her breath and jumped again.

Leslie came over, as naked as she. Their bodies touched and jostled for an instant as he took down each valise, but without affection. He set them on the floor, the round one and the square one.

"And I want my pants back," she told him. "I'll trouble you to give them back, please."

"What pants?" he said.

"You know, my knit pants."

"I don't know any knit pants."

"Yes you do," she said. "Remember? My blue-green winter pants? I had them in New Hampshire. You said you wanted them for a souvenir."

He snickered through his nose and she reddened darker.

"Where are they?" she said.

"I don't know."

"You don't know? You mean you haven't got them?"

"I don't know." He seemed full of innocent amusement, as though her question were both unexpected and absurd. "Honest, I don't know where they are. I haven't any idea."

It seemed the most insulting thing of all. Apparently he had never thought of those pants again, after asking for them and taking them from her room. He might even have left them in New Hampshire.

She knelt and snapped open the valises, agitated and becoming tearful in her anger. She opened the drawers under the counter where she kept her underwear and began to pack.

"You're a conceited, overweening coxcomb," she said.

She had chosen her words with some care, but they seemed to have no effect on him except perhaps to amuse him more. He was sitting on the edge of the bed, apparently untroubled.

"You are," she said as she packed her things. "And I'm not coming back until you admit it. And not even then. Your great claim to fame is that you happened to be born male, that's all."

"What did I do?" he asked innocently.

She was surprised that her packing did not jar him into some humility. His failure to make any effort to talk her out of leaving seemed spiteful.

She glanced up at him. He sat there gazing at her, his knees innocently apart, without a stitch of clothing, and some slight motion of his eyes reminded her that she was as bare as he was. She pulled on some underpants. Then she put on a bra. She resumed packing. She was nervous and inefficient but she tried to do it quickly. She got some dresses from the wardrobe.

"I'll be out of your way at last," she said.

"I didn't say you were in my way."

"Do you want me to leave?"

"It's up to you."

"Well, I mean it," she said. "This is good-bye."

"Good-bye," he said.

She was sorry she had given him the satisfaction of asking him if he wanted her to leave. He was too self-centered to concede anything, or ever admit to his own rudeness, or to admit that he didn't want her to go.

She put on socks and shoes, her hands shaking. Then she found a half-slip and a denim skirt, and pulled a sweater over her head.

"I thought you were different," she said while she put her clothes on, "but you don't respect me at all, do you."

"Sure I do."

"No you don't. Women aren't people, are they. They're just for your amusement, aren't they. Well I'm tired of being a garbage pail for you to dump your needs in. You can go spill your needs somewhere else, in some other receptacle."

She pressed one of the valises shut. It was overstuffed and she had to put a knee on it before the latches would click.

"If your glands have to be drained every so often that's your personal problem, Leslie Hollander. Because I'm not going to make it mine any longer. I don't exist for the purpose of meeting your needs. I'm not a bathroom. And I'm not a laboratory for your experiments, either."

She squeezed her alarm clock into the other valise and got it closed. Her shoulder-strap bag flopped about her. He sat watching. She picked up both valises, the square one and the round one.

"Come on, Theodore, we're going out," she said to the cat.

The cat was wandering about under the tubs. Millicent opened the door, put one of the valises out in the hallway, and picked up the cat with her free arm.

"I'll come and get the rest of my things tomorrow when you're not here," she said to Leslie. "So don't think I'm keeping the key just as an excuse to come back."

"Okay."

She was certain that his insulting show of indifference was one more aspect of his conceit. It was infuriating. She stood with the cat in one arm and a valise hanging from the other. She wished the door opened outward so that she could have kicked it shut in his face while he sat looking at her.

Instead she turned her back and let the cat down to the floor, and started to the stairs with both valises, speaking gently to the cat again and nudging him with her foot to show him which way to go. She went down the stairs, gripping the valises, the cat preceding her, and did not glance back at Leslie's open door. She could see no choice but to teach him a lesson, and show him that he could not forever play lord and master and insult her besides. The cat went down, arching its body, a step at a time.

She was glad she didn't meet the landlady. When she got to the sidewalk she was weeping.

The street sloped down in a direction away from the early morning sun, and it was cool, though the roofs and tops of buildings were sunny. She wished she had taken her coat instead of leaving it for the next trip. She wondered where to look for a cab—whether she should climb up over the top of the hill or go all the way down to the wide street at its bottom.

She decided to go up. She kept looking about to make sure the cat stayed near her. It sniffed at things, and explored as it went, but followed. There were chilling breezes. But as she rounded the State House she came at last into sunshine. The golden dome above the graceful brickwork was shining like a second sun. There was still dew on the lawn.

But she carried the valises some distance down the brick sidewalk, past the green expanse of the Common, without finding a cab. They had grown heavy and she had to rest frequently. There was no traffic, and no one on the sidewalks yet. Theodore went in and out of the iron fence, and in the trees she heard birds.

At last, when she reached a traffic light that blinked, a lone taxi parked far down the intersecting street spotted her and approached.

She dropped her valises into the cab with an exhausted stumble and reached down to nudge the cat. She told the driver the address of the girls' apartment. She heard the metal slam of the door and the motor accelerated with a terrible grinding. She sank back and low, smelling the cab's old leather. She massaged the fur about on the cat's shoulders. The driver was skinny and old and wore a large, bulging, soft cap. His neck was cracked and shaven.

She closed her eyes, and felt the motions of the cab and smelled its engine. She slumped far down. Tiredness filled her.

She tried to reconstruct the argument with Les, and understand how he had come to say such nasty things. It simply wasn't true that living together had been her idea.

She recalled having borrowed his place when he was on call, because Barbie was crowding the apartment, but she was sure that he had suggested it before that.

When the cab stopped the driver reached and pushed open the door.

She thought he would help her drag out her things, but he didn't. He didn't even watch, but sat waiting, elbow out the window, staring ahead, his lower lip tightened over the upper one. He seemed to have no teeth.

She paid him, gathered up the valises again, and set them down once more when she hauled open the heavy door of iron and glass. She guided the cat with her foot. "Go in, kitty," she said.

In the dirty white lobby she collected her breath and her strength. Her name was still on the mailbox as she had added it in pencil. She began the climb. The valises knocked on the steps, but she rounded the landing without pausing. Outside her own door she set them down on the hard floor. The cat went in as soon as she turned the key. It seemed to head for its favorite spot in the kitchen.

She put the valises inside, one at a time. Barbie Chisholm was asleep on the studio couch in a messy tangle of bedclothes, breathing so heavily it was almost a snore. The blinds were shut and the light was dim.

There was a sound of flushing and Ella Jane came from the bathroom, leaning on her cane. She stared at Millicent and the valises.

"Hi," Millicent said.

"Well, for goodness sake," said Ella Jane.

"I'm home," said Millicent.

59

She went to Leslie's place on Monday, while he was away at the hospital, and got the rest of her things. She kept a taxi waiting downstairs while she brought down her coat and her umbrella, and the cat's box, and some pillowcases and quilts that belonged to her, and the afghan her mother had made, and Malcolm's big box of paper hats, and whatever articles of clothing had not fit in the valises the other time. She checked the drawers and the wardrobe, pushing his sheepskin jacket and coat and shirts aside, to make sure she had forgotten nothing. She even took hangers that had been hers. She checked the bathroom and the medicine cabinet, to be certain she had not even left a tweezer.

At last she laid the shiny brass-colored door key he had given her conspicuously in the middle of the counter, where he would be certain to find it, and departed.

The closets at the girls' apartment and the drawers in Natalie's bureau that she had used to have had grown quite overstuffed, and it had been with difficulty that they had made room yesterday for the things she had taken from her valises. Not only were there Barbie's things, but the weather had turned warm and some of the blankets had been put into the closets. For the time being there was not much she could do about the additional things she now brought, except that she did manage to get her coat onto a closet bar that was already jammed full.

Late at night, when she returned from the city room, the girls were still up, and they helped her put away a few more things, but she had to leave most of them rolled up in a sheet on top of everyone's shoes on the closet floor.

Then she sat for a while on the edge of Ella Jane's bed, conversing with Ella Jane, and confiding a little, while she waited for the bathroom to become free.

"The trouble with living with an intern is that they've got no time for you," Ella Jane said after a while. "Try one of your reporter friends next time. They've got time on their hands."

"Those oafs? No thank you," said Millicent.

Natalie seemed to want to talk to her too, but she felt less inclined to talk to Natalie than to Ella Jane.

"I thought he was nice," Natalie said to her.

"Well, I thought so too for a while," Millicent said. "But he needs to grow up a little, I guess."

Millicent slept on the floor, on the long cushion taken from the studio couch. She felt entitled to the couch itself, as she was one of the prior roommates and Barbie had come later and been supposedly temporary. But she knew Barbie had gotten used to the couch, and as Barbie did not offer to give it up and sleep on the floor Millicent said nothing.

She had had a kind of nervous insomnia the night before, which had been her first night back here, and she hoped it would not happen again. If it did the lack of sleep would give her sneezing fits. Besides she had begun to have a thick feeling in her throat that made her keep giving empty little coughs. There seemed to be always a coughable layer on her throat; yet when she coughed there was nothing to cough. The coughy nervousness extended all the way down into her stomach.

She could hear Barbie's deep breathing.

She was surprised that her parents had not phoned or bothered her lately. Apparently they had decided that they could not change her mind and that it was useless to make trouble. She had not expected them to come around to such a sensible attitude so quickly.

They would be relieved to know that she had left Les. Still, she was not going to go out of her way to inform them. They would see it as an admission of guilt, probably. As proof of their Victorian rightness. It was useless to talk to them at all.

She had come to feel while living with Les that her life was making no sense; actually, though, leaving him had not made sense of it. If anything, it made still less sense now.

He had of course not called. Undoubtedly he would go off into the Army at the end of June without calling, and she would never hear from him again. She had hoped, in walking out on him so angrily, to teach him a lesson. But it had really been too much to hope.

She heard Barbie cough in her sleep. The breathing became inaudible a few moments, but then resumed.

She remembered the system by which she had slept in Natalie's room when Natalie had a date. She wondered how they could work that now, if Natalie should want to bring home a date again. It was no good to move two girls to Natalie's room.

Lying in the darkness in this close air, smelling Barbie, it seemed that the possibility of love was too much to hope for. So was the possibility that one's life could make any sense. This blackness was the reality, and she was hardly better off than Charles.

By day, when she tidied up the place, she was aware of the silent telephone. It sat on the floor usually, pale lavender, next to the drop-leaf table. Toward suppertime on her day off it rang at last, and she snatched it up. But it was for Barbie.

She called Barbie, who squeezed around the ironing board in her slip and fat brassiere. Barbie took the phone from Millicent and said hello but paused only a moment. "I'm not in, creep," she said, and hung up.

She returned to her ironing.

"Which creep was that?" Ella Jane asked. She was lounging in the armchair. "The one we had the pleasure of the company of at breakfast?"

"The gall of that guy," said Barbie. "Okay, a one-night stand is a one-night stand, but then he doesn't even call up for a week and a half. And now he's got the gall to think I'm still available. I mean—the brass. I mean, all right, you can't win 'em all, but when a guy doesn't even care enough to phone the next day, I get the message. I'm not dumb."

Millicent was shocked.

It must have showed in her face, because Barbie suddenly looked at her and the iron stopped. "You don't have to look at me so blue-nosed," Barbie said. "For a girl that's got secrets of her own."

Millicent looked away.

Barbie seemed to her a stupid person. She had quit the saleslady job, or lost it, and then had talked again of being an airline hostess, but the airlines had not hired her because she was too short and chunky. Now she was studying to be a dental technician, but Millicent was sure somehow she could not be a good one.

Besides, Barbie's sloppiness had been particularly irritating these past few days. It seemed to have grown worse. She had even left a pad on the bathroom floor instead of throwing it in the basket.

Especially when the apartment was so overcrowded some neatness was in order, Millicent thought. But she would find Barbie's things over her own, doubled up on hangers, and sometimes her own things in a heap on the floor, hangers and all. It was not fair. She had been assigned little enough space. Barbie seemed to have no system—girdles, stockings and whatnot were in every drawer, sometimes unfolded and sometimes unwashed. It seemed to Millicent that it was the disorder rather than the amount that made all the drawers so overstuffed. You could take nothing from a drawer without pulling and wrinkling something else. But she knew it was useless to make Barbie understand that, though she would have liked to try, as she had not even been able to unpack many of her own things.

Barbie's long black hairs lay on the sink or floated beside soaking cigarette butts that discolored the toilet bowl. Meanwhile Barbie walked around completely naked sometimes for an hour or more, with flopping fat and with shapeless buttocks.

Millicent's anger came near to boiling when she discovered her big bottle of perfume on a kitchen shelf, behind the baking soda, the stopper gone and the perfume all evaporated away. She knew that only Barbie would have been so careless as to leave the stopper out, and Barbie did own up to having used it.

"That was a terrible thing to do," Millicent told her. "Do you know what that cost?"

"I only used a drop," Barbie said. "I didn't think you'd grudge a lousy drop."

"That's not the point. You left the stopper open."

But Barbie denied leaving the stopper open. It gave Millicent a feeling of tragic waste. She remembered Charles's estimate that Malcolm had paid a hundred dollars for that perfume. And she had used it only one time, that very last date with Malcolm.

"I never heard of such carelessness!" Millicent said. "That stuff costs a fortune!"

"It was practically empty anyway," said Barbie.

"It was not! It was practically a full bottle. I used it exactly once."

Twice Millicent stepped barefoot on sharp slivers of toenail paring on the bathroom floor. There was no question that they were Barbie's. It had never happened before Barbie came to live there.

In her free daytime hours, when the other girls were at work, she tried to keep up with the cleaning, as she had used to. But it was much harder now than formerly. One of the filthiest of Barbie's habits was throwing crumpled papers and cigarette wrappings and butts into the green tile fireplace. It might have made sense in a fireplace that was in frequent use, but this one had never even had fire irons, at least in Millicent's time, and the tile had been kept shiny and clean. Tossing crumpled papers there only made a junk pile in the living room.

They had already quarreled while preparing for bed, because Barbie had left a tangle of stockings on the studio couch and Millicent swept them to the floor in taking the long cushion off. Then they quarreled about which of them had used a disagreeable tone first.

On the morning of her second day off Millicent awoke as Natalie shut the door on the way to work. In the past she had often slept through the noise of breakfast and the girls' leaving, but this week she had not been able to. She lay there, feeling exhausted, and trying to fall asleep again. At last she rose, in her white pajamas, and got a grapefruit from the little refrigerator under the stove. Barbie was there in her slip, sleepily watching coffee percolate. They said nothing to each other. She'll dump the coffee grounds in the toilet, Millicent thought. She just doesn't care. It had happened before, and several flushings did not quite get rid of them all.

Millicent sat with a half grapefruit at the drop-leaf table. The toaster was already on it, and a plate and some crumbs from Natalie's breakfast. In a moment Barbie sat opposite and sipped hot coffee gingerly.

"Do me a favor," Millicent said after a while, "and don't throw rubbish in the fireplace. Like your olive-oil bottle. Do you think it just disappears? I'm the one that cleans that. We need a little consideration, you know, when things are so crowded."

Barbie said nothing. She looked sour. Ella Jane appeared, wrapped in a bathrobe, her eyes scarcely open. She muttered a good morning and began to make toast.

Millicent got up to make cocoa and Barbie shut herself in the bathroom meanwhile. When she came out of the bathroom Millicent went to use it, but sprayed it with a deodorant first, and from a glance that Barbie gave her she realized that Barbie took the spraying as an insult.

When she came out of the bathroom Barbie had put on a dress and was standing before the mantelpiece mirror, tilting her head and combing her hair with long downstrokes. Ella Jane sat hunched with coffee, looking not quite awake. Barbie's eyes in the mirror looked at Millicent.

"You barge around here like you're the queen of the May," Barbie said. "Who asked you to move in, if you think it's so crowded."

"Well, you have a nerve!" Millicent told her. "It happens to be my apartment, if you remember."

"You left it," said Barbie.

"Now just a minute! There was a clear agreement!" Millicent was standing by the table, and she poured cocoa from the pot to a glass. "You're the one that was just bunking here temporarily."

"Oh no! Oh no ya don't," Barbie said. "You're not putting me out on the street." She was pulling some long hairs out of the comb.

"Don't tell me it's not my apartment then," Millicent retorted.

Barbie resumed combing. "Who pays the rent?" she said.

"I do—I expect to. Now that I'm back."

"You were living with a guy and he threw you out," Barbie said, "and you come barging in here like you owned it."

"He did not throw me out!"

Barbie faced her. "You can't come in and go out. In and out and in and out, whenever you please. What do you think this is? I've been paying the rent. You moved out and I moved in."

"Watch the toast," said Ella Jane. She took the smoking toast out herself.

Millicent looked at the toast confusedly. She sat down to the table, furious and shaking. She began to butter the toast.

Barbie stopped combing and stood with hands on hips, one foot before the other. "My name's on the mailbox," she said. "Not yours. Until you scribbled it in."

"Who gave you authority to put your name on?" said Millicent. Her voice quaked.

"What do you mean, who gave me authority! I live here, that's who."

"Who's right, Ella Jane?" Millicent pleaded.

"Leave me out of it," said Ella Jane. She scarcely took her face from the coffee cup.

"Anyway the furniture's mostly Natalie's," said Barbie, "and Natalie's my friend."

"She's my friend too," said Millicent.

"No she isn't," said Barbie. "She's my friend a lot longer. And who said you could bring that cat in here? Messing up the joint, and scratching everybody's stockings."

"That cat lived here before you did! And he does not mess up the joint! It's not true."

"I want him out," said Barbie.

"It's not true!" Millicent persisted. "It's a lie! You arbitrate it, Ella Jane. I'm willing to let Ella Jane arbitrate it."

"Oh no! No arbitration," said Barbie.

"Don't involve me," Ella Jane said. "You settle it among yourselves." She took a sip of coffee without looking up. "Four's kind of a crowd around here, that's all I've got to say."

"That's right, we'll settle it among ourselves," Barbie said, going to the closet. "Four's a crowd around here."

In an instant she dragged out Millicent's valises, with scrapes on the floor, the sheet full of unpacked clothing half rolling out with them and coming untied, and threw the valises to their sides.

"Hey!" Millicent shouted in a high-pitched voice, jumping up to protect her things, but Barbie had already pulled out the sheet further, shoes sliding and tumbling before it. She threw some clothing on the valises in a heap.

"Ooh!" Millicent shrieked.

Barbie grasped a bunch of clothing from the closet, hangers and all. Millicent tried to wrest them, but Barbie elbowed her in the chest and pulled the fabrics hard. Millicent let go lest they rip.

"Ooh you—ooh you—" Millicent exclaimed, and fell into the closet against the hanging dresses. Barbie yanked and the flying hangers battered Millicent's fingers.

"Ella Jane! Call the police!" Millicent cried out.

"It's your battle," said Ella Jane. "You fight it."

Barbie gave Millicent a thrust of her shoulder and hip to shove her deeper among the dresses. She had already stooped and clicked open Millicent's valises. Millicent scrambled beside her and their hands struggled in the cloth, but whenever they both seized one garment Barbie was willing to wrench and yank, risking any damage, until Millicent let go. Millicent kept shouting for her to stop, but Barbie worked grim-faced. "I'll kill you!" Millicent cried out. Ella Jane sat with her coffee, scarcely watching.

Barbie sprang up and tossed the alarm clock onto the mess of clothing she had thrown into the round valise. It bounced from the soft clothing to the oriental rug, apparently without damage. Then she snatched up Charles's ivory piece, that had been on the mantel beside the clock, though Millicent tried to stop her, and pressed it down into the tangled clothing with the clock.

"Look out! That's fragile!" Millicent squealed.

Barbie shut the round valise, forcing it, and pressed the latch closed even though clothing stuck out. Millicent opened it.

"You broke it!" Millicent said. An ivory arm, holding its tool, had come loose from the figure. It made her heartsick.

"It was cracked. I didn't even touch it hardly."

"It wasn't cracked! You broke it! You squashed it in there!"

Barbie shut the valise again.

"You're just a savage!" Millicent shouted.

Barbie opened the door and grabbed the valise, though Millicent tried to seize it. She slid it out onto the landing. Then she grabbed the sheet full of unpacked things. Millicent kicked her, and Barbie punched Millicent in the eye with a powerful arm. Millicent began to cry. Barbie dragged the whole bundle onto the landing while Millicent scurried about weeping and snatching at it.

"I'm coming back with a cop!" Millicent said. "And a lawyer."

"Go ahead," said Barbie. "Somebody's getting out and it's not me." She got the box of paper hats, which was deep in the closet on the floor, and booted that out. She was growing red-faced. She left the door open.

"Where's that cat?" Barbie said.

"Leave him alone!"

She found the cat in the kitchen and gave him a sideways kick.

"Ooh you—" Millicent said.

"Come on, cat! Out! Scat!" Barbie gave the cat another kick, her instep catching it under the belly. Ella Jane looked up as the cat flew nearly to the ceiling, its legs spread out. It landed on its feet and was gone through the door like a rocket. It leapt down the stairs.

Millicent ran blubbering to the landing to look for it but then back again as Barbie began pulling things from Natalie's bureau and throwing them to the floor. She threw the Communist bayonet at Millicent in its scabbard.

"Get out!" she said. "I'm sick of you."

She threw the manila envelope that contained Millicent's clippings.

"Can I get dressed at least?" Millicent pleaded.

"Go on! Get out!"

"Let me get dressed. I can't go out in my pajamas."

"Get dressed." Barbie threw some underpants toward her.

Millicent got the other envelope, that contained Aunt Rosalind's watercolors. She found them uncrushed, in the bottom of Natalie's bureau. She laid them neatly in the square valise. As she did Barbie threw the goggle-eyed stuffed dog with floppy ears and it struck her hard in the face.

"Take your silly-faced dog!" said Barbie.

"That's not mine! It's Natalie's," Millicent said. "And give me back my mother's rug."

"The rug's ours. You left it," Barbie told her.

Millicent stepped out of her pajamas and dressed rapidly, weeping softly. She felt like attacking Barbie bodily, but she was afraid that Barbie was the stronger. She chose a sweater and denim skirt. She was amazed at Ella Jane's silence and nonchalance. Barbie meanwhile threw a pillowcase that belonged to Millicent out onto the landing, and dragged a sheet which she threw against the air in that direction. She flung the shoulder-strap bag through the door with an underhand pitch. Millicent frantically packed her things which Barbie had thrown at her feet and all about her on the floor. She tried to put them into the square valise with some semblance of neatness, but Barbie helped her, snatching pieces of clothing from her hands and stuffing them in every which way, and at last shut the valise suddenly, so that Millicent's hands were nearly pinched. Then Barbie half threw and half shoved the valise over the threshold with a swing of her body and kicked it dancingly with the side of her ankle. She pushed Millicent with both hands and Millicent fell back over a valise. In an instant Barbie shoved both valises and the box of paper hats and the roll of packed sheeting down the stairs. The sheeting did not go far, but the square valise slid bumpily to where the stairs reversed themselves in mid-flight and then popped open, stopping against the wall and spilling perhaps a third of its contents. The apartment door slammed with an echoing bang, leaving Millicent to pick herself up from the hard floor sobbing alone.

She didn't see what Barbie had had to throw the things down the stairs for. Millicent went down a few steps and tried to repack the opened valise and to gather up the rest of the mess into one of the sheets again. The varicolored paper hats, which were everywhere among the pieces of clothing, she did not bother. The flat crepe hats had slid easily, some down to the turn in the stairs, and the shiny pointed ones and drum-major ones still rolled and fell with hollow cardboard noises when her gathering up the sheet or other items disturbed them. It gave her some satisfaction that Barbie or Ella Jane or Natalie would eventually have to clear all those hats and the overturned corrugated box off the steps.

It took her two trips to get the valises and the heavy rolled sheet full of clothing down to the lobby. Then she carried them out through the iron and glass door one at a time, and put the two valises on the sidewalk and the roll of packed sheeting on top of them. She had expected that the cat would be waiting for her down here, but he was nowhere in sight.

"Theodore!" she called as loudly as she could, looking about at the tree and up and down the sidewalk and at the facing of the building with sunshine on its stone sills. Her voice sounded weak and high in her ears.

A tall man who walked rapidly past looked at her strangely. She knew her face must be tear-stained.

She called the cat again, leaving her belongings in the sun and walking a little up and down the block. There was no sign of him.

She came back to the little stack she had made of her things and sat on a corner of the square valise, resting against the stuffed sheet. Her coat was in that sheet, she thought. It would need a pressing when she got unpacked. The arch across the building's indentation cast its shadow on the flagstones that led in to the heavy door. She felt that she had come to love that building, with its massive old sturdiness, even though she had not spent much time in it in the past few months, and it was heartbreaking that things had gotten so out of hand. She had not realized that she had been provoking Barbie that much. She supposed it was partly her own fault. She had been irritable, and maybe somewhat arrogant. She had not realized that Barbie had such a temper. Perhaps the best thing would be to find a hotel for the night and try tomorrow for some temporary reconciliation. And get a lawyer the next time Barbie tried anything. Natalie might help smooth it over for now.

She had scarcely the energy to find a hotel room. She dragged herself up, feeling as she did so the beginning of an inward despairing sob, without tears. She went slowly up the block to look for a cab. She realized that a reconciliation was not really possible. She would only beg and make herself abject and be refused. If Charles were alive and stationed at some air base, she would buy a bus ticket there and live nearby. Charles at least had had a sense of blood, and kin, and love owed. He would not have let anyone throw her out of an apartment. It seemed to her that life was something that grows steadily worse, and that the good part of her own life was already behind her.

The thought of that ivory broken, that Charles had selected with such care, made her sick with fury. She decided she would come back some day when all the girls were out and chuck all Barbie's things out the window. She still had a key. It would serve Barbie right.

At the corner she could still look back and see her belongings. There was more traffic here, as the intersecting street was an important one, and soon a cab stopped. But it could not go down the one-way street, so the driver took it around the block while she walked back to her things. He met her there and helped her load the cab. He was an old man, as small as herself. When she had gotten in beside the valises and stuffed sheet she felt very tired.

"Go around the block a couple of times, and look for a black cat," she told the driver.

He looked at her strangely.

"I lost my cat," she told him.

They started off. There was a sound of grinding that seemed to come from beneath her seat.

She asked him to go more slowly so she could watch for the cat. They cruised past one building after another. She saw him nowhere. Once she called the cat's name out the taxi window, but some people on the sidewalk looked at her and she thought she must seem peculiar.

It might be better to search the neighborhood on foot, she thought. But there was no way to do that and still keep watch on her luggage, unless she hired the cab for quite a long time. The meter was clicking busily, a number changing every several seconds. She wished she had taught the cat to answer to some whistle.

They rode all around the block very slowly twice, and she realized it was useless. The meter kept clicking. She would have to place an ad in the lost and found.

She asked the driver if he knew of any low-priced apartments for rent. She had to ask twice before he heard. He said he didn't, and she asked him to stop near a drugstore where she could get a newspaper.

She brought the paper back to the cab and studied the classifieds. She heard the meter ticking, even though the cab was parked. Most of the listings asked a rent two or three times what she could afford. But she came across a two-line ad finally that offered two furnished rooms and bath for forty dollars. Business-woman, it said. She told the driver the address and they started again. It was only a couple of blocks from Leslie's place, but further down toward the bottom of the hill. She hoped worriedly that it would turn out to be satisfactory and that it was not already taken. The cab fare was already mounting steeply and the paper showed no other good prospects.

"What's that noise?" she asked the driver.

"What noise," he said.

"In the motor, or the machinery. It shouldn't sound like that, should it?"

"Needs a transmission," he said.

They moved slowly in traffic. Besides there were many traffic lights and cross streets. The trembling of the seat and the metal and the windows was never-ending. She had opened the windows but it seemed that she smelled the fumes not only of this cab but of the cars beside her. And smelled them not just with her nose but with her ears, her forehead, her temples. She wondered how the driver stood it, how he worked at this all day.

The meter ticked, and when a number changed it clunked. She began crying softly.

When they got to the address the driver parked but did not look around. He seemed to know she was crying. She composed herself and crossed the dirty sidewalk. The driver sat waiting.

It was a narrow building of brick, squeezed among others. A door with an oval window stood open and there were tinny mailboxes, not matching one another. She could not find the janitor's bell, and her eyes could not adjust to the darkness of the stair well. But then a woman's voice shouted down and asked what she wanted.

Millicent inquired if the apartment was taken. There was a noise upstairs as if a pail had been set down. Footsteps shuffled down, and at last a small, thin old woman looked at her with narrow eyes.

"You employed?" the woman asked.

Millicent told her where she worked.

"I'm particular who I take in here," the woman said. "You can't be too careful." She turned and led the way, and Millicent could look through gray hairs to the pink scalp.

The woman threw open a door. "There's a nice two-room apartment," she said. "Airy. Quiet. And street floor. No stairs to climb."

There was old-fashioned wallpaper, mostly pink but much darkened, an iron bed with chipped white paint, and an oval sepia print of wild-eyed horse heads. A single large window looked out on a collection of little fenced yards behind brick buildings, with weeds growing in them. A curved dresser with grainy wood looked serviceable, despite a broken knob. On the floor linoleum was pressed and dirtied according to the shape and warp of the boards beneath. The kitchen was a separate room, but with no window of its own. The landlady put on the light. Both rooms were small. The bathroom was beyond the kitchen in railroad style, again without a window, and the landlady turned on the light there also. The bathroom door was of gray-painted boards, with hook-and-eye locks inside and out, and within the bathroom another such door, shut but with its hook and eye unlocked, led still further beyond.

"You share with the lady on the other side," the landlady said. "A quiet elderly lady. As sweet as anybody you'd ever want to meet."

Millicent wandered again through the rooms. The one window was large and the weedy space outside gave it plenty of light. An earlier tenant had fixed a board outside the sill and some empty flowerpots still rested on it in the rain-beaten dust.

"I'll take it," she said.

"That'll be in advance. A month's rent and a month's security. And you're not to have any men in your room."

"Don't worry," said Millicent.

The cabdriver helped bring her things only just inside the stair well. The meter had come to more than six dollars, and the landlady stood by while Millicent counted it out. Millicent realized as she did so that she ought to have explained that she could not pay a whole month's rent immediately. But she did explain, as soon as the driver left. She got paid biweekly, and would not have her salary until the week following.

The landlady sighed, and said she should have told her that before. Millicent agreed, but said truthfully that she hadn't thought of it. She was afraid the landlady would refuse her after all.

"Well, I can't afford to make exceptions," the landlady said, "but you seem to have an honest face. But I'll have to hold your luggage until I get the rest. The rent and security."

"Oh, thank you."

The landlady took the twenty dollars that Millicent offered her on account. Millicent said she could give her five more now but it would leave her short for food.

"No, that's all right," the lady said. "You pay me when you get your check." She dragged the stuffed roll of sheeting and the two valises into her own rooms and shut the door.

Millicent went out, thinking she would place ads for her cat. She had held out money for the ads also, but realized as she walked downtown that all her calculations had been close. She checked the purse in her shoulder-strap bag. She ought to have paid only fifteen on account instead of twenty. She had bought a lot of groceries both at Leslie's and at the girls', and had spent a fortune on cabs. It was hard to tell where it had all gone.

She went to each of the four papers, including her own, and wrote out a little ad in the classified office. She also sent Leslie a postcard, saying she had not meant to get in touch with him again but that she would appreciate his letting her know if Theodore went back there. She explained that she had moved from the girls and in the confusion the cat had run away.

She also, after some hesitation, telephoned Ella Jane at Ella Jane's office, feeling humiliated at doing so, and asked her also to let her know if the cat came back.

"Okay," said Ella Jane.

Millicent walked slowly back to her new apartment, thinking she would like to nap. It occurred to her that she ought to have unpacked the changes of clothing and pajamas and towels she would need before giving the landlady her luggage.

When she got there she knocked at once on the landlady's door. There was no answer.

"Mrs. Hoyt?" she said.

She looked up the stair well.

"Mrs. Hoyt?" she called.

There was silence.

She went to her bed. The spring was of a metallic netting that sagged under her like a hammock, but it was not uncomfortable. The sun was on the window now. She resolved to put some plants on its shelf. A colorful spread on this old bed, instead of Mrs. Hoyt's brown one, would also make a difference, she thought, and so would some bright pictures on the walls, and a thorough washing of the linoleum.

She slept.

She awoke in the afternoon, and did some shopping, as economically as possible, including some staple foods, a few cheap dishes, a pan, a pot, a cake of soap, a floor brush, a mop, insect powder, and toilet paper. When she got back she looked for the landlady again and this time she found her.

"Mrs. Hoyt," she said, "I need a few things from my luggage."

"You get your luggage when you pay the rent," Mrs. Hoyt said. "And a month's security."

"But I just need a few things—pajamas and underwear and some changes."

"When you pay the rent and security," Mrs. Hoyt said, and shut the door in her face.

Millicent had a lonely supper of sardines, and in the evening walked down by the river, feeling gloomy. She did not see how she could go a week without a change of clothes. She wondered if she could borrow some money from Maud at work tomorrow. She had never borrowed more than a few cents from anyone before.

Before going to bed she stood naked at the sink and washed her bra and slip and underpants and socks. The water at the sink was not very warm so she heated a potful at the stove. She felt chilly. But she could see no choice. She hoped her things would be dry by morning.

To dry her hands she had to use toilet paper.

The bed had only one sheet, and the single blanket was scratchy on her skin. It seemed to be not wool but one of the new cheap woody materials. She knew that Leslie thought nothing of sleeping bare at this season, but she did not like it. It was quite cold, and she was sure the radiators had had no heat throughout the day. She thought of a hot bath. She wondered how many heatings of her little pot it would take to fill the tub. By the time she could heat the last potful the tub would be cold again.

She thought of her roommates, and of Leslie, and of her family, and of the cat.

She slept quite late in the morning, despite her nap the day before. The apartment was in fact quiet, as Mrs. Hoyt had promised. She had never heard the lady with whom she shared the bath, and scarcely seen any sign of her existence, and the buildings cloistered the weedy back yards in such a way as to shut out noises of the street.

She went at once to the radiator by the big window to feel her underthings and socks. They were still damp. She was nude at the window and glanced up to see if anyone was observing her from the windows opposite. But she saw no one.

There was nothing to do except put on her sweater and skirt and shoes.

She had meant today to begin the cleaning, and also to begin shopping for a nice bedspread, even if she could not buy just yet, and for frames for one or two of Aunt Rosalind's pictures. But for some hours she did nothing. Mostly she lay on the spread, in sweater, skirt, and shoes, feeling depressed. At last, however, she began to scrub the linoleum. She worked with her sweater sleeves rolled, and nothing on below the waist, so as not to dirty the skirt and shoes she would have to wear to work. She lowered the shade somewhat, but not enough to keep the drying clothes from getting any sun they could. Then after some minutes she decided she could not chance working like that in view of the window, and had better confine today's scrubbing to the kitchen, where she could shut the door and put on the light. But once in a while she went to the cold radiator, and felt the wet clothing that lay on it.

She hoped they would be dry enough in time to wear them for work. But the day was overcast and they got no sun.

After the scrubbing she put her skirt and shoes back on, and spread bug poison around the fixtures and around the edges of the linoleum in both rooms. She had seen a few roaches. She put poison down the sink drain also.

When it was nearly time to go to work she sought out Mrs. Hoyt desperately. She found her collecting bags of garbage on the second floor.

"Mrs. Hoyt," she tried, "I don't want the valises—I just want to get something out. I haven't got any underwear on."

"No, not a thing till I get the rent," said Mrs. Hoyt. She looked at Millicent a moment and the skin about her eyes was all in straight lines. She went to another door and bent to a garbage bag.

"But my underwear's still wet," Millicent said. "What am I gonna do?"

"I don't know," Mrs. Hoyt said. She dropped the bag into a burlap sack she dragged and went on.

Millicent made a gesture of confusion. "How about if I give you the wet ones?"

"No, I can't be bothered going into the closet all the time. Once you've had that key in your hand, and once you've slept in that bed, you owe me a month's rent and a month's security."

Millicent stood there an instant. Then her head gave a little shake. She followed Mrs. Hoyt. "I haven't got one single thing on under here," she said. "Not even pants. I haven't got anything to put on."

Mrs. Hoyt continued in her garbage collecting without answering.

"How can I go to work?" Millicent asked.

Mrs. Hoyt paid no attention. It was as though Millicent were not there.

She looked at Mrs. Hoyt, feeling that she would weep with humiliation and anger. But she didn't. After a moment she went downstairs and set out for the city room.

It felt strange to walk in the city with no underclothes. Her skin was raw and the denim was abrasive on her goose flesh. She was conscious of her breasts, especially when she stepped down a curb. It was an impossible situation, she thought. She would have to go to the five-and-dime when she got a chance and get a cheap change of underwear to last her the week. That would still leave her without pajamas. She wished she owned a savings account instead of a collection of Government bonds.

At work it felt even stranger. Whenever she could she found excuses to clutch the papers she carried high in front of her, so that her arms could have a steadying effect. She could not get used to the feel of the sweater and the denim against her. The skirt had rough seams. She kept wondering if the men in the city room could sense that she had nothing on under the skirt either, but whenever she glanced at any they were not paying particular attention. Nor did Mr. Valentino or the others upstairs at the linotypes, nor Mr. Garvey and the other men she met on her errands.

When she returned from her errands Danny McBride was in the city room in one of his jovial moods, so that she at once feared that before long he would give her a spank or feel her in some way. But somehow he didn't notice her, and soon went out.

She had hoped to ask Maud for a loan, but Maud was off and would be off again tomorrow. She could not bring herself to ask any of the men for money.

Mr. Hopkins sent her home a little early. She did not take a cab, as her cash had become very low, but walked, even though she had heard that some of those streets could be dangerous at night. She had always taken a cab to Leslie's.

The night was chilly and blowy, and it was still overcast and damp. She wondered if Theodore had found shelter, and what he had found to eat.

She watched for sinister figures, and she shivered in the cold.

If her underthings were still damp after all this time, she thought, maybe she could hold them to a light bulb. She wondered if that would scorch them. Or she could hold them over the gas range on the mop handle.

She found her new residence, glad to have gotten there. The street was deserted. She took the key from her shoulder-strap bag and let herself in.

At her own door she reached in and clicked on the light. There were cockroaches everywhere. She could see thousands. She gave a gasp, and then a cry. Brown insects ran in all directions on the floor, some many times bigger than others, some quite tiny, and all intermediate sizes, but shaped alike, as though all ages were among them, the young ones miniature replicas of the adults. They were on the walls, with long antennae, and on the bed, and the table, and some even on the sill and the radiator and her clothes that hung in the ribs of it. She shut the door, and some smaller bugs crawled out under it.

"Help, somebody!" she cried out.

They had been thickest on the floor—she knew she could not have gone into that room without hearing several of them crunch together under her shoes at every step. And even in that brief glance she could tell it was worse in the kitchen. They had seemed to be coming from there, and near the kitchen door the floor was black with their milling about. The room had been a horrid sight. They crossed each other's paths in dizzying patterns of straight lines.

She pounded on Mrs. Hoyt's door. "Mrs. Hoyt!" she shouted. "Mrs. Hoyt!" She pounded again. "Mrs Hoyt!"

Mrs. Hoyt opened the door in a nightgown, squinting with sleep and her thin gray hair hanging down disheveled all about her head.

"Oh!" Millicent put her hands to her bosom breathlessly as if she would collapse. "Mrs. Hoyt! Cockroaches! Thousands—millions! I used bug powder and I think it routed them out of where they were. They're all over the place. It's terrible. I should have let them alone. Oh, you wouldn't believe it!"

"Are you afraid of them?" Mrs. Hoyt said as though in surprise. "They won't hurt you."

"I can't stay there. I won't go in there. They're on everything."

"Oh, I see a roach myself once in a while."

"Mrs. Hoyt, you never saw so many. I—can't you do something?"

"I can't do anything tonight."

"But I can't go in there. I can't sleep there. I'll have to find another place. I'll have to move. Or go to a hotel."

"Suit yourself." She began to shut the door but Millicent put a hand to it.

"Mrs. Hoyt," she said, her voice shaking, "can I have my luggage now please?"

"I told you, when you pay the rent and security."

"But I'm moving. I was only here one day."

"I want a full month's rent," said Mrs. Hoyt, "and a month's security. I rent by the month. I told you that. I don't take no transients, fly-by-nights. That ad cost me money. I could have rented to others."

"But I can't afford two places!"

"Then I'd stay put if I was you."

"But Mrs. Hoyt—!" Millicent pleaded.

"Don't Mrs. Hoyt me. What's the idea? Waking me up in the middle of the night." She forced the door shut.

Millicent looked about the dim hallway and whimpered.

"Please, Mrs. Hoyt," she said to the door and rapped on it. "Can I talk to you please?"

There was no answer.

She went out to the glow of the street lamp and sat on the stone step. It was cold. But the thought of her room was terrifying. She got up, and looked in her shoulder-strap bag under the street lamp. She had not quite two dollars left, not enough for a decent hotel. She walked a few paces aimlessly, shivering. It would be unthinkable to knock on Leslie's door at this hour. Especially to have to crawl to him, after what they had said to one another. It was out of the question. Destitute, and shorn of her underwear.

For all she knew there was another girl in his bed by now. Some nurse.

But she couldn't walk the streets all night and freeze like this, or crouch in Mrs. Hoyt's hallway, or sleep on a bench by the river embankment. Even if she did, she doubted if Mrs. Hoyt would give her any more satisfaction in daylight. She wondered if she could complain to the police about Mrs. Hoyt's cockroaches. She began walking, thinking she would find a policeman.

She soon lost her nerve. The only other course was to walk to North Station and wait for the late train to Wilmerding Crosswalk. She did not want to sit in that vast gloomy concourse alone at night without underwear, nor did she want to come without underwear to her parents' house in the middle of the night. But it seemed that she had no choice.

60

Ed waited until the Sabbath was over, and then drove to Boston to get the two valises and the articles rolled in the sheet. Mrs. Hoyt gave him difficulty for only a moment. He told her he was a busy man, and that if he had to come a second time it would be with a search warrant and a health inspector. She led him to the valises, grumbling about the kind of people you get these days, and complaining about Millicent's fastidiousness about cockroaches. "If she thinks that's a lot she should have seen it when I bought the place. I got rid of a lot."

Millicent had left Wilmerding Crosswalk in early afternoon to go to work, so they left the porch light on at night for her return, and also a snack on the unpainted wooden table in the kitchen. Lucinda put clean linen for her on the iron cot in Patty's room.

Lucinda speculated in bed as to why Millicent had left her friend. "Let's not ask," Ed said.

Millicent had told them that she was at home only temporarily, until she could find a satisfactory apartment of her own. Yet she seemed reconciled to commuting until then.

Ed asked her Sunday morning if she would be available to teach Sunday school again if she were needed, and she said she would. However he did not ask her immediately, as Marilyn Prince seemed to be enjoying it.

Sunday night he had been asked to attend a meeting of the congregation's executive board. He and Lucinda had heard rumors that there was some sentiment against renewing his contract, and he knew that the purpose of the executive board meeting was to get him on the carpet. And he knew that Lucinda knew it. Yet she did not mention her uneasiness, but spoke instead as though Ed were in a position to make demands upon the congregation. She told him to insist upon tenure and a guaranteed pension. He had had that in his Brighton assistantship, but not as yet here.

Shortly before going he went up to the bedroom and found Lucinda lying there with her eyes closed, not quite napping. He lay beside her, thinking he would rest before the meeting. He looked at the cracks in the ceiling. Rosalind's portrait of him was on the wall. Then he looked at Lucinda's profile. She had her glasses on, though her eyes were shut.

As he lay there he began fondling her leg in a slow, tickling way, and edging her skirt and slip away. His fingers traced to the frontiers of the nylon, but she rejected him with a twitch. "Don't," she said. "Please, I'm not in the mood. I've got too much on my mind." A quick motion of her hand brushed her clothing into place. Her forehead had become tense and wrinkled, though she didn't open her eyes.

He went to the temple on foot. It was not dark yet. The towering trees of Massapeequit Road had put out new leaves up in their spreading and interlocking parts. In the trees beyond the fields also the leaves were new, undersized and the green still a pale and powdery shade. Some species had put out tiny reddish ones, and some even had odd shades of yellow-green. He knew all those pastel tints would turn a deep green in a week or so, when the tiny leaves got larger. This first moment of early spring is like a little autumn, he thought.

It was just a little more than a year since he'd come to this town.

Ultimately the question of his contract and its terms would rest with the congregation, in a full membership meeting. Still, he wished he felt more certain of the executive board.

He saw cars parked near the temple, under the maple trees that lined the curb, and the light was on in the room called the library.

He found Conrad Bernstein lounging in the presiding chair at the end of the long varnished table. He looked thin and spare, his face almost weather-beaten. He wore a bow tie. The Walkers were there, Phil and Sandy, and Amethyst

Gilbert, and big, gray Roy Herzlinger, and Burton Seligman, tall and young and slightly freckled with hair combed to the side and a mild, one-sided smile and his shirt open at the collar. There was also Murray Spingarn, youngish but quite bald, with a flat nose and black jowls and a fixed scowl. "Hi, Ed," Conrad said. The others greeted him also.

Ed pulled out a chair, saying he was sorry if he was late, but Conrad said they were waiting for Joe Haskel and for Norman Swift and Mrs. Frank. They sat chatting aimlessly.

After a while Conrad looked at his watch and said it looked as if the others weren't coming, and that they might as well get started in any case. Sandy Walker folded back her spiral notebook.

"It's not a formal meeting, Sandy," Conrad said. "You don't have to take notes. We'll dispense with a secretary's report on it."

Ed saw Burton Seligman and Phil Walker smoking cigarettes, Burton casual and bland and Phil with an intense expression. Phil had wide brows that curved up over eyes far apart. Murray Spingarn was biting the tip off a cigar. Conrad cleared his throat and leaned forward, elbows on the table. He coughed, raising a hand to his mouth. His eyes behind the metal-rimmed glasses met Ed's and fell away again.

"Ed," he said, "you know there's talk that some of the new families over in Sparkstown Heights and the Squegantum section might set up a new congregation over that way."

"I know it," said Ed.

"There's been an influx over there," Conrad said, looking at Ed, "and it would be strictly reform. Which of course is the sentiment of a lot of our membership too—we have a cross section here—and some people estimate that a new place like that would pull away half our membership. A third to a half."

"I wouldn't think so," said Ed.

"It could. It's a touchy situation, Ed. It could ruin Beth El. Ed, I built this temple. For years, starting with a little community center in a private house. I spent hours, every day sometimes. I neglected my business for it. We did it for the sake of our children, and we held all factions together. I built it, Ed. You know the story. And I don't want to see it pulled apart. But an awful lot of people have been complaining that if you stay, and a reform place starts in Sparkstown, they'll pull out. Now, that's the story, Ed. What we need is a statesman, that can hold this congregation together. And you're not it, Ed. A year ago, when we started with you, I hoped you were for us. I really did. I thought you were a man that would put the temple first."

"Ed's brilliant," Amethyst said to Conrad firmly, and Ed looked at her.

"Naw, look," Phil Walker told Amethyst, "we need a peacemaker. Ed's too controversial."

Amethyst looked besieged. She stared at Ed as if she were watching a hanging. Her hair was pulled up to a knot, in a way that seemed to show the shape of her skull bones around her ears.

"Can I bum a cigarette?" Ed asked Burton Seligman.

Burton slid the pack and a book of matches across the varnished smoothness to him.

"I don't say anything's settled," Conrad said, "but we've got a few bones to pick with you."

Ed puffed the cigarette. Burton slid the ashtray half across the table, to a position midway between himself and Ed. Roy Herzlinger sat at an angle, his big face solid and smooth and unsmiling.

"For one thing, Ed," said Conrad, "I wish you were a little less narrow, not quite so sectarian." His thin face was pained. "I don't like your attitude that our religion is the best, you know. I don't approve of that."

"Well, don't you think it's the best?" said Ed. "Why are you in it?"

"No, I don't think it's the best," said Conrad. "I just happen to be in it, that's all. All religions are equal."

"Look, I'm sure every minister in town thinks his religion is the best," said Ed. "At least it stands to reason. Don't you suppose Father Donahue thinks his religion is the best?"

"Sure they do," said Conrad. "That's why they're all equal."

"One religion can't be better than another," Roy Herzlinger said flatly. Ed looked at him. "I should hope that in the twentieth century we'd have gotten beyond that," Roy said. "I mean civilized religions. I don't mean primitive cults."

"They all say the same thing," said Murray Spingarn, taking the cigar from his thick lips. He spoke rapidly.

"That's right," said Phil Walker, not taking the cigarette from his mouth.

"What are you talking about?" said Ed. "All this aggravation for four thousand years, only to say the same thing as everybody else?"

"Sure," said Phil.

Ed stared at Phil a brief instant. "Then what's the point?" he said. "Why don't we bust up, and go out of business? I mean it." He noticed that Amethyst nodded solemnly as he spoke. "If after four thousand years we're only saying the same thing as everyone else it's time to quit. Who needs one more people? Aren't there enough?"

"Well that's a hell of a God damn attitude!" Phil said, taking the cigarette out.

"You *are* much too sectarian," Roy Herzlinger told Ed calmly. "It's an occupational hazard of clergymen, I suppose."

Phil put the cigarette back in his mouth. Ed rubbed his brow and his face. He thought Amethyst looked as if she would weep.

"You've got to simmer down, Ed," Roy continued. "We don't want a prophet Elijah raving by the side of the road. You know, you can't have it both ways. You've been complaining that you feel isolated from the congregation, and on the other hand you claim the right not to conform and to criticize everyone else."

"There is such a thing as being a nice guy, Ed," Conrad said. "There are guys that manage it, in spite of having been to a seminary and everything. They mind their own business, and don't feel they have to bother everybody."

"That's right," said Phil. "You move in here, and right away you're knocking yourself out. What gives? Nobody believes in that crap."

"I disagree," Ed told him. "I think modern knowledge doesn't give less reason for observing religion, but more—that is, better. I mean the modern scholarship that backgrounds it. The relevance is increased, not decreased. And as far as different religions, different traditions are concerned, well, sure there should be more than one in the world. Different slants and points of view. None of us have all the answers. Like it says in Job, we weren't there and we don't know beans about it. But I believe that the world has a meaning and purpose, and that we're part of it. And I've studied this tradition and I believe it's still a rich mine that isn't played out. And if only we'd live up to it, bring it visibly into being, we'd be such a light that the world would be transformed. My grandfather believed that, and I believe it, with all my heart. Because if I don't the world is chaos. This is light and sunshine to me. And if that makes me a nut, put me away, lock me up. It's what I believe."

"You're a fanatic, Ed," said Conrad. "It's okay for the rabbi, but you don't try to impose all this stuff on the whole congregation."

"That's right," said Phil Walker. "It's tough enough to be a Jew without being a religious one on top of it."

"I disagree," said Ed. "I think it's easier to be a Jew when it has a purpose. I mean, immerse yourself, and see for yourself."

"Ed, the trouble with you is, you don't want a religion, you want a way of life," Roy Herzlinger said.

"What I want," Ed answered, "is that it shouldn't be me alone. We should all get interested in what we're supposed to be. So that you don't make a nut out of me, and out of my children. What's the sense in isolating the pastor? You make a nut out of the pastor and what have you got? You haven't got a community, that's for sure."

"You lose sight of one thing, Ed," said Roy. "You're an employee of the congregation."

"That's right," said Phil Walker. "You work for us. And we don't like your sermons, boy."

" 'Boy'?" said Ed.

"Yes, you don't call a rabbi 'boy,' " Conrad reprimanded Phil quietly. "That's way out of line."

"It's dreadful," said Amethyst.

"I don't say a man in the pulpit should be muzzled," said Roy. "Or a schoolteacher either for that matter. I didn't mind what you told the ladies that time, about immortality and that, although some people did. But the role of a clergyman is to be a comforter, isn't it? You've had grief—you should understand that. Well, that wasn't comforting. And did you tell the teen-agers that if your religion doesn't change your personality it's destruction of God? Or something like that?"

"Sure," Ed admitted. "Of course I did. If a religion doesn't do that it's not worth anything. It's less than nothing."

"That's not comforting," said Roy. "What kind of an expression is that—'destruction of God'? And this business of referring to the youth group as the Shloomperdik Generation. My daughter cried when you called them that. That club has a name—the Beth El Wilmerdingians or something like that."

"Ed's marvelous with the children," Amethyst protested.

"Not with all of them," said Roy.

"You can say that," Phil said to Amethyst. "You haven't got any."

"I haven't cared for the emphasis," said Spingarn.

"Another thing, Ed," said Roy. "A lot of us don't like the way you've slighted the late Friday evening service."

"Well, these responsive readings, they bore me," Ed said. "I don't like the translations—they're too bland and they're too pompous. They don't say anything. All they say is 'look at us proper respectable churchgoers.' "

"That's because you're a fanatic, Ed," Sandy Walker said in her high phlegmy voice, and had to stop and clear her throat. "You don't want anything translated. You just want to do everything the old way."

"You've practically put the whole late Friday service over on Bill," Conrad said. "In spite of the fact that it would be our main talking point against those that want to pull out."

Ed heard murmurs of agreement.

"And when Reverend Stillman wanted to bring the Congregationalist kids over to see a temple service," Conrad said, "you steered him away from the late Friday service, and you steered him to the Saturday morning service—you told him it was more authentic. And then you called everybody up and twisted everybody's arm to be sure and come on Saturday morning so the Congregationalists wouldn't show up and see a lousy attendance. Now that wasn't right, Ed. A lot of people resented it. It was just a little underhanded."

"As I said, Ed," Roy cut in again, "no clergyman should be muzzled, but you're our representative. In the eyes of the town you're our spokesman. And you should try to play the part a little more. Now we called you here tonight largely to air our grievances, and see if some meeting of the minds can be found."

"That's it, Ed," said Conrad. He was leaning back now, with his hands on the arms of the wooden chair. "A clergyman has to play the part. You're our spokesman, and we want a spokesman worthy of Wilmerding Crosswalk. This is a nice community. I'd like to see a little more of a saintly demeanor."

"A what?"

"A saintly demeanor. Some people say you don't seem like a clergyman. Like you know Reverend Briggs? He has a saintly demeanor. Last winter he went all over the place to make sure the McGoon family had enough firewood, to keep warm. It's in the way he looks, the way he walks."

"That's right," said Phil Walker. "I don't say you should be Jesus Christ exactly, but you should have a saintly demeanor."

"Yeah," said Sandy, "and what about schnapps in shul, for instance? You want to get old man Brill plastered or something?" The pretty face was round and soft, with blond hair lying about it, but the expression was unfriendly.

"Or take the cigarette, Ed," said Conrad. "I don't say you shouldn't smoke, but at least a pipe would be a different kind of an image, you know what I mean?" Ed grimaced and pressed out the cigarette in the ashtray. "Or riding the fire engine in shirt sleeves," Conrad said. "The fireman thing is okay in principle but it makes you a character. It's a matter of dignity. Father Donahue's a character, with his bicycle, but that's different. That has a simple charm. He's a character with finesse."

"Well, it wouldn't really be good to get out of the firemen right now," Ed said, "at least until this danger of brush fires is over. Until the woods get a little wetter. They could need every man. And I've enjoyed it as a way to keep fit. If you believe in reverence for life, a corollary is keeping fit."

"Well, keep fit some other way," said Sandy.

"Ed, I don't object to the firemen," said Conrad, "that's not important. It's your whole spirit, the impression you give. Ed, a word to the wise. You have to play the part."

"Maybe you can straighten up and fly right," said Phil.

"And you wouldn't even let them boil water in the temple for coffee Friday night," said Sandy. "You've got some religion, if you think schnapps is more religious than coffee. I'd like you to show me where it says that." She cleared her throat.

There was a little silence.

"I know you're not happy with us either," said Conrad. "I don't know if you've put lines out for a job elsewhere."

"I haven't, no."

"Well, we've made no decision either. It's just good to get the air cleared."

"I'm sorry if I've hurt any feelings in the past year," Ed told him. "Or offended people here and there."

"Well, maybe some meeting of the minds can still be found," Conrad answered. "I don't know. I hope so. Maybe we should adjourn and sleep on it. I'm sorry we didn't have the full board here."

"Ed," Roy Herzlinger said, still settled back and a bit to the side in his chair in his authoritative way, "is it true that one of our members asked you 'what's the message today,' or something like that, and you told him you weren't a Western Union boy?"

"Well, that was Dr. Yarrish."

"And do you think it's good to be flippant like that?"

"Well, I didn't know what to say to him. Every time he'd see me he'd wave, and 'hi, rabbi, what's the message today?' I'd buy him a copy of the Sayings of the Fathers if I thought he was serious. I don't walk around with a head full of nuggets. These things are in context for me. Let him go look at the today's-special sign in front of Folger's church."

"Let's go," said Burton Seligman.

The meeting broke up with a scraping of chairs. They walked out together into the cool of the dusk, and began to spread a little toward parked cars.

"Well, let's hope it's the beginning of a new and improved relationship," said Conrad. "We haven't been the ideal congregation either. I admit it."

"Good night, Ed," said Roy Herzlinger, with a little wave. He was walking diagonally across the lawn.

Others said good night.

Amethyst Gilbert offered Ed a ride. He said he felt like walking. But he held the door of her car for her as she got in. It was a big convertible with a white roof, and new, not the one he had ridden in before. A branch of maple hung low over it. He heard another of the cars start off.

She looked up at him. Her window was down all the way.

"Ed, I'm just mortified. I don't know what to say. They're such fools. They don't appreciate you and they don't understand you."

He said nothing.

"I'm pulling for you," she said. She smiled up at him sadly.

He smiled back.

"Ed, there's just one criticism I heard from one of the Sparkstown Heights crowd that seemed valid to me, so I'll pass it along. The children spend so much time learning to daven that they can't cover history properly. Don't you think there's a point there? After all, there's four thousand years of history to cover."

He nodded thoughtfully.

She gave him her hand and he felt a little squeeze. Then she started the motor quickly, one white glove on and one off, and put on the headlights. He could not tell for certain in the twilight and behind her upswept glasses, but he thought her eyes seemed moist.

He began to walk home, unhappily. The sky was purplish.

He was not sure how much the feelings of the executive board represented the congregation as a whole. And Burt Seligman was a strange one. He had smiled affably and hardly said a word throughout the meeting.

Ed was dissatisfied with his own accomplishments as a leader. One should be a scholar, and when you become a man with something to say, being a leader should follow from that. But he had done badly.

Should he have thought to fetch loads of firewood like Ralph Briggs? He hadn't known that anyone in this town heated a home with wood. He had always gone out of his way for the crippled peddler, giving him rides to his customers, and telling Lucinda always to buy whenever he came to the house, even if it was hard to find something useful in his satchels that she had not already bought from him before. It was for the man's pride mostly, to let him feel he was working. That poor man must creep with his satchels for hours without making a sale.

How does one play a part? You set an example by being a person, not by playing a part. They wanted him to be a sanctimonious country parson, he thought. A decoration, like the Civil War monument. How could you give in to that? The Law was for the real world, or it was nothing at all. The world in which our daughters get laid.

As he neared his house the branches had grown quite black. A fading tint of day still lingered in the sky but some stars were out.

Even Amethyst's criticism, delivered out of hearing of the others, seemed now not to be valid, though he had thought at the time a reasonable point had been scored against him, and he had not known how to answer.

But he saw it now. She had said learning to daven, he realized, and by using the old Yiddish word, with its acquisition of musty connotations, she had tricked him. She had made it sound obscurantist. If she had said learning to pray, it would have sounded quite different.

And who, actually, were the obscurantists? Men who prayed? Or historians who could not?

That's how he should have answered her. To be able to join men who pray, and recognize where they are in the book, and be at home—that's something. To study history, you have to ask, history of what? But if you can pray, it's your history.

He hadn't been wrong. People want roots, he thought, but roots have to be in the prayer book. What's roots? A house? A homestead? What's a house, when the chips are down? Even when you're safe from flood, war, revolution and the Nazis, where are you? Your career can move you. Or you can beautify the place and rebuild your grandfather's grape arbor, and the Turnpike Authority could come along and bulldoze you out by eminent domain. The prayer book has to be your house.

As for history, when you sing those wild beseechings again, you are history. You were there.

What was so bad about praying, davening? They talk of hypocrites, he thought, but he had known people who kept up with their daily prayers, and they had been good people. The effect of praying, and the purpose of praying, were to bring it home to you that you aren't God.

He walked up the winding dirt driveway. He could see Lucinda waiting for him on the porch. She would ask how the meeting went, and he would have to say not good. And that he'd forgotten to bring up the subject of tenure and pension.

When he got close he could make out that her face was sour. She looked worried.

"Did you insult everybody?" she asked him.

61

Millicent had made her entry into the house as quietly as possible, hoping to wake no one. She had asked the taxi driver from the Sparkstown depot not to go up the dirt driveway, and she went up the staircase slowly in darkness, leaning on the banister and stopping when a stair creaked. The ticking of the carved clock was the only other sound. Even Patty's breathing was silent.

No one woke. There were some pajamas she still kept here, in the curved white bureau. She was not sure she could find them in the dark, but the moon had risen and shone in the window by the head of the iron cot. She pulled open the drawer carefully, lest it make a noise. She tried, squinting and feeling, but could not find her pajamas among Patty's things. She would have to sleep in the nude again. She got onto the cot with the greatest of care, lest it squeak. She pulled the blanket over her head. Her heart was pounding.

Yet she slept. In daylight she was awakened by the quacking from the duck farm and a squirrel on the window sill. The squirrel leapt back to a branch. Then she heard Roland preparing to go out on his paper route, making whistling noises which he punctuated with Bronx cheers. A door slammed downstairs and she heard him outdoors.

She remained still, her head half covered by the blanket.

When Patty wakened Millicent feigned sleep. She heard Patty's gasp of surprise, and when she heard Patty's quick footsteps she knew it was to tell her parents that she was there.

She knew when her mother looked in at the door. She continued to pretend sleeping, hoping to put off conversation and explanation as long as possible.

They went down to breakfast without having bothered her, and after they left for the temple she slept again.

When they came back her mother asked only if she were all right, and she answered yes.

Her family had lunch with her almost in a respectful silence. She was surprised that they did not pry more. She had been prepared to tell them that she had decided to look for an apartment of her own, and that she had decided that the girls' place was much too crowded, and nothing more. Eventually she volunteered this much without having been asked.

They did not mention Leslie and neither did she. She did not tell them that

Barbie Chisholm had thrown her out. But she told about Mrs. Hoyt, and she said her cat had run away.

After lunch she telephoned the Boston newspapers and placed new advertisements, asking anybody who found her cat to telephone Wilmerding Crosswalk collect. She told her mother that the old oriental rug was still at the girls' place. But she was relieved when her mother showed no interest in picking it up. Her mother said it wasn't worth anything anyway.

Millicent and Patty tidied their room together. They worked at opposite sides of each bed, pulling the sheets taut and stuffing them under the mattress. She knew that Patty kept trying to meet her eyes.

"Have you left him for good?" Patty asked in a low voice.

Millicent tucked the sheet with efficiency, not answering. She felt herself redden a little at the ears. As the silence continued Patty reddened also. Patty kept working and did not repeat the question.

Millicent took a walk afterward, in order to be alone. The crab-apple trees had blossomed pink-white, and a few petals came down on the breeze like snow. The yellow forsythia was out and the lilacs were just beginning, their clusters still tight and reddish, not the powdery lavender yet. The flowering crab-apple trees especially caught her eye, but she wanted to be away from the house, so she walked through the woods behind the house and down by the marshes. Especially as the woods got thick toward the water she could hear many birds, though she didn't see any. There was at least one single-noted one that kept calling, and lots of twitterers. The leaves were still small and pale. The mixture of live grass and dead was soft under her feet, but a nervousness kept her from enjoying it.

She looked down between the railroad ties at the water, and pushed pebbles with her foot, making them splash. The brook was slow-moving and black here.

She went back to the house restlessly, but it was not time for the bus to the depot yet. She went up to the iron cot and lay on the spread. Her eye fixed on Patty's torn teddy bear, which sat on the big bureau reflecting in the mirror. Outside her window Bobby O'Shaughnessy and Roland were climbing about and talking on the kitchen roof. She heard a fragment of slate slide down to the rain gutter. She heard Roland telling Bobby that any time he wanted to get even with his father for something all he had to do was sneak over to Bobby's or some place and eat a ham sandwich.

"Isn't it supposed to be a sin though?" she heard Bobby say.

"That's okay—until I'm thirteen all my sins go on my father."

"You mean like the time we busted Slaney's winda?" said Bobby. "That goes against your father?"

"Sure."

"Gee."

Patty came in, and shouted through the window for the boys to get off the roof.

"We weren't spying on ya," Roland said.

"I didn't say you were! But you're not supposed to be there! Go on!"

Millicent heard the sounds of their clambering down, while Patty watched, and at last the thuds as they jumped.

Patty sat on her bed and talked to Millicent, seeming to want to be friendly. She did not refer to Leslie again, but Millicent was cautious.

Patty told her that Lucinda said prayers for Charles and had been to the cemetery a couple of times. She said they had a Gold Star hanging in the living-room window now. Millicent said she had seen it. Patty said they had a Purple Heart medal too, and that it was in Charles's room.

On the little brown bus and on the train she kept trying not to think of Les.

In the city room that afternoon the noises of the place seemed especially oppressive—the incessant jumpiness of the teletypes and their blinking lights, the unrhythmic, patternless clack made by frowning men at typewriters—the unmodulated harshness of the ringing telephones. She kept carrying copy from Mr. Hopkins's basket up to Valentino, reading snatches of it from habit. The stories were about nothing—sometimes there was an effort at folksiness, and occasionally a hopped-up jazziness—yet all of it sounded as though written mechanically by men who didn't care.

It was strange how drab and empty her whole life seemed, now that Les was out of it, even things that had seemed to have nothing to do with him.

She did the routine errands, and had a sandwich for supper at the spa. It seemed to her that eating alone was even drearier than sleeping alone. She was not really ready to have an apartment all by herself, she thought.

She returned to the city room but was sent to the spa again to get a sandwich and coffee for Mr. Hopkins and for some of the others. Mr. Alpert never said thank you to her these days, but took his coke and his change silently, glancing at her sourly if at all.

Mr. Hopkins sent her home a little bit early but not quite early enough, so she had to wait a long time at the rail terminal. The concourse was dimly lit at this hour, and huge and empty. In the bigness, hollowness and silence she thought she felt drafts. Its shops and stands were closed. The wood benches were hard, and when she walked back and forth a little her footsteps echoed. At a distance two Negroes worked with mops and pails.

The train turned out to be lit dimly also. She sat upon a hard convex seat of woven cane, alone in a car that swayed. It seemed never to have been swept. The engine burned soft coal and the air had a taste. From the window she could see only blackness, or occasionally, slow-moving, the side of some long shed that had not been designed for beauty. The train whistle kept mourning.

How do you put meaning into a life that has none, she wondered? Where do you begin? Should she study law? It seemed now only something else to fail at.

When she got home the luggage from Mrs. Hoyt's was by her cot. She thought Patty was asleep, but while she was undressing Patty suddenly spoke to her.

"Hi," Patty said.

"What are you doing awake?"

"I had a date," Patty said.

Millicent kept preparing for bed in the darkness.

"Come and sleep in my bed," Patty said. "With me."

"No."

"Why?"

"Because."

"Because you sleep bare?"

"I don't sleep bare. Just because. I have my bed and you have yours."

Millicent went to the bathroom and came back. She settled in the cot.

"Hey," said Patty.

"What."

"Nothing."

"Go to sleep," said Millicent. The blanket was up to her ears.

"Let's talk," Patty said. "You know. About things."

"No thank you."

"We ought to be able to talk more. Other sisters talk to each other and everything. Confide things. And we never do. We're the only ones."

Millicent didn't answer.

"Your sister should be your best friend," said Patty.

"It's very late," said Millicent, without turning. "It's time to sleep."

Patty was quiet only a moment.

"You'll be sorry. Charles is dead, and you're driving your only sister away, and someday you'll want someone to confide in, and there won't be anybody."

"You'd be a fine one to confide in. After that letter."

"It wasn't my fault," Patty said. "I couldn't help it. What would you have done?"

"I certainly wouldn't have done what you did."

"But what could I do? I didn't know what was gonna be in it. It was so spooky. I thought maybe I should burn it. Slow, you know—like you're supposed to do when a flag wears out? And then I thought maybe I should send it back, with 'expired' or something written on it. Or bury it. I think there's something called the dead-letter office but I didn't know who to ask."

"Your instinct to burn it would have been the best thing you could have done."

"Well, but how could I? It was like Charles's ghost was trying to tell me something, and I wasn't letting him."

"It wasn't even addressed to you."

"I know. That's just it. I didn't even have a right to burn it."

"It was addressed to Dad," Millicent said. "And so you went and opened it and read it, and then you showed it to Mother."

"How could I show it to Dad?" Patty said. "You can't discuss a thing like that with your father. And I didn't know if you were in trouble or what. I was trying to spare him. Shouldn't I spare him?"

"You might have given it to me, if you were so concerned."

"You weren't even home. See, that's what I mean. That's why we should confide. If we'd been confiding it wouldn't have happened. About the letter, I mean."

"You're going to wake up the whole house."

"Oh, they're asleep," said Patty. But after another moment she slipped her feet from her bed and tiptoed in her nightgown to the door. She peered in the darkness. "They're asleep," she said again. But she closed the door. Her bed squeaked as she got back into it.

"Does Roland know?" Millicent asked.

"Why?"

"Does he know?" Millicent repeated.

"I don't know. I don't think so."

"He kept staring at me at lunch," Millicent said.

Patty adjusted herself in the bed and it squeaked again. Then there was a silence. Millicent tried to let herself grow sleepy.

"Were you in love with him?" Patty said suddenly.

"Patty, will you stop?"

"What's the matter with that?"

Millicent didn't answer.

"I think that's your trouble, you know it?" Patty said. "You never confide. You never had girl friends. You're too lonely."

There was another silence.

"You know what?" Patty said. "I'm gonna start telling you everything, just like I tell Polly. Even if you don't ever tell me a thing."

"I'm really not interested."

"You really ought to be an older sister to me, and guide me and everything," Patty said. "So I don't make the same mistakes."

Millicent wondered how she could quiet her. She thought of threatening to tell their parents that Patty wouldn't let her sleep. But it seemed foolish.

"Do you mean to say if I had a question I wanted to ask I couldn't feel free to come to you?" Patty said.

"All right, when you have a question you ask it, but right now let me sleep. It must be going on three in the morning, for goodness sakes."

"Well let me ask just one question then, and then I'll go to sleep."

"What?"

Patty paused only a moment. "Did you do it every night?" she asked.

"Look—Patty—for goodness sakes!"

"Well you said I could ask."

"I didn't mean stupid things."

"Well I didn't know it was stupid."

"For one thing don't go assuming things," Millicent said, her voice quavering. "You don't have to believe something just because somebody put it in a letter."

"Oh, come on. I'm not naïve. I just want to ask a couple of questions, like how he persuaded you to do it, and if you were scared the first time."

"Now shut up!" Millicent said. "I insist!"

"Aw, a fine one you are," Patty said. "You're just a big prude. I didn't think you'd still be a prude after a thing like that. And then you wonder why nobody's ever on your side. You always want to be stuck up and high hat with everybody. Even your own family. You are. You're not a friendly person. You don't have any warmth. That's really true, and everybody knows it. And I'll tell you one thing, I may not be a little genius like you but I'll never cause hurt to my parents the way you did. Especially after losing Charles."

Millicent felt outraged to the point of tears. She wanted to say that Patty had already caused them hurt, by showing them that letter, but she knew she couldn't speak just then without bursting into sobs. She felt like setting upon Patty with her fists. But Patty was bigger and had the worse temper.

"How could you be so weak?" Patty said.

Millicent buried herself in the blanket, determined to say nothing more.

In the morning she found herself unable to sleep late, and went down to share breakfast with her parents. Roland was out delivering the Sunday papers. Patty came down to breakfast too, sleepy-eyed. Millicent avoided looking at her.

Patty said she would probably make about twenty-eight hundred mistakes at the organ and that she hoped Mr. Briggs wouldn't notice. Lucinda said that if she wanted to keep the job she shouldn't stay out so late.

There was talk of Patty's date and of the movie she had seen. She had been with a boy named Paul Wernick, and Millicent gathered that her parents knew the boy's parents. Patty began humming a song in the midst of breakfast, even while she put fish in her mouth.

"You're a sinnin' little bugger,
You're the worst kid in school—"

"Don't sing when you eat," Lucinda reprimanded her.

Patty asked if when she got done at Saint Tim's she could have lunch with Polly Cook and go horseback riding.

"No," said Lucinda. "I've planned a good dinner, and Grandma Annie's coming. You can go some other time. You know how I feel about horseback riding anyway."

Patty muttered a four-letter word under her breath, apparently intending it not to be audible or recognizable, but it was, as though by miscalculation. Ed looked darkly at Patty from under his eyebrows, but kept eating. Patty reddened a little.

"What!" Lucinda cried out furiously. "What! What did you say?"

"Nothing," Patty mumbled.

"Don't tell me nothing! I heard what you said! You should go to your room for the day, that's what I think! Organ or no organ! Where do you get that stuff, I'd like to know. Such language. Do you hear me talk like that? What if Roland walked in just then?"

"He knows worse than that," Patty mumbled.

"Oh yes! I bet he does! And if he does he better not let me hear it. Did you talk like that to Paul last night? He wouldn't think much of you if you did, I can tell you that. Does Polly talk like that? Does Denise talk like that?"

Patty was red-faced. "Nope," she said.

"Aren't you going to speak to her?" Lucinda said to Ed. "Haven't you got anything to say to her?"

"Well," he said, "I think we should have a minute of silence, in solemn memory of the standards of decent speech that used to prevail at this breakfast table."

"You watch your step," Lucinda said to Patty. "You're growing up just a little too fast to suit me, young lady."

"Don't worry about me," said Patty. "I'm not weak." She took another piece of food, finished her breakfast, and left the table.

Millicent went walking again, to avoid her mother. Along the path in the woods, by rocks, she counted in all five yellow-gray translucent skins discarded by snakes. At the swamp some new flowers had blossomed and stood in the water. She made an imaginary conversation with Leslie about them. She found a crawling turtle on the railroad's gravel embankment. It was black and hump-shelled, and nearly as big as her hand. She carried it down to the mud and the moss.

When she got back she saw Grandma Annie's car parked before the porch with its crumpled fender. Yet she did not go directly to the house. She massaged the old dog's head for some minutes in the barn.

She stood on the porch glider a while for a better view of the nestlings.

In the kitchen she found her mother, blowing her nose and red-eyed as though she had been weeping. Grandma Annie was saying she couldn't see how civilized people could live without a television. Millicent greeted her grandmother, who reached up as if to pinch her cheek, without rising from the chair, but Millicent leaned away. Her grandmother gave her a light spank. She found herself a chair. She knew these conversations—her grandmother would say that Ed's salary wasn't high enough and criticize their economies. But this time her mother was saying that Ed was too religious and that the congregation didn't like him.

"Well," said Grandma Annie, "the way I figure it, religion's for the old folks, and I'm not old enough yet." She cackled a flat laugh.

Millicent went upstairs and began to sort and put away the things her father had brought back from Mrs. Hoyt's. The ivory figure and its broken arm she put carefully on the dresser, and allowed no other object within inches of it. But she hadn't finished sorting when it was time to go to her job.

The train ride to Boston, and the slow hours in the clack of the city room, and the cavernous train terminal at midnight, and the night train to the Sparkstown depot were dismal again, and she kept thinking of Les.

She found Patty asleep this time.

It seemed to her now, as she lay in bed, that with Leslie in her blankets it had been much easier to sleep. It was not the lust; what she missed was just the knowing that he was nearby. If they had been tired, or if he had been asleep when she had arrived, she had been able to shut her eyes and drop into a dreamless slumber at will, without having touched him or having been touched by him. Simply because he was in the bed. The presence of the sleeping Leslie had somehow told her who she was, and put boundaries on the world. And now her bed had again a strange insomnia, that she had used to know. Alone in bed, the night seemed boundless, and you started to be uncertain who you are. Alone the night is nerve-wracking, she thought; the body sleeping beside you quiets it.

She admitted to herself wet-eyed that this had been a true love, or could have been, or should have been. And at the first impatience on his part she had angrily let it go to pieces. Or maybe she had had no choice. She had the feeling that to go to him now and apologize would accomplish nothing. It seemed to her that he really didn't want her around there any more and showing up would only make another scene. Would it be good to wait a month, and then try to go to him cheerfully? That probably wouldn't work either. And if it didn't, she would have to accept that she had lost him.

They should at least be able to be polite to each other, and perhaps write occasionally. She did not want them to be enemies forever.

What was better, to marry one's true love and be disillusioned with him later, she wondered, or to lose one's true love, and have to marry a poor substitute years later, and keep the illusion? Her own parents had never really known a true love, she thought.

And she had nothing to remember him by. Her brother Charles had given her that beautiful ivory, and the bayonet. And she still had Malcolm's perfume bottle, even though Barbie had wasted most of it, and the short-eared racing rabbit was still in its hutch out back. It was only Leslie who had given her nothing. How odd it was, that she had not one object from him. True, he was miserably poor. Yet he never brought a knickknack from the five-and-dime, or a curiosity in a bottle from the hospital. Even their little outings had been dutch, and she had bought their groceries and paid the laundry. He had spent more than he could afford in order for them to be happy together—the rent itself, and especially the motor scooter. But on her directly, never a penny that she could remember. It was a peculiarity of his nature, perhaps. Yet she had never given him anything either. It had been that kind of relationship. They gave only themselves.

It seemed to her that on that final morning she had told him she hated him—that he stunk. Where had she gotten such a foul tongue? Maybe he had even taken it literally—that he had some hospital smell she detested. She wished she could remember for sure if she had really said that or not.

And why had her parents had to know? Girls do that all the time, and their parents never know.

She was like her parents, born to be one of these people for whom things never work out, she thought. Look at her father—his career had brought him no satisfaction.

The next morning her mother asked her if she would like to have Charles's room for her own. She was surprised, as Patty had said her mother had been keeping the room as a sort of mausoleum.

It was smaller and narrower than the one she had shared with Patty, but that didn't matter. It also had two windows, and one looked out on the slate roof of the porch. She saw that it had a view of Mrs. Davey's two horses in the pasture. There was no mirror and no chair.

She went through the drawers preparatory to bringing in her own things. There were civilian shirts and socks that had belonged to Charles. But they took little room and she thought she could leave them there, under her own things, for the present. Nor did she disturb the Purple Heart medal that someone had placed on the bureau top, in the middle of a lace scarf. She squeezed his suits to the side of the closet. Below them she saw the cardboard box of his effects that the Air Force had sent. It was opened, but it looked as if nothing had been taken out. Among the contents she could see the binoculars she had given him.

Her mother came with a pail and cloths and said she would help her clean the windows. They set to work, each on a window.

"Be careful," Lucinda said.

Millicent noticed how lined her mother's face was. Her eyes were bloodshot. She looked somehow much older than Millicent had ever seen her before. Not depressed, but busy, with eyes focused on the windowpane—yet lines of sadness seemed to have settled permanently into her face, even though the sunlight fell on it. She opened the window and reached with her cloth to its outside surfaces. A fresh outdoor breeze swept the room.

Lucinda spoke of how Millicent could fix the room with curtains to suit her taste, and so on.

"It's only temporary," Millicent said. "Until I find a decent place."

Her mother didn't look from her work, but Millicent saw the lips tighten.

"I should think you'd have learned your lesson."

"Mother, let's not discuss it, please."

"All right, let's not discuss it." Lucinda concentrated on the window. "I don't know, you've got your own ideas—I can't talk to you."

"Mother, it's different generations. I can't explain it to you."

"What can't you explain? That if a man and a woman want to be lovers, go and live together, it's perfectly all right?"

Millicent said nothing. But she knew she had reddened. For a while there was no sound but the squeak of rags on glass. Millicent adjusted her window and stood on the sill. Her hair hung forward and the air cooled her bare forearm.

"At least the neighbors don't know," her mother said. "And the family doesn't know." Millicent knew she meant aunts and cousins.

"I refuse to feel ashamed."

"No, go out and brag. My modern daughter. You're still in love with him. You just won't admit he made a fool of you."

62

When Lucinda had readied herself for the general membership meeting she looked to Ed more stylish than he had seen her in a very long time, as though she wished to put aside the spirit of mourning and make the best possible impression on the congregation. She had spent much time arranging her hair in a new way, pulled up, with braids woven around in a kind of disc on the back of her head. She had some make-up, and she had worked at the dining-room sewing machine to improve the modishness of a dress from the closet.

But her expression was pensive and cheerless when she came down the porch steps to the old Plymouth. He sat at the wheel, watching her. But she arranged herself in the car almost without looking at Ed, and they rode off saying nothing, down over the pebbles of the dirt drive and then under the soaring foliage of Massapeequit Road.

"Well," Ed said after a while, "this congregation's no bargain. Maybe I shouldn't have come here. I think I overestimated the congregation, or overestimated my own talents, or something."

"You wouldn't like any congregation, and I like this house," she answered without turning. "I don't want to move again."

"I like the house too," he said.

"Don't get fired then."

He understood her feeling. He had gotten used to the twittering of forest birds, and the quacking of Mrs. Godkin's ducks, and the feeling of knowing one's neighbors. To start all over with moving-van men, and excelsior, and a strange neighborhood—it was unbearable; it was to be avoided.

They rode the rest of the way without conversation, around two sides of the common and up Muckanaug Street. There were a lot of cars, parked along both curbs, and more arriving, and all the windows of the temple were lighted.

Ed and Lucinda mingled with other arrivals, on the walk and in the large vestibule, where a buffet supper had been set up on some folding tables, and Ed saw that Lucinda at once became smiling and gracious. He said hello to one or two people and tried to keep occupied with a cup of coffee. People stood around holding paper plates and nibbling and socializing a long time, and again and again he made small talk. But he was intending to ask for the floor in the meeting and speak a little in his own behalf, and his thoughts now were mostly of what he meant to say. He hoped to explain what his purposes had been—that he had tried to convey some inkling of the moral society, and of the role a particular people is obligated to play in helping to bring it among men. He wanted to say that he believed it was not preposterous, but eminently practical and possible.

There were many people, and more kept coming. Some had drifted into the pews, even with their plates and forks. After some time Ed moved into one of the pews and sat waiting for the meeting to begin. He heard some already urging that they get started. Lucinda came and sat beside him. When he looked about he guessed that more than half the membership had shown up.

The little speaker's lectern that usually stood at the side had been moved to the center, and Conrad Bernstein rapped his gavel upon it. He seemed to Ed a tense, nervous man. The forehead that rose high over the long thin face to the brown dry hair had many lines across it. He raised a hand, cleared his throat, and straightened the bow tie. Near him there was a card table, and Sandy Walker sat at it in her careless lounging way, tapping a pencil idly against a notebook. Conrad thanked the committee that had prepared the food, and asked the people who were sitting further back in scattered little groups to move closer.

He asked Sandy to read the minutes of the last membership meeting, and she stood, giving her head a quick toss to move some curling tresses away from her face. She began to read, with many long and troublesome throat clearings. Her voice as always sounded on the verge of laryngitis.

She had a remarkable shape, Ed thought.

Murray Spingarn read a treasurer's report, with a rapid deep voice and thick lips, about the mortgage, and cake sale and rummage sale, and the sinking fund, the salaries of rabbi and cantor, and so many dollars and cents for this and that repair and so on. Ed felt jumpy and impatient and could not listen. Next someone gave a report of the nominating committee and all the officers were re-elected without opposition by a voice vote. Somebody made a motion that Sandy cast a unanimous ballot and this was carried.

"Do you get a gold watch after twenty-five years, Connie?" someone said to Bernstein, and there was mild laughter.

"He gets to keep the gavel," someone else said.

"He gets hit in the head with it," another man joked.

Then Conrad made a speech, fingering the gavel, and thanked various committees, and outlined the progress he expected Temple Beth El to make in the next two years.

At length he paused and looked down woodenly at the page of notes on the lectern. Then he coughed into his hand and said the next item of agenda was the rabbi's contract.

Amethyst Gilbert rose and asked if she might be heard, but Conrad asked if she wanted to make a motion and told her he wasn't ready to entertain motions just yet. He found the faces of Ed and Lucinda and asked if they preferred to leave at this point. Ed answered without rising that they would just as soon stay, since they were members after all.

Conrad coughed again, his face without expression. He asked if there was any old business to come before the meeting. Amethyst rose again but he told her that if she intended to make a motion about Ed that came under new business. Then, looking out blankly over the gathering, he asked if there was any new business.

"I move that Ed's contract be renewed, with permanent tenure," Amethyst said.

Conrad began to say something but meanwhile one or two people said seconded, and a man near the back moved that the contract not be renewed. That was also seconded. Conrad said he wouldn't entertain the second motion as there ought to be a simple motion that the contract be renewed, as it would be easiest to vote on it first in that form, without reference to tenure. He said that and Amethyst's motion could be discussed together. Somebody made the motion and a few other voices said seconded. Conrad asked if Amethyst's motion had been seconded and several people said it had. Someone asked what about the cantor's contract, and Conrad said that would be a separate item of business. One or two other voices had begun interrupting to answer in the same way and ended by saying sure, in agreement with Conrad, as he finished the sentence.

"May I be heard?" Amethyst said, standing very straight. Her hat had a little veil that stopped short of the tip of her nose.

Ed sat looking at his hands, and sometimes at Lucinda's hands, while he heard Conrad let Amethyst come to the lectern to speak on the motions, and while he listened to her speak in his behalf. Amethyst did not speak well, he thought, but there was emotion in her voice. She talked five minutes or more, praising Ed for his sincerity, and saying it was the membership that had let him down. She said he was one of the finest men she had ever known. Next Conrad gave the floor to a man named Garfield, who did not come to the lectern but spoke from his place, about halfway back, hitching up his belt and shifting from one foot to the other. "I think we have to bear in mind," he said, "that we aren't in any position to expect a top-caliber man. You have to remember that if Ed were a top-caliber man he wouldn't be here. He'd be down in New York, or Boston at least, Newton. You want a top man and you have to pay for it. And we can't afford it. For nine grand a year you can't expect the Archbishop of Canterbury." He went on in this vein, seeming to be on Ed's side, yet always in a backhanded way. When he was done Murray Spingarn spoke, outlining some of the general complaints against Ed. He said that Ed was unregenerate and unrepentant, or at least he had seemed so when the executive board had met with him. Then a man named London rose on the far side, speaking in a forceful and angry way. "When a man talks about fighting Arabs," he said, "I know what he's talking about. And when a man talks about building a hospital in Boston for all races and creeds, I know what he's talking about. But when a man starts talking about God, and all that kind of stuff, I don't know what he's talking about." There was a scattering of applause. It struck Ed that almost any view could win some applause if it were expressed with enough vehemence. He turned to look at the speaker, though he avoided looking at Lucinda. It was a man he had seen at services scarcely more than once. The man kept talking. "I'll tell you what I believe in," he said finally. "I believe in Wilmerding Crosswalk. And I believe in Temple Beth El." This brought some more applause, though not everyone joined in it.

"He's right," a little old bald man down front said, without rising.

"You're out of order, Mr. Gottlieb," Conrad told him. "The chair has the floor."

"Joe London has the floor," someone said.

"I'm sorry, I thought Joe sat down," said Conrad. "Have you sat down, Joe?"

"I've sat down," said London.

A stout lady with glasses then talked a while, saying that one of Ed's daughters was the organist at the Episcopal church and that that was very good for public relations. She said that the fact that Ed and Lucinda had lost a son in Korea was also very good for public relations. She sounded to Ed as though she favored him. But then as she went on she said that inasmuch as he had had a tragedy in his family recently people should make allowances, and understand if he tended to be blunt with people. And at last she said that while Ed was free to say what he wants, the congregation was also free to get another man. It was a free market. And that was the purpose of a trial period without tenure. She said in her opinion the fact was that Ed hadn't worked out.

"He has worked out," Amethyst cut in. "The kids love him and that's the main thing."

"It's not the main thing—" the stout lady began.

"No, it's not," said Ed.

"You're all out of order," said Conrad, rapping the gavel. He asked the stout lady to cut her remarks short, and asked everyone to keep it short and give everybody a chance.

"May I be heard?" Amethyst said again, rising.

"Not now, you've had a chance," Conrad said.

Joe London stood up again, his mouth open, and Conrad told him also to let others have their say, but then the man next to London rose, addressing Conrad as Mr. President, and said a point of order took precedence and that this was a point of order. He said he wanted to raise the question of whether it was right for Ed and Lucinda to be here, in this discussion. "It isn't fair," he said. "In any shul I ever belonged to the rabbi cleared out, to give us a chance to rip him up the back. Anything we say here he's gonna get wind of it anyhow, but at least people should be able to talk."

"He's a member," said Conrad.

"He's not a member," said the man. "He's an employee."

"Regardless of employment," said Ed, turning in the direction of the man but not rising, "I live in the community, I attend services. I'm a member."

"Mr. President, I make a motion the vote should be by secret ballot," Mr. Brill said in his accent and his phlegmy voice, rising.

"Nah, we'll be here all night," someone said.

"Sit down," said someone else.

Mr. Brill looked about him. Conrad rapped his gavel. "You're out of order," said Conrad.

"Do you pay dues?" the man with the point of order asked Ed.

"Let's not split hairs," somebody said.

"I get free dues as part of my salary," Ed answered the man.

"Naw, naw," said another man.

"Let's not bicker about that," said Conrad. "Actually I didn't expect to see Ed here, but I'd say technically he's a member. And Lucinda. The question before the house is whether they should sit in on a discussion of this kind."

"I make a motion he don't sit in," said London.

"Seconded," said someone else.

"Please, let's not get carried away," said Amethyst. "That motion's not in order, is it?"

"Let's blow," Ed said to Lucinda in a low voice, putting his hand on hers.

They rose and found their way sideways along the pew. He kept his head down. He knew Lucinda was red-faced. There was applause, which spread, and he knew that it was intended in support of him in a general way, that it was not directed at his leaving. But he looked at no one, and outside in the night he could scarcely look at Lucinda.

In the car she wept, nearly silently. He said nothing. He felt that he was another of those who had let her down, who had disappointed her, like Charles and Millicent. He sensed that she felt his humiliation but was also angry with him, and that she would not want his comforting. He did nevertheless try once to take her hand but she withdrew it.

She made herself some tea when they got home. Ed wandered restlessly outdoors. There was a moon. The breeze carried the swamp noises to him, the high-pitched chorus of young frogs. The grass grew rapidly in May. He had cut it Sunday and it was beginning to feel long again. A mosquito sounded near his ear.

He returned to the house, thinking he ought to be the one to answer the phone if it rang.

Lucinda had gone upstairs to lie down. A forearm rested across her eyes, as though she had a headache. He asked if she wanted anything. She said no.

He tried to busy himself in the study, with books. It seemed a very long time, but at last he heard the kitchen telephone and went to it.

Amethyst told him they had voted not to renew his contract. She sounded very upset and there were tears in her voice. The vote had been extremely close, and they had needed a count of hands. But a miss is as good as a mile, he thought. The closeness surprised him; before the meeting he had expected renewal, but he had come away from the meeting feeling that sentiment against him had risen shockingly high. Amethyst said it was perfectly horrible, and that the way some of the members had spoken in his presence was disgraceful. She said they were rude. She burst out blubbering and he tried to soothe her on the phone. She said he was so misunderstood. He told her that everyone is misunderstood.

She said they would never again have such a capable man, and that her heart bled for him. And for Lucinda and the children also, she added. Lucinda came into the kitchen and looked at him questioningly while he stood with the phone at his ear. He pointed with his thumb downward. Lucinda's lips parted a little and she nodded ever so slightly. He saw her eyes moisten. In the receiver at his ear Amethyst's voice continued. She began to tell him who had spoken for him and against him after his departure. Fox, Raphael, Bookbinder, Robinson, Brody, Tobias, Citron, Thau, Marder, Sonnenschein, Diamond, Springer, Wise, Rottenberg— Lucinda turned and left the room. It was striking, he thought, as he listened to Amethyst, how many strong opinions were held by people who never came to services. Some had complained of little incidents he had nearly forgotten or could not remember at all. One had accused him of having said he did not believe in the supernatural, and Ed did recall that he had said that whatever is and whatever happens is natural. And yet those who said he was too old-fashioned and took religion too seriously and those who said he was too atheistic seemed somehow to agree with one another, or at least to approve of one another's remarks, as far as he could tell. Amethyst kept him on the phone a long time, giving her opinions of his detractors, and recalling more and more details to tell him. Some had mentioned the possibility of a split and said they weren't big enough yet to afford competition, and someone had said the Squegantum crowd were mostly very young and didn't have enough money to start a temple, and someone else had said don't be too sure. Somebody had called Ed a wise guy. Somebody else said he was going to be frank and let the chips fall where they may. Someone bawled out the congregation for poor attendance and for not giving Ed support, but it was someone who never attended either. Mr. Brill had made a speech in his favor, which surprised him, but apparently had been very excited and difficult to understand. Ed felt particularly bad on hearing that young Wisebard, Munk's son-in-law, had told the meeting that Ed was a good man and ought to be retained, but that he was going to vote against him anyway in the interest of unity.

And after the vote they considered the cantor's contract, but there was very little discussion. They retained Bill Prince with a raise in salary.

Ed thanked Amethyst finally, and went upstairs. Lucinda was on their bed, weeping face down, not loudly but not as inaudibly as in the car. He sat on the bed. He put a hand to her back and patted her.

63

No one answered Millicent's ad. The cat was apparently lost for good.

She disliked the train, and especially the waits at North Station in the middle of the night, but in some ways it was good to be living at home, and have her own room, and have her laundry done with the family's, and the country roads to walk in. Sometimes she took Roland's bike.

Sometimes she took books from her father's study, not the religious ones but the general ones, and one on the Age of Pericles kept her occupied in her room for hours.

She saw from her window that the birdhouse was tenanted, and once or twice a bird went in while she watched.

Meanwhile she had gone through Charles's things in her closet and drawers. It was mostly clothing. She found in his wallet a photograph of herself.

His portrait still stood on the piano downstairs. She remembered how her mother had asked the funeral-parlor men for a lock of his hair, but the blond hairs would not stay together because his crew cut was so short. There was a childhood lock, though, from his first haircut, that her mother still had in a celluloid box somewhere.

But the family would be leaving in another three months, whether to another town somewhere near Boston or in New England, or whether they would even quit this part of the country entirely she did not know. Her father's contract was only until September and the congregation had decided not to renew. If the family went to another part of the country she thought she would stay behind in Boston for the present, though she was not sure. If she had found no apartment by the time her family left she could perhaps move in with Aunt Gwen temporarily, and make up with free baby-sitting for the inconvenience she caused. And in any case she must think through by then what to do with her life, and what additional schooling to get. She felt she was in a rut, and that if she were not becoming old maidish she soon would.

The only prospective offer her father had had so far was from a congregation in Needles, Arizona. They had written him that they would pay his plane fare if he would come out for an interview.

"Would you like living in the desert?" she had heard him ask her mother.

"Are you crazy or something?" her mother had answered.

Meanwhile he kept as busy as ever with his duties in the community and at Temple Beth El.

Her grandmother visited, and said her mother had been out of her mind to run off at nineteen and marry that nut. Her mother had a crying jag.

Her mother also began economizing, as though she feared Ed might not get another job at all. But her economizing seemed to Millicent like erratic gestures, not like the dogged penny-pinching of Leslie's mother. Her mother drove great distances to look for bargains in farmers' roadside stands, not counting the cost of the gasoline, and said she had heard of a farmer who sold chickens very cheap if you slaughtered them yourself. She made Millicent and Patty and Roland come strawberry-picking with her, in a hectic and frenzied mood, but it turned out the berries weren't ripe yet. The field beyond the barn was golden with thousands of dandelions and she said she was going to find out how to cook them like the Italians did. She dug a lot of them, getting somewhat sick with the effort one morning, but she did not find out how to cook them and they rotted meanwhile. She increased the size of her vegetable plot, spading and turning earth and buying fertilizer. She also bought some new clothes, which she said were for her morale, and went to Boston to meet Celeste and Gwendolyn for lunch and shopping.

Then one afternoon she drove up with a chicken in the car. It was one of Millicent's days off, and the children were already back from school, and from her room upstairs Millicent heard the clucking, and heard Lucinda shout to Patty to catch it, and Patty's surprised voice and her footsteps as she left the porch glider. Millicent ran to the window but they were close to the porch and the slate roof cut her view. She ran downstairs.

The chicken was still in the car, and Roland and Bobby O'Shaughnessy had run up from the direction of the barn or the fruit trees in the field beyond, asking what was happening. Lucinda had stepped out of the car, looking sweaty in her shirt and shorts, with a strand of hair askew down her face, and had shut the car door and stood confusedly with Patty. Millicent saw the chicken lift itself flapping from the back seat and descend again.

"Boys! You have to help me catch him," Lucinda said.

Roland opened the rear door and the brown hen flew excitedly past him, brushing Millicent's jeans so that she jumped. It scurried across the cut grass, over a little rise in the ground. The boys chased it shouting, one on each side. Lucinda stood panting, and pushed aside the strand of hair.

"The legs were tied, but it got untied," she said.

"What are you gonna do?" said Patty.

"Kill it."

It tried to fly up between the outspread arms of the two crouching boys but Roland seized a leg. Bobby gave an elated yell.

"I got it for practically nothing," Lucinda said.

Roland grimaced, holding the leg as the squawking bird flew upward. It could not get away from him. He tried to catch the other leg. "Ouch!" he said. Bobby's hands were trying to catch it also. Roland caught the other leg. Bobby fell back and lay down on the grass and laughed. A couple of feathers floated in the air. Millicent noticed how freckled Bobby was. He kept laughing even when he sat up. Roland, still grimacing, managed to get both the legs into one hand. The chicken was cackling and the beating wings looked big. He swung it down but it kept beating its wings on Roland's bare legs and turning its head up.

"What are we gonna do with it?" he asked his mother.

"Kill it," said Lucinda.

"What did you do, steal it?" Bobby asked. He was sitting on the grass, holding a long grass in his mouth.

"No. I bought it from Mr. Lorenzo," Lucinda said. "Roland, get the ax."

"Get the ax, Bob," Roland said. "It's in the cellar." He swung the chicken up and tucked it in his arm. It calmed. The head looked this way and that, jerkily.

Bobby raised the bulkhead door and went down.

"Who's gonna kill it?" said Patty. "Not me. Ugh."

"I'm gonna do it," said Lucinda. "I don't want anybody to get hurt. Mr. Lorenzo told me how. We have to find a flat stump."

"There's stumps out back, where Dad cut trees," Roland said, "but they're not so flat."

They went there, Roland carrying the chicken in his arm and holding a leg of it for good measure with the other hand. Millicent could smell it. Bobby joined them with the ax. But the stumps were all small and rather pointed. They showed each cut and blow, and chips still lay about some of them.

"Let's just forget the whole thing," Patty said.

"What do you mean forget it?" said Lucinda. "What am I gonna do with it?"

"The bulkhead's a flat place," said Bobby O'Shaughnessy. "Or the step, at the door. That's a good place."

"Ya, that's a good place," said Roland, and started over there with Bobby, the girls and Lucinda following.

Roland knelt in the grass, holding the bird's legs in both his hands and trying to lay its neck upon the wooden step by the kitchen, but it cackled and flapped and kept turning its head up. Bobby got down behind him, watching over his shoulder.

"Hold your head still," Lucinda said to the chicken. She had taken the ax from Bobby and crouched with it, a long disheveled lock of hair hanging before her face again. "Make it keep still," she said to Roland. She held the ax over the neck with two hands, her eyes concentrating and her lips wide, showing her clenched teeth. The bird kept twisting and croaking, with little flops, and sudden strokes of its wings, and Roland held it against the step with his arms stretched out before him, his head back. Millicent made a face, standing back and watching through her fingers. Her mother's crouching thighs looked strong and the ax moved up and down a little with a slow limberness.

Suddenly it came down hard as the bird squawked. It stuck in the wood against the staring head and Lucinda and Roland fell backwards. "Did you get it?" Bobby cried out. The chicken flew headless upward toward Millicent with a croak, so that Millicent gave a cry, running backwards, and fell down. Patty and Lucinda screamed.

It kept flying, with a noisy flapping of wings, though the severed head lay bloody and still, pinned by the ax. It flew higher and turned. Then it curved against the ground. It ran crookedly from the shade into the sunny part of the yard, its wings still flapping. Lucinda and Patty kept screaming. Patty, the only one that hadn't fallen, ran away awkwardly, looking behind her. The bird passed completely under the wheelbarrow and Millicent caught sight of it next running dizzily over the mowed grass in a different direction. It hit the log pile and fell over. Its wings and legs stirred a little, its feet in the air.

"Oh my God," Lucinda breathed hoarsely, one hand to her chest and one to her stomach. "Oh my God."

"It was like a ghost!" said Patty, her eyes wide.

"Is it dead?" said Roland. He was still sprawled back on Bobby, both the way they had fallen.

"Boy, was that spooky," said Bobby.

"The ghost walks," said Roland.

Millicent was breathless, her heart pounding, but she picked herself up. The odor of chicken was stronger now.

"Is it alive?" Bobby said, "Or dead? Or what?"

"Somebody go see if it's dead," said Lucinda.

"Not me," said Roland.

"Me neither," said Bobby

"Millicent, go see if it's dead," Lucinda said.

Millicent walked slowly over and looked at it. Where the head had been the hole was bloody. It seemed scrawny now, though it hadn't in life. She touched it with her foot. Then she picked it up gingerly by one of its toes.

Lucinda and Patty and Roland and Bobby came toward her a little as she carried it toward them, but moved aside to let her go to the step. She pulled the ax out of the wood and dropped it. Then she picked up the head by its red comb, between thumb and forefinger. Some mucous redness hung from it and the eyes were half closed. Millicent put down the chicken and pulled the cover from the garbage barrel.

"Are you gonna put it in the garbage?" Lucinda asked.

"Just the head," said Millicent. She dropped it in and put the cover on. She picked up the chicken. "Do you want this in the kitchen?" she asked.

"I guess so," said her mother.

"If you think I'm gonna eat that you're nuts," Patty said.

"That's what I say," said Roland.

"It's too scary," said Patty.

Millicent pulled open the screen door and led the way into the kitchen. It seemed rather dark after the outdoors. She put the chicken in the sink.

"That chicken isn't kosher anyway," Roland said.

"Yes it is—I know how to fix it," Lucinda said.

"No, it felt pain, and you can't eat it," said Roland.

"Why not?" Lucinda asked sharply.

"No animal is kosher if it felt pain when you killed it," he said.

"Who said so?"

"Dad. It felt pain. You saw it flying around and squawking. It has to die instantly."

"Well, don't tell Dad," she said. "Don't you dare tell him this chicken squawked."

Roland said nothing.

"Are you gonna tell him?" she asked.

He still said nothing.

"Are you?"

"No," he said.

"Because I'll go along with this monkey business just so far," Lucinda said, "and after that it gets ridiculous. I can't afford to throw a chicken away."

"It was just like something supernatural," Patty said. "Wow."

Lucinda took a basin from a hook and put the chicken in it on the table. It smelled quite strong.

"You understand?" Lucinda said, looking at her son darkly. "Mum's the word. If you tell him about it squawking and flying around I'll knock your block off."

"Don't think you're gonna eat my short-eared racing rabbit," he said.

"Nobody's eating your rabbit. And you learn to keep your rabbit out of the garden, by the way."

She turned the chicken over in the basin and spread its wings.

"Do you boys want to make some money?" she asked. "I'll give you ten cents apiece to pluck the feathers out."

"The heck with that—no thanks," Bobby said, sliding from the chair where he half knelt and half sat.

"I was just gonna get my papers anyhow," Roland said, and both boys started to the door.

"You just wait a minute!" Lucinda told him. "It's not time for your papers yet! You can help your mother once in a while."

"I don't have to do it," said Bobby.

"You don't have to, but Roland has to, and Patty and Millicent have to. Millicent, see that they do it, will you? I want to pick up some fabrics before everything's gone."

Millicent remembered that her mother had spoken of a sale of remnants at a knitting mill in Sparkstown.

"Do you really think it's worth it?" Millicent asked.

"Oh, they have beautiful stuff."

"The chicken, I mean?"

"We're not gonna throw it out, if that's what you mean. Now you see that they do it. You're in charge. It doesn't take long. I want it ready to clean when I get back." She threw her hair back from her face with her hand.

"Do you know how to clean out the insides and everything?" Millicent asked.

"Oh sure. In my day everybody did that. That's the hard part. I'm doing the hard part." She went to the sink, took some aspirin from a bottle on the shelf over it, swallowed them with some water, and left. The screen door slammed.

They stood looking at one another.

"Is Mother going insane or something?" Roland said.

"I don't know," said Patty. "I was wondering that myself."

"I think she is," he said.

"Really?" said Bobby. "You mean she'll have to go to an asylum?"

"Now stop it!" Millicent said. "Roland!" She stared at him a moment. Then she pulled out a chair. "Now let's make a start on it anyway," she said. She sneezed, and felt the next sneeze forming.

Patty started to sit down but Roland snatched away the chair and she fell down violently on the floor in an awkward position, shaking the room so hard that Millicent thought she must be hurt, or might even have broken something. Roland and Bobby laughed. Millicent sneezed again. Patty pulled herself forward, with tears in her eyes. "Ooh you!" she squealed at Roland. "Ooh you!"

She got up and he danced away from her. Bobby did also. Millicent sneezed again. Patty chased Roland around the table. He grabbed at Millicent's chair as he ran past behind it, and then threw down an empty chair against Patty's shins. She yelped and hopped a step. Bobby ran out the screen door and Roland began to dart that way, but Patty was nearer to it than he was. He ran through the dining-room door and tried to slam it in her face but she caught it. Millicent followed them, more slowly because her eyes watered and she had to stop and sneeze. In the living room Roland threw over the tall rocker into Patty's path. She cried out but dodged it. Millicent saw them run out the peaked double front door. They left both parts of it wide open and scrambled noisily down the porch.

When she next saw them Patty had the rake and was running after Roland through the high grass in the field beyond the barn. Patty's skirt was flying about her knees. Bobby kept pace easily alongside at some distance, as a kind of spectator, but she paid no attention to him. Roland allowed her to get fairly close and danced about.

"Patty the fatty, slightly batty," he sang.

"This time I'll kill him!" she shrieked.

She swung the rake up and brought the teeth down into the ground nearer to him than he seemed to have anticipated and he jumped back. He clambered into the apple tree. He raised himself swinging and his shirttail came out. He went still higher and Patty swung the rake up at him. It did not have much force in that position and the branches slowed it, but it nicked his ankle. "Ow!" he said.

Millicent jogged through the high grass. "Put that rake down," she panted.

Patty was panting too, and staring up between the wide branches at Roland with the rake poised. It was a many-branched tree but the lowest was too high for Patty in her skirts. He climbed as high as he could and crouched there, looking down. Millicent sneezed. Bobby O'Shaughnessy stood watching at a distance and had again put a long stem of grass in his mouth.

"Why don't you go on a diet," Roland said to Patty. "So you could run faster. You big tub of lard."

"You're just a little son of a bitch! That's what you are."

"Ooh, what you said."

"You are."

"You heard her," Roland said to Millicent. "She called Mother a bitch."

"Now cut it out, both of you."

"It's not fair. I can't hit a girl." With one of his hands he held to a small branch above, like a monkey.

"She won't hit you. Come on down. Patty, give me the rake."

"No. I'll keep him up there all night. And I'm gonna tell Mother you upset a robin's nest, too. With four eggs in it."

"Go ahead."

"I will." She had lowered the rake a little, as though because of its heaviness.

"You're a fat slob."

"You're fat between the ears!" she answered. She became tearfully furious again and poked in the leaves with the rake. He swung a foot up out of the way.

Millicent had approached meanwhile and now she seized the rake with two hands, but Patty held on.

"Let go," Millicent said.

"No."

"Patty! He started it but you're at fault too if you don't stop. Roland, come down. And go in the house."

"She's gonna murder me. With that rake."

"She's not gonna murder you."

"I am too," Patty said, giving the rake a tug, but Millicent tugged back.

"You're not murdering anybody," she said. "Don't be childish. Give me the rake."

"No." She gave a yank and Millicent lost her grip on it.

"Patty! I can't do anything with him unless you stop. And Roland, you started this. You promise to leave her alone."

"I never touched her."

"I mean not pull any chairs out, or anything like that."

"And never call me Patty the fatty again as long as he lives."

"Do you promise?" Millicent asked him.

"I don't mean promise," said Patty. "You have to swear it."

"Okay," said Roland.

"You have to say 'I swear to God,' " Patty said.

"Okay."

"Say it," Patty told him.

"I swear to God."

"I swear to God what?" Patty said.

"I'll never call you Patty the fatty."

"As long as you live," said Patty.

"As long as I live."

"All right, let him come down," said Millicent. "Put the rake back."

The teeth end had been lowered to the ground. "Okay," Patty said, looking up into the tree. "You remember—you swore it now. On God's Name. You better not forget."

"I won't forget."

"Okay then. Because you better not."

"Come on," said Millicent.

"And there's two witnesses. You're a witness too, Bobby."

"Come on," Millicent said again.

Patty started with the rake toward the barn. Millicent walked with her in the high grass. Bobby approached the tree. Roland swung and stretched from a branch, so that his shirttails drooped away from him and his trousers hung below his navel. He dropped to the ground.

"Patricia the pisher!" he called out.

Patty swung around with a shriek, so that the rake handle thumped Millicent in the back, and when Millicent turned they were already far away from her, tearing through the grass. Bobby ran ahead of Roland. Roland leaped onto a boulder of the wall and over into Massapeequit Road. Patty followed in her wide skirt, rake and all, in such a way that Millicent was struck by her agility. She thought of shouting to her, but it seemed useless.

Millicent ran tiredly after them. She became winded on the bumpy hillocks. She had come home from work as usual in the early morning and had not slept late. She walked a little and ran again. When she had clambered over the wall she saw them already far down the road, where it turned sharply before swooping downhill. Patty also had slowed to a walk and Roland danced ahead, shouting some taunt. Bobby kept pace with him, sometimes turning backwards. They disappeared around the bend.

But on the steep downgrade after the curve Millicent found it easy to go faster and she saw Patty running down wildly after them, the rake high. Beyond where the road turned into the covered bridge the river edge was full of lily pads, grasses, dead cattail stalks and the rising leaves of new ones, all the way to where the duck-farm fence ran into the water, and a square raft lay in the reeds, a corner almost on dry grass and a corner tilting down into the stream. Bobby helped Roland shove it out and Roland seized a pole that had lain near it and leaped aboard alone. The raft glided, seeming barely to support him. He stood with feet apart, but it was awash a few inches at the deepest part and the water flowed over his shoes. He changed his stance and the low part rose, but another side went awash. He pushed with the pole and drifted into the wide part of the stream, where he planted the pole against the current. The dam made a steady noise. Roland reached down and took off his shoes and socks with one hand, though they were already wet.

"You're not gonna get away with it this time!" Patty shouted.

"Help!" he said. "I'm a cruiser pursued by a blimp!"

Patty stood on the bank, red-faced from running, her hair askew, the rake dragging.

Millicent brushed past Bobby, who was standing back now on the road, but Patty paid no attention to him and looked only at Roland.

"Go pick on somebody your own size!" Roland shouted from the raft. "The fat lady in the circus for instance." He tossed his shoes with socks in them to the rocks that rose up in forest on the opposite bank.

"Come on, Patty," Millicent said, approaching. "Don't stoop to his level."

Patty swung the rake furiously at Millicent. "Get away!" she said. Millicent jumped back.

Patty turned and threw the rake at Roland, the heavy teeth end first. But it fell into the water, the handle out. A line of bubbles came up. Both boys laughed.

"Get your hoss and come after me on hossback, why don't ya!" Roland shouted.

"You should have been dead instead of Charles," Patty shouted. Her voice was full of agitation. "I wish you were killed instead of Charles. You're not fit to live."

"She's the fattest hoss rider in town," Roland shouted to Bobby. "It looks like one hoss riding another."

Patty was kneeling, taking off her shoes and socks. "I'll get you," she said.

"And you know what size dress she wears? Size five hundred."

He had glided a little downstream, and she ran barefoot along the grass, almost to the fence. The cattails were somewhat thicker there. She stepped down into the water, and stood uncertainly on the muck and dead reeds of the bottom. Green grasses grew out of the water around her, and thick stems with hard knobs of buds, not yet blossomed. Patty moved out beyond the cattails, pulling a foot from the muck and setting it down again, and the water rose on her legs. She raised her skirt a few inches. A small blue dragonfly hung in the air near her knees, moving this way and that. There was a quacking of ducks.

"Even the ducks are laughing at ya!"

"They are not!"

A school of dark fish moved past her legs in the brown water.

"Can those fish bite?" she asked.

"No," said Roland.

"I asked Bobby—I wouldn't ask you."

"No," said Bobby. "You better watch out for bloodsuckers though."

"Patty! You're gonna catch cold," said Millicent.

"They might suck some fat out," said Roland.

The bottom was ooze and stalks and roots.

"Catch!" said Bobby, and threw one of Patty's shoes with its rolled sock inside in an arc over the water to Roland. Roland raised a hand and caught it near his chest, but he stepped back and the raft tipped deeply, drippings pouring from the high end. He stepped forward and it righted with a smack. Bobby laughed.

Patty gave a screech, turning in the water.

"Hey!" said Millicent, as Bobby reached for the other shoe. She ran up and he backed away. She picked up the sock and the shoe. It was soft buck with a rubber sole. "You keep out of this, Bobby O'Shaughnessy," she told him.

"Rollo and I happen to be allies," Bobby protested.

"It's none of your business," Millicent said.

"Anyway I didn't even get it wet," Bobby said. "A perfect shot."

"He's my bodyguard," said Roland. "I'm his bodyguard and he's my bodyguard."

"We're partners," Bobby said.

"You give me that shoe!" Patty yelled to Roland.

"Come and get it. Try and make me."

She moved two steps forward uncertainly in the water.

"Look out, Patty," Millicent said. "You better come out of there."

A frog jumped in front of Patty but it didn't faze her. She turned and pointed a finger at Bobby. "And I'll fix you later!" she said.

Roland leaned and thrust on the pole, moving closer. He had Patty's shoe tucked in the waist of his trousers. He leaned on the pole again. The water rippled over his feet and the bottoms of his trousers. He crouched, letting one side of the raft submerge deeper, and pulled up a rubbery green lily plant. Patty stepped deeper, raising her skirt and petticoat. Roland stood and flung the lily plant over the cattail stalks toward Patty. "Here," he said.

The muddy stem that dangled from it struck her across the face, spattering her with black. Roland and Bobby laughed. Patty wept. With quick gestures she hiked her skirt and petticoat higher, rolling them inward and tucking them into the leg bands of her underpants.

"Get undressed why don't ya!" Roland said.

She stepped out deeper, crouching and feeling about, splashing helter-skelter in the water for something to throw at him. She threw two handfuls of rotted sticks and mud at one time, one with each hand, but they did not go far. She stepped nearer the fence, where the water was shallower, and groped on the bottom for stones. Hairs on her legs that had been invisible before were muddy black now. She pulled up a dripping mucky clublike root, plastered with black rotting leaves, and flung it overhand, so that black drops fell across her blouse in a straight line. It splashed into the water short of the raft.

"'Plump,'" Roland shouted. "Even the stuff you throw is calling you plump."

Bobby laughed.

"My sister's behind is so big you could paint a map of the world on it!" Roland continued. "Eastern hemisphere and western hemisphere!"

She took a wobbly step toward him again, weeping, but her skirts on one side had unrolled nearly to their proper length and dragged in the water.

"Be careful, Patty!" Millicent said.

"I hate you!" Patty screamed at Roland.

"I hate you too!"

"I hate you worse than poison snakes!"

"I hate you worse than the whole German army! And the Chinese army!" He tossed the shoe. "Here," he said.

She tried to catch it but it hit her stomach and fell in the water. Bubbles came up. She bent down and felt for it in the mud. The back of her skirt and petticoat rose coated with blackened water.

"Yeah, one side of your behind is big enough to take up the whole circle in the toilet! She needs a special toilet!"

She retrieved the shoe and went splashing toward him through the reeds. Bobby was laughing and slapping his knee, but she persisted, weeping tears, one step plunging her down several inches deeper and the next lifting her a little.

"Help!" Roland said. He was dancing on the raft and ripples slid back and forth over it. His feet splattered in water on the boards. "I'm Dr. Livingstone and I'm pursued by a hippopotamus!"

She stumbled, as though she had stepped on something sharp, and tried awkwardly for a new balance, but her other foot sank deep and she fell sideways with a splash among the flowerless lily stalks. Roland hugged himself and Bobby fell on the grass screaming with laughter. Millicent ran forward laughing. Patty managed to get up. Water rained from black clothes that clung to her, but she still clutched the shoe.

"Patty got her panties wet! Patty got her panties wet!" Roland sang.

She made her way toward the shore, sobbing and blubbering.

Millicent tried to make herself solemn. "Come on, Patty," she said.

Patty extended a hand for Millicent to help her. She seemed crushed.

"Patty got her panties wet, Patty got her panties wet," Roland kept singing, poling nearer to shore, and Bobby took it up too.

Patty did not look at Roland or Bobby. On the bank she turned up her foot and looked at it, with Millicent, but there was no mark. She started limping barefoot toward home, with Millicent.

"Don't you care," Millicent said.

"You gonna leave Dad's rake there?" Roland shouted after Patty.

Patty was shaking irregularly with sobs. "He's the worst kid in the whole world," she managed to say.

"I know it," Millicent said.

"You're so big your big sister is really your little sister," they heard Roland shout.

Patty seemed heartbroken.

"You laughed too," she said to Millicent.

"I'm sorry."

They walked together, up the hill.

"When you laughed," Patty sniffled, "that meant you were on his side."

"I'm sorry. I shouldn't have laughed."

64

Early Sunday morning she thought she heard a motor-scooter. It stopped as she came awake, and she thought she had perhaps dreamed it. She lay rolled up, squinting at the sunlight on the blue wallpaper. The painful tiredness in her face told her she had awakened too soon.

She did not move. There was no more motor scooter sound. A bird twittered just outside. Dreamy images floated before her and she let herself sink back into sleep.

She must have slept for a time when there was a knock at her door. She stared confusedly from the bed and the knock was repeated.

Her father looked into her room. He was dressed, but without coat or tie, and his eyes were on her with an unsmiling fixity.

"There's a friend of yours downstairs to see you," he said. "On the porch."

"Oh? Who?"

"You'll see," he said. His face was sour.

"What time is it?"

"Seven-thirty, thereabouts. I don't know. Seven-twenty, seven-thirty."

She began to push herself up. Her father left, shutting the door. It seemed impossible that it was Les. She tried to think of girl friends out of the past or from college who might have stopped by unexpectedly. But she hoped it was Les. She dressed and washed very quickly, and combed her hair at the bathroom mirror.

She came downstairs frowning, her hands in her jeans. If it were Les she would lecture him for coming unexpectedly at such an uncivilized hour. She went out to the porch. Leslie rose from the glider. He wore a sweat shirt and gabardine trousers.

He looked wonderful. His height stooped a little toward her, and the bulb of sandy hair lay across his forehead. His eyes smiled through the tortoise-shell glasses, and the smile curved his mouth, cautiously first at one side.

"Hi!" she exclaimed, smiling broadly. In spite of having known it was he it was a surprise actually to see him, even so.

"Hi," he said.

"Just a minute," she said. She checked back in the house to see where her father was, leaving the front door ajar. She glanced up the staircase, and toward Roland's door down the hall, by way of checking her impression that no one else was aware of Les's presence. Then she looked through the open door of the study, which was quite close to the open front door. Her father was there at his desk, a book before him, but his eyes met hers at once.

"Dad, I'm taking Les for a little walk," she said. "I just want to show him the neighborhood."

She was not even out of sight or earshot of Les as she spoke. She came out again at once, smiling at him.

"Okay, let's go," she said.

They went down the porch steps to the dirt drive. The gray scooter was not there but parked far down, on Massapeequit Road. She could see it beyond the stone wall, resting at a tilt.

"Did my cat ever show up at your place?" she asked as they walked.

"No. I never saw him."

She sighed. "He just disappeared," she said. "I hope he's found a nice home."

She felt the pebbles of the dirt roadway through her sneakers.

"Let's take a spin on the scooter," he suggested.

"No. I said we're taking a walk and that's what we'll do."

They said nothing more until they were down by the gate.

"Down this way there's a covered bridge and a duck farm, and that way," she said, turning and pointing, "there's Sachem Hill and you can see Sparkstown from the top of it."

"Okay, I'll take the mountain view."

They began walking slowly. Mrs. Davey's horses were already out grazing, and there was an odor of wild flowers. But she kept her hands in her pockets and looked down at the road. She was not smiling now.

"Les," she said, "do you think seven o'clock in the morning is a civilized hour to go calling on people unannounced? On a Sunday morning? I ought to be very angry with you. And I am."

"Well, I'm sorry."

"Really, the more I think about it the more preposterous it is. You have some nerve. Ringing doorbells at that hour and waking up the household."

"I didn't ring the doorbell—"

"You didn't?"

"No. Honest I didn't. I just sat on the porch. And I purposely didn't ride the scooter up to the house so it wouldn't wake anybody."

"You seem to have roused my father."

"He was up. He was in the living room saying his prayers, and I was sitting there and he looked out and saw me."

"Well, even so."

"I told him not to wake you. Did it wake anyone else?"

"I don't know," she said sullenly.

"He made me come in and daven with him. He gives me a tallis, and tefillin and everything, and hands me a book open to the page. I just followed along silently, you know, in the translation. And he sort of showed me the place once in a while. And then he went up and woke you up, I guess. I told him not to. I told him I'd just wait on the porch until you woke up yourself."

They walked silently a few steps.

"Even so," she said again. "What's the idea of prowling around here anyway."

"I wasn't prowling around. I got up early, and I was out riding on the scooter, and then I realized I was somewhere near here, so I thought I'd wait until you got up and say hello, that's all."

"Well I wish you wouldn't do it again. You'd be home catching up on your sleep if you had any sense."

"Well, I went to bed early last night," he said, "and I got up early. I couldn't sleep."

The road continued a slow upgrade. Millicent picked up a dead branching stick that lay among the bachelor's-buttons and tall grasses. As she walked she peeled bark from it and broke off its twigs.

"How are your mother and brother?" she asked.

"They're fine. How's your family?"

"Oh, we're all in reasonably good health, I guess. You'll be going into the Army soon, won't you?"

"Next month."

"How do you feel about it?"

"Well, it's an interruption. But it's medicine—it's not a total loss. You know how I feel about it. At least it's some money for a change."

"What'll you be? A captain?"

"First lieutenant."

"Do you know where you'll be?"

"No. I report to Fort Sam Houston in Texas—after that it could be anywhere."

"Well, I guess it was nice of you to stop by and say good-bye," she said.

She snapped off one of the branching twigs. She could hear him breathing as they walked.

"Millicent," he said, and she thought his voice had grown a little huskier. "I've missed you."

"Oh? Well that's nice."

"I mean, we shouldn't have busted up."

She colored a little and began to shake her head as though to disagree.

"I mean it," he said.

She shook her head quickly. "Les, I've tried the love-affair routine, and I found it wanting."

"Millicent, I want to tell you something. You happen to be the greatest thing that ever happened to me."

"Well, I'm sure you can manage. You'll find someone else."

"That's not the point. I don't know how to say this. But you're very unusual, do you know that? I've been very depressed since we separated."

"Really? Well, I'm sorry to hear you've been depressed. I didn't think you were capable of being depressed."

"Well, I am."

"I've seen you tired but I don't think I ever saw you depressed."

"Millicent, listen—"

"You've probably been working much too hard."

"Listen, I'm trying to tell you something. I love you. I'm in love with you."

"You are?" She still walked without looking at him, working at her branching stick. She thought he sounded awkward.

"Yes."

"No you're not. For one thing if you were in love you'd want to get married."

"Well, that's part of it. Of course. It includes that."

"Is that a proposal?"

"If you like."

"Well, I don't accept. Les, you've been working much too hard. It's embarrassing—it's absurd. I ought to be mad at you for waking me up with a stupid idea like that."

"What's stupid about it?"

"It's not even realistic. You're going into the Army, for one thing."

"So what. We could be engaged in the meantime."

"I don't want to be engaged. You can't afford to get married anyway. You've got your mother and your brother to support."

"I don't support them."

"You help them."

"Well, I've helped a little when I could, yes."

"You owe it to them."

"I don't owe them that much."

"Les, I don't mean to be cruel. But I think the prospect of going into the Army has affected you. And my answer is negative. It's nice of you to come and say good-bye."

"I didn't come to say good-bye."

They walked some steps in silence. They turned off Massapeequit Road onto the road that went up Sachem Hill, and the grade was at once steeper. The way before them now was winding, and they could not see a great distance along it. The trees were not so towering as on Massapeequit Road but the woods here were thick on both sides and shut out much light. Millicent broke the rest of the branches from her stick. She walked holding it before her, letting the end of it bounce and scrape occasionally on the road surface.

"Why the sudden interest in marriage?" she asked without looking at him.

"It's not sudden. I've always had it in mind that you and I might marry eventually. I even thought of it that very first time I laid eyes on you, on the Common. That it could be you."

"No you didn't."

"Yes I did. And I shouldn't have let this breakup happen. I needed a little time to think, I guess."

"You didn't let it happen. I decided I'd had enough."

"Well, have it your way. I'm just trying to explain why I want to marry you."

"Why?"

"Because you're the best girl I ever met, that's why. And there's just too much chance that in a few years I'll be kicking myself for letting the best girl I ever met get out of my hands, that's why. I like to look at you. And I can have conversation with you. And because other girls bore the hell out of me compared to you."

"Not all of them. They shouldn't."

"Most of them," he said. "I've seen enough to know what the percentages are."

"Les, it's out of the question. I'm not going to start sleeping with you again for a month and then at the end of a month have you go off and disappear, for two years at least. I'm not going to start and stop."

He didn't answer. They walked slowly up a curve in the road. She watched the point of her stick.

"It just wouldn't make sense," she added. "It just wouldn't. We'd be together again for I don't know—three weeks?—like before, and then it would end again. It ended once, and endings are painful, and one ending per love affair is enough."

"It wouldn't be an ending."

"It would."

"We'd be engaged."

"Les, you're out of your mind. You're going off to I don't know where for two years. Or some place."

"But you'd be here when I got back. That's what I want to establish."

"You're talking like a child," she said.

"Why?"

"Because I don't know what I'll want in two years, and you don't know what you'll want in two years."

"I'll still want you in two years," he said.

She made no reply.

"Millicent, I can't believe there'll ever be anybody like you." He made a despairing gesture as he walked.

"This is silly." She stopped and faced him. "I think you better go back and get on your motorcycle and go home. I mean it. You better leave. You're gonna go off and leave me for two years, so you might as well start now."

"I'm not going off for two years voluntarily. I can't help it if I owe the Government two years."

They were standing in the road looking at each other. She watched his face sternly and steadily, but his expression seemed to falter. Somehow they began walking slowly again side by side up the road.

He seemed pensive.

"Well," he said, "would you feel differently if I weren't going to disappear for two years?"

"But you are."

"Well, I mean, suppose I weren't."

"You are, and let's not talk nonsense. You're going into the Army and that's that."

"Suppose instead of an engagement I'd said let's get married now, for instance. Before I go into the Army. Would you have felt differently about it?"

"I don't think so."

"I was thinking of you when I suggested an engagement instead. I mean, apart from Korea, suppose I'm stationed in West Berlin, or Alaska, or some Godforsaken place in Kansas or something—would you want that? Army camps, knocking around, being an Army wife, one place to another?"

"I wouldn't mind that, if I loved a man. But two-year engagements are ridiculous. They're for children." She still didn't look at him. She flung some bark from her stick and felt the knobs and smoothness of the exposed wood.

"It needn't be a full two years."

"I don't believe in engagements," she said. There was still vehemence in her voice, though the uphill walk had begun to make her feel winded. "If I wanted to marry you I'd marry you, period. Without the formality of an engagement. I didn't need any formalities to sleep with you."

"Suppose I were sent to a combat zone?"

"Yes, suppose you were."

She walked more slowly. The curve had begun to straighten, but they could see a further upward curve beyond. The forest was all about.

She heard him sigh, through his nose.

"Would you have married me a couple of months ago?" he asked. "You used to talk about it."

"I thought I was pregnant. Fortunately I was mistaken." Her voice shook a little but she kept an edge of anger in it.

"I don't mean then. I mean a couple of months ago."

"I don't know." She put an irritable preciseness into the words. "It's water over the dam anyhow," she added. "I don't want to marry you now."

"Do you want time to think about it?"

"I've had several months to think about it. And I think we'd better just say good-bye, Les."

Again they were silent for a few steps.

"Will you answer if I write?" he said.

"I'll see, if I have time. How do I know? That's a juvenile question, Les."

"Listen," he said, "I mean it. Let's get married and the hell with it. Tomorrow, or however long it takes to get a license, or any time in the month I've got left. You name it. I've got through the thirtieth."

"That's even stupider," she said. "There wouldn't even be time to prepare a wedding."

To the side of the road there was a dash of motion in the dead leaves that lay beneath the underbrush. They looked toward it but the greenery was everywhere and thick. They could see nothing.

"What was that?" he said. They kept walking up the road. "A rabbit?"

"Probably. Or a raccoon. My father said he saw raccoons around."

"Raccoons come out at night, don't they?"

"Do they? I don't know. I guess it was a rabbit then."

"What other wild life do you have around here?"

"Oh, I don't know. Chipmunks, squirrels, blue jays. Some people say there are woodchucks. I don't know too much about it. Snakes. Skunks. Frogs. Bobwhites."

"Foxes? Possums?"

"I don't know. You could ask my brother. He'd know."

She held her stick in both hands as she walked, and tried bending it slightly.

"I'll tell you what we could do," she said. "We could get engaged now, and marry in a couple of months, as soon as you're settled in the Army. I could go and join you there."

They kept walking, at the same pace. He said nothing. She tossed the stick aside.

"All right," he said at last, still walking. "We could do that."

He stopped, and turned to look at her. She stopped when he did and looked up.

He took her by the shoulders, gently, and kissed her on the lips. It was not a violent kiss, but a slow one.

Their faces separated, and he kept looking down into her eyes. "Like in two or three months, you mean?" he said.

"Whenever you're settled," she said. "When you send for me."

They began walking again. He held her hand, in a casual way, by a few fingers.

"I'd say about two months from now would be right," she said. "So I could give them notice on my job, and buy clothes and stuff, and plan everything, the invitations. Would they give you a furlough so we could get married here?"

"It's possible, I guess. It seems to me I've heard of such things."

"Yes, I think I have too. And I'd want my father to marry us. Would that be all right with you?"

"Sure."

"He's always wanted to do that."

They walked further, hand in hand.

"There's a path along here," she said, "where you can cut through and see the view."

"Would that be it?" he asked. A footpath led from the road into the woods.

"No, I don't know where that goes."

"Well, let's see," he said.

He led the way under the trees, kicking through slim bushes of oak that slapped about his legs. She followed. He held aside branches so they would not swing back into her face. One of them had the gray house of a tent caterpillar.

But the path faded into the undergrowth, as though no one had used it for a long time. They stopped.

"It doesn't go anywhere," he said.

However in one direction bits of sky showed between tree trunks quite far down, as though there were a summit. They went that way. The underbrush thinned, and pink lady's-slippers grew among it. There were more pine trees as the ground became higher. She climbed beside him, panting.

All at once the brim of a cliff was at their feet. It sloped down away from them. They stood at the forest edge, above flowered grassy fields that rolled away lower and lower. There was a road far down that wound past cultivated fields and a white farmhouse and farm buildings, all seeming quite small, but yet not small at all compared to the exquisite details in the broad panorama far beyond. It seemed quite a height.

Leslie stood behind her, with his hands upon her arms. A breeze was fresh upon her face, and stirred her shirt. On low distant ridges innumerable buildings clustered as if in miniature, and some unidentifiable window or shiny spot among them reflected back the sun with a great gleam. Still further away the buildings thinned and scattered toward the bumpy horizon, which was an ascension of blue-green woods.

"What town's that?" he said.

"Sparkstown."

He asked about a construction site that he could see, but at first she thought he meant the lumberyard, and he had to point, and direct her gaze, and mention steeples and brick buildings and tiny landmarks. His cheek came quite close beside her face, and his hand guided her shoulder. Then she saw the sandy clearing he meant, and its little steam shovel and bulldozer. He straightened again, still behind her, though his fingers locked together on her belly. She put her hands on his.

He asked what the distant hills were called, but she did not know.

"It's nice," he said, gazing at the view.

They stood a while looking, without moving. She had one foot before the other and her back was against his chest.

She guessed that the clearing was for the new elementary school.

"Give me a kiss," he said.

She turned and gave him a quick kiss and turned away again.

"Oh come on," he said.

She gave him a better kiss, and his embrace tightened. His hands made her jeans tighter.

He did not stop her from breaking away, and she walked back among the first big trees. He followed, giving her a spank. She went faster, with a little laugh, into the woods, not in the direction from which they had come but rather among the pines where the underbrush was thinner. The pine grove went down into a hollow and he chased her there, further from the cliff, but when the ground began to rise again she sat down, laughing. He came down beside her and kissed her. When he stopped she sat up and picked a small treelike grass from a dry tuft, to put in her mouth, but he took it from her, and threw it away, and pushed her down again. He lay embracing her on the soft pine needles.

"Are we really getting married?" she said. "It's sort of scary, isn't it. It's a big step."

He kissed her hard on the lips, pushing her head into the needles. She drew her knees up. The kiss continued. When he had unbuttoned her shirt she turned in the kiss so that he could reach the clasp of her bra.

Their lips separated and came together again. She moved the pieces of pine cone and sticks from beneath her and settled back, giving him her lips once more. He used her shirt slowly like a polishing cloth upon her breasts.

Sometimes her eyes flickered open but closed again. She wondered how far he meant to try to go out here.

She heard her jeans unsnap. "Les, no," she said.

She felt him lowering the jeans around and around her. She tried to squirm and press her buttocks to the ground to pinch his fingers, but he was strong.

"Les! What if somebody came by?"

The underpants seemed very flimsy to her. He was already testing their stretchiness.

"Let's get slippery," he said.

"Please," she said. "You can't strip me naked here."

His fingers went plunging. She twisted and rolled to let him slide the pants away. Her brows were knit and her eyes shut tight as she tried to embrace him. He sat up and quickly yanked off her sneakers. The wrinkled fabrics were shoved free of her. The snaps of his own trousers popped in series like a machine gun and she raised all her limbs to enclose his impatience.

Sometimes he almost seemed to lift her, though she lay beneath him. At times it was as though he stirred her like a cauldron.

She felt meanwhile the air, and the soft depth of pine needles beneath her, and past his head she saw low pine branches sloping down over them in merging layers.

She fell into a rhythm of titillation with him.

How well she knew him now, she thought. She saw the dizzy tottering in his face, and the indecision, and then his slowing and resumption. She slowed, and resumed when he did. She made a tight internal contraction and saw his delight at the squeeze. She did it a few times in a row. She heard a mosquito's hum and thought it would be amusing to slap it on Leslie's bare behind.

It hummed near her ear on the other side. She made a pass at it and did not catch it, but it disappeared. Leslie made her catch her breath. She played her fingers along his backbone. She wiped the soles of her socks on his hairy legs. At last she felt the spending, and his surrender to helplessness.

He lay quiet in her arms. She heard the mosquito again.

Leslie set up, dully. She could smell him, and smell herself and the strong odor of pine besides. She put a handful of pine needles over the thing he discarded.

"We're awful," she said.

"No we're not."

"I think we're terrible. Out in broad daylight like this. Like a couple of animals."

She was still lying flat, naked except for her socks and open shirt and disarranged bra. He sat with one knee out to the side. She saw him look at the breathing of her abdomen and navel, and then his gaze moved up. When it reached her face it stayed.

The air sounded in the branches, sometimes softly, sometimes with a touch of force.

"I'd really forgotten how fantastically beautiful you are," he said. "I thought I remembered. That face, extremely beautiful. But I didn't. I just had to see it again to remember. It's incredible. You have the deepest, most—I don't know eyes I ever saw. They have to be looked at continuously—they're so unlike anything you can't keep them in mind. As soon as they're out of sight your mind scales them down to something believable. I'm telling you. They fix you like the eyes of a lunatic or something."

She closed them, and opened them again, and smiled as if amused.

He was still staring at her eyes.

She sat up. She brushed away the scattering of pine needles, some single and some in twos or threes, that had stuck to her buttocks. Looking down she saw that besides the few that had clung some had made pink impressions in her skin.

"You sat in some pine pitch," he said.

"Where?" She moved, searching herself.

He showed her where.

Then he held her and kissed her again, sitting beside her. The mosquito sounded. But Leslie's fingers had an extraordinary loveliness.

"We better go or you'll get mosquito-bit," he said. He rose and offered her a hand. He pulled her to her feet. They dressed, without saying anything. He watched her put on her pants. When she had fixed the bra he buttoned her shirt for her, and they tucked it in together.

They walked hand in hand on the carpeting of needles, in the direction where the road ought to lie.

"This is the path I was looking for before, I think," she said after a while.

It was not exactly a path, but rather an impression of vehicle tracks through the woods. They walked along it. Pine cones lay about, and here and there a fine grass came up green through the needles. Low vines hugged the ground.

They came out of the woods onto the same road as before, but not at the same point at which they had entered the woods. There was a big metal oblong sign there on an iron post—black raised letters on a silvery background. She stood leaning against Les, and they read it. His arm rested about her waist.

> NEAR THIS SPOT STOOD THE HOUSE OF WILLIAM SPARKS, FIRST SETTLER IN SQUONKAMESSET, NOW WILMERDING. IN 1640 SEVEN FAMILIES UNDER THE LEADERSHIP OF SPARKS PURCHASED THE LAND THIS SIDE OF MASSAPEEQUIT BROOK FROM MUCKANAUG, SAGAMORE OF THE PIGS GUSSET INDIANS, FOR THREE BOLTS OF WOOLEN CLOTH AND A STIPEND OF TEN SHILLINGS PER ANNUM.
>
> 1630 MASSACHUSETTS BAY COLONY TERCENTENARY COMMITTEE 1930

"Let's go back down and have breakfast," she said.

"Okay."

She started walking, but he stopped her and they kissed.

They began strolling down the road, their fingers locked.

"Do you still want to marry me?" she said.

"Yes."

Their locked hands swung, and she took a skip to get in step with him.

"Massachusetts has the ugliest name of any state in the union," she said.

"I guess it has," said Leslie after what seemed a reflective pause.

"Wyoming is the best," she said.

The walk back seemed much quicker. She stopped once to gather flowers.

"Do you want to ask my father for my hand in marriage?" she asked Les as the house and its big yard and trees came into view.

"No. It's too Victorian," he said.

"I know it, but go ahead. He'd love it."

"I wouldn't know what to say."

"Anything," she said.

They came near the gate.

"Well, do you mind if I tell him?" she said. "Can we tell them?"

"Okay."

They passed the standing scooter and the gate squeaked as they moved it. There was nobody on the porch. She wondered whether to tell them all at once, or to tell her mother alone. She felt a tingling excitement. They walked through speckled light that shone down through a tree.

She led the way into the house, and through to the kitchen. Her mother and Patty were having breakfast and looked up. Patty was dressed and her mother was in a robe.

"Les is having breakfast with us," Millicent said.

"I really don't want to disturb anybody," he said.

"No, that's all right," said Lucinda, rising. She asked if he wanted eggs or cereal. Patty sat staring. He began to say it didn't matter but Millicent said she would get his breakfast. She put butter in the pan, telling him to take a chair. Lucinda poured him some juice.

Millicent broke eggs, and heard her mother beginning to make some faltering small talk about the hospital.

"Les and I are getting married," she cut in, with her back to them.

There was an instant of silence. "Well!" her mother said. "I'm very glad."

Patty made a little grunt of surprise. "Gee," she said. "Shall I get Dad?"

"He'll be down," said Lucinda.

Millicent cooked the eggs. Her mother again made small talk, asking when it had been decided, and asking politely about Leslie's family. Leslie seemed uncomfortable. Patty took some cereal now and then, but mostly stared.

They heard Ed's feet on the staircase and he came into the kitchen, in suit and tie, as if ready for Sunday school.

"Millicent's getting married," Patty told him.

He didn't smile. "When?" he said.

"Les, I've just had a brainstorm," Millicent said, turning at the stove. "It could be the day before you go into the Army. June thirtieth. It gives us a whole month practically and I don't mind rushing a little—I'll get everything done. And then you don't have to worry about when, or where you're going to be. Whatever base you're at we'll find a room or something."

Everyone was looking at Les. She saw his Adam's apple move.

"Okay?" she said.

"Okay, I guess."

"June thirtieth?" said Ed, squinting toward the calendar that hung on the pantry door. "What day of the week is that?"

"There won't be time for a honeymoon," said Patty.

"That's all right," said Millicent. "We haven't got money for a honeymoon trip anyway."

"Well, shake hands with him at least," Lucinda said to Ed. "And I forgot to kiss him." She rose from the chair and went around the table to Les, her eyes moist.

65

Ed's contract had still three months to go, and he kept working as conscientiously as ever, but word that he would be leaving spread in the town. The other clergymen particularly asked him if it were so, and expressed regret. Caleb Folger seemed personally sorry, as though he had looked forward to a long friendship. Young Ralph Briggs, whom he met on the street in Murphy Square, still wearing his surgical collar, asked if it were true his congregation had sacked him.

"Yeah, I've been canned," Ed said.

Briggs seemed to think it was because Ed had preached religion in action, but Ed said it was nothing like that. He said it had been just a conflict of personalities, mainly. Plus the fact that it was only a short-term try-out contract anyway—after looking him over they had decided to shop around further, that was all.

To Father Donahue Ed explained that the congregation had wanted him to be more nonsectarian, and Donahue laughed.

Meanwhile Bill Prince had confided to Ed that he did not want to stay, in spite of the congregation's having offered him a salary increase. But now Bill told him he was going to stay after all, because his psychiatrist forbade job changes during analysis.

The hurt of having been fired deepened in Ed. He was in his middle years, when a successful clergyman should be aiming for the twenty-five-thousand-dollar-a-year bracket, with tenure and a pension. Not getting fired after a year at nine thousand. By ordinary standards he was a failure. Certainly by the standards of Lucinda, and of his mother-in-law, and of his own brothers. And he was a failure by his own inner standards. He had run his career all wrong; he had waited too long to settle in a congregation of his own, and then had fallen flat on his face and failed to win them over.

What percentage of it was his own fault? He had made his sermons brief and informative, his classes fairly lively, not dull, and kept the services streamlined and rapid. But he had been left with a feeling of getting nowhere—everyone was indifferent while he thrashed about. Was he just not the kind of man who could persuade, who could get to people? Or could nobody do anything with this bunch except to agree with them, and abandon all effort to influence them?

He did not want to be a man paid to be the sole example of old-style ceremonial piety in the community. Like a man paid to dress as an Easter bunny. It was too bad, he thought, for children never to see piety as the norm. A pastor works toward the anticlimax of pastor emeritus, and is exposed at last for what he is—a mute old man sitting up there like they had stuck him on a stick.

He had known beforehand that the pulpit was like that; he had taken the risk that his life might turn out like that. But when he was young he had thought it must be possible to meet that challenge and lick it. It had to be possible, or life wasn't worth living.

But he felt no confidence now that he could be more persuasive with the next bunch.

Maybe the approach taken by Peter Donahue's church was more realistic. Your flock sinned, they confessed, and you railed at them. There was not this mad illusion that an entire folk—men, women and children—could be welded into an order under vows.

Lucinda gave a party so that all the relatives could meet Leslie. Grandma Annie looked up at Leslie and said he looked frightened. "What's the matter?" she asked him. "You look scared. You look blue. Who you scared of? Me, or the girl?" She pinched his cheek. She turned to Millicent and nodded her approval. It struck Ed that his mother-in-law did look rather frightening, with her mascara and her big mole. "Have a baby the first thing, and name it after Charles," she said, with another nod. "That's what you should do."

Grandma Annie gave Ed advice about his job, what he should have done and what he ought to do, and so did his brother Maxwell. Ed mixed drinks.

Maxwell wrote a check, which he called an engagement present, saying the wedding present would come later, and pressed it on Millicent.

Watching Maxwell talk and laugh with Celeste's husband and Grandma Annie's husband and chew his cigar, it occurred to Ed that his brother was a happier man than he was, even though he had always considered him an insensitive and unreflective sort. It occurred to him that perhaps people like that, who have no awareness of history, no feeling of past or future, were the ones who were the real people. These people who don't see, who live immersed in the fashions and narrow viewpoints of their time and place, using the latest slang—those were the ones who really belonged to the human race. They don't think, they react to the stimuli of the little environment, and in this manner they make the villages and the cities. They live the trends, they live the fads. To see, and to know, and to think, and to consider society, was in a way to detach yourself from it.

He fetched Leslie a drink.

He watched Millicent serving hors d'oeuvres, and he could see her already as a matron, as though in a home of her own. How was it that he had never really gotten around to talking to this kid?

Ed had begun as soon as possible to address Leslie as "son," to develop the right atmosphere, and on the phone when Leslie called he said "this is Dad."

There had already been talk about whether the wedding would be big or small, and they had spoken of a caterer who handled a hundred and fifty or two hundred guests at house weddings by the use of tents. There would be long tables with tablecloths under tents, and there would be no sides on the tents if the weather were nice, except on three sides of the serving tent.

Ed found himself beginning to like Les somewhat, as another male with whom he needed an alliance against female obtuseness. And Les like himself was working for the betterment of the human species; each was doing God's work. Medical discovery was revelation too.

He had also told Millicent that he liked Les, and that he hoped to guide him into a little bit of religious study, as Leslie's childhood training had been very scant.

"Dad, Les hasn't got time for that," Millicent had answered. "Do you realize the vastness of medical study he'll never catch up with? It's an age of specialization. A doctor can hardly keep up with all the publications in his own special branch of medicine."

He supposed that was true. Still, just as everyone should know a little about health, and about the human body, so should he know a little about the best moral code God had put into the earth. And especially if it was a tradition he was born in.

In her job Millicent was put onto a split shift because of someone's vacation and worked daytime hours now for three days and her old hours for two, so she had begun to be out with Leslie more, often quite late. Sometimes she phoned to say she was staying in town to talk to him all evening at the hospital if he were on call. And Leslie came out to Wilmerding Crosswalk often for supper. Millicent and Leslie would sit on the porch glider sometimes far into the night, and the rest of the family would keep away and let them alone. Or Millicent and Leslie went for walks after supper, and once Ed looked out from an upstairs window and saw them returning in the moonlight, Millicent walking lazily beside Les and almost leaning on him.

Meanwhile Lucinda found out by accident that Patty had had Paul Wernick keep her company baby-sitting. The fact that Lucinda and Ed approved of the Wernick boy made Patty's failure to mention it seem all the more underhanded, and Lucinda told her she could not go out for a week. Small things like that seemed to depress Ed these days. He had a feeling that he was losing touch. He asked Patty about a phenomenon he had noticed lately on the sidewalks and at the drugstore—two girls and one boy going about together in threesomes. Patty told him it was called odd-balling and that it was the latest thing. There was safety in numbers, she said. And anyway boys were always working or studying; this way the girls went out twice as often—they went out another night with the boy that would have been there if there had been a foursome. Ed could think of nothing to say. But somehow the combination of one sheepish pimply boy in dungarees and two healthy-looking laughing girls in brief shorts was disturbing.

Then one night he had a dream in which Charles was alive, but three years old, and had been struck by a rare illness that ruined his brain, leaving the child utterly mindless, the most vegetable kind of idiot. It was a dream so harrowing, so ghastly, that it was a relief to awaken in a sweat, but what he awakened to was a terrible emptiness. Charles was like an ulcer in him. And it would gnaw incurably forever. For all the rest of his life he would have to say to himself, how old would the boy be today, if he had lived, and what would he be doing now?

Ed had sleepless nights often now, and by day he was tired. He kept looking for a pulpit. He inquired discreetly whether his old assistantship in Brighton was still open—he had heard it was unfilled for a while after he left. It was not open. A congregation in Newton was looking for someone; it was a location Lucinda would have loved, and he wrote to them, but they showed no interest. He heard afterward that it had gotten to them that he did not get along with people. However an interview with a congregation in North Adams seemed to go very well. It was an old established congregation, that had not lost its spirit altogether, and they seemed to want someone to pep things up and seemed to like him. He set his heart on it. The city was in the Berkshires, smallish and self-contained, too far to run into Boston for an afternoon but yet Lucinda could keep some sort of touch with her sisters and mother. But another man had been interviewed also, and soon Ed got a letter that the other man had been chosen.

Lucinda told him that if he took the Needles, Arizona, offer she would remain with the kids in Wilmerding Crosswalk and get a divorce. Meanwhile the Colby & Dill real estate people came around once or twice with prospective buyers who looked at the house with indifference. He was disgusted with Colby & Dill. They had praised the house enough when he bought it, but now they said to hope for his money back was unrealistic. The market was brisker last year, and they had expected him to hold on for twenty years until values appreciated. There was no turnover in seventy-year-old stuff in the outskirts, new ranches were overproduced, and anyhow nobody seemed to be buying or moving this year. It seemed as if he might have to take a loss.

Lucinda was gracious and flustered when the house was shown. Ed knew she was miserable at the prospect of moving, especially if it should turn out to be very far. She made arguments with him about offers he didn't even have. She seemed to feel that if there were an offer in a nice town convenient to Boston he might still turn it down because he disliked the congregation, or some such reason. And he knew that as a matter of fact it was true. He could not afford to keep jumping around; he had to choose carefully now a congregation for life. A clergyman like a professor or a lawyer or a doctor had eventually to settle down somewhere. This was it. And he was tired of congregations that couldn't care less.

Once she even asked if they could keep the house and he could commute to work if a nice congregation turned up in a fifty-mile radius. He told her clergymen didn't commute. She said that was stupid, and that he could rent a room for the Sabbath if that bothered him.

Once she said he was just a man who couldn't hold a job. She said she hadn't known he was going to be a rabbi when she married him—she had thought he was going to be a professor—and he had gotten worse as he got older. "All you know how to do is give me babies," she told him. She said Patty and Roland needed a town to call their own. Children needed a place and a community.

But he knew how Lucinda felt, because he himself had no stomach for moving. In the little more than a year that he had been here the house and its surroundings had grown on him.

He stepped outside. Beyond the barn tall grasses blew, pale waves moving across the field.

He had spent a month making repairs in the house after his arrival here. Fixing the gate down at the bottom of the winding dirt drive, so that it hung straight and swung again, had been especially difficult. The huge spreading tree out front had given him pleasure with the sight of its abundant greenery, and abundant shade to park the car in. The other day he had counted a flock of seventeen little birds, patterned black and white and a rusty color, all twittering together on the roof of his barn. He had described them to Roland and Roland had told him the species. And he had been watching the strawberries ripen that grew alongside the road. It had taken this long to get to know the town. He knew his congregation and he knew the firemen. The firemen still had Averys, Babcocks, Underwoods, Yerxas, the same local names that were on the Civil War monument and the greenish War of the Revolution tablet. Lucinda was in the Crosswalkers and the Garden Club, and when Muckanaug Lodge held a Third Degree he was second ruffian regularly now, and Caleb Folger was chaplain, and he enjoyed the sociability. And to deal again now with moving-van operators, to pack all the books, the glassware and the china—he had no stomach for it. Things got busted in moving. And lost. And another house, the insurance adjusters, the aggravation, the putting up of shelves, mirrors, the hundred minor repairs. He felt as if he had just recovered from the last time. And getting acquainted again in a strange town, and a new dentist X-raying you all over again.

It would have been good to stay put, if only the congregation had worked out better. Lucinda had put such emotion and sweat into her flower gardens and vegetable plots. It was too bad people don't live in a house for generations —then you could really have a garden. He had even thought of making grape arbors, like his grandfather's. And where the yard was flattest, on the side away from the barn, he had meant to build a permanent sukkah for use each year in the Feast of Tabernacles, but with walls mostly removable so that it could serve in summer as a rose bower.

He had even had thoughts, before she died, of eventually persuading Rosalind to live here with them. The more members of one family you could squeeze into a house the better off you were.

He walked slowly toward the barn, thinking he would get the lawn mower.

He would have the problem of selling the Model T, he thought. If he moved, where would he keep it? That and the station wagon he had rebuilt from a wreck were all that Charles had left to the world. The Sunday school and the afternoon classes were still using that station wagon. It still ran well.

As he walked he saw the rusty harrow, and beyond it the spot where he and Roland had decided to bury the old dog Roger. The dog still lived, but he did not see how it could hang on for many months more.

He went into the barn, on its uneven floor. In the sun by the opening the dog slept. Two swallows flew in curves in the brown dark interior, high among the lofts and the tie beams and struts and posts. He did not take the mower, but sat down on a couple of worn tires that lay there, one upon the other, his knees up. He stared at a cobwebby saddle that hung on a peg and had belonged to he did not know whom.

Roland and Patty had spent the past year making new friends, he thought. Well, they could make new friends again. They would have to.

Patty said kids still talked of the sweet-sixteen party she had had.

The thought occured to him of quitting the rabbinate, and remaining here in town and in the house in some other business. He could still teach, without compensation, if they would have him, and could offer lectures for whoever would come. For a living he could run a filling station, and fix cars. Except for the pulpit cars were the only business he knew.

Why not? Maybe people would listen to him more readily if he were not a rabbi. The men who made the Talmud had been carpenters, cobblers, so why should not Ed Gordon run a gas station?

One thing he had always disliked about the rabbinate, and that had made him hesitate about that choice of career in the first place, was the modern idea of the rabbi as clergyman, set apart, living off the community. Maimonides had supported himself by working twelve hours a day as a physician, and Rashi by the manufacture of French wines. Ed had used to hope Charles would be such a part-time scholar, supporting himself as an inventor and engineer.

It had been a mistake for rabbis to follow the fashion, he thought, and become at last, in modern times, a clergy, like other clergies. Because clergymen did not sweat out their own livings and their families' livings by economic labor, as mechanics and traders and artisans like other men. Rabbis had used to, until modern times. But clergymen did not. Clergymen were supported. And that gave rise to the notion that clergymen were impotent.

He would assist and volunteer in the congregation in any way he could, and would continue meanwhile to try to live as piously as possible, as an example to others. Whomever they hired to replace him would be delighted to have such a man in the congregation. Maybe pious laymen were needed more than clergy. One or two nights a week he would join some study group in Boston, if one could not be gotten together here. He would rather teach adults than children, and the adult he most wanted to teach was himself. He craved to be part of a circle who studied together.

What was important was not to be on some congregation's payroll but to spread light, to strive to make oneself as fine as possible an example of this tradition, and to struggle for its growth. This he knew he would do, regardless of how he earned his keep.

He could not let it deteriorate, because it wasn't just his own. You don't keep the festivals and Sabbaths, the statutes and prayers, for your personal salvation, he thought. You do it on behalf of all, that this Law in our midst may not be dead yet. Even the unreligious like to feel that there's somebody religious still around somewhere. If the irreligious did not have the religious to jeer at they would have to be religious themselves, and all mankind would pay for their awkwardness.

He had to carry the religious instincts of all his relatives, that they could not admit. And by his practice make their religion visible.

Once you entered God's service, you could not get out. You knew too much. And once you'd accepted this tradition and had taken a stand for it, there was no more question of how desperately it needed you. From the inside you had seen the fewness—you knew that ultimately you could promise only this: that as long as I'm alive it won't come to an end, even if I stand alone.

The only trouble was that he had no money to buy a gas station. He thought about the banks. The banks would not back him when he had nothing for a down payment. Gas stations were expensive.

Maybe he could make ends meet with a bunch of part-time jobs. There were men in town who did that. He knew one who greased cars part-time at Moon's, and drove a school bus part-time, and wore a uniform as a special policeman part-time, and collected unemployment compensation part of the time, and waited meanwhile for the factory that had laid him off to call him back.

There must be a garage or a filling station that needed a reliable grease monkey. Ed wondered if Giles Littleton would consider him for a special policeman. He liked the little white clapboard police station.

Then it struck him suddenly that the answer might be to go into farming. This property had been a farm once. There was considerable land with it, especially if the woods were cleared, and if you arranged with the Daveys to graze animals on theirs. You grew your own food; you got along. Lucinda might prefer that to Needles, Arizona. Seeds cost practically nothing. Newborn animals could be bought cheap and raised in a year. The Government gave pamphlets, and price supports, and even paid for what you didn't grow. And in the winter he would have lots of time for study.

But no. It wasn't practical. It was all preposterous. It would mark him as more of an eccentric than ever. If he quit the rabbinate now it would be seen as a whim, a private indulgence, an instability. He could visualize how upset Lucinda would be. His was not the profession she would have chosen, but she felt the whole family had sacrificed to put him in it, and were entitled to share in whatever prestige it had.

Besides, he could not bankrupt the tradition in his children's eyes by becoming a failed rabbi. Maybe he shouldn't have gone into the clergy in the first place—a religious man yes, but making his living some other way. But that choice was gone. Having made the mistake, he could not now compound it, and besmirch the whole tradition by demonstrating in his children's eyes that the rabbinate was impossible.

Sometime in your forties, he thought, the realization sinks in that we're condemned to death, and then you either drift down to skid row if you think you can't make it, or if there's something you must get done you find new ways to work harder than you thought you could.

He filled the secondhand mower from the jerry can. He took it out of the barn and started its rackety motor with a yank of the cord. The place had to look decent in case Colby & Dill brought people around.

When he was finished perspiration dripped on his hot face. He went in to supper and washed. Lucinda gave him leftovers, which he did not mind, but she explained it with some sarcasm about his being unemployed. He told her he was not unemployed.

"No, not yet," she said.

"I'm a lame duck, but I'm not unemployed," he said.

Patty came in, late for supper, and slamming the screen door. She went to the refrigerator, singing.

"—In words of one syllabubble
You're gonna get in trouble—"

He watched her take her supper.

That night he awakened in the small hours. He was cold, and he had a headache. Lucinda had turned in such a way that she had most of the blankets. He pulled the edges that scarcely covered him, but they held fast, so he stopped. He didn't want to wake her.

His headache hurt like a crack in his skull. He got some aspirin and returned to bed. He lay huddled and uncovered and did not sleep.

The difference between youth and age, he said to himself, is that in youth you can believe in the possibility of your life being straightened out in its main particulars, so that it can be called happy and successful. When you're young you can work for yourself—call it ambition, wholeness—a whole world you're going to put around you.

But there comes a time when your life is such an unrepairable, unfixable thing that you know you're working for those that will come after.

Even though not very well, to judge by the visible results.

What's a career? It crumbles in a man's hands as he grows older. A parody of something he used to dream. We call some people successful, but everyone is at least half a failure. You die like Charles, or you die at ninety, reconciled to failure. Everything ends but nothing is finished.

The death of Charles, the death of Rosalind, and the deaths they recalled, were unfixable. What you love flies apart in your face.

Living his life over again, he thought, he would do much differently. He would have had eight children instead of four, he would not have married so young, at least not to a woman who considered him a nut, he would have gotten more education earlier.

He wasn't young now; life was not a challenge but a lost war, from which you try to salvage the best terms possible.

At this age, he thought, you know the decades will gallop quickly. How long did a man live? He felt he wanted nothing for himself any more, but to do as much as he could of what he was supposed to have done.

If your life changed nothing, what were you doing in the divine plan?

Just when you're ready to live your life over again, to improve upon it, you're snuffed out. If God were a gentleman He'd let a man live twice. He tries you out, you flub along, and you're on the junk heap.

He lay awake until daybreak.

The next night he did not sleep well either. Long after the house had grown quiet he heard Millicent and Leslie come in from somewhere. He heard their muffled voices downstairs, but did not make out what they said.

It became quiet again. But he didn't hear the front door again, nor the sound of the scooter buzzing off, and Millicent did not come upstairs. A dim yellow light continued to rise in the hall from downstairs. Once in a while he again caught a trace of their murmuring voices.

He heard two o'clock on the town clock, and then on the carved clock downstairs.

For stretches he heard nothing, except the tossing of Lucinda beside him, until he would wonder if they were still down there, but then he would hear a soft snatch of voices, though he could not make them out.

He was aware after a while that Lucinda was awake too.

"Are you awake?" he asked her.

"Yes."

"What are you thinking about?"

"Charles," she said.

He had gotten that answer at other times, but he had not expected it just now. He thought the wedding had begun pretty much to fill her thoughts, since she spent hours now in preparation for it, in helping Celeste arrange a shower, in shopping, in discussing the pattern for silver with Millicent and whether linen should be monogrammed.

They lay silently a moment.

"They're down in the living room," he said. "Millicent and Les."

"I know it."

"What's she doing with him down there, necking?" he said.

"I don't know," said Lucinda.

"You think I should go down? And tell them what time it is?"

"I don't know," she said.

"I don't like it," he said. "I don't like this system. We're supposed to stay up here, and play dumb, so they can be alone down there. We can't go down. Privacy. They should have a little privacy from each other, if you want my opinion. They're not married yet."

"Well, even so, maybe you shouldn't go down," said Lucinda. "Why don't you just holler from the stairs."

"Why? It's my house, isn't it? I have to be afraid to go down, because she might have her pants off?"

Lucinda gave a miserable-sounding sigh. He knew she was as disturbed as he was.

"I don't know," she said. "At least they're in the house. Maybe if we drove them out she'd be in Boston, spending the night in his room or something."

"All right," he said bitterly. "They count on us to keep out. Why don't we make their bed for them? Invite them up here. It's all in the family."

He rolled in the blanket, away from Lucinda.

"Maybe they're not doing anything," Lucinda said.

"No, maybe not. Meanwhile we're supposed to close our eyes. And feel lucky that if they do it, it's in our house and not some place else."

He wished he could put them from his mind and sleep. The yellow glow from the hall bothered him.

A few nights ago he had waited up for them when they had been out, and on their return had sat around with them, but Leslie had showed no sign of leaving, until at last Ed had felt awkward and had had to retreat upstairs.

Well, at least they were engaged. Some parents had to stay out of sight like that when there was not even a semblance of an engagement, and guess what went on.

And what was engaged supposed to mean now—that anything goes? What these kids didn't realize was that the ceremony of a gold ring on the finger, that people today called a wedding, had in Bible days been the betrothal. The sleeping together had been the wedding. But engagement and marriage tend to merge, he thought, and then new, redundant engagements were set up to go before. The two rings on a woman's finger were a redundancy historically as well as to the eye, since each represented the one betrothal ring of the Law. And now the new redundant engagement was beginning to merge too, because kids slept together during it. And in time people would set up a still more redundant engagement before that, and that too would merge, and so on.

We don't control the times in which our children live, he thought. We don't choose the epoch or the age they must live in.

Maybe when you've passed the halfway mark of your life you should try to make peace with your God, since you can't with your wife or your children.

Suddenly an icy feeling came over him that he had not succeeded in passing on his values to his children. And if not to them, then certainly not to all those kids who had come to Sunday classes and to afternoon classes.

It seemed to him that others had in the past influenced him very much, but that he himself had had little influence on anyone. Not on his family, not on the congregations with whom he had dealt.

He had wished once to be a professor of history, with religious scholarship a magnificent side line, but neither his education, nor his marriage, nor his career had been done right. And perhaps it would turn out that way with his children too—that would be the ultimate failure.

A son already dead, and as for the living children, he suspected he had not gotten through to them anyhow. If he had not gotten through to Millicent in twenty-odd years, then probably not to the others either. Patty too at sixteen was already developing into an unhappy kid. Perhaps this was the truth, that he had been a damned fool all his life, getting through to nobody. His life was not a sanctification of the Name. People did not look at him, and at his situation, and think, "I'm impressed by this guy, his God must have something." They did not.

It seemed as if his failure was at last confronting him, like a deathly insight. To fail and still hope that one day you would be the person you wanted to be, and could respect—that was one thing. But to perceive that you will never, never approach that picture in your mind, but always be what you are now? And that your children would have lives as unhappy, as mismanaged, as wanting in true success as your own? Their failure would be his all the more. His ancestors would not have the descendants they deserved, neither in him nor in his children. He had not the ability to do his task, or to maintain a house of the sort he would aspire to, or to educate satisfactorily the children whom he loved. It made you feel as if the godless were right, after all, he thought, that the universe really was just a secular mess. All this strewn space, like a dump, with its fires and crawling things. And meanings were only the flickering of dreams, from which you wake fitfully in darkness, to find that God has vanished.

He sat up in bed, nervous and distraught.

"What's the matter?" Lucinda asked him. "Are you going down?"

"Yes, I'm going down," he said. "I'm sick of this."

He went to the closet for his bathrobe.

"They count on us to keep out," he said. "They depend on it. And the whole family's careful to stay upstairs, and mach dich nit vissendik. It makes me nervous." He looked at Lucinda's face on the pillow. He could tell in the dimness she was looking at him. "If they're not doing anything like that," he said, "what's so terrible if I walk in there? You tell me, why am I excluded from part of my own house? Because they're liable to have their pants down? I'll kick him the hell down the porch. And throw his pants after him. I'm not gonna lie here like a damn fool and condone it. Do you condone it?"

"I don't condone it," she said.

"When she was living with the guy I tried to drag her home and I couldn't, but to go make their bed for them and give them my blessing, it's too much. I'm still a father. She's not a wife yet."

"Shoosh," said Lucinda.

He tied the cord of the bathrobe. He stepped into his slippers.

The door made no noise when he widened it, and he went down the steps quietly. As he suspected, the French doors were shut.

The stairs brought him to the doors from the side, but he seized the glass knob and opened quickly. Millicent and Leslie looked up at him. They were properly clothed. Leslie was stretched on the couch, his head propped, and Millicent sat curled a distance away in the tall rocker. Her feet were up beside her, her shoes off but socks still on. Ed knew he had interrupted some conversation.

"Hi," he said.

"Hi," said Millicent.

"Hi," said Leslie.

Ed wet his lips.

"I just wanted to remind you to lock up," he said to Millicent.

"Okay."

"Can I get you a drink?" he asked Leslie.

"No, I've got to get out of here. I've got to be up in the morning."

"Okay. You won't forget to lock up?"

"No," said Millicent.

He closed the door. He glanced at the carved clock.

He returned to Lucinda and took off his bathrobe in the near darkness.

"So?" she asked.

"Nothing. Talking."

He dropped the slippers. He got under the blanket.

"Well, are you satisfied?" she asked.

"Nope."

66

Mr. Killian told Millicent that the copy boy Zucchino had broken a leg pole-vaulting in his back yard, and that until he returned to work she would have a change of schedule, working early daytime hours until four o'clock three days a week and her old late-afternoon-and-evening shift two days.

It was a godsend to her, as it was so important now to have evenings to see Les, and go visiting, and make plans for the wedding. Les came on his motor scooter to Wilmerding Crosswalk almost every evening that he wasn't on call, and had supper with the family. He said the food was better there than at the hospital. Besides there was nothing he and Millicent could do in Boston of an evening without spending money, and they wanted to save as much as they could.

She even talked of hanging around Boston after work until six-thirty, so as to ride home behind Les on his scooter and save the train fare, but her parents said no.

After his proposal she had gone to work almost in a state of dizziness, uncertain whether she had even wanted things to happen quite so rapidly. And that night she lay awake till the first twittering of birds. It seemed crazy how the pattern of her life was changing so abruptly, how she would give up her family and her job all at once, how she would live in various parts of the country or the world, as the Army sent him about, and then in whatever city his career took him to afterward. She would look for a job on a local weekly newspaper near their Army camp, so they could start a savings account. Or she would try to sell a magazine article on being an Army wife, or perhaps even travel articles if he were sent abroad. It seemed now somehow as though it should be quite easy and natural to do such things. And yet how recently the effort to become anything better than a copy boy had seemed to her impossibly difficult.

She enjoyed the party her mother gave for all the relatives to meet Leslie, and she was amused by his blushing shyness when Grandma Annie pinched his cheek. Aunt Gwendolyn, whom he remembered from the time they had baby-sat, kissed him. "I'm very happy," Aunt Gwendolyn said to them.

"Can I kiss you too?" Aunt Celeste asked him, and she did.

Grandma Annie told Les he looked skinny and hit his stomach with the back of her hand. She asked him what the matter was, and said her granddaughter would fatten him up, and told Millicent she was smart to marry a doctor because she'd never starve.

"Yeah, you can always fry up an old appendix," said Uncle Maxwell, and blew some cigar smoke.

"What doctors charge these days—it's a crime," said Grandma Annie.

The party lasted long, and Millicent found herself feeling quite grown up, in a way she had never felt till now. Her cousin Jill confided in her, and told her she had changed her mind about marrying the Hindu, because she had decided she would not look good in a sari after all. Someone asked whether Millicent's early wedding date allowed a decent period of mourning for Charles, and her father answered that it was all right. Leslie gave Roland and then Patty a ride on his scooter, and then the gaiety of the evening had become such that Lucinda took a little ride on it also. She had to hold her skirts in the wind, and Grandma Annie called her a flapper.

Within a week a surprise shower was given for Millicent—she went to Aunt Gwendolyn's one day directly from work, thinking she was needed to baby-sit, and all the aunts from both sides were there, as well as her mother and grandmother, and Patty, and some old friends of her mother's, and a couple of cousins of the older generation. The little apartment was quite full of ladies.

The two aunts by marriage on her father's side gave her a forty-piece set of steel tableware, and she was told the shower gifts were not wedding gifts—the wedding gifts would follow. She could find no words to tell them how she felt. There were so many shining articles. It was a warmth that brought her to tears. She fondled a Dutch teapot that had bright, crude, modernistic flowers.

There was a buffet supper and Aunt Gwendolyn brought her some of it. Someone suggested that her first baby would probably be named for Charles, especially if it were a boy, and Millicent said that everyone had been saying that. Actually she and Leslie planned not to have children until Leslie's brother had been put through college and medical school, she said. But after that she hoped for a large family, with at least two boys, one to name after Charles and one to name after Leslie's father. One of the ladies said maybe she'd have twins. An aunt on her father's side said she'd think Millicent would rather have postponed the wedding until Leslie got out of service, instead of shlepping around Army camps for two years, and Millicent explained that Leslie had suggested waiting for exactly that reason, but that she did not mind shlepping around Army camps. Several ladies said that Millicent was right and that shlepping around Army camps was nothing if you were young. Especially if your husband was an officer. And she told them that she and Leslie had decided against an engagement ring, because she was against extravagances and it was going to be such a short engagement anyway. They said she was very sensible.

At work she told Mr. Killian of her marriage plans, by way of making sure she would have the wedding day off. She did not give notice yet, but said she would when her husband was settled. Within a day or two word had spread around the city room. Maud Dickinson caught Millicent's hand, when Millicent passed her desk, and looked up with a smile that turned her whole face to wrinkles. She looked as happy as though she herself were getting married. Her eyes narrowed to slits under the gray bangs, and all the metal reinforcements of her old teeth showed.

"So you finally hooked him," she said.

"Oh, it happened very suddenly," said Millicent.

Later in the week Maud called her to her desk again, at just about quitting time, and drew a large block-shaped package from the deep bottom drawer. The wrapping was printed all over with big wedding bells and little brides and grooms and churches.

"Oh, you shouldn't have done that!" said Millicent.

"Don't open it now," said Maud. Her eyes were merry and narrow amid the wrinkles.

"Gee," Millicent said. "Thank you. But you shouldn't have. I don't know what to say."

"Don't say anything," said Maud.

On the train Millicent undid the package. It was an electric coffeepot that mirrored her face in an elongated way. She displayed it that evening to her family and Leslie, and told them she hardly knew Maud—she was just somebody in the office.

Natalie telephoned her at the city room, and offered congratulations and said she was sending a gift. Millicent wondered how she had heard, but she explained it quickly enough—all the roommates had been invited to the shower, but Natalie had had a parent-teachers' meeting, and the others had been unable to go for one reason or another. She was glad to hear from Natalie, and told her all the reasons why she felt she and Leslie were perfectly suited.

In the evenings there was constant discussion with her family of the wedding arrangements, whether Leslie was visiting or not. They had determined on about a hundred and fifty guests, and there was talk of having it catered in Boston, as the temple had no social hall as yet. Patty said she thought Bingle's German & Yankee Cookery could set up a kosher luncheon if her father gave them the recipes but Lucinda said Bingle's had ashes in the potato salad. It kept falling off Bingle's cigar when he made it. But at length they hit on the idea of engaging a caterer that Ed had heard of, who supplied tents for outdoor buffets, and having a house wedding. Millicent liked the idea of being married at home. With rows of folding chairs the guest could be squeezed into the living room and dining room for the ceremony, if most of the other furniture were taken out. Then lunch would be in the yard. The caterer usually set up several tents with no sides, over tables, and another over the bar, and another over the hors d'oeuvres table, and a serving tent, except that they all had sides if it rained. During lunch the folding chairs would be cleared from the house for those who wished to go in and dance afterward. They talked about whether to hire a three-piece or four-piece orchestra, and Patty said they should get one that wasn't too cornball. There was some argument over where the canopy should be erected for the ceremony—if it took place in the bay window, away over at the side of the living room, some people in the dining room would not be able to see.

They talked about the different menus the caterer offered, and Lucinda said she had heard from someone that the chickens were small and tough.

Ruthie Meyers, the cousin of Leslie's who had introduced them, telephoned Millicent at home and Millicent chatted at length, telling again why Les was right for her.

Leslie's mother and brother were of course coming up for the wedding, and so were others of his relatives, not only from Connecticut but from Glens Falls and other places. Ed and Lucinda and Millicent and Patty had all spoken to his mother long-distance. They had insisted one night on Leslie's calling her from their house, and had taken turns at the phone.

It was not long after that Millicent asked Leslie in one of their walks how his mother was taking it, and what his mother had been writing him. He told her his mother had written a letter with all the reasons against marrying too early. But he said not to worry, his mother was very mixed up. In the same letter she had told him to do as his heart dictates, and that she wanted him to be happy, and so forth.

"Maybe I should phone her again," Millicent said. "Or make a trip down there on my days off. I've never even met your brother."

"Don't," Leslie said. "She'd think you were extravagant." He said the one long-distance phone call had been enough and that long-distance telephoning just wasn't part of his mother's world.

Millicent said that perhaps while she was waiting for Les to get settled in the Army the whole family would drive down to his mother's for a visit. And if she and Les ever settled near New Britain she would help out in the store.

Some days later he said his mother had written it was too bad he would have to spend money for a suit just when he was going into uniform, and had suggested that perhaps he could get married in his uniform instead. So he had written his mother that he would have use for the suit again.

Millicent thought often, when she was alone on the train, or lying in bed, how she would make a point of getting along with his family, and how his family and hers would become friends, and how their children would have two uncles and one aunt. And she would borrow his mother's recipes.

She asked Les how he liked her parents, and her relatives. She told him that everyone admired him and liked him. He said that her father seemed to be a man with a wide diversity of interests.

She noticed that Les was shy about calling her parents Mother and Dad. They spoke of it once, and she told him he'd get used to it. For a long time he called them nothing.

Her mother proudly showed Leslie the mounted butterfly collection in Roland's room, and also some things that Charles had made, and the Model T that he had half restored in the barn. Millicent followed them to the barn. "Poor Charles," Lucinda mused to Leslie. "Whenever it's good weather, I think 'what a perfect day to work on that car.' "

Millicent noticed too the rambling, elderly way in which her father spoke to Les. All at once her father had begun to sound older-generationish. The invitations had scarcely been sent out when he began bothering Les almost every day about which of his friends and relatives were accepting and which he had not heard from. He said he had to tell the caterer. He also sat and talked about seating arrangements, making Les listen to him and okay things. And he kept reminding Les of such things as getting the license, and the ring, which had to be of gold and of a plain design. It irritated her that he kept after Les in this way. There was no need to. She and Les had already been to a jeweler's together after work and had her finger measured, and put a deposit on a seventeen-dollar band in a hammered design, plain enough to suit the purpose. Her father asked Leslie whether he had a dark suit. Leslie said he was buying one.

And her mother asked Leslie what color his mother and his aunts planned to wear. His brother was to be best man, and Patty was to be maid of honor. Patty argued with her mother about her gown, and about her hairdo, and wanted a green dress because green went well with red hair.

Millicent went shopping with her mother on her days off and before work on the days when she still worked late. She would wear the same wedding gown that Grandma Annie and her mother had worn. But it needed altering, and she needed satiny white shoes to go with it. Her mother and Patty also needed satiny shoes to match their dresses. They chose a pattern for chinaware.

It was no use to choose furniture as she did not know where she would be living, but she and her mother looked at some in passing. The shopping trips were endless and tiring, and she and her mother became footsore. They talked about the bridal bouquet, what flowers it should contain, and about corsages and boutonnieres.

"I hope you and Les haven't started being intimate again," Lucinda said to her, out of the blue, as they sat waiting for their train at North Station. "You'll have plenty of time for that later."

"Mother—" Millicent began testily, coloring.

"Well, I know the wedding isn't far off," Lucinda said nervously, "and I don't mean to pry, but your father and I are concerned. It's just not right, and I still don't think it's the smartest thing in the world, either."

"Mother, I'd rather not discuss it. I didn't ask for your advice."

"I went with Dad a whole year before we were married, and we never did anything like that."

"Is that how you got him to marry you?" Millicent asked sourly.

"He was very anxious to marry me, if you'd like to know. But we waited until the wedding."

"Until the first wedding, or the second?"

"And you're altogether too fresh," Lucinda told her. "I don't like your attitude about the whole thing." She sat more huffily, to show her displeasure. "The second," she added, after a moment. "We didn't know if it was going to be annulled or not."

For a while there was no conversation, only a strained silence. But on the train Lucinda began to talk about the dress Aunt Celeste was making for Nan, as Nan was going to be flower girl.

Millicent had in fact not slept with Leslie since their walk up the hill on the day he proposed. But she was irritated with her mother nevertheless, both for assuming the contrary and for intruding at all. She had seen her mother show an oblique flustered concern in various ways, but she had thought her mother would have the decency at least to try to mind her own business.

Actually she and Leslie had been so busy that there had not been the occasion for it. The preparations for an early wedding made the atmosphere quite rushed and different, and there did not seem to be the same opportunities as before. Dr. and Mrs. Mahady were back from their semester in Buffalo, so Leslie no longer had an apartment. Most of his evenings when not on call he spent with Millicent and her family and he usually had supper in their kitchen. They did get away for an evening but only to visit Ruthie Meyers and her husband, who showed them slides of Europe. She had begun to think they might not have an opportunity to sleep together again until the wedding night. Then she even found the idea appealing. She hoped it would turn out that way, so as to give the wedding itself a freshness and make it a new beginning.

Leslie did in time begin to mention that they hadn't been to bed in a long time, and she remarked on how busy they'd been. She said she'd scarcely had time to think about it.

Then after several more days he suggested that they get together in the interns' quarters. But his roommate would have to be told, in order to be certain of the roommate's absence, and the circumstance of the roommate having to know made her uncomfortable, so that she refused. Leslie's next suggestion was that they could borrow the Mahadys' apartment for an evening when the Mahadys were going to be out. But she made the same objection. "I'd feel funny about it," she said. "That woman knowing I was coming there to have sex. I don't know what nights she has it."

"So what," he said. He was sitting on the log pile in darkness by the barn, and Millicent was on the seat of the rusty harrow. "If they know they know. They assume we do it some time. What's so awful if they're decent enough to accommodate us with a room?"

"Because it's none of their business," she said quietly. "And then Mrs. Mahady would put the sheets in the wash. No thank you."

"We don't even have to do it on the sheets. We can leave the thing folded."

"No. And try to keep your voice down," she said. It was late and the house was dark.

He was silent a moment. "Do you think they heard any of that?" he said finally.

"I don't know. Probably not. Mine's the only bedroom on this side."

"Their windows are open over there though."

"I don't think they could have heard," she said. "I just want to be careful, that's all."

"Listen, we need some kind of setup where we can have privacy. This house is all eyes, for Christ sake."

"It is not."

"You've got the nosiest parents in the world."

"I do not."

"If we go out your father waits up, and if we sit in the living room he comes cruising through. Snooping."

"He only came in that once. He came down to lock up or something."

"Or something. He's just a peeping Tom, if you want my opinion."

"Oh, you're not fair. And I thought you said you liked him."

"Well, parents shouldn't go poking around like that. It would have served him right if he'd caught us in the act. It'd be his shame, not ours."

"He's just a father who's concerned, that's all. How would you feel, if you were a father, and you had a daughter?"

"I'd expect her to lead a normal life."

"Maybe you would and maybe you wouldn't," she said. "Men tend to want these things both ways."

"Not me."

"Men like to have their cake and eat it."

"Well, he can have it, but I want to eat it. Can't you ask them to go out to a movie and give us a little privacy? And take the kids along? Other parents do, for Christ sake."

"The average parents don't have a daughter that lived with a man."

"The hell they don't."

"Or at least they don't know about it. Les, it's natural for parents to worry."

"Why don't we baby-sit for your Aunt Gwen again?"

"I can't just ask her if we can baby-sit."

"Doesn't she ever ask ya?"

"Well, she hasn't lately. And I couldn't do anything with Sharlene in the next room."

"She'd be asleep."

"She could wake up. And she'd have a trauma."

"No she wouldn't."

"Les, please. Let's not argue about it."

"I'm not arguing. I'm talking."

"Please, Les," she said. "Relax."

He blew a long, irritable sigh. He clapped his knee. "Well," he said, "I think I'll go home and get some sleep."

"A good idea," she said.

They rose and walked slowly around to the front of the house and the dirt driveway.

"Walk me down to the gate," he said. "And I'll kiss you good night and give you a feel at least."

"Not so loud."

"See what I mean?" he said. "We can't even talk privately."

They walked on the sand and pebbles of the winding drive. He took a short cut over the piled boulders of the wall, because his scooter was not parked directly at the gate. She followed him. The scooter was in tall grass between the road and low wall. He turned to her. She kissed him. She embraced his neck, and he embraced her buttocks, fondling her, pressing and lifting her flesh. He rubbed her body in fistfuls, kneading it like dough. They stood rocking.

His hand came round to her front and popped open the coppery snap.

"No," she said.

"I don't want to feel a bunch of denim. I want to feel you."

"Well you content yourself with denim. What if a car came along with headlights on?"

Later she dawdled in the kitchen, reading a scrap of newspaper, in order to give him time to get to the hospital so she could phone him. She thought it would be nice to tell him she loved him, and that she wanted to make sure he had gotten home safely.

The next night he was on call, and she didn't see him.

The night after that Ed and Lucinda went to a special town meeting, and Patty went along to watch and to help the high-school girls who sold doughnuts. Leslie and Millicent sat in the kitchen. Roland was about in pajamas for a while, but he went to bed, and when Leslie and Millicent went to the porch to sit on the glider they passed his room and saw him sleeping.

The glider squeaked under them. Millicent began to talk of a hospital case that Leslie had been describing at supper, but he pulled her to him, rounding a hand on her breast, and they kissed.

He began to explore her thigh.

"Now don't get yourself all excited," she said, pushing his hand away.

"Let's go up to your room," he said. "Now's our chance."

"No."

"Come on. They've given us an opportunity for a change. You don't think Roland's gonna wake up, do you? He's out like a light."

"No. Les, I couldn't. Not in my parents' house."

"They won't be back till eleven."

"Even so. Not in my parents' house. Not right in their house. Whether they're there or not. I have a certain amount of sensitivity to how they feel."

He sat back in the glider, staring before him across the moonlit slope of grass.

"Why don't you move out again?" he said. "To a rooming house or something for a few weeks."

"That would be pretty obvious, wouldn't it."

"Well, we have to find some place," he said. "We'll have to get a hotel room."

"Goodness no."

"Well, where then?"

"I don't know."

"This is getting ridiculous," he said. "How about under the stars, over there? In the high grass?"

"Like animals?"

"Well, we did it up on the hill, under the pine trees."

"That was different. It just happened."

"Well, look, if we want it we find a place. If you don't want it under the stars, a hotel room then."

"You'd spend money on a hotel just like that?"

"Why not?" he said. "What else is there?"

"It'd be extravagant."

"You sound like my mother."

She wished he wouldn't make these suggestions. It didn't seem fair to ask him to do without until the wedding, if he really felt deprived, but she wished he would just forget about it.

"'Extravagant,'" he repeated. "It's important. In all this talk about gowns and caterers and satin shoes you're forgetting to get laid."

She kissed him, hoping to put an end to the conversation. They lay down together on the glider, and she felt the breath of his nostrils on her cheek.

"It's too bad that old car in the barn doesn't have a back seat," he said.

It sounded as though he were teasing her now. She didn't know how to answer him. She made a little sound of disgust, against her teeth.

"Hey, what about the barn itself?" he said. "Isn't there a hayloft or something?"

"No," she told him. "There's a hayloft but there's no hay."

"Oh." He kissed her, pressing down.

"It's stinky in there anyway," she said.

Then she sighed, and gave herself to the kiss for a while, and began stroking his ears.

"Les," she said, "do you know what I wish?"

"What," he murmured.

"I wish we hadn't done it yet."

"Why?"

"So we'd have the first time still ahead of us."

"Well, that's a sweet sentiment."

They lay cuddling. For a long time they didn't speak. His hands moving on her clothing found the projections of her nipples. She kept a foot on the glider frame to maintain the swaying. Already she could hear the spring noises of the swamp. Past the porch roof she could see the stars, and ruffles of high clouds mottling the night sky. Each column of the porch had a gray side merging into black. There was a moon, not full, but larger than half. His hands submerged themselves in her clothing. She made a slow defense but he was quick.

His fingertips were rough-textured, yet they moved with gentleness, making themselves at home in her underpants and stirring warmly and lazily. Her hand rode on his to slow him. In a while she suggested that they take a walk. She restrained his fondling and struggled up.

They walked down the dirt drive.

On Massapeequit Road they turned toward the brook and the bridge and walked slowly, not saying anything. She could see that he was frowning.

"There's an advantage when the first time is the wedding night," she said as they walked, "because if it's a wedding night they can openly plan for the best possible circumstances, and reserve the bridal suite in the Ritz-Carlton, and she can have the most aphrodisiac underwear under her wedding gown, and they can dance around naked all over the Louis Quatorze furniture, and in and out of the hangings, and have prepared themselves mentally with all kinds of tricks, and roll around on a thousand-dollar rug, and the bed has a canopy and rich silks, and room service on a tea wagon of silver and teak, and they hang their underwear on the marble statues in the bathroom—but if the first time is the start of an affair, they can't do that. Because they have to pretend to each other that it was completely unforeseen, an accident. And that limits them. They have to have the most drab and dreary possible conditions, to make it seem unpremeditated."

He walked beside her silently. She saw that he was frowning even more.

"Do you see what I mean?" she said.

For a couple of steps he didn't answer. "No," he said.

"Oh, Les, you know how people start affairs these days. A girl calls up a boy, and says she just happens to be in his neighborhood, and she drops over to his apartment in slacks with a bag of lox and bagels from the grocery, and he answers the door in his bathrobe, and they sit around talking, and they end up in bed. Because they have to pretend it's spontaneous."

She kept glancing up at him. But he walked looking at the road before them.

"The most beautiful first time in the world can be on a beach under the moon," he said. "Do you realize that?"

"I suppose it can."

"Of course it can."

"But it takes money and planning to get to the right beach. That's what I mean, Les. And time to find it. You don't have the freedom to arrange it if you can't be open about it. It limits you when you have to pretend you're surprised, and make it look like it wasn't planned. It's inhibiting."

The road had begun to turn downhill a little, toward the curve, and their footsteps sounded different. She swung hands with him a little. But the hands bumped his leg and it stopped the swing.

"Well," he said, "maybe as people get more liberated, they'll be more open with themselves about starting affairs."

She shook her head. "No. When a girl picks out a boy to lose her virginity with, it's a very special thing, Les. It's a milestone in her life. And if she can't have a special lovely place and circumstance, that does justice to it, nicer than could just happen to be there, she at least needs to have that pretense, that it was a great big tremendous overwhelming passion, that surprised her all of a sudden. It has to be at least that special. There can't be just nothing special. And girls know it, and boys know it. And that's why they pretend. Like the way we went to New Hampshire."

"What about New Hampshire?"

"We didn't go there to ski."

"We didn't?"

"No," she said.

"We skied, didn't we?"

"Yes. That's how much we had to pretend."

"Look, I like skiing. And when I can afford it I'll go again. Maybe you were pretending to yourself, I don't know."

"We skied all day," she said, "and then you screwed me as an afterthought."

He seemed to be searching for an answer. She could already hear the gurgling of the brook beyond the opaque black slope of forest. Their feet sounded on the downhill road.

"I didn't mean it that way," he said.

"Les, what I mean is, a bride deserves a chance to get off on the right foot, you know, and show you how nicely she can play the whore, to best advantage. I mean, a girl's first time deserves not to be an accidental thing. It deserves to be preciously groomed. And when you make her ski all day, and then get into a squeaky brass bed when she's exhausted, you rob her of it. I was even too tired to bathe. And I had those scratchy woolen drawers on. And kids running around downstairs. You couldn't even stay all night. And it all had to seem like a sudden impulse, on the spur of the moment. I couldn't just happen to have a transparent nightgown along."

"You couldn't have anyway. You never had a transparent nightgown in your life."

"All the more reason why I needed the Ritz-Carlton. The honesty of a wedding night has that advantage, that you can go right out and set it up right."

"How do you know so much about the Ritz-Carlton?"

"I don't," she said. "I just imagine it."

They came down to where the road turned into the covered bridge.

"That's how a wedding night should be," she said. "You'd lift up my chemise inch by inch."

One side of the entrance of the bridge was damaged, more so toward the bottom than the top. Splintered boards hung at angles. Leslie and Millicent slowed and paused, and Leslie fingered the end of a spear of broken wood, seeming to study it. A corner of the peaked roof extended over the broken part. Deep inside the tunnel of the bridge there was a cavernous dark in which she could see no details, except the gray square of the opening at the other end and a little moonglow on supporting beams down there. Leslie was idly breaking bits of wood from a thick sliver.

"It just came to me when Aunt Gwen gave the shower for me, when I was sitting there with all the presents and all those ladies and my grandmother and everybody—I mean, what a sexy thing a wedding is when the bride's a virgin. She's in white, and everybody knows that tonight he's going to take her clothes off—it's just sexy. And she's anticipating, and he's anticipating, and everybody's anticipating—tonight her pants come down—that's a wedding."

Leslie tossed a piece of wood into the water. It made a musical splash. He seemed to watch the current take it under the bridge, but she could not see much down there in the grayness. When she looked at him he was still looking absently toward the black water. The moon shone on the frames of his eyeglasses.

"Do you know what the word for bride is in Greek?" she said.

"Noodnik," he said.

"Nymph," she told him.

"The first time isn't the last," he said.

"No, I should hope not—it should be a growing relationship, and maybe there can be real spontaneous times just happening on the right beach, like you said, or like the way we did it under the pine trees up on Sachem Hill, but what I mean is, those spontaneous times can be just as good *after* the Ritz-Carlton thing. I think maybe the older you get the more wonderful they can be. But the Ritz-Carlton thing can't ever be real except as the first. It's just lost."

He had stepped a little into the bridge and tested a board that hung askew in the smashed wall. It fell off.

"What happened here?" he asked.

"The fire engine did it," she said. "That's what they're having the town meeting about. The new hook and ladder. It's too sharp a turn for it here."

"Oh."

"They want to tear it all down and put up a plain junky one with pipe railings and everything. Just a plain iron span."

"Do I hear a dam or something?"

"It's just down there a little ways. It makes the duck pond."

He turned idly, and they began to stroll back the way they had come.

"You've got this wedding-night mystique all of a sudden," he said, "but if that were true, what you say, how would you expect a completely virgin bride without any previous experience to start off like such an expert all of a sudden?"

"It doesn't matter," she said. "It's not that hard. I wasn't so terrible once I got started, was I?"

"No. You caught on fast."

"And even if she's a little awkward the first time, the awkwardness can be cute too, you know. It's not like learning ballet or something. And besides there's something intrinsically sexy about virgins, anyway, isn't there? From everything I read there is. My father even stares at teen-age kids."

"Your father's an old reprobate."

"Les, even a child knows how to make up to a man. Little girls even. They know how to be coy and cute and sexy. And even if she didn't the girlie magazines are all over the drugstore. Girls aren't dumb."

The hill rose before them. She caught his fingers as his hand swung, and they held hands. They walked a while without saying anything. The road grew steeper and she panted a little.

"Les," she said, "let's salvage what we can of our wedding night."

"What?"

"Let's not do it any more until then. Let's make it as much like a wedding night as possible—"

"Are you out of your mind?" He looked down at her. He almost stopped walking.

She felt embarrassed, but her ideas had grown as she spoke, and she found she felt more strongly about it than she had realized. "Please, Les, listen. I just want to salvage what we can. All those people are going to be there, and food, and music, and what's it all for—just to celebrate the signing of a legal document? What good's a wedding party if the bride and groom are just like an old married couple? And when the party's over and everybody goes home, and the musicians go home, and you and I are alone, what are you and I gonna celebrate with?"

"With sex! What we always celebrated with!"

"I don't want it to be a chore."

"It won't be a chore!"

"It might be," she said, looking up at him. "If we've been doing it right along. It might just happen to turn out to be a night when we don't happen to feel like it, and we'll feel that we still ought to do it anyway because we got married that day. Honestly, Les—" She held his hand more firmly. "You don't mind, do you?"

"Millicent, you're crazy."

"Les, we'll hire the bridal suite in the Ritz-Carlton and I'll come slithering up your front with grapes in my pubic hair. And we'll do it like it's fresh and new." They had stopped walking and stood in the middle of the road.

"Where did you get this big ambition to get laid in the Ritz-Carlton, for Christ sake? You wouldn't even wear lacy underwear when I asked ya."

"Well, I've changed my mind about that."

"And you mean not a thing until the wedding? You're gonna send me off with one night and a pat on the head?" She tried to speak but he kept on. "What *is* this? We're not even gonna have a honeymoon, for Christ sake."

"I know we're not, Les. That's all the more reason why we should have a real wedding night. And then you'll be sending for me, and we'll be together again, and we'll have that to remember. I'll quit my job as soon as you have a place for me to stay." Her voice was quavering. "Oh, Les. What can I do? Don't you want a wedding? We'll come together fresh. If you insist, in the meantime, I'll do it, but I wish you wouldn't insist. You think about it, and try to see what I mean. So we'll have a wedding night."

He shook his head, not negatively but confusedly, as though she were mad.

"Les, honest," she said. "You'll be glad."

67

The life of the congregation went along busily, as though Ed's impending departure did not matter to it. The Sisterhood again entered a joint rummage sale and carnival with the First Parish Ladies' Auxiliary and the St. Timothy's Ladies' Guild, under the trees in Murphy Square, and like last year they complained that the other two groups put crummier things in the rummage.

Yet, once it was established that he was leaving, people seemed friendlier, and more cordial to him than ever. He still gave a Monday night course for the few ladies that had stayed with it, and now a couple more came that had never been before. Then the congregation gave a cocktail party in his honor. It was held outdoors, on the Gilberts' lawn, but the congregation itself sponsored it, as a kind of testimonial. Very many attended, and even people who had voted against him seemed amiable.

A few nights later he had a fair turnout of teen-agers when he gave his fourth and last talk to the youth group. There were eight or nine kids at the beginning and about eleven including latecomers. It was to be about sex and intermarriage, and it was held in Dr. Tobias's rumpus room so they could dance afterward. Ed straddled a chair backwards and talked to kids who sprawled in various postures on the couch, on the low-slung chairs, on the hassocks and the floor. He told them after a while that a congregation had to be an educational venture, and that too many people had a kindergarten notion of religion.

As he spoke his eyes kept fixing themselves, as they usually did in these meetings, on a strikingly beautiful girl named Nicole. She was fourteen, with an average figure, and with diction that left something to be desired, but her face was extraordinary. Even Lucinda had remarked once to Ed on Nicole's attractiveness. The fact was that with scarcely any make-up, and no affectation at all, her face had a traffic-stopping beauty. None of her features seemed to have uniqueness that he could analyze, but somehow they went together with a dazzling richness, and even on the High Holy Days, when she had sat in the congregation with her parents, it had taken almost more self-discipline than he had not to stare too long at a time.

To marvel at that face was a joy in itself. But as he talked now he looked at the other kids too.

He told them that what he wanted was to make them love this tradition so, that they could not leave it, but would have to stay and enrich it with their love. He said he wanted them to need it so, that when they went looking to fall in love they would fall in love within it, and want to build upon it, and make it something living, not just something talked about.

"Nicole," said, on a sudden impulse, taking the risk that it might be a bad error of judgment, "I don't mind telling you you're the most beautiful woman I ever saw." He saw her redden. "Whenever I look at you," he said, "it takes my breath away. I want you." Still astride the chair backwards he put forth a hand palm up, his fingers curling loosely, in a sort of grasping gesture. "I want you for this tradition. It needs you. And if you should grow up someday to leave this tradition, or marry out of it, or let it go, I would personally be heartbroken. I want you to know that. You're an adornment to the Sabbath. You're what it needs, and you're irreplaceable. I need everybody here." He looked at the others. "There's nobody here I don't need. We all need each other."

Everyone's eyes were on him silently. Nicole had remained red-faced throughout.

"Well, maybe I've been a rotten rabbi," he said. "It's true, I have. And I'm leaving, in September, but don't think my leaving will cure anything. Because the fact is that you're a rotten congregation. That is, your parents are, for the most part, and to the extent that it rubs off on you. And as long as it's a rotten congregation, you're going to keep on having rotten rabbis, in one way or another—that's all you'll ever get. It's a fact. You can tell them I said it—you may be nice people, but as a congregation you're fourth-rate, and you'll always get the punk rabbis you deserve. You can fire rabbis, but you can't fire yourself."

He paused. His hands were resting on the back of the chair. No one said a word. Then he asked one of the kids to go up and tell Mrs. Tobias it was okay to bring down the refreshments.

He did not stay for the refreshments or the dancing, but left Mrs. Tobias to chaperone and drove home. He already regretted having indulged the impulse to talk freely. There had been a mixture of emotions in him, and he had gone too far. He had particularly embarrassed Nicole, and probably also Patty, who had been in the group, though when he spoke she had been sitting where his eye did not take her in. Word of it would spread through the congregation by tomorrow and he would be in trouble again.

He put the car in the barn.

When he entered the downstairs hallway the carved clock said half-past nine. He called Roland, and then found the boy in his room working at the bug collection. He brought Roland to the study, drew the Morris chair over beside his own at the desk, and opened a volume to a chapter of Isaiah in the original.

"Okay, read," he said to Roland.

Roland began, giving each phrase its proper singsong. In late August Roland would be old enough to participate in services as an adult, and on a Sabbath morning he would be the one called upon to read the congregation the weekly portion from the Prophets. He would also be one of the seven called during the reading from the Law, and after the Law and the Prophets he might even lead the congregation in the remainder of the service.

Ed listened to him rehearse the fifty-fourth chapter of Isaiah. It belonged to the Sabbath that would follow Roland's thirteenth birthday. His voice had not yet changed. The cantillation rose sweetly, and wavered where it ought, according to the tiny markings in the text. Not even Bill Prince could make it sound better, Ed thought.

Roland had not finished when Millicent entered, in pajamas and bathrobe, and began to search the bookshelves.

"I'm looking for something to read," she said.

Roland continued without a break. He had scarcely looked up. Ed listened to him, and sometimes watched the text and sometimes Millicent. Her hair was pulled up and back with a ribbon, in a way unusual for her—whether because of the heat or because she had washed it he did not know. He loved the small unruly hairs sticking out softly behind her ears. Roland finished the text, with its last descending flourish. Millicent had taken a book from the shelves and was looking inside it.

"Okay, good," Ed said to Roland, and gave his head a little push.

Roland pushed back the Morris chair and left quickly without a word. Millicent closed the book she had taken and Ed saw it was the one on The Mind Of New England. She started out. Her bare feet sounded on the wide boards.

"Millicent," he said.

She turned at the door.

He was still at his desk. "Shut the door," he said.

She closed it and looked at him again. "What," she said.

He cleared his throat. "Have you and Les resumed sleeping together?"

He could see her stiffen angrily. Her nostrils widened and her lips tightened. "What's it to you?"

"What's it to me?" he repeated indignantly. "What do you mean, what's it to me. I'm your father, what's it to me."

She kept her voice controlled, and he noticed that she scarcely blushed at all. "Les and I happen to be an engaged couple."

"Yeah, engaged couple. You're not married. Now will you cut it out, please? What's past is past, but from here on, I don't want it, not until after you're married. I don't care whether you interpret it as religious or moral or Freudian or jealous or old-fashioned or however you rationalize it but that's how I feel about it. I don't want it. Not in my house. And not under my nose. Please. And I'd just as soon you didn't anywhere else, either."

"Will you please do me a big favor?" she said. "Mind your own business."

She seemed smug. He thought he saw a cruelty in her face. He could have slapped her had she been a child, or if he had not felt the need to maintain some dignity. He felt too much fury to contain himself entirely.

"God, will I be glad when you're married and off my hands," he said. "God, will I be glad. I wish you were married and gone. I want to forget ya. You and Patty both."

"Oh? Is your imagination working on her too?"

"My imagination isn't working on anything. I'm just fed up. Tired. Damn it."

He sat hunched and turned his gaze from her. But when he heard the click of the knob he looked up.

"Wait a minute," he said.

"I'd just as soon go upstairs and read, if you don't mind."

"Close the door a minute," he said. "I want to talk to you."

"I'd rather not continue this. If you don't mind I'd like to be excused."

"Because I asked a personal question?"

"You had no right to ask it." She was becoming red-faced now, belatedly.

"Oh, I had no right, huh? Are you sore?"

"I'm appalled."

"Appalled, all right. Well, come here. Sit down. I want to tell you something."

"I'd rather stand."

"Come on, sit down. I'll only keep you two minutes, that's all. I want to tell you a story."

She looked at him uncertainly. "What kind of a story?"

"About a man at Abbottsford. A true story. A man that was in the congregation there. A man and his wife."

She came as though reluctantly to the Morris chair, which was still catercorner beside Ed at the desk as Roland had left it. She sat cross-legged, arranging her bathrobe. Her face was still pink with embarrassment and did not look at Ed. The book about the mind of New England was on her lap.

"Millicent," he said, "I won't tell you the guy's name. It was in Abbottsford. This guy used to sleep with his wife before they were married, and then they got married. He told me the whole story himself. And when they were going together, she was always the one that said women are liberated, and all that. The same rights to all the premarital this and that. And boy, was she liberated. She'd go for every trick in the book. Whatever he suggested, she was johnny on the spot. Couldn't get into bed quick enough. She was free, you know—down with restrictions."

He saw Millicent becoming more red-faced.

"And then they got married," he continued, "and in the course of two or three years she got more and more frigid. First of all, certain things were disgusting all of a sudden, things that were okay before they were married. You know, there were certain special things he liked, and before she was married it was go ahead, you know, anything goes, wild, the whole gamut. But after they were married it was 'Oh no. No you don't. None of that. I have rights.' And even as far as just plain normal sex went, it was gradually less and less, in a couple of years. She'd always be too tired, or too this, or too that, and she'd say 'leave me alone! I'm not your chattel.' And if they did have sex once in a blue moon it was like she forgot everything she ever knew—before she was married she was an expert. And now he had to beg. He could be going crazy and she'd say, 'oh, go away, let me sleep. I have my rights. I'm not your chattel.' She was liberated."

"That's crazy!" Millicent said. She was blushing deeply, not looking at him.

"All right, but it happened. And you know what that poor guy said to me? He said, 'if these new ideas made women half as sexy after marriage as it makes them before marriage, that would really be something.' "

"How stupid," she said, red-faced. She looked harassed.

"Oh, it's not so stupid. The time to say 'I'm not your chattel' is before marriage, not after. Only a lot of girls are getting it backwards."

"Are you finished?" she said. "May I go now?" She sat forward stiffly with her book.

"Wait a minute."

She got up. "Dad, really. I don't want to hear about your crazy friends in Abbottsford. I'm sure other fathers don't talk to their daughters about things like that. It's embarrassing."

"Well, my daughters have been on my mind a lot lately." He had risen with her.

"I wish you'd put something else on your mind."

"Well, I know. It's all unmentionable. I shouldn't talk about it."

She had moved to the door but he did too, putting his hand on the knob so as to block her. He looked down into her eyes.

"I want you to have a happy marriage," he said.

"I expect to have."

"Millicent," he said, "keep it holy. It's sexier holy, because it's lovelier holy."

"I really don't want to talk about it. Excuse me."

He moved from the door and let her open it. Patty's record player could be heard upstairs.

"Millicent," he said, touching her arm as she began to pass through the door, "as one of my wedding gifts, I'm giving you that big arty edition of the book of Psalms."

She paused and looked up at him warily.

"You know the one?" he said. "Just the Psalms alone, great big pages and big modern artsy drawings. You've looked at mine. It's on the shelf there."

"I think I've seen it," she said.

"Well, you're gonna have a copy of it. It's a work of art. A beautiful book. And I want to call your attention especially to 'Happy are they that dwell in the Law of the Lord.' You know it—it's in the prayer book too. And you can think I'm a square, or you can think what you want, but that line—I used to accept it as brilliant poetry, without thinking too much about it, but the fact is, it's true. So help me. I can tell you that in recent years I've found a deep personal truth in it. Even when things have gone wrong, I've seen that I was happier in the Law than I would have been outside it. At any time you care to name. And that's a fact. In big things and in little things. And I want to commend that phrase to you, that statement. It's my legacy to you and to Les. Tuck those words away in your mind somewhere, and maybe someday they'll speak to you."

She made a little shrug of embarrassment and exasperation, as though there were no way to reply to such stuff.

"People died at Auschwitz whether they dwelled in the Law of the Lord or not," she said finally.

"Well, even there. Even if I died at Auschwitz, I'd rather die with a trust in my heart that the Nazis were doomed, and that none of it's the end of the tale—someday justice has to evolve. It'll be my world, not theirs. Rather that in my heart than just terror, or meaninglessness. It would be less ignominious, I think. Even on the ash heap."

"Religion didn't open up any escape hatches in the gas chamber."

"Well, did atheism open up any escape hatches in the gas chamber? Look, why does it say dwell, instead of some more obvious word, like follow, or believe? It means people who see the world from the Law's viewpoint. You see the world from your dwelling place. That's what it means. And I think maybe it turns out to be so. The Law's view is the only view of this world you could call a happy one."

"What if your mind just can't accept it?"

"If you can't, you can't. The gas gets you anyway. Millicent, I don't say a life without pain. But the difference between one life and another is in how you meet pain. You know the Psalms aren't meant to be taken exactly like universal statements, like the word of God—they're more like personal testimony. Do you know what I mean? Like in a Methodist Wednesday-night meeting."

"I don't know anything about Methodist Wednesday-night meetings."

"Well, individuals tell about their own experiences. And I think the Psalms are like that. And as far as 'happy are those who dwell in Torah' is concerned, it's true, sweetheart. It's true what I said. I've seen families that dwelled in it, back in the days when I was more in touch, and I've seen people grow serene and fine. In so many ways, it works. That's why a religious man is supposed to read the Song of Songs every Friday night. Or hear it. Because after that, all those sexy phrases, he might get next to his wife and say something nice. Even if she's a dog."

The anger seemed to be gone from Millicent's face.

"Well," he said, "good night."

"Good night," she said.

He watched her go upstairs. Her feet were bare and she carried the book about the mind of New England. Patty's record was still playing.

He turned and went out into the night, shutting the double doors behind him. His slow footsteps sounded on the porch, and then on the pebbles in the drive, and became silent on the grass.

He heard the little noises of the night. There was wind in the trees. Two of the crab-apple trees had become diseased, but he thought there was little point in spending money on them now if he wasn't going to remain here.

He looked at the sky and saw that it was clear. The stars were not always the same. Sometimes, as now, the sky was awash with them, but sometimes they were brilliant and cold in the black.

Near the hugest of the elms he urinated. You're not really in the country until you can piss in the yard, he thought.

He resumed walking. What these kids don't understand, he said to himself, is that you should enjoy the frustration, savor it, just as you enjoy the chase, and just as you enjoy prolonging the act itself.

Frustration too, while you know it will end, is a source of enjoyment, and you must know how to appreciate it, or you've lost a big hunk of life's richness. That full testicles sharpen your appreciation of beautiful women there is not the slightest doubt. Frustration excites. It lights up every twist of a hip and bobbing breast for you. There's a tension, and there are girls in your eyes. Satisfaction brings peace, but it's the peace of impotence and slack, and you must wait then anew for the slow filling of eagerness.

Call frustration by its other name, desire, and don't hurry so to be rid of it. Let them make the most of it, and take a big load off their minds, and do without. What do these kids think sex is, their daily prayers?

It's just about come to that, he thought, when young people who prefer traditional morality are made to feel that their subconscious is therefore out of whack, and that their thoughts are not their true thoughts.

He wandered restlessly by the barn. The log pile was smaller than last fall. He climbed into the high small metal seat of the rusty harrow. Millicent, he thought, the sensitive child who had once seemed his soul made flesh. If he could not communicate with her he was really alone.

His thoughts went to Charles. Eighteen years, what an age to be wiped out. Just when a man's ready at last to begin to think, to be a person, to begin to leave some mark upon the world.

He had been named for Ed's favorite grandfather—there was no one to bear his name now.

We philosophize about ways of death, he thought, dying young, dying old, but it's a pastime of healthy men. The dying man is desperate to stay alive. His own grandfather at ninety-one was frightened of the dangerousness of the age he had reached, as a young soldier is of bullets. He could not imagine where the years had gone. Ed had tried to encourage the old man with newspaper clippings about men who lived past a hundred, and one about a man in the Caucasus who was supposed to be over a hundred and fifty. But his grandfather quoted unhappily the Talmud's comment that seventy is old age, eighty is white old age, that a man of ninety is already bending over the grave, and that a man of a hundred is as though he had passed from the earth. So Ed had replied to him that in that case there were still nine more years of bending ahead, and anyway "as though passed from the earth" only meant removed from active production. Titian painted at ninety-nine; at later ages you made no contributions. And in his grandfather's last illness, when he lay with an oxygen tube in his nose, Ed told the doctor not to shrug at the old man's age but to try to save him as he would struggle to save a child. He died anyway.

And Rosalind has been dead half a year. Certain deaths recall others, he reflected. There comes a time in your life when everybody you loved in your childhood is dead. Charles at least never knew this. He died with his family intact. His childhood over, but not yet destroyed.

Ed looked up from the harrow. Millicent's bedroom was lighted. At the back of the house he could see the glow from Patty's bedroom upon the slate roof of the kitchen. He knew from having walked about before that every bedroom in the house was lighted.

He got down from the harrow, as if at loose ends, and went into the house.

The door of Roland's room was partly open, and Ed went in. He found Roland busy at a table with some insect specimens. The lamp on the table was the only light.

"Hi," Roland said without looking up.

"Hi," said Ed.

He stood watching Roland. There were a lot of dead bugs on the table, mostly beetles. Several were as tiny and brilliant as gems, round, or elongated, and some of the larger dark ones had a pink or purplish iridescence. There were also a couple of dragonflies, one small and one enormous, almost too big to be an insect. A shallow cardboard box had been spread with cotton, from an open packet that was on the table too, amid boxes and jars. Roland was selecting certain bugs and arranging them on the cotton.

"I thought you read beautifully tonight," said Ed. "We're all going to be proud of you."

Roland said nothing. Ed looked on, over Roland's shoulder.

"Have you got any this year yet?" Ed asked. "Or are those all last year's?"

"Some."

"Do you know the name of every species, every one you've got there?"
"Yup."
Roland worked as though Ed were not there.
This boy was remarkable, Ed thought. Whatever he undertakes he does well. Only recently Ed had done the paper route one morning when Roland was confined to bed with fever, and Roland had written it all down for him from memory—who took a Post, a Globe, a Herald, a Record, who left the money on the sill or under the mat, whose dog might steal whose Christian Science Monitor.
The lamp on the desk made shadows in the room. There was an old brass mariner's compass on the low bookcase, beside a pile of cards showing portraits of baseball players. A hunting knife hung on the wall. The walls also had three large charts in full color, picturing birds of many kinds. The bottom of one chart had a row of staring owls.
"Well, study everything you can," Ed said to Roland. "You're a smart kid, and you're going to be a scholar. Your curiosity's a gift. And keep it broad, whatever you specialize in, whether it's zoology or whatever it is."
Roland arranged the smaller bugs toward the top of the cotton rectangle. Ed sat on a corner of the bed.
"For one thing," he said, "it all has a bearing on your understanding of religion. You know who Maimonides was?"
"Ya."
"Well, Maimonides said you had to study all the sciences you could get, if your perception of God is going to be a reasonable one. Insofar as the mind is capable of having any. He said physics, logic, math, medicine. Astronomy—open your eyes and whatever can be learned go out and learn it. And naturally you'd add all the newer sciences. Psychology, biochemistry. It's as challenging as that. If you're religious you must have a passion for science—in the first place you can't speculate about God without becoming curious to know what can be known. You can use anthropology and sociology even, and archaeology, in your appreciation of this religion. Along with the religious literature. Even while it's the most advanced, it keeps its ties to the most primitive."
"Why?" Roland said without looking around.
"Because it's human. The human experience is tied up in it. A good religion has to take in the whole business of being human, and that means anthropology, and poetry and argument and torts. Lots of things. Love and marriage. And history. How can you think intelligently about God in history, if you don't know history? You have roots, Rollo. That chapter in Isaiah that you're gonna read, it's been read just like that every year on its proper Sabbath—do you know how long? It's not something that died out and was restored. It never stopped. In Charlemagne's day and Haroun al-Rashid's, down to Napoleon and the present—you name it and we were there, and somebody got up in the congregation and read it, against the background of that day, like you're going to. It's unbroken, year by year."
"I know it," Roland said.

From where Ed sat, somewhat behind and to the side, he could not quite see Roland's profile. It crossed his mind that each of his children somehow had been a little less neurotic than the preceding.

"Rollo," he said, "what does 'Israel' mean?"

" 'He wrestles with God.' "

"That's right—'he wrestles with God'—'he contends with God,' " said Ed. "That's right. And do you know why it says 'wrestles'? Why doesn't it say 'he boxes with God,' for instance? Or just 'he fights with God'?"

"I don't know," said Roland. He didn't interrupt his work.

"Well," said Ed, "because wrestling is strife, struggling, contention. But at the same time it's an embrace. It's like when you wrestle with a problem. You have to love the problem, or you don't wrestle with it."

68

Millicent finished work at four in the afternoon and then went to exchange some soup bowls for bread-and-butter plates at Jordan's, because among the wedding gifts so far there were too many of one kind and none of another. She also had gloves to exchange for another size. Then she went to the hospital and had supper with Leslie, because he was on call.

He looked haggard and spent, and the white jacket and trousers were rumpled. His eyes were squinting and bloodshot.

"You poor man," she said.

He had been up practically all night, he told her, and had removed part of a woman's kidney. Then he had worked all day and his left eye was developing a tic.

"It's stupid the way they drive interns," Millicent said. "And they expect you to be on call again after that?"

"Well, you can't plan emergencies," he said. "I'm young—I'll survive it."

He went to his quarters and she took the train home.

The next night he came to Wilmerding Crosswalk for supper. Patty smilingly modeled for him the green gown she would wear as maid of honor. Lucinda was still altering it. The talk was of where the flower arrangements would be stood, and what music would be played, and the menu they had chosen. Leslie said little. He looked weary. Ed thought that even though it would be a buffet with tables under tent tops there should be placecards, and he sat down next to Leslie and explained at length a diagram of seating arrangements. He asked Leslie if he had any aunt and uncle he wanted to put at the head table to balance it out, as his family was smaller.

In time Leslie said he would like a breath of air, and Millicent walked out with him to the cool and darkness of the porch.

"Go up and put on your jeans," he said, with a gentle slap on her behind. "We're going for a ride on the scooter. Unless you want to ride sidesaddle."

"Where are we going?" she asked.

"For a ride."

She went in again, and the spring clapped the screen door shut behind her. In her room she put on jeans and a shaker sweater. She came down and told her mother she was going for a spin on the scooter.

She walked down the curving dirt road. He walked silently beside her in the night. He seemed jumpy and restless, she thought. They went downhill around the big curve, and she felt the pebbles through her sneakers.

"We're gonna get laid," he said.

"Oh, Les." She paused in her tracks, but then had to walk to keep up. "Is it really necessary, if we're getting married in a week?"

"Yes. I'm gonna normalize this relationship." There was no break in his walk.

She was following half a step behind. "Les, please! I wish we wouldn't. Let's not spoil it."

"I'm not spoiling it. You're spoiling it."

"Our wedding night, I mean."

"Millicent, what do you think you're doing? You can't become a virgin retroactively. Look, kid, I'm sick of this. And I'm gonna take you to a motel and take your damn pants off. You said you would if I insisted, and I do insist."

"We've done it before—why do we have to do it now? We know we're compatible."

"Are you serious?" He had arrived at the gate and as he spoke he widened it for her against the high grass. "Now get on," he said.

She climbed silently onto the back of the scooter.

"I'm sorry, kid," he explained, looking into her eyes. "It's just too stupid."

He turned from her and put a leg over the scooter. He balanced it, one foot on the road. Before her his jacket lay rounded on his hunched back.

"It's the healthy, normal thing for an engaged couple," he added. "And anything else is sick. You don't stop screwing because you're engaged." He started the motor and clicked on the head lamp. "Your whole attitude's sick."

The scooter became loud, and turned in a leaning U-curve that circled the width of the road. She held his waist. They set off in the direction of the duck farm and the brook.

"I just wish we wouldn't," she said. "I'm not in the mood."

"What about my mood?" he said.

The breeze pushed at her eyes and face. Where the road turned downward the forest was black about them, but in front the scooter made brilliant greens and browns among the pines. It coasted downhill and the motor eased. She heard frogs.

The scooter swayed and they entered the broken bridge. She had never been through it on the scooter before. It rode bumpily on the worn knotty flooring. The motor was loud in the enclosure.

They came out. A bump jolted her. She held to the knob with one hand and grasped his belt and trousers with the other. They accelerated into the wind.

"Let's just go some place and have an ice cream," she said.

"Millicent, listen," she heard him say. "Maybe it would make sense if we'd never done it, and then okay, you could say save it a little longer. But just because we're getting married you seem to want to imagine yourself a virgin, and you're not. And it's absurd and inappropriate. You're too young to go moaning over your lost innocence. It's silly. We're an old married couple, for Christ sake. This ceremony's just a legalism—"

"And what about our wedding night?"

"We'll have champagne."

"Champagne isn't what makes a wedding night."

"And we'll make love, for Christ sake," he said. "Lots of love. We're practiced now. We're all the better for knowing each other. And this last week should be full of love—all we can get. Sure, I'll be sending for you—soon, I hope. And in the meantime one night's too short a ration."

The scooter sped, and she felt the road's bumps.

"I don't know," she said. "I'm all mixed up. I can't even think it through. I wish you and my father would both be quiet and leave me alone long enough to think things out for myself."

"Your father—were you talking to your father?"

"Well, he had a talk with me, and it strengthened my resolve, as a matter of fact. Les, I really don't think we should. He said a lot of things in line with what I was thinking."

"I might have known. Don't you think you're along in years to be consulting your father about your sex life? It just isn't done. You're twenty-two. You're engaged."

"I didn't consult him."

"I could see talking with your mother, but not your father."

"Well, I couldn't help it." She kept clinging to Leslie in the wind as she spoke. "I told him that not everything's healthy to talk about. But he did say some things. I mean, like keeping it holy. Let's make the ceremony a little bit sacred at least. If we love each other our being together is something that deserves to be sacred, isn't it?"

"What does that man do? Lie awake nights, thinking up reasons why his daughters shouldn't get laid?"

"Well, it's a question of what you want to associate things with. Don't you want sex to be associated with our marriage? Instead of with nothing in particular?"

"Millicent, whose girl are you? Mine or your father's?"

She was holding to his waist. The road was smoother here, and faded pieces of a broken white line kept coming to them out of the darkness. "My own," she answered him.

For a moment there was only the sound of the scooter.

"I didn't think marriage was that individual a matter," he said.

"Well, my father did say some good things. He said you should try to be as sexy as possible after marriage. And I think that's right. And if I ever have a daughter that's the way I'd bring her up. To be a virgin beforehand and go all out after the wedding. And then a wedding would be a wedding. I'd teach her to wait, but not be inhibited."

"And how do you expect her to make that sudden switch? After she's been raised as a demure little prude all her life?"

"Well," said Millicent, "I'd tell her everything I know, about all the crazy things men like, but I'd tell her to save it. I'd have her know whatever there is to know. From books, and foreign movies, and what I could tell her, and buy the sexiest trousseau in the world, and she'd save it all up for the big blowout."

"You'd show her obscene training films, maybe."

"Maybe," she said. "I might." Her voice was growing uncertain.

"And she's supposed to save it all up for the big blowout."

"Yes."

"She'd blow up before the blowout."

"Maybe not—"

"Well, her boy friend would. And you'd go down in history as the biggest nut since Fanny Bloomer."

"Well, I wish I could explain it the way my father said it. I wish you could have heard it the way he said it. Or I wish you'd have a talk with him. He can explain it better than I can."

"Are you out of your mind?" His voice had risen. "What am I supposed to do—talk to my prospective father-in-law about whether I should screw his daughter or not?"

"Well, I'm all mixed up," she said. "I wish I knew what the answer was. I don't know. I'm of two minds about it, I suppose."

"Isn't there something in the Bible about a girl leaving her parents and cleaving to her husband?"

"Yes."

"Well let's go somewhere and cleave. You've got to get them off your back. It's terrible, and it just isn't healthy. They're sick in the head, both of them—not just your father. And they're making you sick. My parents were sick too—I give credit where it's due."

Basically Les was right, she thought. After all it was the healthy and normal thing to do. Certainly people didn't stop doing it when they became engaged. She felt confused. When her father had said happy are those who dwell in the Law of the Lord she had pictured a bride happily losing her virginity in the richness of the Ritz-Carlton, and it had seemed a truth, but now, behind Leslie on this scooter puttering in the night, it was harder to make sense of it. It occurred to her that her father had tried to dwell in the Law of the Lord and instead of making him happy it had gotten him into trouble with his congregation and gotten him fired.

She leaned with Les when the scooter did. The yellow head lamp explored before them, seeming to turn the road's mild curves into an adventure.

She wondered if he meant for them to remain at the motel the entire night. She thought of her parents. If they gave her wounded and disapproving looks the next day she would just have to ignore them.

It would be better not to spend the night, and get home at a reasonable hour. But if they checked out after a couple of hours, the motel manager would know what they had come for, and would know that they weren't really married.

She wondered if they would arouse suspicion by having no luggage. She wished she had at least stayed in her skirt and ridden sidesaddle. There seemed something tough and hardened about going to a motel on a scooter in blue jeans.

She wondered whether the clerk confronting them at the desk would be a man or a woman.

"If we go to a motel, we'll have to register as Mr. and Mrs.," she said.

"So what," said Leslie.

"Nothing."

"As a matter of fact, I don't think we do," he said. "I think one person registers and just puts down the number in the party."

"Oh, hotels aren't like that, are they?"

"No, I think in a hotel it's Mr. and Mrs., but in a motel you put one name and the number in the group."

That's interesting, she thought. It saves a certain amount of embarrassment, anyway. But then she was not sure if it did. It seemed a left-handed discreetness that admitted the motel to the conspiracy.

"How do you happen to know that?" she asked.

"I heard it. What's the matter? Do you suspect me of taking girls to motels?"

"No. I guess I just don't like your having such lore."

She felt she was being disagreeable.

She wanted to restore warmth and rapport between them by assuring him that she was going along willingly, after all. But it was hard to find a way to say it.

"What motel are we going to?" she asked.

"There's one in Pingree."

At the crossroads he left the road to Sparkstown and turned north. Glancing over her right shoulder she saw what for an instant seemed a forest fire, but then she saw it was the rising moon, remarkably huge and orange.

She should perhaps tell him to look at the moon. But she wondered if it might be dangerous to tell him to take his eyes from the road.

I know exactly what my father would be saying if he were here, she thought.

He'd be saying that the full moon tells us that on the religious calendar we're at the fifteenth of the month.

For a long time she rode the bumps, feeling the chilly wind about her face and on her eyes, and feeling self-conscious.

The road merged with a wider straight one of yellowish concrete instead of black, with crosslines of tar giving the scooter a little jolt every several yards. There were modest frame houses, none of them new, their porches making angles amid shrubbery. Leslie drove slowly, and she could hear the leaves rustle in the big branches overhead.

"I'm not exactly sure of directions," he said.

They passed a liquor store, a little wood building with a peaked roof. A glass sign with lights in it hung over the sidewalk.

"Shall I ask in there?" he said.

But he didn't stop. They passed between opposing blocks of stores, which led to a crossroad where a traffic light blinked yellow. Everything was closed, even the gasoline station, and there was no one on the streets, except for a middle-aged policeman standing at the left-hand curb, and a lean elderly man in coveralls who stood passing the time of night with him.

Leslie parked the scooter. "Wait a minute," he told her.

She saw him walk across the street toward the two men, who watched him. There was no sound but his footsteps. The traffic light put its periodic yellow over everything except a pair of street lights themselves.

She tried not to look at the policeman and the other man. She had seen them look her over. In a darkened store window beside her a hand-lettered cardboard bellied against the glass, advertising a clambake at the Congregational Church.

"Are we in Pingree?" she heard Leslie ask.

"Yup. You're at Four Corners. Poor House Road and County Way," one of the men answered.

"Is there a motel around here?"

"Right on ahead."

Leslie came back, put a foot over, and started the engine. They motored through the intersection. It had surprised and shocked her a little that Leslie so boldly asked a thing like that, while she sat on his scooter in plain view. There might even be a law against fornication. She glanced back, to see if the policeman had hurried to one of those telephones on a post. But he was only still standing with his friend.

The village petered out, and after some swamp and underbrush she saw the word Vacancy in blue neon.

The scooter swung in on a wide apron of gravel. She thought of suggesting that they change their minds.

He got off. "Come on," he said.

The building and the area before it were floodlighted. Walls of green stucco extended around a great semicircle, and the architecture was a bland modern, bright and new, with a flat roof extending outward as an overhang. There were rows of doors in either direction, and in the center picture window the manager sat beneath a bluish fluorescent tube, looking at her. He looked bored, and was flabby and dark-complexioned, Middle-Eastern-looking she thought. There were very few cars.

"I don't like the looks of it," she said, without getting off.

"Why? Do you want to look for a different place?"

"I don't know. I'd rather do it out in the woods or some place."

"Come on, we're here now. 'Out in the woods or some place.' At night. Then you'd squawk about mosquitoes."

She followed him to the main door. It was a slab of extremely grainy wood, but shiny, and it had a fancy brass doorknob. She tried to straighten her hair, which had become wind-blown.

Inside the manager scarcely looked at her. He was low behind a high desk that had a barrier of pigeonholes, and handed Leslie a card over it. She didn't watch Leslie fill it out.

She kept a hand covering her wedding-ring finger. It occurred to her that Leslie had already bought the ring and that he might have had the consideration and foresight to bring it.

She looked at the floor, which had big squares of colored linoleum, and at the flowered upholstery on the low chairs. There was indirect lighting. She thought she must look like a delinquent in her heavy black sweater.

She heard the man say ten dollars. She was aware of Leslie paying him from his wallet, and then the man directed him to cabin four down on the left.

"Come on," Leslie said to her.

She followed him out, and along under the slanting overhang, past doors and curtained windows. He held a big key.

Their door squeaked open, and they came into a room furnished in the same style as the lobby. She glanced at the wall mirror and ran her hand through her hair again, and Leslie drew the curtains. Then he lay down on the bedspread with a sigh, shoes and all, and tucked his arms under his head. She sank into the chair.

"Ten bucks—that's a hell of a price," he said, looking at the ceiling. His eyes shifted to her. "Do you want a drink for a change? If we're gonna have champagne on the big day you might as well start getting in practice."

"No."

"Some food?"

"Do they have any?"

"I don't know. We could find out."

"No, never mind," she said.

"Well, come on, come to bed." He drew up a foot to unlace the shoe, and began to undress where he lay. "You wanted a wedding night, so this is the dress rehearsal."

"Can we just talk a while first?" she said.

"Sure."

"We're not gonna stay all night, are we?" she asked.

"Why?"

"I'm just asking."

"Well, I was planning to get you home at a reasonable hour. Knowing how worried you are about what your parents think."

"I mean there's no need to hurt them unnecessarily, if that's how they feel."

"They're looking to get hurt."

"But I have some sensitivity to how they feel," she said, her voice becoming quavery and tense. "I don't want to hurt them."

"Okay, okay. Don't get excited. I said we'll go early."

Millicent rose, and tugged at her shaker sweater, but it was hard to remove, so she unsnapped her jeans instead and stepped out of them. Then she began again to hoist and tug at the sweater.

"I could have worn lacy underpants," she said. "I have some, for the wedding. I never even thought of it. I'm sorry." She was wearing very plain ones.

"That's okay."

He had on only his argyle socks and his undershorts, like a tight loincloth, cut high. She saw the bulge in them. He pulled the bedspread away. She saw him take a contraceptive from a pocket of the rumpled trousers he had taken off and slip it under the pillow. He looked round-shouldered. Her sweater had hardly budged, and she stopped for breath.

"I hope you didn't buy that in the drugstore at Wilmerding Crosswalk," she said.

"No, don't worry. And I'm sure even if I did they wouldn't print it in the local weekly."

He came to her and helped her with her sweater, and then with her shirt. She reached down and pushed off her sneakers and socks at the heel. When she came up he wobbled her breasts in her bra. He embraced her and helped her undress, all at once.

Their underpants were a cushion beneath her feet. His embrace grew warming.

"Why did you have to drag me along to the registration desk," she asked him. "I could have stayed outside."

"I know, I just didn't think. I'm sorry."

"I didn't have to go in there. We have a separate outside entrance anyway, and only one person registers, like you said, so why couldn't I have just waited outside? I'd much rather."

"Well, I've never been in a motel before. I didn't even think about it."

He embraced her harder.

"I think you better put that thing on," she said.

"No, there's time."

He embraced her some more, and then gave her a spank.

"Let's lie down," he said.

They clambered and rolled onto the bed and pulled the blankets back.

"Take off your socks," she said.

He drew off the argyle socks. She thought it was gauche of him to have left the socks for last. She could smell them.

He turned and clasped her. They lay quietly.

Her legs pinched his hand and then relaxed. She returned the caressing, with a gentle upstroke.

The patterns of hair on his belly and chest were symmetrical, like the bones of a split-open fish when the entrails are removed, she thought.

He rolled onto her and kissed her, and she responded to the kiss. She felt him encroaching. Her feet stirred upon the bedding.

"Please, Les. Try to remember I'm not made out of rubber."

He became less insistent, but not for long. She did not intend to put him off, but she found she had to. He caressed, doggedly, but there was a nervousness in her, and the caress was like a rubbing. Excitement seemed to evade her.

"I don't know what's the matter with me," she said.

"It's all in your head."

"I know it. I can't seem to get in the right mood. Maybe we better let it go till another time."

"Just relax," he said. "You'll be all right. We already paid ten bucks for the room."

He gave her his lips, slurpily, first upon her nipples, but then he slid his face wetly down her body.

"Now what," she said. She was startled. "I told you I don't want that. It makes me feel like a spittoon."

But he persisted, as if with devotion. It seemed a kind of loyalty to her, as though he were determined that she receive some pleasure.

"I guess it does work," she said after a while. She thought it somewhat surprising.

His face approached again to her own face, lazy-eyed. She felt him sinking, heavily, and she raised her knees about him.

He was both light and heavy, forceful but delicate. His face was serious, his eyes never moving from hers. He became motionless, but his tautness remained.

"There," he said, "now is that so bad? Why'd you fight it so hard?"

Slowly he began moving. She moved too. In a while she stopped moving. He continued.

"It hurts," she said. "Wait a minute."

"What's the matter? Are you out of the mood again?"

"I think we're a little out of adjustment," she said. She squirmed a bit, and used her hand a little, and he also tried to adjust. "Let's just rest for a minute," she said. "I'll be all right."

They remained still, but he did not separate himself from her. He kept watching her eyes. There's another thing in favor of a wedding night, she thought. If it's a real wedding night, and it goes badly, everything is forgiven and understood, because it's only the first time. But if it's the hundredth time, and then it just happens to go badly on the night of the wedding, it's a disaster.

He moved a little.

She tried not to wince. It was as though she could feel a wrinkle of the contraceptive.

"No, not yet," she said.

"I have to move a little," he said.

"No, please. I'll be all right in a minute. If you move when it hurts I get more unrelaxed, and then it's worse."

He waited again. She felt his fullness. She tried to accomplish an old trick of tightening herself, to squeeze him in a way that had sometimes pleased him in the past. But this time she could not manage it. He looked a little irritated. Then in time he moved a little. "Okay?" he asked.

She said nothing.

"Does it still hurt?" he asked.

She didn't answer.

"Does it?"

"Only a little bit."

"What's the matter with you?"

"I don't know. I can't help it. I was all right for a while but I couldn't seem to stay all right. You better just finish."

"I can't, if every move is gonna hurt you."

"No, you go ahead. When you get going I'll probably get stimulated."

His rhythms began again. He was looking down at her. She kept her features calm. He paused often. She knew he was being cautious and restrained. For an instant a shudder would jolt him, but again and again he seemed to make himself be leisurely. He meandered. She appreciated that he wanted to cajole her into melting. He would swoon and awaken, and send her an arrow. Yet it was as though the touch of him grated and dragged. She wanted to press him instead into a cooling stillness, that she might allay her nerves and trick them into an unguarded peacefulness.

At length he was spent.

"I'm sorry," he said.

"No, that's all right," she told him. "It was my fault."

"I don't know, maybe you're out of practice."

He sat on the edge of the bed, staring absently at the rug. They had not turned down the lights, and there was a shininess on his back and arms and shoulders.

"You know, we could spend the night, and try again later," he said. "The room's paid for."

"No! You said we wouldn't! You said you'd get me home early!"

"It's just a suggestion."

"Well, Les, I just know I'm not in the mood, and it wouldn't be any better later. And my parents would know what we're doing, if we stayed all night. Even Patty would know it. I bet even Roland would. It's not that I care what they think but I like my privacy. I don't like having the whole world know when I have sexual intercourse." She had propped herself on her elbows.

He still sat there, staring at nothing, looking burdened and tired.

"We could stay an hour or so and try," he said.

Maybe they should, she thought. She probably owed it to him to concede him that.

"Oh, the hell with it," he said. Then he rummaged around for his clothing. She left the bed and picked her underwear from the floor.

They dressed in silence. He sat on the edge of the bed and bent poking about for his shoe. The absence of conversation seemed very long.

She turned her back on him and struggled into her thick sweater. She straightened the bottom of it, which was tight about her jeans.

He unlocked the door.

They went into the night, and walked under the lighted overhang toward the scooter. He was half a step ahead of her.

"That was the lousiest lay I ever had in my whole life," he said.

"So go to the desk and ask the man for your ten dollars back," she answered him.

Leslie stopped, and turned to stare at her. "Now, was that necessary? I ask you—was that necessary?"

She looked away from his censoring eyes.

69

He shook his head. He turned, and she followed him onto the gravel.

She mounted behind him, and the motor battered the air. It made blue exhaust.

They curved to the right and the left, onto the road. The road was straight, and though he did not go fast the cooling wind made her realize she was sweaty about the neck—the motel had been warm.

"Your parents really made a mess out of you," he said.

She looked at the back of his head. Around the dark mass of his shape she could already see the far-off yellow flashing of the blinker.

"I wish you wouldn't be so sullen," she said. "It just happened to work out badly."

"It didn't just happen. It was your God damn mental attitude that made it work out badly. You just had your mind made up that all your guilts and resentments had to come along for the ride. So they could be justified."

"I did not!"

"Yes you did. Subconsciously anyway. I don't know why I didn't foresee it. I should have foreseen it."

"So you could have saved the ten dollars."

"Will you shut up about the ten dollars?"

"And you leave my subconscious out of it. You don't know one single thing about my subconscious. You better worry about your own subconscious."

"I don't know," he said, "when it was completely illegal we had a good sex life. Now we're engaged and it stinks. What's it gonna be when we're married?"

"I hate you," she said.

They went through the intersection, past the blinker. The policeman and the other man were not there now.

She was surprised at having said what she did. But she did not like his ignoring it.

"Hey," she said.

"What."

"Did you hear me?" she asked.

"I did."

He did not look around, but continued driving as before. The brick buildings ended and frame ones began. They passed a shadowy repair shop where a tow truck stood.

"Les," she said.

"What."

"I didn't mean it."

"Do you still want to marry me?" he asked.

"Yes."

"You still hate being a woman, don't you."

"With good reason," she said.

Suddenly she felt an impulse to weep. In a moment she let it go, sniffling and sobbing, without a handkerchief. The scooter gave a periodic little jounce whenever a line of tar ran across the yellow paving.

"You're still woman enough to use tears when all else fails, though."

There was an urge to weep louder, but she checked herself. I won't give him the satisfaction, she thought. She caught her breath and held on with one hand only, reaching to her hip pocket for a handkerchief.

They had already passed the liquor store and forked from the wide yellowish road onto the black one. There were patches of woods. It struck her how much shorter distances seemed on a return trip than on the way out. She blew her nose, sniffled, and wiped it.

"But don't tell me in a couple of weeks you've missed another period," he said. "That would be too much."

She swung back her foot and gave the back of his leg a sharp kick. The scooter swerved sharply and wildly far over the white line, the headlight brightening the tree trunks across the road, and in an instant leaned crazily again the other way. It wobbled and bumped and he brought it to a stop in the gutter, on a mixture of hairy grass and a moist layer of last year's leaves. He put a foot on the ground and panted, his hands still spread on the handlebars. She had clutched the scooter with two hands and had lost the handkerchief.

"Well, for Christ sake," he said, almost quietly.

He looked half around at her.

"Don't ever do that again," he said. "There was almost a funeral instead of a wedding—do you know that? There would have been another funeral in your family."

She was crying.

He partly turned in the seat, while still straddling it, one leg in the leaves and one a few inches in the air. She remained in her seat, though the scooter leaned, and put one foot to the ground too.

"What the hell is the matter with you? What if there'd been something coming the other way? Of all the idiotic—are you dumb?"

"There isn't a kind word in you," she said, her voice breaking.

He was looking at her, and his expression was clear in the moonlight. The anger modified a little, and he looked worn.

"What do you want from me?" he said.

"Protection."

"Oh, that's fine." He shifted his footing, and the scooter tilted under her. "I want protection too. All this crap you gave me about objecting to phrases like 'women and children,' and you still want to be protected like a child. That's what marriage is to you. Isn't it. The man does the protecting, so the woman can be protected and doesn't have to bother growing up. You're a woman to the core, all right. Self-centered and full of double talk."

"There's no kindness in you at all," she said, sobbing.

"I heard you the first time." He began to turn, as if he would start the motor. But he paused. "You're not so full of kindness either," he said, "with all that 'I hate you' stuff."

She kept sobbing.

He heaved a sigh. He half turned again.

"I don't know," he said. "What am I gonna do with you?"

She asked him for a handkerchief, and he found one in his trousers. She blew her nose and it sounded bubbly.

"When I first knew you," he said, "you seemed sort of depressed, and cold. For months. And then for a little while you were warm. Hot even. And now—I don't know. You've got your moods, and your problems, and I don't have the feeling I could always count on you, for warmth, and for understanding of me."

"You mean you couldn't dominate me."

"There, now that's typical of the kind of hostility you're full of. You think you're manning the barricades against me. We're in a war, or something."

She kept making gasping fitful sobs, although she tried not to, and wiping her nose. He sat heavily and patiently, not speaking now, but not looking at her and offering no comfort.

"Speaking of domination," he began again after a moment, "you're the one that always tries to take over the timing and the decisions. And I wish you'd quit pushing me around."

"I'm pushing you around? You're pushing me around!"

"You tried to take over the timing that time when you thought you were pregnant, and when I came looking for a reconciliation you did it again. And now you want to decide whether we're allowed to go to bed or not."

"You decided—I didn't." There was a catch in her voice.

"You didn't exactly go along with good grace. I don't know—you were deceptively soft for a brief period when we were living together and you were sort of courting, but whenever you think you have the upper hand you try to take over."

"That's unfair! That's the most distorted thing I ever heard." Her face was soaked. "You pushed me around, and I did everything to make you happy. I gave you everything—and you tried to make me destroy myself, manipulate me like a dishrag or something. Wring me out and drain me."

"What?" he said.

She sniffled and blubbered.

"What are you talking about," he said.

"You know."

"I wanted you to have an abortion, I suppose."

She wept without answering.

"I did not," he said.

"You did."

"I did not. I never said it and I never wanted it."

He seemed to look at her with disgust.

"You're a lunatic," he said. "You're raving." He opened his mouth as if he would say something more. But then he turned away, as though it were useless.

He started the motor with a racket. She heard it echoing back from some hill. They shot into the road with a jolt, and she held tight, the handkerchief around the knob in one of her hands.

The motion and the wind stopped her crying.

He drove far on the right, and if she were not holding so tightly she could have put out a hand to be slapped by foliage. The moon was before them now, high and white, and when they got to open country it illuminated fields and she could see far. It seemed strange that the moon could so soon become normal again, after such outlandish size and redness.

She thought of commenting on how little traffic there was. The roads were empty. But she had not the courage to begin a conversation.

"I don't blame you," he said. "I blame your parents. They've imposed this outworn morality on you that belongs to another age—your father out of his ideology, and your mother I guess out of stupidity. And their jealousy of the young—I guess that's always a factor."

"Maybe you're right," she said. "I don't know. I'm all confused. But I tried to get into the mood, Les. I really did try."

"You talked yourself into something."

"I didn't mean to."

"Well, it's just one of those things, I guess. I suppose I minded it more because we hadn't done it for such a long time."

He stopped talking, and so did she, and for a while the only sound was the popping of the motor. The phrase that stuck in her head was his remark about her parents making a mess of her.

It gave her a gloomy feeling that her own opinions and inclinations had been grafted on her, willy-nilly, and she could no more change them than the blue of her eyes.

It was certainly true that her affection for the old morality was rooted in her whole upbringing. In her mother even more than in her father, she thought—it hardly mattered which Bible verse her father had popped up with. She had simply known since childhood how vehemently her parents would disapprove.

Once she had heard Patty ask her mother where you get morality from, and her mother answered sharply that she didn't know but you get it. Her mother might think the Bible was obscurantist and stupid, and her mother might fancy herself in shorts and a halter, but chastity was as much a part of that woman as her hipbone.

"I need about a week of sleep," Leslie said.

Then there was silence again, except for the buzzing of the motor. On her calves she could feel the fluttering of her jeans.

She wished she could think of something interesting or agreeable to speak of.

"The moon's full," she said. "That means it's the fifteenth of the month on the religious calendar."

"What month is it?" he asked.

"I don't know," she said.

There was nothing more she could say about that. She saw a barn and a silo. There was a scarecrow in the moonlight, the first she had seen in a long time. She thought of speaking of that, but she did not want to divert his attention from the road. She felt ill at ease.

The scooter turned sharply, with a scrape on sand and gravel, and she leaned with it. The road became smooth again.

"Would you like to go some place for ice cream?" she asked.

"I thought you wanted to get back early," he said.

I wish I were married so I could stop being a mess, she thought. Single, you had to sleep with the guy and be a mess, or not sleep with him and be a mess.

70

For close to a week Millicent hardly saw Leslie, except for a minute when they got the license, and he was solemn and harried then and had to rush back to the hospital. Even their phone conversations were brief and few. They both were busy with final preparations. She had begun to feel tired with all the rushing about. Besides Leslie was on call a lot, and when he did have a free evening it was one of her nights to work late. Another evening he was tied up selling his scooter. Gifts kept arriving. Her mother talked her into having her hair done in a beauty parlor for the first time in her life.

Saturday night, the night before the ceremony, there was to be a rehearsal. Leslie's mother and brother and his Aunt Gert were already lodged at a hotel in Sparkstown, and they drove over with Leslie to the house for the evening, in Aunt Gert's car. Others of Leslie's relatives were to arrive in the morning, setting out from their homes at dawn, and some had gone to hotels and were weekending in Boston. Aunt Gwendolyn and Sharlene had also been invited to Wilmerding Crosswalk for the evening and had brought their wedding clothes and were to spend the night. Millicent saw her mother doing the last nervous straightening up of the house before the Hollanders got there, and saw her straighten the Gold Star that hung in the living-room window. But Millicent herself was upstairs helping to put Sharlene to bed when Leslie and his mother and brother and Aunt Gert arrived.

She wrapped her ivory carving in tissues and put it in Patty's dressing table, so Sharlene would not damage it. The little broken arm had been glued by a German refugee who did restorations for museums.

She came down the stairs without having dressed up, in her jeans and her brown-and-green plaid shirt. It occurred to her that she would have to address Mrs. Hollander as Mother, and it did not seem easy or natural. She saw the two families down there. Les was making introductions and Patty was smiling and wide-eyed. Leslie's little mother put out her hands toward Millicent. There was also the smiling round-cheeked woman with hair pulled back who must be Aunt Gert, and Jack, a staring, pale, skinny teen-ager with freckles and black hair. Millicent said Mother to Mrs. Hollander, not loudly. They embraced and exchanged kisses. She felt Mrs. Hollander's tenseness, but saw moisture in her eyes. There was something moving in the way everyone stood in attendance, smiling, even Roland, and for a moment it almost brought a lump to her throat She said Aunt Gert to the other lady, feeling warmth toward her at once because of the radiance of her smile. "This is Jack," said Leslie. She grasped the limp wet hand. Jack smiled on one side of his mouth, showing teeth.

They all moved to the living room, Aunt Gert explaining that she was late because she had gotten lost in Sparkstown, and Ed explained that Lucinda's directions were always cockeyed. Millicent sat on the sofa, between Mrs. Hollander and the aunt. Roland brought extra chairs from the dining room. Aunt Gert asked Millicent if she had quit now for good, and she said no—she would give notice as soon as they knew the Army would permit Les to have her with him. Sitting back on the sofa in jeans and shirt she felt somehow childish and squeezed, and much the center of attention, even though Mrs. Hollander was quite small and Aunt Gert was kind and affable. She saw Leslie standing near the wall opposite and looking quite as ill at ease as herself. Aunt Gwendolyn came in, from upstairs, and gave her hand to each of the newcomers, smiling gushily and leaning coyly. She sat on the piano bench, telling gaily how she had gotten Sharlene to bed. "You have to say, pink baby bunny go to the bathroom, pink baby bunny lie down under the blankets, nighty-night pink baby bunny. She's a pink baby bunny today, and you better remember it or she won't do a thing. Yesterday she was a puppy. You had to say, drink your milk, puppy, do this, puppy, do that, puppy, or it's no go." Aunt Gert was laughing. Millicent saw Jack poking about and examining objects on the mantelpiece. His posture was terrible.

Lucinda explained to Mrs. Hollander and Aunt Gert how the folding chairs would be set up in the room where they now sat, and in the dining room, and cleared away again while everyone was out on the lawn getting lunch under the tents so that people could come in again afterward and dance, and how the musicians would play at the ceremony and then outdoors and then indoors again. Aunt Gert said the forecast was for perfect weather. There were murmurs of approval and thankfulness. Aunt Gert said that the morning wedding was a nice idea, as it would give a longer afternoon and night together, especially since he was going into the Army the next day.

"Do you know where they reserved a room?" Mrs. Hollander said gravely. "The Ritz-Carlton. You'd think they were millionaires."

"It's once in a lifetime," said Aunt Gert.

"Well, it's what they want," said Lucinda.

"It's an extravagance," Mrs. Hollander said. "I don't know what they did that for. Such an expensive one." She told about Leslie selling his share in the scooter at a loss. She talked slowly, sometimes in a murmuring way, hardly opening her mouth. In contrast to her sister's affableness there was a graveness about her. In the introductions she had seemed apprehensive. Leslie bit at his unlighted pipe. Ed asked him if he had the ring and the license. "I even got a haircut," Leslie answered. Mrs. Hollander began talking meanwhile in her slow way of the arrangements she had made at the store for the weekend—she had been uncertain whether to close it, but at length had hired a neighbor, so as not to lose trade and not have the cream cheese spoil at the sandwich counter. But she was not making any money on it.

Patty wanted the rehearsal to get under way, and wanted to go upstairs and change into her green gown for it, but Lucinda told her to keep the dress nice for tomorrow, and Patty began to argue. "Patricia Jane," Ed said. "Behave yourself."

"I suppose you'll be marching down the aisle yourself in not too many years," Aunt Gert said smilingly to Patty.

"They won't even let me bring my steady to this wedding," Patty said. "It's a disgrace."

"Who's your steady?" Aunt Gwendolyn asked her.

"Paul Wernick."

"Are you in love?" Aunt Gwendolyn asked.

"I'm not sure," Patty said sullenly. "I don't know. I haven't decided yet."

"You're not going steady," Lucinda told her. "Nobody goes steady at sixteen."

"When then? How old do I have to be?"

"When you're eighteen. It's time enough."

"When I'm eighteen you'll say when I'm twenty."

"Who'd ever marry you," said Roland. He was slumping in the tall rocker with his legs spread.

"Lots of people," said Patty. "And when I get married you're not even gonna be invited, because you don't know how to behave."

"That's enough," Ed told them. Lucinda said the children were very badly behaved.

"Oh, no, you have a wonderful family," said Aunt Gert.

Somehow they talked more and more about the children. Lucinda began to talk about Charles, and how devoted he had been, and mentioned the insurance money he had left to Millicent, which would come in handy for the newlyweds someday. Mrs. Hollander recounted the history of Leslie's achievements, and Millicent's parents began to counter with similar tales about how bright she had been all through school. Millicent felt an embarrassing contentiousness in it, almost as if each were trying to prove that the other's child had got the better bargain. Leslie tried to light his pipe. Jack was sitting now opposite Millicent, straddling a dining-room chair backwards, and his eyes were fixed on her in an absent-minded stare. The eyes were like slits, in a pale, narrow face. She would glance away and back again, and once in desperation she even covered her own eyes with a hand as though resting them a few moments, but he kept staring.

Patty kept asking when the rehearsal would start, and in a while the others rose to begin. Lucinda showed where the marriage canopy would be set up in the morning and also told Mrs. Hollander and Aunt Gert and Gwendolyn how other things would be different in the morning, how the florists would set up flowers around the canopy, and how some interns would be ushers. Ed tossed skullcaps to each of the boys. "Nan will be flower girl—my sister Celeste's little girl," Lucinda said. Millicent noticed that her mother tended to address her remarks more to Aunt Gert, though she tried to include Mrs. Hollander.

Ed asked Leslie his Hebrew name, so as to have everything ready for the signing of the contract in the morning. Leslie had forgotten his Hebrew name, and looked to his mother. She answered, but Jack corrected her.

Then there was some fussing and arranging as to where everyone should stand, and Millicent said she wanted to come down the stairs alone, not on her father's arm, because it was silly for her father to run around playing two roles, and besides she would need one hand to hold the flowers and might need the other to keep her hem from dragging on the staircase. She thought it was unnecessary to come down the stairs in the rehearsal anyway, as she could come downstairs without a rehearsal. But Patty wanted to come down the stairs, as maid of honor, and she did.

Roland began singing, leaning through the French doors as Patty came down.

"Here comes the bride,
Big, fat, and wide—"

"Shut up," Patty told him.

"Daa dum da deeee da—"

"Shut up," Patty said again, descending in a stately manner, some fingers on the banister.

"You shut up!" Lucinda said from the living room. "Both of you shut up!"

Patty came into the living room, and Lucinda showed her where to stand. Roland had seated himself, sprawling far back on the sofa, and was swinging a foot.

"Bob O'Shaughnessy's gonna be best man at my bar mitzvah," he said.

"You don't have a best man at a bar mitzvah, stupid," Patty told him.

"We're gonna have a new system," he said.

Millicent and Leslie stood together before Ed, in the place where the canopy would be raised in the morning, and he touched their arms as though arranging them for a photograph. In her flat shoes she was small, and she knew that in heels tomorrow it would feel different. Patty and Jack stood behind them and were placed each a little to the side. Patty towered in heels.

"There, that looks nice," Lucinda said.

Ed did not go through the ceremony, but instead explained to Leslie and Millicent how he would do it. He lifted Millicent's index finger, on which Leslie would place the ring at first, in accordance with the ancient betrothal ceremony, and he said the words that they would repeat after him, and showed them the wine cup they would both sip from, and the tumbler that Leslie would crush beneath his heel. Then he went through it all again. Afterward Lucinda asked everyone to come to the study to see the presents.

"Let's get some air," Leslie said in a low voice to Millicent as his mother and aunt moved off toward the study.

She opened half the front door and slipped out with him. They went down the porch steps. The night sky still had color in it—it was not gray but of a dark and metallic blueness, the few stars brilliantly incandescent and yellow.

"I had to get out of there," he said. "I couldn't listen to them any more."

They walked slowly past Aunt Gert's car. It was cream and green and unwashed, with a sagging rear end, and was parked at a deep tilt in a gully of pebbles. They began strolling down the winding driveway.

"And my mother's been a pain since she got up here," he said. "Really in rare form. First she gets to this place where your father made the reservations in Sparkstown, the Webster House or whatever you call it, and she decides the rates are too high, so we went to the only other place in town, and it turns out to be a real flea bag, a flophouse for bums practically, and it would have been just fine for her—I should have let her stay there—but Gert and I talked her out of it, and I had to lug the dresses into this dump and out again—they have these dresses that can't be folded. So then she made us drive all around pricing all the different rooming houses, and Gert started to get fed up, and we ended up at the Webster House again, and then she made a scene with the bellhop because he tried to pick up the suitcases. The poor slob didn't know if she'd gone crazy or what. Jesus, I could have gone through the floor. She was afraid she'd have to give him a tip. And then she wanted them to put up cots for me and Jack in her room—she says we can go out when she undresses and she can hide in the bathroom. I wouldn't do it. I insisted on my own room. And Gert wanted a room to herself too, and she's hurt on account of that. I'm telling ya, she drives ya crazy. She can make anybody nervous."

"Well," Millicent said softly, "I'm sure she means it for our good. To save as much money as she can for our benefit."

Leslie didn't answer. They walked in silence down the long curve of the dirt road. Twice in the long grasses she saw the brief spark of a firefly.

At last they passed through the open gate.

"Did you catch up on your sleep?" she asked him.

"I'll never catch up," he said.

He walked as though deep in thought. She walked across the paved road with him. He sat on the loose boulders of the stone wall that bordered Mrs. Davey's pasture. She sat beside him. She felt the tufts of long grasses on her bare calves. Les plucked a tall stem of grass. They could see the lighted porch far before them, across the road and up the broad rise of field, partly behind the big elm, and Aunt Gert's car parked in front. Les tasted the end of the stem of grass, and took it from his mouth.

"I'm not just tired," he said. "I'm bushed. And this marriage is bearing down. I wish we had more time."

He broke another stem of grass, and she watched him wrap it around a finger.

"What do you mean?" she said.

"Well, I don't know how you feel, but I'm scared. I'm kind of mystified by how we got into this. It's all happened so fast. It crept up on me so fast somehow. We're actually tying the knot tomorrow. There's no time to even think about it. Although I do have the feeling that my doubts would very likely disappear if I had more time. It's not a lot before I'm ready. It's just a little before I'm ready. I don't know—maybe I haven't had enough experience to make that kind of a quick judgment. But do you know what I mean when I say there's such a thing as feeling you haven't met your ideal, and at the same time feeling that a certain girl is pretty good, and the best one you know, and for all you know better than any others you might happen to meet later."

Her eyes had been blurring as he spoke. He was not looking at her. She could see him unwind the grass from his finger and wind it tightly in the other direction. She tried to wink the moisture from her eyes. Her breathing deepened.

"Maybe it's natural to fall in love with whoever you've been sleeping with, when you're overworked," he said. "I don't know, I get these awful thoughts."

"It's because you feel you can't afford it—" she said, but her breath failed at that point and she had to stop.

"No, that's not it. That wouldn't bother me—"

"If it's just the economic problem," she began again, "I'll be working—at least till we've got Jack through school—we'll cut corners—"

"That's not the point. It's not that. It's—I guess part of it's that I'd like time for a little living. If it were possible."

"Isn't living with me living?"

"Well, it's just that I'd like my life to include a year or two unburdened by responsibility for a change. But don't get me wrong—I think if I did have time to think about it I'd still come to the same conclusion, that you're too good to lose. So that's why I said okay, actually."

"What do you have doubts about?"

"I figured maybe this is all there is to life, and that marrying you is the mature thing to do."

"You said you have doubts."

"Did I?"

"Yes."

"Well, it's silly, actually. But sometimes I think we don't have the same values. And I suppose basically I like the soft, warm, feminine type. You're pretty sexy at times, but sometimes you seem sort of hard and intellectual. You're not consistent. And I need warmth, understanding. I used to be attracted a lot because I thought you were very smart, and I'm not so sure now it's the most important thing. We argue. You're an arguer. I don't know if I really know you—if we know each other yet. It's gonna be for a lifetime. And sometimes I think crazy things like maybe you're too little for me. The soft hefty type seems sexier to me. I've always sort of seen myself eventually with somebody taller, softer. More pliable, sort of. Blonder. And I also planned my life with a lot more playing before marriage. I've been cheated of my play time somehow."

"You didn't plan the Army."

"Well, I planned around it. Saying yes to you was the first really unplanned thing I ever did. I planned the apartment. I planned an affair. And it seems very possible that eventually I'd have planned marriage—with you, I mean. You maneuvered me into a quick sudden decision, that's all. When I would have liked to think it over longer. I sort of said okay that day—I meant okay to tell them it's in the talking stage. And the next thing I know—well, in my life, in the big things, I've always called the shots. Like the time you thought you were pregnant, I just didn't want to have a baby that way, by accident. I think more of my sperm than that. When I have a child, I want my child to be intended. That's why I was always so careful. But you're sort of too masculine sometimes. You want to take over. Even in bed. You tell me no, you tell me yes. And you've taken over the timing. The wedding, I mean. I don't know, maybe it's characteristic of the eldest child to be bossy."

She leaned forward, sitting on the rock, and covered her face with her hands.

"If you really had doubts, why didn't you say it sooner?" she said in a strained voice.

"I didn't see how I could. Preparations were going so fast. And your parents rushing to make an honest woman of you before anything could change our minds. It got away from me. I know, you're right, I shouldn't have waited so long to talk about it. But at the beginning I sort of thought there'd be time to think it through. I meant it's in the talking stage, but then you told your family it's set, and there was no way to explain I hadn't meant that without sounding —it would have sounded awful—your family shaking my hand and kissing me and me saying hey you misunderstood. So I said okay, and I thought, all right, let it be that way, it'll be a little faster than I intended, and so I'll hurry up and think it through faster. And arrive at the same decision anyway probably. Eventually I've got to marry, and you're certainly not gonna be surpassed in all departments at once, and since I'd eventually come to the conclusion that you're the girl to marry I might as well come to it a little sooner. I just wanted a little time to accept the idea, kind of. But I meant, tell them it's in the talking stage. And then all of a sudden your father's shaking my hand, and there was nothing I could say, I realized you were right—if I was gonna marry you it was beyond the talking stage. It was a fact of life already, and I had to grow up and accept it. I was mature enough to realize that if I didn't want to lose you it was the point of no return. And I thought maybe it's for the best. I was sort of glad the decision was made for me."

"I didn't make it for you."

"Well, you did, or circumstances did. Or in a sense, once I'd taken the plunge and made it, it was made for me. Only it was as if every time I meant to advance things a foot, they advanced a yard. As a matter of fact I did ask you if you wouldn't rather wait until I got out of the Army. I did ask that. And the way things were going, preparations so fast, I didn't see any way to say it any stronger. Unless I wanted to sound like I wanted to kill it. And I don't want to kill it. I'm not ready to kill it. You've got a lot that would be too hard to replace. Look, if I wanted out I'd say I want out. I haven't said that."

"Do you want to marry me?" She kept her voice as steady as she could. She did not look at him.

"Yes. I made my choice. When I was forced to make a choice without thinking it through, I made it. I made the best choice I could. And I've been trying to think it through ever since."

He tossed away the piece of grass he had been winding. He ran his fingers clutchingly through his hair, and rested his forehead and eyes on the heels of his hands.

"I'm engaged—I should be enjoying it," he said. "And I'm not. I'm scared to death. All these people are here, and they think I'm happy, and I'm not."

He gave his head a quick shake, as if to shake away confusion. He grabbed another long stem of grass. The root came up with it. He began tearing bits off one of its long narrow leaves.

"Do you think we should postone it, or something?" she asked, her voice shaking.

"No. It's set—let's not get confused any further. I think it'll pass. The way I feel just now, I mean. We've got no choice at this point anyway. At this point we can't get out of it any more. I've had thoughts of what it would be like to break it off four days before, three days before. Two days before. I kept thinking every day I'll decide the next day. And then I think, the invitations are already out. And your father after me constantly with details about who's gonna sit next to whom—I couldn't think it through, let alone break it off. And then what a damn fool I'd look like if I did break it off now. And then when the day would come that should have been your wedding, you'd cry your eyes out." He ripped the leaf off. His thumbnail began rubbing away grains from the tuft at the end. "Plus the fact that I don't think I want to break it off anyway. I tried a nurse again for a little while after you left, and it was just no comparison. It was such junk compared to you. So I'm really sure that if all this hadn't been so rushed all my doubts would be resolved in your favor."

She watched him play nervously with the strand of grass. He had picked another and was twisting them, not looking at her. There was a lump in her throat and she was breathing through her mouth.

"Probably if you were about the tenth girl I was involved with instead of practically the first one I'd be able to make a judgment now a lot more easily, without being bothered by all these damn doubts. I should have made it my business to get more experience before."

"I don't see what good that would do," she said. "You still might fall for the first one and not know whether to marry her or not."

"I should have had more premarital stuff," he said wretchedly. "I should have realized the importance of it. It's my own fault. I started late and slow."

"It wasn't your fault," she told him. "You couldn't help it. You were too busy studying and working."

"No, busyness was also a cover for a certain amount of shyness, or laziness. I should have made myself find the time. I should have appreciated how important it was."

"You never seemed shy to me. Or lazy either."

"You probably thought I was pretty debonair when you first met me."

"No, I didn't think you were debonair—I thought you were very earnest. I still think so. But you were always very self-assured. If you were shy it didn't show."

"That's because you were shyer still. But that's one aspect of my life I just didn't run right. I never found out how to run it right, not early enough—frustration became a habit with me. When I was an undergraduate I literally didn't have a nickel to buy a girl a coke. Or buy myself one. And I didn't have an evening to spare, between bucking for A's and working at two jobs, or I thought I didn't. I used to write down my masturbations on a calendar, trying to control that. I was a senior in college. And when I was at Johns Hopkins I went to one of these joints where there were supposed to be easy pickups, one of these Baltimore joints—I heard you could feel a waitress for a quarter, and that kind of stuff—and so a girl fleeced me out of five bucks. She was supposed to get me a sandwich from the kitchen and bring me change, and she disappeared. Vanished. With the five bucks. Whether she was hiding in the kitchen or the ladies' room I couldn't tell you, but nobody saw her, nobody heard of her, she didn't exist. I sat, I waited. It was all the money I had. I'm telling you, it took me a year to live that down. That five bucks was in my mind for a year. I felt so stupid, that I could be so frustrated, that I could be taken advantage of like that. Do you know when I first got laid? I was in my third year of med. When I was the age you are now I was a virgin."

"So what," she said. "What does it matter, Les, if you can be happy now?"

"A life with no spice in it, that's mine. It was just starting to turn. It was only a few months before I got together with you that you could actually say things started to pop a little bit. And at last I get a decent affair going, and then a wedding date's set, and the family's involved, and all of a sudden everything's so regulated, and according to Hoyle, and fixed. It's all system now. All system, and coldly making plans. Your mother yakking about matching tableware, and your father with his seating arrangements—and you don't seem to mind. You don't seem to miss it. You sit there making plans too. Look, I love you, and all that, as far as that goes, and I've always seen myself getting married, about the age I am now. A man needs a wife, for Christ sake. But I wish you were the fourth or fifth girl, instead of almost the first. So I could have done a normal amount of playing around first. Things haven't worked out right for me. You're the girl I should have met last, not first. And what bothers me is that it's really my own fault. There were girls I could have had. Even without any money for dates, and all the other excuses I had, there were still some available. And yet I was timid, or inhibited or something. I had a very narrow upbringing, somehow, even if there wasn't much Sunday school in it, and I took a long time growing up. Real slow. You were the first really decent thing that ever happened to me. Or that I let happen to me. I was thinking the other night, back through college, and jobs, all the different girls that I'm positive I could have laid, if I'd only been ready. And I could count eight. Eight definite. Maybe nine."

"Les, it's stupid going to the past and regretting things like that. I don't want to hear about it. I don't want to know who you slept with. Or didn't sleep with."

"Don't you ever regret things?"

"Yes, I suppose I do."

"It *is* my fault," he said. "It's my fault for not starting younger. And now marriage means my youth has gone down the drain. I never had any. And you know every girl's different. A man's entitled to a little broader vista before he settles down."

"You'll see enough examining patients."

"It's not the same thing. And I don't mean just bodies—the whole girl, her style. I just wish I'd had more affairs and then met you about fourth."

"Oh, you and your damn sex. You've got sex on the brain." The sound of her voice had a quality of grief.

"No, on the contrary. The trouble is that I didn't have it on the brain enough when I should have. If I had we wouldn't be having this trouble now."

"I'm just as glad you weren't sleeping around all those years."

"No, Millicent, it's healthier. This proves it. If we'd each had a few affairs we'd be ready for each other by now. What do you suppose my conflict comes down to, basically—I want to recapture the youth I should have had, but I know I should be mature enough to admit I can't. I can't, that's all. And now maybe they'll send me to Alaska, and there'll be no women at all. Or maybe they'll send me some place like Japan or Germany, where you can get women as easy as a stick of gum. And yet on the other hand it would be silly to ditch you for that junk, because I still want to marry sometime and you're too good to lose. So that's why I'm stuck. I'll have to forego the playing around, that's all."

"Chasing sex is just a dead end."

"I know. In my mind I know it. You're still the best girl I ever met. I've just, I've just had too much nose to the grindstone, and I wish I could have my cake and eat it. For a while. If it made sense."

"Do you wish you hadn't met me?" She could hear a tearfulness in her voice.

"No."

"Do you wish you hadn't asked me to marry you?" She wasn't looking at him.

"That's not the point," he said. "Maybe if we'd decided before to be friends for a few years and then get married we could have done that. It would have been possible. To take it slow, and go off and come back, and marry you later. But anyway you convinced me that it wasn't, and now that we've come this far it isn't."

"I didn't know you were full of all these doubts."

"I know you didn't."

"You always used to seem so strong-minded. That's what I mean. As if you always knew what you wanted."

"Well, that's it—that's how women are. They have this myth that men should always be strong and decisive, but you can't be decisive about everything. Some things are complicated—we're complicated, you're complicated—and coupled with your insistence that we set up the wedding date—well, the pressure from you to appear decisive is one of the pressures. It makes me feel like I've got a problem and no room to maneuver. I have to sit on my doubts, and not talk, and not think, so I can look decisive and masculine. You know an affair can be ended, but I don't want to go into marriage that way, thinking it can be ended. Marriage is for a long time, and I want it to be on more than a guess, more than a hunch. Although my hunch was to go along with it, if I had to decide right then. But we had an affair, and there was no question that I needed the affair. I needed it. I'm twenty-six. And then we broke up, and I thought maybe I'd loved you, and I was depressed and lonely, and I thought maybe you were the nearest I'd come. That you had so much, that maybe I'd never even find that much again, let alone more. And then we got together, and the bickering resumes, and I remember the bickering from before. If we get married we've got to do better than we have in the past. Because the fact that people can quarrel, even before marriage, and even look for imaginary issues—it's not a good sign. You went and left me on that abortion issue even after facts proved that the issue hadn't been real in the first place, which was all I'd ever said. The fight seemed to mean more to you than the issue, as if you wanted an excuse to fight. And I hate fighting. I hate bickering. I saw this Reader's Digest article the other night—it gave a test, and it said if you answer yes to any question she's not the right mate for you. And so one of the questions was 'do you ever have doubts.' I'm right in the middle of trying to work out my doubts and I have to see a damn stupid thing like that."

"You shouldn't worry about a Reader's Digest article. You should have put it out of your mind."

"I did."

"Do you love me?"

"Well, that just begs the question. That's what I wish we had plenty of time to be sure of. But the world isn't set up right—I suppose realistically that if you spend the kind of time on women it would really take to find the one you'd be sure was just right, then you can't spend the kind of time it takes to really get somewhere in a career. That's what I tell myself. And meanwhile my hunch is more yes than no, and at the same time this has been handled in such a way that any delay now would kill it. I mean that's what its effect would be on you—that's what my thinking has been. I could end up wishing I'd grabbed you when I could. You gave me a perfect affair for a while, and I never would have predicted it. You're the last person I ever would have predicted would have turned out like that, when I first knew you. So maybe you'll turn out to be perfect in other ways too."

She felt for a handkerchief without finding one. There was moisture in her nose. She sniffled.

Far off on the lighted porch of the house the front door opened and a figure came out.

"Leslie!" she heard Mrs. Hollander call. "Leslie and Millicent!"

They sat without answering. Mrs. Hollander called again.

"What," he answered loudly.

"Don't you think you'd better get some sleep?" Mrs. Hollander asked. She did not seem to be looking in exactly the right direction, as if she were not sure where they were. "You have a big day tomorrow."

He didn't answer and made no move to go.

"You better come in," his mother called. "Aunt Gert wants to go back to the hotel. Everybody's tired."

"A couple of minutes," he said.

They saw Mrs. Hollander turn and go back into the house.

They sat without speaking. Far off she could hear the treble young frogs, punctuated now and then by an old one. It occurred to her that soon the mosquitoes would be about.

"Well, I guess I shouldn't have told you so much," he said.

"It's all right."

"I've been in this turmoil, more and more—I thought it would get less. I thought you could help me talk it out."

"I can't give you strength, Les. I'm not strong enough myself." She felt again for a handkerchief.

"Listen, it's not that I'm not strong. When a man's indecisive it's because there are reasons, so give me some sympathy. Maybe I shouldn't have let you know I had any doubts. But if a wife can't be a confidante what good is she? We're in this together, and I assumed thoughts could be shared. Look, I must be in love with you. The fact that I've had all these doubts and still decide to go through with it proves something, doesn't it?"

She said nothing.

"Look, I'm all entwined with you," he said. "I'm sentimental about friendships, I guess, but there's never been a time when I wanted it to end, actually. Maybe complete sureness isn't possible."

She couldn't make any answer.

His mother came out and called again.

He cursed in an undertone. He gave Millicent a friendly slap on the knee of her jeans.

He rose sluggishly, and Millicent rose with him. "Okay, okay," he said.

They walked across the road.

On the dirt driveway she asked Leslie for his handkerchief, and he gave it to her. She blew her nose. They continued walking, silently. He gave her his arm, in a comforting way.

As they mounted the porch steps the others began coming out, amid chatter, and Aunt Gert was laughing at something.

"Come on," Mrs. Hollander said to Leslie. "We're all going to need a good night's sleep."

Millicent kissed Mrs. Hollander, and again took the limp moist hand of Jack. She stood amid the good-byes, nodding and speaking without hearing her own voice. Slowly the party went down the porch steps, talking sociably. At last the Hollanders were in the old car with Aunt Gert, and there were more of the cheery good-byes.

She watched the pair of red lights curve down the drive, pause at the gate, turn and accelerate. Then she followed her family into the living room. She saw the portrait of Charles on the piano. Lucinda and Gwendolyn and Patty were chattering. Emptied teacups and saucers of half-eaten cake were on the sills, the piano bench, and the floor. Roland made a disgusting noise of forced air by putting a hand to his armpit and pressing his arm down on it. "Dad," Patty said, "Will you speak to that boy of yours?"

Millicent sat on the sofa. She felt ill. There was a cigarette butt in the fireplace. It was amazing, she thought, how soon after the close of the Sabbath her father could mess up the house with those.

"Do you think you could go for Jack?" Aunt Gwendolyn was asking Patty.

"He's an ick," Patty said.

71

At the Webster House in Sparkstown Aunt Gert said a smiling good night to her sister and the boys and went to her own room. The boys however did not go at once to the room they were to share, but went instead with their mother to her room to keep her company for a while.

It was a small room, and the ceiling bulb was dim. Mrs. Hollander told Jack to be sure and shine his shoes before he went to bed. Then she checked some detail of her gown, holding it out on its hanger with one hand and holding another part of it toward the light. Jack sat spread in the one chair and slowly turned the big pages of a magazine. His exposed bony ankle rested on the opposite knee.

Leslie sat on the radiator cover, his back to the darkened air shaft and reflecting windowpane. "Well, tomorrow I'm a married man," he said.

He rose to walk about a little but his mother turned with the dress she was holding and they bumped. He retreated to the tight space between the foot of the bed and the dresser, but his mother came there too, carrying the dress, and started to open the bottom drawer against him, so he went back to the narrow dead end between the radiator cover and the side of the bed. His mother started down there too, and sat on the edge of the bed to thread a needle. Leslie squeezed out again past her legs.

The least crowded spot was an area about four feet square in front of the chair on which his brother sat, and he stood there aimlessly. He moved the pipe from his pocket to his mouth, but didn't light it.

His mother stared down at her sewing.

"I think I'll go out for a walk," Leslie said. "I feel like a little walk."

"Anything rather than sit and visit with your mother for a little while," Mrs. Hollander said, not interrupting the sewing. "Your mother, that you're not gonna see for two years."

"He's nervous," said Jack, without looking up from the magazine.

"Yes, I know he's nervous," said Mrs. Hollander.

"So what," said Leslie. "It's natural."

He started to examine his nails but abandoned that.

"I wish I had my scooter," he said.

"No, I'm glad you're rid of that," said his mother. "It gave me heart failure, that thing."

"It was good for me," he said. "It had a real calming effect."

"Well, why don't you go to your room then and try to get a good rest for tomorrow, if you're so anxious to be out of here."

"I don't want to go to sleep. I want some exercise. Jack, do you feel like a little walk?"

"You're nervous—I'm not nervous," Jack answered him lightly, still looking idly at the shiny magazine.

"That's right—both of you go out," Mrs. Hollander said bitterly.

"I just wanted to work off a little surplus energy," said Leslie.

He traced the grooved decorations of the dresser and its mirror listlessly.

"Would you rather we all went down and sat in the lobby?" his mother asked. "There'd be a little more room."

"I'd rather not face the bellhop again if I don't have to," he said.

His mother broke a thread, and rethreaded the needle.

"Jackie, you might offer your mother the only chair in the room," she said.

Jack moved to the bed and sprawled on the tufted spread with the magazine. His mother sat on the chair with a sigh. She kept sewing the hem. There were pins in it.

"I should think her parents could have put you up at least," she said to Leslie. "In a big house like that."

"They've got Gwen and the baby staying over," he said. "And anyway that would be nice, wouldn't it. In the same house with my bride."

"I didn't say in the same room."

"It still isn't done," he told her. "Now cut it out. All that stuff. Like asking the hotel for an extra cot. What are we? A bunch of gypsies?"

She gave her head the slightest shake. "I hope you don't intend to talk to your wife the way you talk to your mother," she said.

"No, I don't. I certainly don't."

"Well, I hope not, for both your sakes. Because if you do she's liable to walk out on you."

"I'm sorry," he said. "It's just that sometimes you haven't got any pride."

"No, you think I don't, the way you talk to me."

He wandered restlessly to the window again and looked down toward the dark courtyard. He leaned his forehead on the glass.

"You don't look very happy for a boy that's getting married in the morning," his mother said.

"Leave me alone, will ya?"

"Is something troubling you? Did you and Millicent have a disagreement or something?"

"No, no. Nothing like that."

"Well, something's troubling you. I can see it."

He remained looking out the window a moment, and then half turned, one hand fondling the window sash.

"Listen," he said, "I've got things on my mind. That's perfectly normal, isn't it? It's a big step I'm taking. There's things I want to think through." He sat again on the radiator cover. It came out only a few inches from the wall. He threw one leg over the other and clasped an ankle.

"I should think you would have thought it through before now," said his mother.

"Well, it's just that things have happened awfully fast. My thinking hasn't had time to catch up, that's all."

His mother was looking at him steadily from the chair. Between them Jack lay on the bed, propped on an elbow, and turned a page of the magazine. "I don't understand you, Leslie," she said. "Do you love her?"

"I think so."

"You ought to know so."

He made a gesture of frustration. "Mother, you don't understand."

"No, your mother's stupid," she said.

"Mother, I don't want to go into it."

"I should have known there was something bothering you, the way you've been nasty to me ever since I got here."

"No, no, Mother, please, let's not go into it."

"Well, if you're not sure, Leslie—" she persisted, and then paused, with a little shake of her head. "You just find out now, instead of when it's too late. Even if you find out the day before, it's better than finding out the day after. I just assumed it, that you loved the girl. I assumed that it goes without saying."

Jack glanced up at Leslie, and down again to the magazine.

"Well, what can I do?" Leslie said to his mother. "I'm sure in any case I could do a lot worse. A majority of my mind is still in her favor, so to speak. It's probably the right thing to do. It's just that I sort of got propelled into it before I could think it through. By events, I mean. The Army."

"You don't marry somebody just because it's the right thing to do," his mother said. She wore a troubled expression. She took pins from the dress and stuck them in the upholstery.

"Well, I meant right in that sense, in the sense of wanting to. I mean if I had time to think it out, I think I'd still decide to."

"What's the matter then?" his mother said. She looked up from the sewing. "I can't make you out."

"It's a lot of things. I think basically I'm undecided between two types, as far as my ideal of a wife is concerned—"

"Leslie—" she said earnestly. "I want whatever's best for you. I came up here expecting a wedding—I've been preparing ever since you wrote me a month ago. And I thought you're a grown man and you know your own mind. But if you're not sure—"

"I don't want to break it off," he said with some firmness. "Because maybe I do want it—maybe I do want this girl. It's just that ideally I want another six months to be sure. There's things I really like about her a lot, very much."

"Why don't you ask her for more time?"

"I can't do that!" he said irritably. "Not once a wedding's planned. It would seem like breaking off. And what then? What do people do in a situation like that, when they've postponed a wedding? Do they go out with others meanwhile? Maybe I'll want her and I'll have lost her."

"I think you've been working too hard. What you need is a rest." She resumed sewing. Her eyes glistened with damp. She rose, putting the dress down by Jack on the bed, and went to the dresser, where she took a handkerchief from her pocketbook.

Leslie rose from the radiator cover, and took a step, as if he would walk about pensively. But after a step he sat back down again, his hands in his pockets. Jack glanced up and fixed his eyes on him. He avoided Jack's eyes and addressed his mother, who had sat on the chair with the dress again and was dabbing each nostril with the handkerchief. "Anyway I'd be a heel to call it off now," he said.

"You might be a bigger heel if you went through with it," said his mother.

"No. I told her I'd marry her, and I'm gonna go through with it. Damn it. I've got to know my damn mind. And stick to it. I've got to be decisive."

"Well, I agree with that," said his mother, stitching again, "but breaking it off at the last minute isn't necessarily weakness, if there's something bothering you. It can be strength, too, you know."

Jack was turning pages of the magazine again.

"No, having come this far I have to go through with it," Leslie said. "It's too late to back out. It's gone too far."

"What do you mean, gone too far?"

"It's just gone too far."

"Let me ask you something," said his mother. Her tone was different. She paused, but did not exactly look at him. "Have you been sleeping with her?"

Jack glanced at Leslie only for an instant and back to the magazine.

Leslie reddened. "That's not what I meant," he said. "I meant the guests are all here, and they've hired the musicians—how can I change my mind now, after her father's had the whole thing catered and everything. People have sent gifts and everything."

"Well, Leslie, you're very softhearted." She blew her nose softly, and wiped it. "You didn't answer my question, Leslie."

She turned and looked at him.

"I asked if you two have been having an affair."

He said nothing. There was color in his face. Jack kept staring at a page of the magazine.

"Well, you don't seem to deny it," his mother said, "and it explains a lot." She gave a sigh. "Is she pregnant?"

"Of course not! Nothing like that."

"Look me in the eye, Leslie."

"Oh, for Christ sake! She's not pregnant. Believe me."

"Well, it still explains a lot." She sighed again, looking away heavily. She looked drawn. She shook her head. "Well, that's how they hook them these days."

"She didn't hook me."

"I know you're very fine and sensitive," his mother went on, "and you've never wanted to harm anybody. But you have to think of yourself, too."

"I am thinking of myself."

"Well, I know these things happen," she said. "Especially nowadays. But I'm sure that if the girl hadn't been willing it wouldn't have happened. I'm a little disappointed in her, too, frankly."

"Oh, Mother, for God's sake—" His hand brushed his hair.

His mother wiped her nose. "Boys often do develop a feeling of responsibility for a girl under those circumstances," she said. "Especially boys of the fine and sensitive type. See, Jackie," she said, and Jack looked around innocently. "This is a lesson for you. When you get older, only go out with girls you can respect. My boys don't have that kind of callousness, to let a girl down, so you have to be very careful of temptation."

"Leave Jack out of it," Leslie said. "I don't see why Jack has to hear this."

Jack's eyes returned to the magazine.

"For his own good," Mrs. Hollander answered. "He's of an age when he'll be meeting girls too. Especially as he'll have years of study and hard work before he's a doctor, and there'll be plenty of girls that'll have their eye on him."

"I shouldn't be talking to you," said Leslie.

"You have to talk to somebody," his mother said.

He rose, beside the radiator cover, and turned to rest his face and hands on the top of the lower half of the window. It fell a few inches until it was shut and he momentarily lost his balance.

"Don't you have boys at the hospital you could talk to when you're upset?" his mother asked.

"I didn't want to blow it up into a big thing yakking about it. I had to straighten my own mind out first."

"Well, if you had doubts, you might have been better off talking it out with someone."

He turned, putting his hands in his pockets, and cursed under his breath. He turned again, and sat down heavily on the soft bed, his back toward his mother, and jarring Jack momentarily.

"Who says I don't love her," he said. "You don't know how I feel about her. The very first time I laid eyes on her it crossed my mind that this could be the one to marry someday, do you know that? Something about her. Even though we waited months before we started dating. I just didn't think I wanted to get married for a while, that's all, but every time she'd turn up she'd look good again."

"Well, if you loved her you wouldn't have waited months. And another thing, I don't know if the ceremony will be legitimate anyway. Her father's getting through, you know."

"So what. He can still perform a marriage. He's losing his job but he's not disordained."

"Well, I don't know. I heard he's getting through. That's all I know. He isn't liked."

"Don't worry about it."

"That girl's been taking advantage of you. You said she was beautiful, but I don't see it. I think she's a little odd-looking. Cross-eyed, if you ask me."

"She has beautiful eyes."

"Well, I know the Army seems long," his mother said. "Two years. But it's not forever, it'll go quicker than you think. And you can meet nice girls even in the Army. I think they even have dances for the officers."

"Oh, Mother, it isn't that—"

"Well it's true," she said. "Officers get invited to nice places. And people's homes. It isn't so lonesome."

"Stow it. Please. You don't get the point."

"You don't have to be nasty, when I'm trying to help you."

"You're not much help."

"No. No, that's right, I'm not much help." She brushed her eye with a finger. "I never struggled all alone to raise two boys, and put you through four years of college and four years of medical school, and scrimped and saved and held off the bank and mended the clothes to do another year. No, I'm not much help. I never opened the store from seven o'clock in the morning to eleven at night, Sundays, holidays—"

"Oh, Christ—"

72

Millicent went to bed in Patty's room, on the iron cot, so that her own room could be used by Aunt Gwendolyn and Sharlene.

No matter how she turned she could feel her pajamas, the sheet against her cheek, the beginning of aching tiredness in her eyes. When her eyes were open she saw a three-quarter moon, beyond the foliage and the billowing window curtain. Patty's breathing was sometimes audible, sometimes not.

The steeple clock at the common—its slow, hollow count of the hour gave distance to the stillness. Each time she heard it told her she was still awake. The bone-white moon had crept higher. She lay sprawled. She was too uncomfortable to relax, and too tired to be comfortable. She heard also the solitary bong of the half-hour, knowing each time she heard it what hour had preceded. And after a minute the ting of the carved clock downstairs always followed.

She tried to fog out thoughts, and to relax, knowing the importance of a good night's sleep. This house—she had known it only a year, and lived in it but a fraction of that. And soon it would be sold, house and barn, yard and woods, and her mother and Patty and Roland would follow her father God knows where. It crossed her mind that all along she had been assuming unwittingly that some sentiment attached to her marrying in it, as though she had played here in childhood, as though her grandparents had dwelt here. She wondered if the Army would send Les where she could follow, and what city they would be near when her father found his next job. She told herself once that maybe marriage was what Les needed to steady him.

The whole roundness of an eyeball ached. At dawn the winds breathed in the high branches. With aching despair she saw the trace of blue beyond the window curtains assert itself more and more into daylight. The indoors was grayer, but already she saw the drab green and brown of the plaid shirt she had worn last night and had thrown with her jeans beside Patty's old torn teddy bear on the bureau. All the hours of darkness had escaped from her.

She lay this way and that. Her left nostril was pregnant with its old sneezy feeling, that she had not had for some time, and it hurt the eye near it, even though it didn't sneeze yet. It dripped, but her nose was not blocked, and sniffling made the sneezy feeling sharper. Now the heavens were the beautiful color of day. She had not known that daybreak was so early. The bird twittering irritated her.

She blew her nose, but there was nothing to blow. Still it dripped. That whole nostril felt pickled. The clock bell of Folger's church was beating out its spaced notes again, and their quality was somehow different in daylight, as if their overtones were higher pitched. Five o'clock. The tangled coverings were half over her head. She kept a crushed handkerchief to the nostril. Patty's even breathing continued.

After the stroke of six she began to hear sounds of Sharlene talking to herself, but for a long time the rest of the house remained quiet.

But in time trucks came into the yard, and she heard the voices of her parents and of Aunt Gwen, and the sounds of the bathroom and of feet. When she heard Patty get up she lay with eyes closed, the blanket half across her face, and pretended to sleep. She heard shouts of the men raising tent poles, and from downstairs the bumps and scuffling of furniture being moved.

"Is she asleep? Let her sleep," she heard her mother saying close to her. "If she can in this racket. I'll bring her breakfast in bed."

She heard her mother tell her father to ask them to be quieter downstairs. It sounded as if they were filling the living room and dining room with folding chairs, and it was an endless clattering and banging. She opened her eyes to slits and saw Patty at the dressing table. All her thoughts of the long night merged in a gloomy feeling that this marriage would trap her in a mistake.

She shut her eyes quickly, lest Patty see them in the mirrors. Even when Patty had left the room she still lay immobile, because no course of action seemed attractive. The door was shut, but it closed off no sounds. She hardly knew how long she had been lying here, in the night, and in the long morning daylight hours. There were even the sounds of cars arriving. Her stomach felt as though she were falling. Footsteps went up and down the stairs. Doors opened and closed. Sharlene ran the length of the hall. Roland was singing the wedding march in the upstairs hallway, and now and then making his disgusting armpit noise.

"Daa dumm de aa—
Daa DUMM de aa—
Daa dumm ba DEE aa,
Ba dumm diddle de aa—"

"Shut up, you idiot!" Patty told him in a subdued voice.

"Isn't she up yet?"

She pressed the eye that hurt to the pillow, and the crushed handkerchief to the tingling nostril, and breathed through her mouth.

With one squinting eye she saw her mother come in, maneuvering the door carefully so as not to drop the tray of food she carried. "Time to get up, morning glory," her mother said. "Nine-thirty. I don't dare let you sleep any longer."

Her mother had on a house coat, but her hair was fixed and she had make-up, and Millicent could see the satiny high heels and the stockings. Her mother set down the tray upon the dressing table and lowered the shades, but not all the way.

"You've got beautiful weather," she said. "A perfect day to get married."

Millicent buried herself in the blanket and whimpered.

Her mother put her hand on the blanket, over Millicent's buttock, and shook her a little. "Come on," she said. "People will be here in an hour. Have some breakfast and you'll feel better."

"I don't feel like it."

"What do you mean you don't feel like it. Come on."

Millicent sat herself up in the bedclothes, tiredly. Her mother went out. Millicent got out of bed, barefoot, and went out toward the bathroom, her eyes nearly shut.

"Hi," said Patty.

When she came back she looked at the breakfast. Patty had come into the room with her, gowned in layers of gauzy green, and her auburn hair resplendent upon her height.

"Want some breakfast?" Millicent said.

"I had mine," said Patty.

Millicent tasted the orange juice, but not the eggs on toast or the milk. In the dressing-table mirrors she could see three haggard images of herself.

"The tents are up," Patty said.

Through the window, below the half-drawn shade, Millicent could see the fluttering elm leaves and the top of a circular tent, radiating sections of yellow and green that sloped sharply and then less as they spread and widened.

"I've got an awful headache," she said.

"Oh."

"See if there's some aspirin. There's some in the bathroom."

Patty went for them. Millicent began to dress. She put on the panties, which were completely patterned in lace, and the bra. Then she sat on the edge of the bed doing nothing, looking at her spread feet.

Patty came in, and Millicent took an aspirin with some orange juice. Her mother came in, this time completely gowned.

"She didn't eat a thing," said Patty.

"I really don't want anything," said Millicent.

"Well, she's nervous," said Lucinda.

Millicent's eyes met her mother's with a kind of suddenness.

"I'm frightened," Millicent told her. As she said it the word terrified her.

"Well, it's natural," Lucinda said. "But don't be. You don't have to be. I'll put the tray on the bureau. You can take it or leave it, whatever you want."

Millicent watched her mother take the tray.

"I think I'm not feeling well," she said.

Her mother paused at the bureau, still holding the food. "Oh," she said. "Well, it'll straighten itself out in a couple of days. I've heard of cases of that—girls get irregular all of a sudden right on their wedding day. It's nerves. It's caused by nerves."

"No—"

"Les is a doctor—he'll understand."

"I don't mean that. I mean I'm just exhausted. I heard every hour and every half-hour."

"Well, it's the excitement," Lucinda said.

She put down the tray and went out. Millicent lay back flat on the bed with a forearm over her aching eyes. She made a little protesting whimper. "I wish I could sleep," she said.

"Boy, you better get ready," Patty said.

Millicent dragged herself up on an elbow. She shut her eyes and wrinkled her forehead.

"Come on!" said Patty.

Patty brought her the stockings, and helped her into the rest of the underclothing. There was a matching garter belt, and there were special skirts to go under the gown. The stockings were straightened, and buckled to their suspenders. She felt strange in these clothes. She sensed Patty's excitement. At last Patty took the gown itself from its hanger, splendidly white and brocaded, and when it was on she buttoned it up Millicent's back.

"You look scared to death," she said. "You look as white as a sheet."

"I've got a headache," Millicent said.

"Isn't it any better?"

"No."

"It's nerves," said Patty, as her mother had before.

Patty fetched the box that contained the veil down out of the closet. The babble of voices downstairs was fairly continuous now, and there were strange footsteps on the stairs, like middle-aged fat ladies in heels, and the bathroom sounded as though in constant use, its door opening and shutting and water running. Music began to play downstairs. Patty was laying the veil out upon the iron cot.

"I don't need that yet," said Millicent.

"Comb your hair," said Patty.

Millicent seated herself on the little carved white bench that faced the dressing table and looked at the three white-gowned images that looked bewilderedly back at her. Her eyes were half open and bloodshot. She almost had to sneeze, but she avoided it by opening her mouth and contorting her face in a grotesque way. There was a constant awful feeling in her left nostril. Patty began to do the combing for her.

"What's the matter?" Patty asked her.

She didn't answer. She relaxed the grotesque expression and sniffled cautiously, still without sneezing. The membranes of the nostril were as though lined with vinegar. The window was next to the dressing table and she could see more than one of the tent tops, sunny beyond the shadiness of the nearby elm branches. Patty's gentle combing jostled her head. She did not like what the beauty parlor had done to her hair.

Even while Patty combed, Millicent's head rolled and nodded once as if she would doze off sitting there, but jerked straight again. "Hey," Patty said.

Millicent put a hand over the eye that hurt more, and massaged it slowly with her fourth finger.

"I'm gonna give you some mascara," Patty said.

"I don't want that stuff," said Millicent.

"You need it."

Patty opened the drawer against Millicent's stomach. She began to work at Millicent's face, with lipstick first, and Millicent parted and firmed her lips to oblige.

"I've got some eye drops that will open your eyes up," Patty said.

"Let me alone," Millicent answered, but her voice was weak.

Lucinda came in, shutting the door behind her, and said the lipstick shade was no good, so they began anew.

"Leslie's downstairs," Lucinda said. "He looks just scrumptious." She made Millicent stand and turn and admired the fit of the gown again. "Grandma Annie will be so pleased," she said.

"Let her sit down—she needs some eyebrow pencil," said Patty.

Millicent sat down. Her mother went out to see about something and Patty worked a while with the eyebrow pencil, once or twice telling Millicent to look at her and to hold still.

"There," she said after a while, sitting back onto the cot and admiring her in the mirrors. "You'll be all right."

Millicent sat brooding over the dressing table, allowing her forehead to sink and slide in her hands.

"Let your hair alone," Patty said, starting up. "You're gonna louse up your permanent."

There was a rap on the door. "Millicent?" Leslie's voice said.

Patty hurried to it and Millicent turned. Patty looked up into Leslie's face.

"Hi," he said, smiling at them both. The sandy hair lay across his forehead as informally as ever, but the effects of the haircut showed about his ears, and his flannel suit was well-fitting and splendid, nearly black. He wore a deep maroon tie and was holding a large bunch of white flowers. "One of your aunts was bringing your bouquet up," he said to Millicent, "so I said I'd do it." He handed Patty the bouquet, and she pressed it to her nose and face. Then she laid it gently by the veil. "How are you, sweetie," he said to Millicent.

"I'm fine, I guess."

He sauntered past the back of Millicent's chair to a window sill and sat. It was not the window that faced the elm and the tents but the one over the slate roof of the kitchen.

"I'd like to talk to Millicent alone a minute," he said to Patty agreeably. "Would you mind?"

"Oh," said Patty, suddenly hasty and flustered, as though she ought to have realized it. She left, shutting the door.

He sat facing Millicent's stare in the mirror. He moved as if he would put his arms about her but she held him off. He sat back on the sill.

"I feel a lot better about things," he said.

He was still smiling a little, though he didn't look at ease. Her tired gaze drifted away from him, down to the table.

"Is there any chance your sister's listening at the door?" His voice was low.

"I don't know."

He glanced from Millicent to the door doubtfully, then rose and opened it a few inches. He shut it and returned to the sill.

"I took a long walk last night," he said. "I left my mother and everybody at the hotel, and I walked for hours. I walked all over Sparkstown. You know there's this old cemetery up on a high hill—it overlooks the whole town. Have you ever been up there?"

"No."

"Well, you should. It's a real peaceful spot." He no longer had any trace of the smile.

She wasn't looking at him. Her hand played absently with a rounded comb of Patty's that lay on the dressing table, and she looked toward the mirror, but pensively, as though she saw nothing.

"I just wanted to think everything out," Leslie continued, "and actually I do feel a lot better about it." He paused, and studied her profile. "I really do feel a lot more at peace about it."

One of his hands slowly massaged the other, with visible slow tension, and he watched for her reaction. But she gave no sign.

"I'm sort of relieved," he said, "that the wedding's here. There's no more choice about it."

"Why are you telling me this?" she asked, without looking up.

"Well, I feel better, and I thought you'd want to know. After all the talk. I just thought you'd feel better knowing I felt better about things. I didn't want you to tie the knot thinking I was feeling like last night."

"When you say you feel at peace you sound like you're accepting death."

"Aw, no, no. I'd been having this terrific turmoil all week, and finally I just thought maybe I could share it with you, that's all. I just assumed you could understand. Maybe I shouldn't have, I don't know. You can't dock me for sharing my feelings. Even my innermost feelings. I don't know—"

She said nothing, and didn't move.

"Well, anyway," he said, "here we are. It's just got to be right, that's all."

"You're a pain, do you know that?"

She seemed tired, but she still didn't look at him. In the silence he swallowed.

"All right. I'm a pain," he admitted. "But I want to marry you. Okay?"

"You don't have to do me any favors."

He made himself smile, rose, and massaged her shoulders, standing behind her. He massaged the base of her neck languidly.

"Don't," she said.

"Don't be sore," he asked her, massaging gently. "You still love me, don't you?"

"I guess I still do. But I'm starting to hope I'll get over it."

"Okay, so I shouldn't have thought I could confide. People should keep these things bottled up, I guess."

She took his hands from her shoulders.

"You're always analyzing yourself," she said. "Why don't you analyze me for a change?" She looked around at him. "I'm going to have to follow you to wherever the Army sends you. And after that go and live in whatever city your career takes you, and subordinate my whole career to yours. Anything I choose to do has to be limited by what fits in—what advances your work. Just like children have to pull up stakes and move to another city if their father decides to. My whole career and everything I do has to be dependent on you. Like a child vis-à-vis a parent. Just like my mother has to follow my father around, and just like my sister and brother have to follow my father around. He gets himself fired, and wife and children have to follow him. And did it ever occur to you that if I'm gonna be in a position like a child again, I've got to be loved and cherished, just like a child needs it? That's the compensation. Being dependent without being loved—it isn't tolerable. A child couldn't take it and I couldn't either. I've got to have either love, if I'm dependent like a child, or else be independent and on my own and take care of myself. At least one or the other."

He sat on the cot. "Well, I've—"

"Don't sit on the veil."

He moved. "I've given you a hard time," he said. "I'm sorry. I've had a hard time myself."

"Les," she said, half turning on the backless seat to face him, "when you first used to say let's go to bed I asked you to give me a code. Remember? Rules. I asked you for rules, so I could know what I was doing—know where I was, so to speak. And you wouldn't. You just wouldn't. You said the new morality hasn't got rules. So then I asked you to love me. After that I asked you to love me, and you wouldn't. You wouldn't do that either."

"I do love you."

She was staring at him with some intensity and he was staring back. There were the noises of the house and yard. A man laughed heartily downstairs.

"I'm not going to marry you, Les," she said quietly.

They continued staring. A muscle twitched in his jaw and became firm again.

"I just now realized I'm not going to," she said. "I've decided."

She watched his face but his expression scarcely changed. A brief narrowing of his eyes and a widening of his nostrils were almost imperceptible.

"Are you relieved?" she asked, her voice suddenly quavering.

"No. I'm not relieved. Look, I couldn't help it. I had problems—maybe I should have kept them all to myself, but I couldn't help it. Isn't a wife supposed to be a confidante, for Christ sake? Who am I gonna talk to if not you?"

"Don't worry, Les," she said, almost in a whisper. "I'm not gonna cry my eyes out."

Both their faces had softened. They sat looking at each other.

"I know you're sore," he said. "But bawl me out tomorrow. Tomorrow morning. This isn't the time."

"You are relieved, aren't you." Her voice still quavered.

"No, for Christ sake. I'm not relieved. Now cut it out." He rose. "Let's have a decent wedding day. You wanted a decent wedding day. Wedding night. Whatever it was."

He looked at her somewhat pained. He sighed and turned.

"Where are you going?" Millicent asked.

He looked at her again. "I'm going downstairs. To get married. Where do you think I'm going? Take it easy, will ya? They're gonna start pretty soon." He put his hand on the doorknob but turned to her once more. "I know how you feel," he said gently. The corner of his mouth twitched into a little smile. "Take it out on me some other time. All right?"

As he went out she glimpsed some old friend of her mother's in the hall, and it occurred to her that the location of the only bathroom in the house brought traffic past her door.

The door shut. She continued looking at it, and then turned and looked through the fluttering leaves at the tent tops. A shudder rose in her like the beginning of a sob. The door clicked open and Patty entered, shutting it behind her.

"There's a million people here," Patty said. She took the veil from the bedspread with both hands and shook it a little to make its folds hang cleanly.

Millicent rested her brow on her hands and let her fingers run into her hair. "Patty—" she said.

"What."

She didn't say anything.

"What," Patty repeated.

"Nothing."

"Do you know you're wrecking your hair?"

"What if I didn't marry him. If I changed my mind."

"Oh boy," Patty answered lightly. She lay the veil down. "We're gonna need bobby pins." She pulled open the dressing-table drawer against Millicent's stomach.

Millicent stared at herself in the mirrors, allowing Patty to work at her with bobby pins. There seemed a triteness about the veil now. She did not like the way it was truncated. It seemed a compromise with the full classic one that descends into a train, but the full classic one of course would have been impossible. And trite also. She remembered she had wanted the beauty of this gown of Grandma Annie's, the moving loveliness of a ceremony full-blown—the fiddlers, the toasts—the feel of here am I, here she comes, to wed and make a new generation, the flowering bride with her white-girdled loins. Yet now she wished she had decided instead upon a tweed suit, and as few witnesses as the State permits.

And even that would be trite. Hackneyed. Wherever you fled, there was corniness. For a moment she wished Leslie had been right in the first instance—that people could just go to bed together and forget each other when they were fed up.

She stared at her thumbnail. It occurred to her that everyone expected her to be happy with this man. In a little while they would be crowding around her, kissing her, smiling with joy for her.

Patty brought her the veil. "I don't know if we can get this on," Patty said. "Maybe we better wait for Mother."

Millicent brushed it aside with her wrist. "I can't," she said. "I can't do it."

"Want me to get Mother?" Patty asked. "Come on, we have to get going. They'll play here comes the bride and I'll look pretty silly running in. I can't stand around."

"I'm not going through with it," Millicent said in her throat. "Tell Mother."

"Oh come on, you're not that scared."

A sob burst from Millicent, jarring her. Once it began it seemed uncontrollable and she buried her head in her arms on the dressing table, shaking. She heard Patty make a click in her mouth and the swish of Patty's dress as she left. The door hung open and she heard the musicians.

Even if she did go through with it she couldn't go downstairs bawling like that. It was imperative to control it, she told herself. The three selves before her in the mirrors looked terrible, with reddened eyes and wet cheeks. She would have to get Patty to fix her make-up all over again.

Somebody shut the door but she could still hear the music drifting above the voices. The music stopped. She hoped they were not about to play here comes the bride. The musicians resumed. It was not here comes the bride.

Her mother rushed in, with Patty following, and Millicent turned on the little seat and flung herself weeping onto the cot.

"What's the matter!" Lucinda said, sitting down half over her and protecting her with her arms. "What *is* this!" she patted her.

Millicent felt ashamed and ridiculous.

"There, there, now," her mother said. "You've got to pull yourself together."

Patty sat on a corner of the cot too, watching them with an alarmed expression.

Millicent did pull herself together somewhat. She rolled to her side and looked at the sober, authoritative expression her mother had put on. She saw Patty sitting just beyond her mother, looking alarmed. "I'm not gonna marry him, Mother. We don't love each other, and we're calling it off." Tears remained in her voice. She let her mother take her in her arms. "You have to go down and apologize for me."

"You're not calling anything off. A last-minute panic is perfectly normal." Her mother patted her and told Patty to get some tissues. "I had the jitters too when I got married."

"Mother, you don't understand—he doesn't want me, Mother. He doesn't love me."

"Don't be silly. If he didn't love you he wouldn't be here."

"He doesn't love me. He hates me."

"Have you two been having a fight?" Lucinda's voice rose. "On your wedding day?"

"He's been trying to get out of it for weeks. Ever since he proposed he's been trying to think of a way. He thinks he's trapped. Mother, he doesn't want me, and I'm scared to marry a man that doesn't want me. It's bad enough to have to traipse all over the world after somebody—but I can't go traipse all over after somebody that doesn't want me. I'll be in Korea or some strange place and I'll have nobody in the world except a husband that doesn't even want me."

"It's just your imagination." Her mother took the tissue from Patty and wiped Millicent's eyes and face. "If he's willing to marry you he wants you. And he's down there waiting. We're all waiting."

Millicent blubbered again. She took the tissues from her mother and wiped her nose.

"You mustn't think he doesn't love you, just because you had a little spat," her mother said more tenderly. "Your father and I have had fights all our lives, and the worst fights are in the beginning. You'll fight less as time goes on. If you really love each other."

"That's just the point—if you really love each other. Mother, you can't imagine how he talks. It's awful. He's just marrying me because he thinks he has to. He practically said it in so many words."

Her mother's face was grave, and Millicent felt she was beginning to get through to her.

"Do you think he's happy?" Millicent added. "Has he looked happy to you these days?"

"Well, I thought he had concerns on his mind."

Millicent gave a snort that was almost a sob.

"But you don't all of a sudden call off a wedding just because you don't think he loves you enough—" her mother said, "—just because he doesn't say it just right. I don't care how unromantic he says it. You don't turn down a brilliant, handsome doctor that's all ready to marry you. Not if he's willing with the guests all there, and the ring, and the license. He could have gotten out of it if he wanted to."

"He doesn't know what he wants."

"Well, lots of men have doubts. They aren't always certain when they get married. You have to make them certain, by devotion. Look at me—I married for love, and after the elopement we were apart with our families for three weeks before we got together. That's how uncertain we were."

"I've already given him plenty of devotion."

"He might be nervous, you know. Did you ever think of that? You can't judge everything he says. Don't you think Dad was a very mixed-up boy when I married him?"

"Dad wasn't mixed up about getting married. He made all the plans and he made you elope at nineteen. He wasn't mixed up about that."

"That doesn't prove anything. A few years after we were married he changed his occupation, and he's never settled down. God knows where we'll be next year—"

"If a man started making all the plans you wouldn't do it," said Patty. "You'd be fighting all the time."

"Okay, but at least I'd know what we're fighting about," said Millicent. She began to cry again.

"Now, look, it's enough, Millicent," her mother said. "You have to control yourself. We're keeping everyone waiting."

The crying diminished. Her mother gave her some pats on the thigh and on the arm and a little hug.

"That's a good girl, that's right," Lucinda said. "Get her a glass of water," she told Patty. "And tell them we'll start the ceremony in fifteen minutes."

"I mean it," Millicent said. "I'm not marrying him."

Patty paused at the door.

"So what am I supposed to do?" Lucinda asked, her voice going up sharply. "I can't go down and tell everybody you changed your mind. People are seated already." She caught Patty's eye. "Get Daddy," she said.

Patty started out.

"Patty," Lucinda called her sharply.

Patty looked at her.

"Don't make a scene," Lucinda said. "Just get him quietly." She sighed as Patty left and glanced again at Millicent, who was blowing her nose. "I don't know," she muttered. "I don't know. I just don't know. Crazy."

"I won't marry without being loved," Millicent pleaded. "I won't. I want to be loved. At least in the beginning."

"Love can grow, you know. It can get stronger."

Lucinda sighed again, and Millicent's sniffling quieted, as if both were listening to the sounds of the crowd downstairs. She thought she heard Sharlene cry out. Sometimes the musicians played and sometimes they didn't.

"I suppose you feel he thinks he owes it to you," Lucinda said. "You think he's going through with it to be a gentleman."

Millicent saw tears in her mother's eyes too, and her mother's voice had become as tearful as her own.

"Is that what it is?" her mother said. "I certainly wouldn't hold it against him on that account—I'd say it's very decent. And I'll bet there are fine marriages that started that way, because that shows devotion too. If he didn't think anything of you he wouldn't care. But he respects you and he wants to make an honest woman of you. I admire him for it."

"I'm ten times as honest as he ever was."

"Well, you know what I mean. Give you a good name."

"My own name is good enough. He's not good enough to give me a good name."

"Well, he's doing the right thing. He has character at least. I'd think you'd be tickled. You don't know how lucky you are. It's not every boy that compromises a girl and then comes around and proposes marriage."

"There was no compromise about it."

She saw by the sour look her mother gave her that her mother thought she meant it as a witticism. But she had not. She blushed.

"Well, I resent this idea that a man has the power to make you honest," she explained. "What's a man? God or something? Why don't I make him honest? Women are a lot more honest about these things than men are."

"You're talking like a damn fool. What's the matter with you? You should be tickled to death that he's willing to marry you."

"This whole stupid idea that a man can disgrace you and a man can make you honest," Millicent persisted. "As if he has a magic wand or something."

They heard quick feet at the top of the stairs and in the corridor and Ed entered, anxious-faced, followed by Aunt Gwendolyn and Patty.

"What's this all about—" he began.

"Millicent honey!" Gwendolyn exclaimed, rushing in wide-eyed with her arms extended to seize her as though Millicent had had an accident.

"We decided we're not right for each other, that's all," Millicent answered, her nose in her handkerchief and her wet eyes apologetic. "We're not right for each other."

"What! Are you serious?" Ed said.

"Oh, you're crazy," Gwendolyn said in a tone of disbelief.

"Who decided!" said Ed. "What do you mean. Are you gonna act like a three-year-old? Patch it up, whatever it is. You don't get cold feet in the middle of a wedding."

"It's always bad luck for the groom to see the bride on the wedding morning," Lucinda managed to say. "Before the ceremony." She began crying openly.

It startled Millicent to see her mother break down like that.

"Snap out of it, for God's sake, before he takes you seriously," her father said to Millicent. "You're getting everybody upset."

"We're all wrong for each other—" she tried to explain tearfully.

They had left the door open and suddenly Leslie stood in it. She glimpsed Jack behind him.

"Get out, Les!" Millicent told him, her voice shaking. "Get out while the getting's good. Before I change my mind."

"For Christ sake, what are you so sore about?" he said, coming toward her. He shut the door behind him in Jack's face but it opened again. "You misunderstood me," he said.

"You don't sound like I misunderstood you."

"Can I talk to you? Alone?"

"No!"

"It's a fine time to chicken out," Ed told Leslie sourly.

"He didn't chicken out," Millicent said. "I chickened out."

"I didn't chicken out," said Leslie. Jack had not come in, and she saw some curious strangers in the hallway.

"Everybody get out," Gwendolyn directed, sweeping the air with an arm. "Everybody get out and let me talk to her." Her arm almost hit Mrs. Hollander, who came in just then. She tried to push the door shut against Mrs. Hollander as though she had not recognized her, but then let her in and shut it.

"It's true—" Lucinda wept meanwhile, appealing with her arms to Mrs. Hollander. "They shouldn't see the bride in the morning, before the ceremony. It's always bad luck. I tried to keep him down but he insisted. She didn't look good this morning. A bunch of nerves, and circles under her eyes. She didn't sleep a wink all night. The excitement. It's the anticipation, the night before."

"Millicent," Leslie said. "Millicent. What are you trying to do—"

"They were quarreling," Lucinda told Mrs. Hollander, "but she doesn't mean it. She's all upset."

"Well, I guess they have to decide," Mrs. Hollander said.

Leslie was hunching his shoulders, almost as if dodging the others, and opening his mouth as if trying to speak to Millicent. "Les," Ed said, putting a hand on his shoulder and turning him somewhat, "listen to me. Are you honorable?"

"Let him alone!" Millicent told her father. "I'm not in any shape to get married anyway. I was up all night, and I look awful."

"Go through with it. Go through with it, darling," her mother begged her. "I know it's crazy but get through the day somehow and I'm sure you'll forget what a crazy wedding day you had. Someday you'll laugh about it."

"No I won't."

"Your father and I had a crazy wedding day too."

"Listen, son," Ed told Leslie, "I don't know what's bothering you—"

"Oh, Daddy," Millicent cut in, "for goodness sakes—"

"They should certainly do what'll make them happy," said Mrs. Hollander. "They're both very young after all."

"Sure they're young," said Ed.

"It isn't as if she were pregnant, after all," Mrs. Hollander said.

"Mother," Leslie said, "shut up. Just shut up."

"Well, I want you to do whatever will make you happy," his mother said.

"Sure you're young—you could stay a bachelor for years," Ed told him. "But when you look at it, what good is the bachelor's life? It's not so simple. You start feeling sordid about all the breakups and the broken hearts—I got married young and got it over with."

"Dad, for goodness sakes," Millicent said bitterly. "You're running off at the mouth."

"What do you say, Millicent?" Leslie said.

"Just go!" she answered, with a strain in her voice. "Will you please go?"

"Everybody clear out," said Aunt Gwendolyn. "Everybody. I'm gonna have a talk with Millicent. Go on, everybody out. There's too many people."

"Everything was all right until her family got into the act, do you know that?" Leslie said to Gwendolyn.

"No it wasn't," Millicent contradicted him.

"That's what started it," he told Millicent. "We were happy together. We could have gone on indefinitely."

"No we couldn't have!" She reddened.

He colored also. "I mean we'd have gotten married."

"When you got around to it?" Her voice was angry but it shook badly.

"Do you want to put it off temporarily?" he asked her.

"Oh shut up! Shut up! I can't stand it! Get out of my room!" She threw the box of tissues at him and he dodged with his arm.

He had stepped back and the box had fallen to his foot. "Do you want to postpone it?" he said to her.

"What do you mean postpone it—" Ed shot at him.

"You're so confused you're getting him confused," Lucinda told Millicent, her face wet.

"Do you want to think about it?" Leslie asked Millicent.

"No! I don't want to think about it and I don't want you to think about it and I don't want to be thought about! It makes me nervous." She gave a hysterical sob.

"You're the one that's giving the whole thing an unhappy ending," he told her.

"I don't care! That's what I want."

"We're not calling it off. We're just putting it off," Leslie said to Ed.

"No!" she shouted. "It's the same thing. It means finished."

"Well, that's what I was afraid of," Leslie said to her. "That's why I'd rather go through with it."

"Go! Will you go?" Her voice shot high and squeaky.

"Take it easy—" He took a step backward.

"She's crazy—what can I say?" Lucinda said desperately to Mrs. Hollander, her face contorted.

"She has to make up her mind," Mrs. Hollander said.

Leslie was half out of the room. "We'll keep in touch," he said quietly.

"No! I don't want to see you again!" Millicent said loudly, her voice quavering.

"Tell your people not to go yet," Ed said to him. "She might come around."

"No!" said Millicent.

Leslie narrowed his eyes, but seemed to decide against saying anything. His face was red. He left quickly.

For an instant of silence they stared at the door he had shut behind him.

"All right. All right. What's the use," said Ed. "Let her alone. Leave her alone. Go on, Patty."

"It's my room," Patty protested.

"Go downstairs," Ed told Patty. But she didn't go, and Ed did not press it. No one else left either.

"If they're not sure, they don't love each other, that's what I say," said Mrs. Hollander.

Millicent sat crying aloud without using her hands or making any effort to wipe her tears. Lucinda was not sobbing but her eyes were full.

"Go away," Millicent wept.

Aunt Gwendolyn looked at Ed. "Do you want me to talk to her?" she asked.

Ed shrugged. Gwendolyn sat beside Millicent and put an arm about her.

"Shut up," Millicent blubbered.

Gwendolyn dropped the arm and looked at Ed confusedly. But Ed was looking at Millicent sourly.

"Brilliant," he said. "Absolutely brilliant. My genius."

"I could wring your neck," Lucinda said, wet-faced. Millicent looked at her mother with large wet eyes and her crying halted a moment, but then quieter sobs resumed. "Stupid," Lucinda said to her. "Like a three-year-old."

"Well, I don't want to be stuck all my life in a mismatch. I couldn't stand it."

"It wouldn't be a mismatch!" her mother answered her sharply.

"Yes it would," Millicent sobbed.

Aunt Gwendolyn began to say something but Ed cut in. "I've got news for you, Millicent Audrey," he said. "The whole world's a mismatch. God and man are a mismatch."

"You go marry him yourself if he's so great," Millicent sobbed to her aunt.

"I have to go down," Lucinda said tearfully to Ed and Gwendolyn. "What are we gonna say?"

Ed shrugged. "I'll go down," he said. "I'll make an announcement. She got sick. She took sick. She's in no condition right now anyway."

"And what are we gonna do with all that food," Lucinda muttered, dabbing her face with a crushed handkerchief.

"You could say he got a telegram from the Army and got called away immediately, and couldn't wait," Mrs. Hollander suggested.

"Or how about that he got transferred to some special part of the Army where they don't let them get married," said Aunt Gwen.

"Yes, that's good," said Mrs. Hollander.

"Or he got a call from the hospital," said Aunt Gwen. "An emergency. Some patient's dying."

"That sounds reasonable," said Mrs. Hollander.

"No, I'm going down to explain," Millicent said, rising, her tears gushing wetter. Ed and her mother pushed her down to the cot but she rose again. "It's my fault," she said.

"Don't make it any worse," Ed said, forcing her down again. Aunt Gwen was pulling her down by the arm.

"You're not going down looking like that!" her mother said sharply through her tears.

"Don't make a scene!" Aunt Gwen was saying.

"Maybe we can put it off till this afternoon," said Ed. "How about it, Millicent?"

"No!" Her voice came as an uneven bleat.

"I wish they had decided before," said Mrs. Hollander. "It cost money to get clothes and come up here."

"I'll say it cost money," said Ed. "Gwen, you stay with her, will you? Come on. Get out. Let her get some rest." He made wide sweeping motions with his arms.

Millicent saw them go out. She sat weeping, looking at the closed door, not giving in to the gentle arm and stroking hands of her aunt. She started up.

"Millicent!" said Gwendolyn.

Millicent went out to the hallway. Her mother was sobbing and talking to someone at the head of the stairs and her father had Leslie cornered against the railing.

"She's too high strung, that's her trouble," she heard her mother say.

"She's gorgeous, she's beautiful, she's brilliant, what do ya want?" her father was saying to Les. Patty saw Millicent and seemed to blanch. Then her father saw her. "I ought to take you over my knee, you know it?" he said, advancing on her. "Your mother suggested it once. In another connection."

Aunt Gwen had her by the arm and she was pushed and pulled back into the bedroom and the door was shut.

"You're going to lie down and get some rest," her aunt said.

Gwen undid the hooks of the gown. She helped her out of her things. "You got married and then you got divorced," Millicent blubbered to Aunt Gwen. "We got the divorce first." The door drifted open of itself. In the moment it was open Millicent saw some middle-aged man with a mustache glimpse her in her underwear. Aunt Gwen shut the door. At last Millicent lay crying tiredly in chemise and stockings.

"There, now. I'm going to get a cold washcloth and sponge your face," Gwendolyn said. "And you know what else I'm going to get you? I'm going to bring you a drink, for once in your life. You need it. A stiff drink."

Millicent saw her aunt go out. Her crying subsided. She remained on the cot, an arm over her face. The bouquet rolled against her. She knew the door had swung open a little and that she ought to close it, and also that she lay on the folded veil and was crushing it. She wished she could find a way to humiliate Leslie further. At the same time she contemplated what had happened with a kind of stupefaction.

She heard the music start a new tune but it stopped after a few bars. Nothing about the hum and babble downstairs told her what was happening. But she listened, and in a while some female voice she did not know rose above the others. Then she heard her grandmother exclaiming "How do ya like that!"

Millicent sat up nervously on the cot. She raised herself a little and looked through the window at hats and balding heads. Men and women had begun to come out to the yard and to mill about here and there among the tent tops—people of her parents' generation she knew vaguely or hardly at all. Beyond the tents she saw cars parked on the grass. The tents had no sides on them and she could see some tables laid out beneath them. She recalled her mother asking what would become of all the food and she was struck by the thought of the enormous expense. What a vicious person Leslie was, she thought. He used his so-called problems as a consummate sadism. He ought to be made to pay for all this.

Patty came in. Millicent glanced at her only an instant and looked out the window again, but she felt Patty staring.

"Why'd you turn him down?" Patty asked. Her tone was one of complete mystification.

Millicent made no answer. She refused even to move her head, but she felt her eyes fill again.

"Mother said to see if you're all right," Patty said. "Where's Aunt Gwen?"

Millicent held still, without answering. At last Patty made a little noise with her tongue and teeth and left again, shutting the door. But the sound of voices had already grown louder. "What do you know about that!" she heard a female voice exclaim. "Can you beat it?" said another one. Occasional male ones from below and from outdoors rose more loudly, and someone laughed. She heard the door of a car. She stood up, not knowing what she intended to do. Then she drew both window shades to the bottom and hid curled under the blankets in her underwear. Even her head was covered, and in the dark of the blanket sounds were softened. She wept into the pillow.

Les ought to have had more sense than to let this happen, she thought. What a fumbling, incompetent boob he had made of himself. Lean on him for two minutes and he croaks.

There was a rap at the door.

Her weeping stopped. She was breathless a moment. "Stay out—" she said.

No one entered or spoke. There were footsteps in the hall of various persons, not all together. She wondered who had knocked, and if it had been Leslie. She decided it wasn't. Apparently it was no one special.

The level of noise in the house was like a party. It annoyed her that people hung around and didn't have the grace to leave.

Then the thought occurred to her that all those people down there were angry with her, and that they were right. She did owe them all an apology and an explanation. She rose from the cot. There were all those gifts to be returned to stores, and all those people who had traveled distances. No wonder they were all furious. She snatched her plaid shirt from the bureau. The door opened and she ducked, expecting some stranger to see her again in her lace underfrills, but Patty entered and pushed the door shut with her hands behind her. "Boy, you sure made some mess out of this," Patty said.

Millicent pulled the jeans up over the stockings and the lace.

"Grandma Annie took a whole plate away from Mrs. Hollander," Patty said. "A chicken leg and squash and it spilled all over the place. And they're fighting about the presents and everything."

Millicent choked a sob. She was buttoning the shirt as quickly as she could. She caught a glimpse of herself in the bureau mirror beyond the teddy bear, and saw she was still in mascara and that her rouge was tear-stained, but there was no time to fix it.

"Are you going down?" said Patty, suddenly alarmed. "What are you gonna do?"

Millicent pushed past her. Patty had been leaning on the door and almost fell into the hallway. Millicent rushed out to the stairs in her stocking feet, tucking in the plaid shirt, with Patty following, but she got away from Patty in pushing past a stout lady who asked her if there was a second bathroom. She dodged someone else and hurried down. She had to slow herself for a couple of violent sneezes. Her left eye felt as if she could hardly open it.

Near the bottom of the stairs she met Aunt Celeste in a shiny pink gown, with Jill behind her long-haired in a bell-like one. They were both in tears and their eyes filled even more when they saw her. Aunt Celeste flung her arms about her. "Oh, my poor child," said Aunt Celeste. Jill looked on with a fixed expression, tears running down. Their crying made Millicent sob too.

"Forgive me," she pleaded in Aunt Celeste's arms. "I'll pay for everything. I'm to blame. I thought I was sure but I wasn't—" She saw her mother, red-eyed, at the door, saying good-bye to people. Millicent sneezed, and the sneeze broke the sobbing. She had no handkerchief.

"There she is! Oh!" Grandma Annie said with hoarse excitement at the foot of the stairs. Sneezes kept exploding in Millicent. Her whole sinuses hurt and one sneeze seemed to wrench her back muscles. "I want you to have it. That coffeepot's from our side. It's yours—I don't care if you're married or not. The nerve—some nut walks right off with it—I saw it. She'd a walked off with the whole shootin' match. Some crazy woman. I know what's our side."

Millicent remembered she wanted to apologize to Mrs. Hollander for Grandma Annie. The sneezes slowed. She kept a hand over her left eye.

"Are you all right?" Lucinda asked, starting toward Millicent.

"He's rotten, you're well out of it," Aunt Celeste wept.

"The hell with him, the rascal," Grandma Annie said. "They're crooks, I seen it with my own eyes. And you can put that in your pipe and smoke it."

Uncle Maxwell put his hands on Millicent's shoulders and sang a dirge, grinning at her. He wore a skullcap at a clownish angle. "I don't know, what do you do with a wedding feast, you eat it," her big, florid, mustachioed Uncle Franklin was saying. She pushed through their hands and arms, looking for Mrs. Hollander, but her father moved toward her scowling. "Now what!" said Ed. "Have you changed your mind?"

She saw Ruthie Meyers with her husband in the entrance hall near the door and called to her. She had to contort and wrinkle her face to keep from sneezing, and covered her left eye again.

"Oh, Millicent. You poor kid!" Ruthie said. She was visibly pregnant. But she moved recklessly through the crowd to Millicent and they embraced.

"I made a mistake," Millicent explained to her. "Please don't hate me. We thought we were right for each other but we weren't."

"There isn't any right one," Ruthie said with sad appealing eyes. "You have to marry one of the wrong ones."

"Those stupid kids," Ed said, coming over. "They decide to have a lovers' quarrel. I could knock their heads together."

"I'll pay for it," Millicent told him, crying. "Out of my salary. I don't care how long it takes. I'll pay for everything. Patty's dress too." A sneeze stopped the crying.

"You want to pay me back?" said her father. "Marry the guy."

She saw Aunt Gwendolyn, and Nancy, and Patty holding Sharlene. "I'll pay for Sharlene's dress," she said.

"Oh no," Aunt Gwendolyn said.

"Yes I will. I'll pay for Patty's dress too." She sneezed, but she had held it off too long and again it hurt the middle of her back.

"I don't know—Lucinda!" a lady said, pushing in at the open front doors. Millicent recognized her as an old friend of her mother's but the lady pushed past her without recognition. "Do you want to tell the caterer to go or what? There are people eating."

Millicent went out to the porch in her stocking feet and down the steps. There was a confusion of people standing about, especially near the front of the house, and cars pulling out. They did not follow the winding dirt road, but crossed the grass every which way and got onto the dirt road anywhere. She saw one driver motioning the right of way to another. Little groups of people were at tables under tents munching away, and a few were at the hors d'oeuvres bar, but the caterer's men in tan coats were almost as numerous. She saw Leslie standing in the grass amid cars as though in a parking lot, and shaking hands through a car window with young men in black suits. They were interns—she recognized a couple of them. They had white boutonnieres. Though Leslie's back was toward her she could see an embarrassment in his whole stance. The car pulled away and he stood hunched, as though he would rather not have been visible. He seemed to bite a hangnail.

A bald man she knew as a lifelong friend of her parents recognized her and touched her arm, though she tried to avoid him. "Well, what do I say?" the man said. "Good luck—condolences—what?"

She ducked away from him and hurried toward Les, feeling the grass through her stockings. "Les—" she called.

He turned and watched her steadily as she came near. She did not look back as she ran, and she knew he shared her hope that nobody much watched them. She came among the cars, not looking to the right or left, but she sensed that some people getting into a car glanced at her as she passed.

"Hi," she said to Les as she came near.

"Hi."

His face was unsmiling, but with a softness of expression. She stopped, and there was a feeling of awkwardness, though their eyes remained fixed on one another's faces.

"Have you got a handkerchief?" she said.

He pulled one from his hip pocket. She pressed it to her nostrils, breathing through her mouth. Her eye still hurt.

"I'm sorry about my grandmother," she said.

"Oh. I'm sorry about that," he said, and his regret and confusion seemed genuine, as if he felt the fault was on his own side.

"She pushed your mother or something, Patty said," Millicent told him. "With a chicken leg." Her eyes filled again.

"No no. It wasn't like that." He colored a little, glancing away.

She did not pursue it. Their eyes met again but they shared one another's awkwardness. He put both hands in his pockets. His face seemed somehow fine, even though uncomfortable—his features for some reason were at their best, and the maroon tie and the charcoal flannel suit became him.

"Well—" he said, with a vague finality.

She glanced about. There were some people moving and talking among the cars, and others beyond, but no one just now seemed to notice herself or Leslie.

"I'm sorry about everything," she said to him. "It's not much of a send-off to the Army."

"That's all right."

Her nose was less raw now and she was able to lower the handkerchief. They stood there silently, looking at the grass and at the fat dusty tire of a car. It was as if they communed there a moment, sharing the wreckage of their wedding. The place where they stood was nearly through the collection of cars, away from the house, and the low wall of loose stones that bordered Massapeequit Road was nearby, with high grass near it. The sun shone on the wall and on the grass.

"Maybe we should still get married," she said, as if thinking aloud.

"Maybe we should," he said. "I don't know."

They still gazed throughtfully, not looking at each other. She scratched the sole of her foot through the stocking by rubbing it slowly on the stiff grass.

He leaned back on a car.

"I don't know," she said. "Do you want to elope?"

"I don't know," he said tiredly.

"I know—I'm all confused," she agreed. "Maybe we should think about it. Do you want to think about it? And discuss it by mail?"

"Look, I can't even think."

In a moment he seemed to give a start. He rose suddenly, looking irritably in a new direction, and Millicent saw Mrs. Hollander carrying a high-piled armload of boxes of various sizes, with Jack carrying more behind her. Their wrappings were open and crushed paper and ribbon stuck out.

"Mother," Leslie said, approaching her, "just where the hell do you think you're going with those?" Millicent followed him.

"She's loading up Uncle Bernie's car," said Jack. "Aunt Gert's car is full of food."

"These were all from our side," Mrs. Hollander said, and a bundle of colored towels in cellophane slipped to her feet. She tried to stoop and a long striped box dropped.

"I don't care whose side!" He was red-faced. "They all belong to Millicent! They're all gifts to Millicent."

"No, they all have to be returned," Millicent said.

"There, see?" said Mrs. Hollander, squatting on the grass in her gown and trying to collect her load again. "She's very fair. And there are some things that aren't returnable. Millicent hasn't got all the addresses."

"Well put 'em back! Jesus Christ!"

"I don't mind doing it, Mrs. Hollander," Millicent said.

"You don't know what's from who," said Mrs. Hollander. Unbalanced boxes tumbled from Mrs. Hollander as she squatted there, more rapidly than she could get them together.

Leslie stooped to help her, with a noise of angry disgust through his teeth. "Jack, get everything out of Bernie's car," he said.

"Are you kidding?" said Jack. "You help me then. She's got it piled up to the ceiling."

Millicent had an impulse to squat also and help gather the boxes that had spilled around Mrs. Hollander but at once realized it would only multiply everyone's confusion and discomfort.

"Honest, Millicent, I was talking to people. I didn't know she was doing this," Leslie said without looking up.

Millicent tried to slip away. She dodged around a moving car. She was still holding the handkerchief. Her shoeless feet were uncomfortable now. She pretended to brush a lock of hair, and raised the crushed handkerchief to the irritated left sinus area, but mainly to avoid catching the eyes of parting guests. She saw Aunt Gert leaning into the window of a car to say good-bye to someone on Leslie's side. Then she had to hang back a moment to let another car pass, and studied the litter on the ground. She heard Jack call her, and when she turned he was hurrying toward her, still with his armload of ribboned boxes. He had a loping gait. He was thin-jawed and a little sweaty, and he panted.

"My mother wants to know if you have any containers, for stuffed cabbage," he said.

"I don't know," said Millicent. "I'll ask my mother."

73

Millicent took to her bed, in her own room. She slept for much of the day, but fitfully, and was aware at times, in a kind of twilight sleep, of the voices of men taking down the tent poles and the clatter of the folding chairs being removed. When she awakened she remained there, the sheet and blanket nearly over her head. She knew her grandmother and her aunts were still downstairs, though most of the guests had gone. She lay for hours, with angry fantasies of Leslie. She imagined him writing her letters, begging her to believe that he had grown up and knew his own mind now.

But in the evening the sense of aloneness struck her. She had forgotten what a horrible thing loneliness was. Now that it was back it was familiar. She had known it before. It was as if it had been the basic fact of life, just under the surface all along.

She was glad the family had the considerateness to let her alone.

The next morning she stayed in bed late to avoid the family. She had arranged with Mr. Killian long before to have that day off anyway. But during the morning her mother phoned the city room and told them Millicent would be ill for several more days.

"They think I'm married," Millicent said, when her mother told her.

"No, I said the wedding had to be postponed because of sickness," said her mother.

Millicent hung about her room. She wondered if she should reimburse her father for the caterer out of Charles's ten thousand dollars. But it seemed wrong that Charles's insurance money should have to be spent for anything so foolish. The task of returning presents seemed huge and dismal. She wondered if she was expected not only to return them but to send letters with them. That seemed impossible. She considered delaying a while, on the chance that a letter from Leslie and new wedding plans might still spare her that.

She went down to lunch, and her mother kept talking about the way Mrs. Hollander had behaved the day before. "I never saw anything like it. Buckets of food in that car—I hope she has a freezer at home. Knishes—you should see the rolls she took. Paper bags full—I haven't even got bags left for garbage. You'd think she was going to the north woods. And then she sends Jack asking for containers. For the stuffed cabbage. I told him ask the caterer—I don't have any containers. And she says she's doing me a favor—it would go to waste anyway." Lucinda made a click in her mouth and shook her head. "And in the middle of it she sits down at the table to eat. She and Jack. She had plenty of appetite too. You'd think she didn't eat for a month. I could have stuffed it down her throat. Stuffing, sweet potato, there was nothing she didn't eat. I don't know where she puts it."

In the afternoon Millicent took Roland's bicycle, to avoid the house and family. But at supper, and in the evening, she heard more stories about the wedding. Lucinda and Patty kept talking about it. They said the expression of Leslie's face had looked all weekend as though he were going out to face a firing squad. Apparently even one of Leslie's uncles had admitted it. And Uncle Maxwell had been disgusting afterwards, pretending he was at a funeral, as if it was a big joke, and when he was reminded that there had been a death in the family recently he said he had forgotten. There was a story about Aunt Gwen reprimanding Mrs. Hollander for taking a present, and Mrs. Hollander had told her to try and get it.

Millicent went upstairs, so as not to hear any more stories. But Patty followed her and told her more. She told her of all the conflicting rumors that had spread among the guests, including that Leslie had gotten a Connecticut marriage license by mistake. "Mother kept contradicting herself about a dozen times," Patty said, "and Uncle Max said you just found out you weren't pregnant. He thinks he's so smart. And he isn't funny a bit. And he said you didn't pass the syphilis test, and somebody even believed it."

Millicent went to work the next day, even though her mother had phoned them not to expect her. She came into the city room with an uneasy dignity, inwardly embarrassed, and avoiding faces, but in general it turned out as though nothing had happened. Mr. Killian apparently was too basically ill at ease himself to begin a conversation about such a thing. She had pictured Danny McBride as making some awful wisecrack, but Danny was not there, and the others worked as usual, as though they had not heard or had forgotten. Apparently they cared less or were better bred than she realized.

Maud Dickinson looked at her tenderly once or twice, and when Millicent came near her desk Maud remarked quietly that she had always been a great believer in the idea that things happen for the best.

"Well, I don't know," said Millicent.

"You're young. You've got time," Maud assured her.

On the train home she tried to calculate how long it would take to hear from Les. He would certainly write, in one way or another, because they had not parted angrily. But she could not make up her mind as to what his tone would be.

By the time her days off came her mother was no longer letting her alone. Her mother called her a damn fool again.

"He was a catch," her mother said. "There was a beautiful marriage handed to you on a platter, and you threw it out the window. It's natural for a bridegroom to get cold feet, you know. And if he's willing to go through with it you don't hold it against him. You don't get panicky and ruin everything."

"I wasn't panicky."

"If you weren't, then you're a lunatic. If he was willing to marry you to give you a good name that shows love too, for goodness sakes. That's a kind of love too. And if you loved him, and he was willing to marry you, you should have had less pride about it."

"How would you like it if I'd said okay and then we got divorced in six months," Millicent said.

"Yes," her mother retorted. "Yes. Because you wouldn't get divorced. I'm sure he would have stayed with you and his love would grow. Because if he was willing to marry you he wants you."

Her mother's words fanned the spark of hope she had that she might still get together with Les somehow, after all, but at the same time they deepened her feeling of remorse.

She tried to deduce from her mother's words that Les would surely write to her, and thus leave the way open to a new beginning. Even so, she had no real certainty that he would ever get in touch with her again at all.

Sending him away at the very moment that he struggled to resolve his doubts seemed now a ridiculous thing to have done. The fact was, they were suited. As her mother had said, he had been ready to marry her. They had been happy before, and they would have conquered their doubts together, and they'd have been happy again. The fait accompli would have conquered their doubts for them. Doubts were just something that plague all highly intelligent people, and she should have had common sense enough to ignore them. Les was a man who labored round the clock, taking the lives of others in his hands, even if his own flesh were destroyed by lack of sleep. The wonder was that he managed to open his eyes day after day and work on and on, and have strength left to talk to her a little. A man in work like his hasn't got time to worry about who's insulting who and all that kind of nonsense. It occurred to her that maybe he had wanted to feel forced, so as to solve his dilemma without having to think about it, since his busy schedule left him no time to think it through.

She told herself she had no common sense. How could she have been so neurotic and stupid? In a moment of self-centeredness she had probably ruined her life. It could take twenty years now if she waited to meet another man as peculiarly suited to her as that one was. Congenial souls were not found in directories. Life was a lonely business.

It had been a disaster, and she would have to struggle to right it, beg him to let her right it, no matter how much humbling was involved.

Maybe she was out of her mind and should see a psychiatrist, she thought.

What she had done was idiotic, and she was left now with a feeling of utter aloneness. It was a black world of aloneness. No one was talkable to. Except Leslie—what they had been through together made him talkable to.

And besides he was a smart person, with a mind like hers. To have some day to marry a dumb person would be the permanent, ultimate aloneness, a prison.

She wandered in and out of the house, and behind the barn. She wanted to write to Les, yet she was not sure what effect it would have on him right now. She lay on her bed for hours, a forearm over her eyes.

When she returned to the city room after her days off Maud mentioned to her that Heustis Garvey had died suddenly that morning.

"Now's your chance," Maud said quietly, sitting at her typewriter, looking up from under her brows. "Ask Dexter for his job."

It seemed wrong to Millicent to seek to take advantage so quickly. But it excited her.

She went about her work. It would be a marvelous promotion. It would give her a lot more money, but that was the least of it. The opportunities it would open up were limitless.

But she was also afraid that Mr. Killian might consider it preposterous. And even if he didn't, and gave her the job, she was afraid she wasn't quite ready for it. She kept at her duties, but in a state of tension. She tried to work out in her mind how she would manage if she did get the job, and how she would present her request to Mr. Killian.

Then Mr. Killian told her she had a phone call. She took it at one of the back desks. It was Freddy Winkler, the mathematician she had once interviewed. He said he wanted to have a drink with her after work and tell her about a job she might be interested in. She cut the call short, but said she would meet him at the spa.

It was a strange thing to have happened. She wondered what kind of a job he could possibly have for her.

When she met him at the spa he smiled at her in the same bright-eyed way he had the time she had seen him in his office. She ordered cocoa. He asked if she wanted whipped cream or marshmallow. For himself he ordered coffee. He was lanky and casual, and he seemed to relax almost to the point of double-jointedness. But the job he had in mind turned out to be of no interest. He himself was flying to Europe the next day, to study in Switzerland over the summer and to do some mountain-climbing, but he knew a professor who was taking his family on the grand tour, and who needed a girl to help look after the children. She would get all expenses and be paid besides, and see London, Paris, Venice, Florence—the works.

She told him she couldn't. "Why did you think of me?" she asked.

"I just did."

"I have a job," she said. "I can't just go and leave my job for a thing like that."

"Maybe you could ask for a leave. Have you ever seen Europe?"

"Really, I'm not interested. It's quite out of the question."

"The kids are seven and ten. It's an easy job."

"I'm not a governess."

It was a while before their cocoa and coffee came. They sat talking about Europe. He had been there before and had climbed mountains before. He was due for a new research fellowship at M.I.T., but he had had two offers from the new electronics firms near Boston, and he thought he might leave M.I.T. in the fall. One company wanted to give him his own research laboratory.

"Do you know you have remarkable eyes?" he asked her.

"Yes, I'm aware of that," she said.

In time he wrote down the professor's home and office phones, and said she could phone the professor or the professor's wife if she changed her mind. He thought they were leaving in about three weeks, and he knew they had engaged no one yet. Then he said he had to be going.

She stood by while he settled with the cashier. She asked if he were really flying to Zürich tomorrow. He said yes and that he had to pack. Then he said good-bye and left her.

What an odd person, she thought. It had been a pleasant interlude, but unrelated to anything.

She threw the professor's phone numbers into a sidewalk rubbish barrel.

Over the weekend Mr. Killian was away, so she had no chance to approach him about the police headquarters job. On Monday she thought she had better act. She had even thought of confiding her intentions to Mr. Hopkins and asking for his good offices with Mr. Killian. But when she came into the city room Mr. Killian at once beckoned with his head, and when she came to his desk he told her she would have the day shift only henceforth, no night work at all. Lyons was being shifted to police headquarters, and Zucchino would replace Lyons, as a general-assignment reporter, and she would have Zucchino's old hours. Dawn would have the night hours, at least until he had someone new.

Zucchino was already back at work, swinging himself slowly and stiffly along with his broken leg in a big dirty white cast. It was logical, she realized now, that an experienced man like Bob Lyons should be chosen to replace Mr. Garvey. But why was Zucchino chosen for promotion to Lyons's old job? Zucchino had written nothing. As far as she knew, Zucchino had never shown any ambition to be more than a copy boy. Mr. Killian sat working scowlingly.

At home that evening she went down to the kitchen in her bathrobe toward midnight, unable to sleep. As it turned out her father was also up, and he sat with her.

She prepared warm milk. They sipped it, and she told him of her disappointment at the office. She said she did not know whether she was passed over because she was a woman, or whether it was because Mr. Killian was still mad at her and convinced she had no ability. Either way, it was discouraging.

"It's difficult to be a woman," she said. "It's so much easier for a boy. All my life I've just never known how to be a girl. From about the age of nine."

"What do you mean?" her father said.

"Well, boys always have certain definite things that make them a boy. Like football, and baseball, or tools and things, or cars, or science, or keeping rabbits, or guns—there's always something. And being a girl is okay up until about the age of nine—she's a child, she can play with dolls, for instance, or skip rope, or she can run around and climb trees and there's no pressure—and I suppose after you're a wife and a mother it's possible to feel female again, but the years in between, say from nine up until marriage, are just limbo in a girl's life. A boy can be a wizard with a slide rule, or a genius, and get all kinds of scholarships, and it's masculine. Or he can try to sleep with every girl in town and it's masculine. Or he can shine in Hebrew school and lead the synagogue at prayers, and it's masculine. Even if he robs a store and goes to prison, even that's masculine. But there's nothing corresponding to be feminine, really. Not in our time, anyway. There's just shadow things. From the age of about ten, or certainly from twelve, it's just limbo, waiting. That whole time from then to marriage is just waste in a girl's life. Lost years. Until nine or ten she's a child and after that she's under pressure, just waiting to be a woman. That's what's expected of her. There aren't all these worthwhile ways to be masculine like a boy has meanwhile. A boy isn't just waiting to be married. But whatever a girl does, it's not the way to be a girl, somehow. I remember my contemporaries used to pin up pictures of Frank Sinatra, and try on lipstick, and it never seemed to me they were enjoying it, really. They were just in limbo, groping for some way to be girls. And as far as I could see they never found any. What are they supposed to do? Bake cookies? I don't know how to be a girl. I never did. I still don't."

"Well, I don't know how to be a rabbi," said her father.

During her lunch the next day, and for some few days thereafter, she looked at the employment ads, thinking she should perhaps change jobs. But the ads offered her nothing.

Maybe she should make the real break and try politics. Some districts were so strongly Republican or so strongly Democrat that they were usually not even contested, and perhaps the minority party would let her wage a token campaign in such a place. Why shouldn't they? She could ask either the Republicans or the Democrats to let her run for the legislature in some district that belonged so completely to the other side that they never even bothered to put up anybody.

But that too, when she thought of it more, seemed a lonely task—fighting an impossible battle in which no one was interested, and with nobody's support, She would cut an absurd figure—a ridiculous old maid. And she would lose, and then what?

Perhaps she should make the rounds of the other newspapers, and start afresh on a different one. But newspaper jobs were very difficult to get, even for men, and doubly so for women. She would never find another one. And how strange it was, she thought, that only a short time ago, when she had expected to marry Les, it had seemed to her then as though it would be an easy thing for her to find a job in whatever place the Army might send him.

She had begun to doubt more strongly now that she would ever hear from Les at all. More time had already passed than she had thought would. He had not even sent an address at which she could write to him.

She accepted a date with a man named Wayne, who had been given her phone number by a lady in the congregation. He worked for the Internal Revenue Service. He seemed to give himself airs as a man of the world, and after a while began struggling to fondle her, so that she had to wrestle irritably. He asked if she were inhibited and she said she might as well turn her inhibitions to advantage. She was glad to get home. It left her very depressed.

Day by day she was edgy. She fought with her mother. Her father was still looking for a new pulpit, and seemed melancholic, and her mother was irritable. Her job was like an endless shuttling. Up the stairs to the linotypers and down again, back and forth from one end of the city room to the other, all to no purpose, among people leading their own lives, to whom she could have nothing important to say. Following Leslie from place to place in the Army, that was the exciting thing that would have had continual newness. The train to Sparkstown made her dizzy with its swaying, and its soot was gritty on her hands. The little bus from the depot stank, and its bouncing made her nauseous. She hated each morning to open her eyes. She had a bitter argument with Patty that got all out of control, because Patty had borrowed her slippers and crushed the backs of them. Twice she walked away from the table in the midst of supper, claiming she could not stand Roland's manners. Once she gave Roland a tongue-lashing for a remark he had made to Patty, and called him a lewd, filthy-minded little ragamuffin, but it turned out she had completely misunderstood what Roland had said, so that she felt like a fool. The family must think she was the filthy-minded one, she thought.

It seemed to her to be a fact that nobody could be under the same roof with her long without finding that she was awful to live with. Apparently even Leslie, despite his pathetic struggles to feel in love, had realized he couldn't stand her.

One day her mother said someone had told her the Harvard Summer School was coed and a good place to meet boys. Millicent answered that it was a dreadful idea.

On the train she thought of it again. But she could not go to the Harvard Summer School without asking Mr. Killian to switch her back to nights, and she was afraid to do that. Maybe in the fall she would take law classes at night somewhere, out of desperation.

She would have to do something. She was a disappointment to her parents. Not only had she made a terrible mess of her love life but she had found no job commensurate with her university education.

It seemed clear by now that she was not going to hear from Les. Yet it was hard to believe that he had wanted to cut her off so completely. Maybe he had not, but maybe her behavior at the wedding had convinced him that he should. She ought to have suggested a postponement, since that was what he really wanted.

She wondered too if perhaps he had had a nervous breakdown.

She visited Aunt Gwendolyn. She told Aunt Gwen she was afraid there was something neurotic in her that would always stop her from marrying. But Aunt Gwen answered that if she had lived with the guy and actually washed his socks she was clearly marriage-minded.

"Why is it so hard to get married?" Millicent asked.

"Look, you're still a kid," said Aunt Gwen. "You'll get married and you'll forget how hard it was."

Millicent wondered if each man she would meet would be progressively worse, until she would end up past thirty marrying someone awful in desperation. It would be better to stay single than do that. Except that she would want children someday. Watching the way little Sharlene sat on the floor putting her pajamas on right now she knew that.

Even if Mr. Killian should promote her after a while, she wondered if she would only end up like Maud Dickinson. Or worse still, like the fortyish spinster in the circulation office, who worked with petty details and had come to think the world depended on them.

"How can a man who's so right for me in some ways be so wrong in others?" Millicent said to Aunt Gwen. "Why does someone who's just perfect in so many ways have to be no good in some way that spoils it? It's such a waste. If that's how life is it's cruel."

"Well, even so," Gwen said, "I think if you know what you want, chances are you'll fight your way to something like it, eventually."

Millicent confided her thought of sending Leslie a going-away present. Yet she feared that if she did his answer would spell out finis all the more sharply.

She could write to him at the Massachusetts General Hospital for forwarding, or at his mother's for forwarding, but it seemed a queer thing to do, if he hadn't even bothered to send an address. Not even a postcard. It looked as though he didn't want to be in touch.

She hoped that Aunt Gwen would deny that and urge her to write. But Aunt Gwen didn't. Later on, though, Aunt Gwen suggested that Leslie may have started a letter to Millicent fifty times and thrown it away.

Finally, toward the end of the evening, Millicent broke down and wept, and said that if Les were a man and weren't so wishy-washy he'd have dragged her downstairs and made her go through with it. Aunt Gwen sat patting her.

She visited Leslie's cousin Ruthie Meyers in the Back Bay. Ruthie mentioned in passing that she didn't know where Les was stationed, and had not heard from the New Britain branch of the family, although Millicent had been careful not to ask. Ruthie's belly was very big now, and they talked about that. Ruthie was gracious, and Millicent avoided any mention of Les. She knew she was depressing company. She said she had thought of learning to drive a car. If her brother were alive he would teach her.

Ruthie's husband Justin gave her a lift to North Station, and she rode beside him through the night streets finding nothing to say to him.

She thought of locating Les through the Army somehow by long-distance telephone. She thought of following wherever the Army had sent him, and taking a room there and living with him agreeably, never making herself a nuisance and never mentioning marriage.

She also had a fantasy in which she trained as an Army nurse, to honor Charles's memory, and she and Leslie chanced upon one another in a field hospital in Korea. Only it would have to be Air Force nurse. Did the Air Force and Army have the same hospitals?

When she had a week's vacation she went alone to Nantucket Island. She had never been there. Ruthie had given her the suggestion. The first morning it drizzled, but by afternoon the sun came out, and on the beach that Ruthie had told her to look for near the breakwater many young people lounged about. Boys were eyeing girls, and were welcomed when they intruded on their beach blankets. A boy named Sheldon intruded on her blanket. He was swarthy, dark-jowled, and rather too soft, but she tried to make polite conversation, according to the custom of the place. She was ill at ease and knew she sounded stiff. For a couple of hours he made small talk, or sometimes lay beside her to sunbathe in silence. And sometimes he went into the sea with her. At his request she put a lotion on his back, rather gingerly. But eventually he moved to another blanket.

The next day it rained, and she walked, looking at cobbled streets and stately mansions. Some people she had seen on the beach asked her to a party in a cottage. The party was quite like the beach. People did not know one another. Some were loud and some were silent. The conviviality was depressing. She did not want them, nor did they want her. It seemed to her that her walks alone were the most bearable part of the trip. She went home to Wilmerding Crosswalk, though she was still on vacation.

When she got home a boy named Howard Oster had phoned. He was related to somebody in the congregation. Lucinda had told him that Millicent was on the way home and he phoned again that same evening.

She accepted an invitation from him to a summer theater, to break the monotony. The play was dull and the actors amateurish, but Howard was not as bad as she had expected. He did not have much sparkle or gaiety, but it was as though he did not consider such things necessary, and did not require sparkle of her either, so that even his silences were comfortable. He was shorter than Les, but squarer and beefier, both in body and face. From the lines at his eyes she judged him to be older than most boys she had been out with before, perhaps twenty-eight or twenty-nine or even thirty.

On the way home, in his large old car, he talked more. She knew he worked for a firm of Boston architects, but he was quite interested in city planning, and could discuss in an interesting way a variety of subjects somehow connected with it, including politics, and child psychology, and art. The connection of all these things was quite new to her, and when she had said good night to him her mind still dwelt on the ideas he had explained.

On Sunday he took her sailing off Marblehead. The handling of a sailboat was a mystery to her, and the knowledgeableness with which he sat on its edge, holding the tiller and a taut rope that went to the boom, impressed her. He made it speed on a tilt, in a straight line, banging and beating on the cold sunshiny spray. Its two great overlapping triangles of sail were curved and full, and fluttered a little along their hypotenuses. She watched the beauty of the moving deep water about them. They traveled far, until the towns of the shore were only a soft jagged line, across the expanse, between two shades of blue, and their great round world consisted of sun and wind and the caressing ocean. She wondered how he would find his way back. Way out here they were perhaps not even in the United States, she thought. It occurred to her that she and Howard were more alone now than she had ever been with anyone. Yet it was a convenient kind of aloneness for a friendship that she didn't want to turn into a romance. His hands were occupied, and even when he smiled upon her face, or her knees, or her calves, she knew his mind was half occupied with the direction of the wind.

But when he phoned again, during the week, she turned him down, lest she encourage him too much.

Even so, he called fairly regularly. He took her to a barbecue that his married sister and his brother-in-law gave on the patio, and his other brother-in-law and other married sister were also there. He took her to the beach, and lay on the sand talking, but when a stray ball flew over them he reached up and caught it without interrupting his thought. He let her try his snorkel.

Then for a stretch he didn't call. She thought perhaps he had begun to find her tiresome. But he resumed, and she was glad. He was not Les, but he was adequate company. He was certainly intelligent. She told him she would like to go sailing again sometime, and he said they would.

She confided to him once that she had been depressed, and that she didn't know what to do about her job. He seemed mature, and knew how to listen. He even seemed to sense that she wanted no necking, and did not push it.

She told him of how she had been engaged and had changed her mind at the last moment, and she told him that she wanted to push her career more and romance less for a while.

Yet on their next evening she did let him kiss her, in a dark car, and the kiss grew warmer. She stopped it. She sat in silence. Then she said they were not children and should not begin. He agreed. Then she said gloomily that she wanted to marry young, if only to make sex more manageable. Her own words sounded awkward and unhappy in her ears.

"I hope there'll be other reasons besides that," said Howard.

"Oh, there will, I guess."

"How many children would you like to have?"

"It's not a thing to discuss lightly," she said.

They remained sitting again in silence. He started the car.

"Do you believe in marrying young?" she asked.

"I'm too old to marry young."

"How old are you?"

"Twenty-nine."

Her mother said to her that she had been calmer lately.

Then late one evening when her father was out she had a strange conversation with her mother, unlike any she had ever had before. They were sitting alone at the kitchen table, and her mother had been talking of the house, and then reminiscing, and Millicent somehow asked her how she had decided to marry her father.

"Well, your father seemed to want me very much," Lucinda said, in a slow, remembering tone. "And Grandma Annie was very domineering. I wanted to get away. And he was such an unhappy young man. He seems a lot happier in recent years. But when we were first married I used to think he didn't like me."

"Why'd you marry him then?"

Lucinda made an almost imperceptible shrug. "He used to say if I'd marry him he could do anything. He was going to be a great professor. And then a couple of years later he was saying if he'd stayed single he could have done anything. It was very strange." Her eyes were not quite looking at anything, as though her mind was far away. "We were very young then."

"You know what you should have married?" said Millicent. "What you needed was a nice, stable, businessman type. You're not suited to a queer profession like the clergy."

"Well, I don't know. I haven't minded making sacrifices. When your father's work demanded it."

"You sure look as if you mind it sometimes," Millicent said.

"Well, knowing you're needed can make up for a lot of things."

"You and Dad are really sort of mismatched. That's what I think."

"Do you really?" Her mother looked at her directly now. She sounded surprised.

"Yes I do. You don't have any understanding of each other." Her voice quavered.

"Could mismatched people have such wonderful children? Four such beautiful children, perfect children, could the parents be mismatched?"

"It's got nothing to do with it." Her voice was still quavering.

"Well, it probably seemed better to us than it did to you." Her mother had the faraway look again.

"I suppose you've made an adjustment more or less, but you and Dad are really a pair of strangers trapped with each other. You have nothing in common. None of your interests are the same. His main interest, that he's all wrapped up in, you and he can't even talk about. I know he doesn't share his thoughts with you."

"Well, religion never made that much sense to me, and I suppose it's better to avoid arguments when we can."

"He's willing enough to argue with everybody else in town."

"Well, and even without being able to talk to each other so much, I suppose we've still kept each other from feeling lonesome for twenty-odd years." Her mother looked at her again.

"Marriage should do more than that," said Millicent.

"Well, and once he was definitely in the clergy, I tried to encourage him to look the part and get ahead in it. I always worked for the sisterhoods, and tried to be diplomatic."

"Marriage should do more than that too," Millicent said.

The conversation seemed to end there. She watched her mother sitting thoughtfully. Some of the long hairs about her mother's face were askew. There were lines about her eyes. The carved clock began chiming down the hall. She was glad her mother had not turned the conversation to Leslie. And not to Howard either.

Her mother never asked about Howard.

After a few days Grandma Annie visited, and asked her if she had any new boy friends yet.

"Not particularly," said Millicent.

Her mother said nothing.

But Millicent went out with Howard again that evening. They drove to Boston, and went to a party given by friends of his who lived in an old narrow rowhouse built onto a wharf, over the water. There were unplastered walls and a huge fireplace. It was a crowd she had never met before. Most of the men there were artists, and some of their wives were also. Howard seemed the least bohemian of any of them. But he surprised her by knowing a great deal about trends in abstract art. He explained paintings to her, in ways that made them almost comprehensible to her. There were some she liked.

He took her home very late. On the winding rural roads there were many hills, and the headlights sometimes illuminated the road and sometimes the high foliage.

On the porch he embraced her. At first she returned the embrace, and they stood tightly together in the darkness. His moving hands seemed to want her flesh.

"Stop it, please," she said.

When she went in it was past four on the carved clock. She went upstairs very quietly. She lay awake a while. She was feeling confused.

Very much lately she had sensed Howard's seriousness. Both of his sisters were married, and all his friends were married. And he showed a sensitivity to her feelings that was extraordinary. He never took offense if she refused an invitation, or if she rode silently, or if she sat too far from him for his arm to come around.

She slept for less than two hours, and then rose to go to work. The brown bus jogged along with her, and she watched the trees go past. She felt the effects of sleeplessness through and through, in her head and in her throat. Her eyes smarted. She oughtn't to encourage Howard, she thought. He was going to propose. And marrying him seemed too great a price to have to pay for his friendship. On the other hand, the abyss of friendlessness seemed too great a price to have to pay for giving him up.

It occurred to her that she had reached that unhappy age when all friendships have a mating basis. Even other girls, if they're your friend, make you secondary to that—if they're married you're supernumerary, and if they're single you're only an ally in the mate hunt or a companion in loneliness between men.

74

Ed's search for a new job did not go well. With summer it had begun to seem as though he might be too late to find anything for the next year at all, and he began to have a feeling of urgency and desperation. Selling the house was also a worry. They had listed it with Colby & Dill and with Weiler and with two other agencies, but few prospects were brought.

He filled in as chaplain at the reformatory and at the mental hospital, because the regular man was away, and gave it more than the prescribed amount of time. There was a reformatory kid that he felt he could help steer toward a feeling of conscience. He made frequent visits also to a mental patient who had a record of suicide attempts. However his main object of interest continued to be not these marginal people but the healthy ones as a community, and Congregation Beth El was even more dormant this summer than the summer before. Getting a few people together so that some minimal framework of observance could be maintained was the worst of his ordeals. Arranging a fifteen-minute weekday service took half a day of searching and cajoling, and then there were broken promises and inattention. On weekends he gave sermons but few came to hear. There were many who thought services in the summer should be suspended entirely, but he fought this idea.

In August he entered into correspondence with a congregation in Philadelphia that sounded promising. It was in a poor urban neighborhood, but it sounded traditional and fairly devout, and they promised to pay Ed as much as he had been getting at Wilmerding Crosswalk, though they had been used to paying even less. But they warned they could not afford any raises beyond that, and no pension.

So one weekend he and Lucinda left Patty and Roland and Millicent alone, and asked the Daveys and the Hubbards to keep an eye on the house, and went by train to visit Philadelphia.

Lucinda was apprehensive and depressed at having to explore so far from home, and said little on the way down.

They stayed with a family. Ed preached to the congregation and met a lot of the members. The home where they stayed was run down, and so was the synagogue. The whole neighborhood was of brick—rows of doors and stoops in endless walls that ran down each side of every street. It was dirty. There was no grass. It was a much poorer district than either of them had expected. But the children received instruction five afternoons a week after school, from paid teachers, and a score of men attended daily services morning and evening. A dozen individuals had the skill to lead a service. Even some of the teen-age boys could. He was impressed. In company like that, he thought, a clergyman could be a man among men—a scholar assisting laymen who were their own clergy.

He had rarely seen Lucinda look so miserable.

He asked them at last for a week to think it over. He felt relieved to have found this place, despite its shabbiness, despite the urban dirt. He knew Lucinda saw only the shabbiness and the dirt. He told her he liked the people. They had warmth, and he could talk to them.

He knew that she knew of no alternative. This late in the season there was little to be had. She was withdrawn, almost sullen.

"You're going down, down, down," she said to him.

On the train she said that there must be something wrong with a style of religion that you had to move to the city for.

"Well, it's actually a rural and agricultural religion," he said. "It's only the accidents of history that have driven it to the cities."

But she muttered that she didn't care anything about history. She said religion was bad enough, and if religion and history were going to gang up on her to make her live in Philadelphia she couldn't stand it.

A man in a soiled coat came through the cars selling magazines. He bought her some.

The ride was long. The train took them past industrial plants, past dumps.

With that crowd they had met during the weekend he could do something, he thought. If the congregation inspires the rabbi, it becomes possible for the rabbi to inspire the congregation. And it was time to start inspiring somebody, before he was too old to. Serving people who didn't want to be served was a job he didn't have skill enough for.

I take my whisky straight, he thought, and I like my religion the same way.

Still, it was too bad that to have a traditional congregation, one that functions, that says the psalm of the day, that watches the new moon and the seasons—to find that, you've got to endure the stink of the city, the exhaust of buses, the unwholesome wind of the subway. And why? Brighton had been too urban, and this Philadelphia neighborhood was a hundred times worse than Brighton.

But pretty rural places had lousy congregations.

How good it would be if you could have both—to have woods and countryside to walk in with your young son, and to have also in walking distance a little group to pray with. That would be the ideal life. He built a little fantasy of such a place. In the fantasy he put Charles alive.

Why couldn't ten traditionalists from Boston or Brookline and their families be transplanted out to Abbottsford, and say their prayers where the air is fresh, to the tune of cows lowing? To find neighbors who prayed, did you have to go live in apartment buildings? To recite twice a day, *and I will give grass in thy fields for thy cattle,* did you have to live where there was no grass?

Yes, because it takes a hundred men before you find one that gives a damn. And a thousand before you find ten. That was why it was no good in a small town. You were a minority of a minority, and that was why you were forced to go where the population was densest.

Besides, he considered, a scholar needs to keep whetting his understanding against that of fellow scholars—that's how the whole field grows. And for scholars to come together you needed the city, no matter how much your soul craves the green grass.

He glanced at Lucinda, who sat between him and the train window, reading a magazine. He felt sorry for her—she had become as attached to country living as he had, and for her there was no compensation. She had put so much effort into those vegetable gardens. In Philadelphia there would be no gardening. She had even begun bird-watching. He felt the loss of these things with her.

Millicent would not go to Philadelphia, he thought.

Colby & Dill would have to look after the house for them, until a buyer was found. He had been stupid to buy it.

Roland and Patty—they'd have to adjust to new schools all over again. But they would. They had before. They'd made new friends quickly.

He thought of Millicent again, and of this Howard she had been seeing so much of. He wondered if they had talked yet of marriage.

He wondered if she had slept with Howard. Or if she would. It worried him.

He had an uneasy feeling that, the way things were done these days, once a girl has given her body along with her heart, she must continue to. Because how can she say no to the man she now hopes to make the great love of her life, when she has said yes to a former boy friend she must now regard as less important? To say no to an importuning fiancé she expects to marry, after saying yes to a guy she did not marry, makes her hard and unfeminine. It makes her doubt which guy she loved the more. And it makes him unmasculine.

A man may sleep with women and then not sleep with a virginal fiancée, without raising this doubt about which one he loves the more. It is taken that he may have screwed the others without loving, but he desires this one so much he is trying to get her the only way she can be got.

Because a virgin's no is understood. It's her lover's excuse for not having made her. A virgin may have her heart broken a dozen times, but if she has said no she is privileged to continue saying no, until a man has put his name on the dotted line and said, in return for giving yourself to me, I shall give myself to you. But once she has said yes. then every broken engagement, every blighted romance, every broken heart must be a boy slept with. She cannot return to merely looking soulfully into the eyes of a man whose proposal she seeks. Having let her pants follow her heart, she must always, for how can she marry a lesser love? Until with luck it ends in marriage, she cannot refuse a suitor she doesn't want to go away. She cannot say, I love you, but don't touch me, though I surrendered to one I loved less than you. His heart would not believe it, nor hers. Having said yes, her no is now too big a no. There is nothing for it then but to embrace the sweat of each man she loves, to withhold nothing from a man she wants for a husband.

Only the virgin can say I love you while withholding.

Ed squirmed and adjusted the backrest, but could not make the seat comfortable. The car was warm. Having slept with the man she was engaged to, she must sleep with every man she gets engaged to. He may try out her warmth and her moisture without obligation. The more she wants to marry him, the more it becomes his privilege to take her to bed while he makes up his mind. And so it goes. You can only hope the guy who marries her arrives quickly and puts an end to it. That's why parents are anxious to see a daughter married once she gets to this point, he thought. Les was her best chance. She should have married him. She would have avoided this. This Howard he didn't know well.

Lucinda held the magazines on her lap but she was not reading them now. The train was in a tunnel. She stared at the blackness and he saw her face reflected dimly.

In the days of Deuteronomy, he thought, a woman belonged to her husband in marriage, because he could threaten to divorce her. Today she belongs to him in the courtship instead, because he can threaten not to make their screwing legal.

Ed leaned his forehead and eyes upon his hand, resting his elbow on the arm of the seat, that separated him from the aisle. He knew he could say none of this to Lucinda, or they would have an awful argument.

I wish life wasn't such struggle, he thought.

I feel like she feels.

It's all a battle. Maybe he should have known how to hang on in Wilmerding Crosswalk, and had been right to move there in the first place—maybe he should go and work where the people didn't care. Maybe that's what he was for. But he didn't feel like it. When you've lost a son, he said to himself, all you want to do is climb in next to God.

He sat up again and looked at Lucinda, but she was staring at the window, looking miserable and defeated. He put a hand on hers, but she didn't look at him.

"You know," he said, "when you have that daily minyan, it's like a village, even in the big city. They all live in walking distance of the shul, and people you pray with every day you develop a bond with. You'll see. I know this. It's real. And in a couple of years you have all these close friends in walking distance. That's how it is in that kind of a congregation. It's like a village. It's a way of life."

"I don't care about having friends in walking distance," she said. "If that's what you want you should have been a mailman."

He looked at her. She was not in a witticism kind of mood. In the reflection he saw tears in her eyes.

What does she know, he thought.

Why do I want a minyan? I want a minyan because I don't want to be alone any more. All my life I've been looking for a minyan. That's the truth. I've been in the Navy, I've been here, I've been there, and all my life I've been looking for nine other guys to pray with. So I don't face God alone. I want people around me who understand this religion, and who have the sensitivity that goes with understanding it.

How can you say that to a woman who has no comprehension of it?

It crossed his mind that perhaps in the long run two people loving one another must become an empty and redundant thing, like seeking happiness, unless the two people were both primarily in love with something else, some third thing. Such as a God, an ideal, a way of life, a cause. Some most-beloved third factor, that makes you a person, and makes you recognize another lover of it as your comrade. What did he and Lucinda love in common? What did they have in common, that each would die for? The children, that was all. Three living, one dead.

He looked at her again, staring at the reflections and blackness of the tunnel. He could see her anger at the whole idea of Philadelphia.

What man is favored by God? The man who is happily married, the Talmud says. It also says you get the wife you deserve.

After returning to Wilmerding Crosswalk he left almost at once for a camp in the Berkshires, where he had promised to conduct some round-table discussions. He asked Lucinda if she would be all right without the car, and she said that if she had to do any marketing she would use the bus or take the bicycle. So he left. He took Patty.

He got home again on Friday. Lucinda met him cheerfully and eagerly. She kissed Patty, and told Ed there was a chance of getting Temple Beth El to reverse itself and renew his contract after all. She had met Sandy Walker in the A. & P., and Sandy said nobody liked any of the men that had been interviewed, and it was so late in the season they didn't know if they'd have anyone at all in time for the holidays. So Lucinda had gone at once to Mrs. Bernstein, and then to Conrad, and begged him to reconsider Ed.

Ed had a sinking feeling. He didn't answer. By now he was looking forward to working with the Philadelphia congregation.

In the bedroom he began unpacking the suitcase he had had at the camp. Lucinda kept talking to him.

"Sandy said nobody liked their names," Lucinda went on. "There was a Bumsky or something."

"It wasn't Bumsky," said Ed, while he unpacked.

"Or Dumpsky, or something like that. Anyway she said you have to admit a name like Ed Gordon sounds a heck of a lot better in this type of a town."

"Sandy said that?"

"Yes. And she said they didn't even like their looks or anything. At least your picture always looks nice in the paper."

"What did Conrad say?"

"He said he'd talk to you, if you'd go and see him."

"Talk to me? And then what? The members voted."

"Well, that's just it. He said he could recommend to the executive board that they call a new meeting and make a new recommendation, if there was grounds for it."

"Grounds for it?"

"Well, like you said, they voted not to renew. He can't ask them to reverse themselves unless he can tell them things have changed."

"I get it. And what did you say to Conrad?"

"Well, I promised you'd do better. He said you'd have to promise to get along with people and not offend people. And stop trying to get people to be religious all the time."

Ed said nothing more then. He was irritated with her. She seemed so happy with this possibility. And yet he felt he would have to say no.

After supper he walked to the temple and conducted a Sabbath-eve service. Conrad was not there. Amethyst Gilbert was, and she knew Lucinda had spoken to Conrad. She was delighted with the idea that Ed might stay. But he said little.

"Conrad said he didn't have the heart to say no to a Gold Star mother," she told him. "And the members are a little wiser now. They didn't go for any of the real New Yorky types. And I think they realize now that everybody has to make compromises. There's lots of congregations that have rabbis they aren't exactly satisfied with."

Lucinda began to discuss it again late at night, when they lay in darkness.

"There's lots of things you can preach about that wouldn't offend people," she said. "What do others preach about? Korea. Communism. There's lots of things that have nothing to do with being religious. Discrimination in the South. Anything. Loving one another, and all that kind of stuff. And Bible stories. You've got the whole Bible. You don't have to always be controversial. There's so many uplifting things that won't rub people the wrong way. Things like that nice Midrash story about angels being jealous of humans."

"Look," he said irritably, "religion involves commitment, or it turns into slop. You live it as a regimen—you need a culture to keep reminding you of commitment. What am I? A third-rate hack?"

"I'll always believe you're a first-rate one. I promise. Ed, you've got all that history to preach about. And human freedom."

He swallowed angrily. "History's only relevant where there's a future. Look, they don't want—the people here don't want—these people don't want a rabbi. They want a stuffed shirt. That's what they want."

"So be a stuffed shirt if you have to. It won't kill you. You have a grown daughter—you can afford to be middle-aged for a change. And if they're willing to give you another chance, for God's sake, go along with it. Try. Ed, it's the one thing I ever asked of you. Haven't I always done everything you want? I just can't bear pulling up stakes again. And starting from scratch all over again now, if we don't have to. I begged him, Ed—I promised. So you don't get your dream congregation—they're not getting their dream rabbi either. You go half way and maybe they'll come half way—maybe they'll talk about tenure next year. You can preach again when you're an old man and nobody cares. Meanwhile the children are happy here. I'm not gonna make them go live in that slum. Doesn't that mean anything?"

"It's not a slum."

"It is too a slum! And Millicent has her job here. She won't quit her job."

"Look, we can't build our lives around Millicent. She could meet some guy next year and get married and settle down in California for all we know."

"Maybe she will," said Lucinda. "And maybe she won't."

"And my career has to follow Millicent, because she has a two-bit job in Boston?"

"You're too old to have a career. And Millicent has to have a home that she can bring young men to—that's the main thing."

"She's not gonna stay in the house anyway. She's talking about an apartment again."

"If she gets an apartment it's all the worse. At least we can maintain a home nearby for when she wants her family. And if we go to Philadelphia what's she gonna do up here alone? Do you want your daughter to slide into another affair behind your back?"

"We have to have a little faith in her, that's all."

"I love her. That's better than having faith in her," Lucinda said, and her voice broke. "There's just one thing I remember you said that's in the Talmud," she continued tearfully. "It says you have to provide for your wife and children first, before you go crusading over the hill. That's in the Talmud. You said that's in the Talmud. Isn't that true?"

He lay in the sheets with his back to her. The best thing was to say nothing and let the matter drop, at least for the present. Or they'd get no sleep. He heard her sniffle. But in a moment, when she spoke again, her voice was clear.

"Ed, you could have a good life here. Beth El will grow, over the years, and it'll be a great temple. They'll put up the upper story, and they'll have stained-glass windows, and marble facing—"

"I don't want to build a building. I want to build a congregation. And I can't do anything here. I don't want to grow old here. There have to be people who say 'we'll do it,' like the people at Sinai. Or there's nothing to work with."

"You can always work with the children. They're the important ones anyway."

"For that you need the co-operation of the parents."

"And what are you gonna do when you get fed up with the Philadelphia people and don't get along? What do we do then? Pull up stakes again?"

"With them I'll get along."

"Oh, sure. Where have I heard that before."

"You haven't heard it before. That crowd there is my type. It was like instant recognition. When I met them I was glad I got fired here. I can put down roots with a congregation like that. It was like the end of a search."

"You don't find roots by searching. You find roots by staying in one place. And you're not really fired if Conrad's willing to reconsider."

"It doesn't just depend on Conrad."

"All this moving around's not good for the children, anyway. You can't wander the country looking for a congregation that understands you."

"Look," he said. "Lucinda—you don't understand. If my impact in this community is as low as it is, I don't belong here. Once a guy has had the brass and the gall to go into a pulpit, he at least owes it to people to make a vocation of it, and follow it where it takes him. If it isn't a calling he's got no business there. He shouldn't be in the pulpit."

"Well, this house is my calling. And I think you ought to put your family first and your God damn integrity second for a change."

He didn't answer that. For a while they were silent, and he thought the conversation was ended. But she began again.

"Don't you start extracting conditions from Conrad either," she said. "I want you to get the job."

"I haven't even said I'll talk to him."

"Ed, you talk to him. Tomorrow."

He didn't answer.

"I mean it, Ed. Tomorrow."

"I'm not gonna phone him on the Sabbath."

"He said he'll be home Saturday night if you'd go over there. Ed, I begged him. You're not gonna just not pay any attention to it."

He said nothing.

"If you tell him all kinds of conditions it'll make it harder for him to sell it to the others," she said. "So don't you dare. I spoke to Phil Walker too, and he said you'd have to promise to toe the mark and shut up and not bother people. And he said you'd have to quit the firemen too. It's not dignified. You're not Fiorello La Guardia."

"You didn't tell me you talked to Phil Walker."

"Phil's important," she said. "I promised you wouldn't ask any conditions. They said the best offer would be the same conditions for another year and you'd be on probation all that time."

"What did you say?"

"I agreed. What could I say."

"You could have left the negotiations to me. I don't appreciate your selling me down the river while I'm off in the Berkshires."

"I get your job back for you, and that's the thanks I get." There was a catch in her voice.

This time she said nothing more.

Actually there were no conditions to ask for anyway, he said to himself. He couldn't ask them for tenure, under the circumstances. And to ask a congregation to promise better attendance—such promises were worthless.

He wished he could tell Lucinda that there was a long view without which human life must at last be a humiliation, and that the long view had to be lived, as a daily system—not just moped about in an occasional philosophic moment. There were people who create society—these were the ones who cared about how it goes—and there were people who just went along with it.

In the morning, after breakfast, he walked to the temple. Bill Prince was on vacation, and he was not able to get more than seven or eight men together, even though he waited a long time and went out to round up a few.

It was not possible under the circumstances to conduct a service as a congregation, but individual prayer was still possible, and he tried to get those who were there to accompany him. But half left at once, and the rest skipped most of it or engaged in conversation. He did not take long, but when he finished he was alone, except for Mr. Brill who sat sleeping.

He walked home. The trees in Murphy Square were full, with a deep green. Past the stone bridge the big old houses had such huge trees before them that more than half of what he saw was foliage. The neighborhood seemed almost a wood.

What bothered him was that he felt he ought to remain here, if it were possible. Though he had said he could do nothing here, he felt that maybe he was needed more here on the fringes. The other congregation could run on its own steam and could always attract a scholar; this one could not. There were children in the town for whom he still wished to set an example.

But he didn't want it to be possible. He resented that Lucinda had made it possible to remain. The comfort of congenialness beckoned him to that neighborhood in Philadelphia. He wanted it to be impossible not to go there.

Remaining here, he thought, meant you could never find your own kind. It meant an end of hopes, at least of those lovely hopes, for peace for oneself within your lifetime. You had to stay among clunks and goons who didn't know what you were talking about. That was a condition of life.

You can't emigrate. There are no more Americas. This is it.

During most of the afternoon he kept to his study, but he accomplished little. Somewhere in the room or the wall a cricket was chirping. Perhaps on the shelves. He could not find it. His thoughts went in all directions. He tried to avoid Lucinda, and when he couldn't he tried not to answer her arguments. Once she said that if he were a more imposing figure people wouldn't care as much what he said or did, and that if he were imposing enough they'd put up with what they disagreed with. Then she said that if God wanted people to have religion they'd have religion. She also said the dog was in no condition to survive the trip.

In late afternoon she napped, and let him alone. He had known all along that Congregation Beth El was not having much luck in finding a replacement for him. Amethyst and a few others had kept him informed of what happened at the special membership meetings. There had been meetings to interview one or two men that they had liked, but the ones they wanted took jobs elsewhere at higher pay. Then lately they had interviewed a man named Barmak, and a Sedrumsky, and a Slobodkin, and a Luxemburg. He heard that one had acne, and another, who wore a pince-nez, was in the midst of getting a divorce and would have to pay alimony and wouldn't consider less than fifteen grand a year. They had also called a membership meeting to interview a man named Botwinnik but he never showed up.

He knew that they had put themselves at a disadvantage by firing him so late in the season, and he had expected that they would end up at best with some kid just out of the seminary.

He had a cold supper, saying little. Then he went outdoors. The fiery color of the sun blackened the foliage that crossed it. The field was a mixture of high grass and flowers. The goldfinches seemed in the habit of circling and swooping low over it at this hour. The light was strange, and affected every color.

He walked, and sat on the wall. The sky kept changing. When it was dark enough for three stars to appear he went to the house, and asked Patty and Roland to assist him in a libation marking the end of the Sabbath. He got the wine bottle and the rest of the gear, and went outdoors again, carrying them. There was no moon. The ground was dark now, but he could see a small toad leap away from his foot. He said the blessings. He passed the filigreed spice box and Roland sniffed it noisily. Patty was in curlers. She shielded the flames of the multiwicked braided candle with her hand.

When it was done he asked the children to take the wine and the other things to the house and put them away. He went in by a different door, and went upstairs and shaved, and changed his clothes. Then he went out again quietly. He walked into the darkened barn and felt his way to the car. He had thought of asking Patty and Roland if they felt very strongly about remaining here, and if they would mind very much moving to Philadelphia. But he hadn't asked them. What could they say?

He ran the motor and put on the headlights. He rode very slowly, over bare places and under a low branch of the big elm. But Lucinda came running out across the porch so he stopped, letting the motor idle. She came to him. His window was down. A strand of hair hung astray down her face and she panted a little.

"Are you going to Conrad's?" she asked. The light from the house and stray reflection from the headlights to the grass and back shone on the edges of her face.

"I don't promise any results."

He could see her smile. "Thanks," she said.

He knew she assumed he had already given in. She reached in through the window to give his hand a squeeze. He thought her eyes were moist.

"Don't worry," she said. "It won't be so bad."

He sat at the wheel, unsmiling.

"Don't feel like a failure," she said. "Do it with style, for the children's sake. You remember how your grandfather looked good to you?"

He made no answer. When he could he let the car roll, onto the pebbles of the winding dirt drive.

He thought of the stone façade of Conrad's ranch house and its velvety lawn, over on the other side of town. He was not fond of it. Conrad would be sitting on the sofa in his shirt sleeves, with that tattersall vest probably, and his weather-beaten face. He wondered how an accountant could get so weather-beaten. Conrad must have the kind of skin that didn't take to the outdoors at all, so that even golfing did it.

This interview would be as embarrassing for Conrad as for himself, he considered, and Conrad would perhaps need a touch of arrogance in some way. Conrad would talk to him as to an employee. And those two kids, the eleven-year-old and the nine-year-old, would look at him blankly, not with impoliteness but not with respect.

He hoped at least that Phil Walker wouldn't be there.

Toe the mark, shut up, and don't bother people. He wouldn't promise. A committed man doesn't get uncommitted. What could you do, except try with God's help to win people's confidence, and hope that some of what rightness, what goodness, what truth there was would get itself communicated.

A religious Jew was married to all the unreligious ones anyway. Let's face it.

And for himself, he thought, he would have to strengthen his ties to the city, and get in to Boston more, in an extracurricular way, and draw nourishment from sporadic association with people more to his taste.

And out here, trust meanwhile that he did influence people more than was apparent. Little by little in that past year here he had gotten to know the few people who were more or less like-minded.

The headlights raised and lowered their aim bumpily on the unevenness of Massapeequit Road. It was dark; the absence of a moon made a difference.

It crossed his mind that they had never jumped on him for embarrassing Nicole that time. He had thought surely he would hear about that. But nothing had happened. No one had ever said anything.

75

Sometimes Millicent did not see Howard for several days on end, and when he phoned she still sometimes refused his invitations, offering little or no excuse. But he was uncomplaining, and easy to get along with. At other times she welcomed a chance to go partying or sailing with him, and once or twice, when she felt in need of company, she phoned him from the city room and suggested a movie after work.

Her family knew him and his big old car but they had no opportunity for conversation with him because Millicent was always ready on the porch and hurried into the car the moment it stopped.

At last she was with him a few evenings in a row. But when he asked about the evening following she was suddenly short with him, almost to the point of discourtesy. He tightened his lips, but said nothing. She did not know what had gotten into her—it happened almost without intention.

He did not call for a while after that. For a few days she was glad not to have him so constantly about. But when a week had gone it occurred to her that he perhaps had no intention of calling her further. It was a little surprising. She had wanted to discourage him from becoming too attached, but it seemed now that he had in fact been less attached than she had supposed.

Finally he did phone. She made an effort to sound especially gracious, to make up for the discourtesy of the other time. He had Wednesday afternoon off, and took her to his sister's summer cottage in Gloucester.

In Gloucester his sister was affectionate toward her, as though Millicent were already one of the family. Millicent found herself being very domestic, helping in the kitchen, and telling Howard's little nephews about the short-eared racing rabbit.

It was very late when they left, but they went for a snack to a roadhouse perched on a rock high over the ocean. They talked sporadically and comfortably, without effort. Their table was by a window. Moon glimmerings rocked on the water, merging to a widening path toward the horizon.

He drove her home slowly, on the twists and hills of rustic back roads, under black spreading branches. She rode hunched down.

"You're going to be proposed to again," he said.

"I know it."

"How do you know it?"

"I just sort of know it." She was not looking at him, but simply forward, where the headlights shone on the road and forest. "You mean by you?" she added.

"By me." She knew that he glanced a moment from his driving. "I'll go into detail when I find the words," he said. "I'm really smitten, Millicent."

There was no question of his sincerity.

"I need time to think," she said. "I don't know what to say."

"That's all right," he said. "Take all the time you want."

She was hunched down by herself. For a moment neither spoke, and she was aware of the noise of the motor.

"How does it make you feel?" he asked. "I mean, the way I feel."

"I don't know. Secure, kind of."

"That's good."

He put his hand on her knee. The conversation lapsed again. Then he made a little small talk. His hand caressed her knee and her thigh when he did not need both hands for driving. It was as though they pretended not to notice that conversation had grown somewhat less easy, and less spontaneous.

The house was quite dark when they got there. The porch light was out. He shut off the motor and the headlights and opened the car door for her, as he always did. They stood kissing by the screen door. There was moonlight, but on the porch they were in shadow. She could hear crickets. She pressed tight in his squeezing embrace. She gave him her lips, then her cheek. His mouth brushed her face. She gave him her lips again. He pulled her even nearer and tighter, pressing her backbone.

It was a long, moist, swallowing kiss, and when they stopped for breath they began it again. The hand on her sweater found her breast and paused there, supporting it lightly. The kiss went on. They breathed in each other's mouths.

Her skirts rose with his hands. She could feel the uneven gusts of breeze behind her thighs. She leaned to him in the kiss, legs at attention, enjoying the exposure. His hands played upon the thinness of her underpants, smoothing their fit. It was interesting and pleasant, and yet it also made her nervous. He caressed the curvature of the skinlike nylon, and explored its edges, its creases, its stretched fullness, as if wanting to know and appreciate the ins and outs of her buttocks.

She put away his hands and let the skirts fall into place. But he lifted her chin with a bent finger and kissed her once more.

It was time to tell him good night. Even in the darkness she could see the gentleness in his broad face. He was holding both her hands.

"Can I see you tomorrow? After work?"

"I don't know—I think I better catch up on my sleep. And Saturday's my brother's bar mitzvah, you know—I have to help my mother with things."

"Well, I'll call you," he said. "Let me know if I can help."

She watched his car go away, and went up to bed, as quietly as she could.

Most girls would grab such a one as Howard, she thought, and get it over with.

And she had been getting to like him better. Maybe she should hold him off for a certain length of time and in the meantime write to Les.

But that idea did not satisfy her either.

Les had showed by not writing that she had been right about his reluctance.

But would it be different if she had gone through with marriage, she wondered? Once that hurdle was over, would it have worked out?

She pondered it, trying to calculate and project intelligently, while she brushed her teeth and when she curled under the sheet, but the more she pondered the more confused it seemed. She couldn't figure it.

Howard was trying not to move rapidly. And yet she did have to make up her mind as to whether it should be seriously considered. She wished there were more time. She understood now how Les had felt, she thought.

She wondered if it was better to marry your true love and become disillusioned with your true love, or to marry someone else and keep the illusion.

Howard was intelligent and sweet. Perhaps he even had more to give her than she him, she thought.

He did not phone on Thursday. Friday he did, and suggested that since she was taking Saturday off for the bar mitzvah they might do something with the afternoon.

"Well, I'm not sure what plans the family has," she said. "But why don't you come around to the bar mitzvah anyway, and have some refreshments?"

In that way she was being polite, she thought. She mentioned afterward to her parents that Howard might stop in at the service. She didn't say he wanted to take her out for the afternoon somewhere afterward.

The family was not planning much of a fuss in connection with the bar mitzvah, just some refreshments at the temple afterward, and not a luncheon. She knew that some people in the town thought it was because of the expense that had been wasted on her own wedding-day fiasco, so that the family could not afford another blowout. And some thought it was because of mourning for Charles. But she knew the reason was neither of these. Charles's bar mitzvah had also been quiet like this. Her father felt that a bar mitzvah was simply the first occasion of a man's assisting in an ordinary Sabbath service. That was all. When he was old enough to he did, Ed said, and he should keep doing it often, all his life.

She spent Friday evening listening to her mother talk about what had been ordered, and whether there would be enough, and about presents. Some people had sent presents, and the relatives had, and the family had also given him things. Millicent had given Roland a cheap watch, and also the Communist bayonet, but she told him the bayonet was to be regarded as a gift from Charles, not from herself.

In the morning she walked to the temple with the family. The paths in Murphy Square were narrow, especially where they went around the Civil War cannons, and she took the occasion to get far ahead and be alone. She wore her blue summer suit, newly ironed. The weather was already hot. She heard her mother say she supposed everyone would be late.

But on Muckanaug Street she could see that there were already a number of parked cars, and she saw Grandma Annie and Krupchick getting out of the one with the bashed fender.

The service began as usual with Bill Prince leading. There were a fair number of people, and more kept arriving, relatives and people from the town. Bill read one psalm after another, his back to the congregation, and sometimes she followed a little in her book. She sat between her mother and Patty. Patty's hair was piled high, and she kept craning and looking around, and sometimes whispering across Millicent to her mother. Beyond Patty Roland sat, looking small in his prayer shawl. Millicent also looked about now and then, and saw before long that it was a fairly good turnout. She saw the Gilberts. They had given Roland a money gift that she thought was rather too large. She saw Bobby O'Shaughnessy, with a skullcap sitting pinched on the top of his head, and some other kids. Then, far back, between heads, she saw Howard. He caught her eye and nodded. She looked at her book again.

When the service approached the more important prayers Roland went up the step to the reading desk and replaced Bill as leader. His voice was musical and clear, and rose soprano. Her father sat near the reading desk, following in his book as at any other service. Millicent somehow glanced again through the congregation and far through the crowd, over by the windows, a young man's lean profile arrested her, as though she had seen someone familiar but not quite placed.

Then she realized it was Fred Winkler. She wondered what he could be doing here. He sat among the congregation, watching the proceedings and looking quite proper. A prayer shawl lay on his neck in a twist.

As though he had felt her stare across that distance and through all those people he suddenly looked at her, and smiled. For no apparent reason she blushed, unsmiling. She turned quickly forward.

She turned pages and looked for the place. Roland was reading exuberantly and his young voice filled the air. She was deeply embarrassed for having blushed. It was a ridiculous way to have reacted, and he must have been highly amused. She determined not to look at Fred Winkler for the rest of the service.

It went on slowly. The big parchment scrolls were laid upon the reading desk and unrolled, and the weekly portion was read, with many interruptions as her uncles and other men were called forward to say blessings stumblingly. There was a collection of several of them standing up there now about the scrolls. She saw the prayer shawls draped on their backs and the wrinkles in the seats of their pants. Roland's head was hardly higher than Bill Prince's shoulder. His skullcap was a circle on the back of it, above his fresh haircut.

She was tempted to steal a glance at Winkler, to see whether he was still looking at her or not. But she found the strength not to. She glanced down at her mother's white gloves, and then up, and saw that her mother's eyes were moist. Her father was very busy, up with the men at the reading desk, following with his eyes in a text and nodding at nearly every word.

She began to enjoy Roland's voice. It had a sweetness. It made her think of

Charles also. It seemed to her that all of them must have thoughts of Charles. She avoided looking at her mother, or at Patty. It was only six years ago that Charles had performed something like this. She had been sixteen. How quickly a present moment flies into the past, she thought. It seemed to her that Charles had not had Roland's ease and facility. Nor had she realized that Roland was endowed with so excellent a voice.

At last Roland was up there alone, and she recognized the characteristic chant that belonged to readings from the Prophets. She found the week's reading, and the translation on the left-hand page.

Sing, o childless, that you bore not. Break into glad song, that you did not have a child.

It was a portion from Isaiah. Roland's voice was bouncing, with a suspense of phrasing.

For thou shalt forget the shame of thy youth. The reproach of thy widowhood thou shalt not remember any more.

She scanned the context. It was not about girls. She read the verse again.

These books had a strange genius, she thought. They found ways to speak to you.

She looked up again at Roland. He worked along, in the distinctive cantillation that he had not used in other parts of the service. Sometimes his voice would hover, rocking on a certain syllable, and then lilt forward. She tried to find his place and follow him in the text itself, on the right-hand page. But she gave up this exercise and returned to the translation, searching out its phrases.

For a small moment only was I wroth with thee and hid My face, but with abundant mercies will I gather thee. For I am the Lord, thy Redeemer.

Roland's voice fell, rose again. Always it seemed to fondle the words. But she could not take her eyes from the book now. She looked at one verse after another.

Even as I have sworn that the waters of Noah shall no more cover the earth, so have I sworn I will not rebuke thee.

She remained with the page, even when she should have put aside the volume of weekly readings and taken up the prayer book again. During her father's sermon she was lost in her own musings.

Roland led the last part of the service, in a loud, singing way. It did not take long, and when the last of the hymns was done people rose, some shaking hands with those near them and wishing one another a good Sabbath. They crowded about Ed and Lucinda with congratulations. Millicent saw both her parents flushed and smiling, each in a different way, and yet each in a way that made happiness and sadness all one. She felt that the complexity of emotion she read in their eyes would move her to tears, and she had to turn from them.

Roland had come down the step from the reading desk and was also in the midst of a crowd, smiling brightly. Millicent heard Bobby O'Shaughnessy tell him something about money under a mat—apparently Bobby had done the paper route. "You were good, you know it? I hate to admit it," Patty said. Ed came and shook his hand, and Lucinda kissed him. Grandma Annie elbowed someone aside and kissed him. Millicent went through the crowd, toward the vestibule, where the refreshments had been set up. She greeted people as she went. Howard joined her. "Hi," she said.

Seeing him reminded her of Fred Winkler. She glanced about but no longer saw him.

The long seminar table had been brought into the big vestibule, and had a heavy white cloth. It was loaded with little sandwiches, cakes, breads, brandies, whiskies, soft drinks, three kinds of smoked fish, paper plates in piles, napkins, cocktail picks. The room was already full of people, on all sides of the table, some of them loading plates or eating, and she heard a jumble of many conversations. Howard was next to her, close by the table, and he entwined his little finger with hers. She saw her Uncle Franklin offering a toast and striking glasses with someone. Then she felt a rough slap on her behind and she wheeled about, snatching her finger from Howard. Her cousin Steve grinned down at her.

She began to introduce them but she was suddenly flustered, and Howard's name fled from her completely. She put a hand to her head, shutting her eyes and beginning to redden. Howard supplied his name, smiling. She wondered what was the matter with her. She thought of making the excuse that she had gotten up too early that morning. But Howard was already chatting with Steve.

Steve hung about, and the two kept talking. She scarcely listened.

She heard Grandma Annie hoarsely praising her grandson, and she saw Roland and his friends reach the table at the far end. She nodded absently to a lady who said something polite to her. She saw her cousin Nan jostled by the crowd as she reached for a petit-four.

As soon as Steve had drifted off Howard offered to fill a plate for Millicent.

"I really don't want anything," she said.

"Well, we can't let you starve, at your brother's party," Howard said, and he began to spread herring salad onto a little slice of dark bread for her. She saw him work at it with seriousness. Even from the side he had a squareness and chunkiness, as though he had no neck. His clothes fitted immaculately, she noticed, and his tie was knotted just so. The room was very warm, and the crowdedness made it close. He gave her the bread and she thanked him.

He did another, and stood beside her eating.

"I was up awfully early this morning," she said. "I think I'll go home and lie down as soon as I can."

"Would you like to sneak out of the crowd?" he asked. "Come on. We'll go somewhere."

"No," she said. "Thank you. I couldn't."

"Shall I run you home?"

"No. I'll just go along with the family. You understand, don't you? It's a long time since I've seen them so happy. And I'm tired, and I just want to be with my relatives for a while. It's sort of a special day. You call me in a few days."

"Okay," he said. "I'll call you in a day or two."

"It was awfully nice of you to drop by, Howard."

"I wouldn't have missed it. Well, I'll congratulate your brother on that remarkable performance then, and I'll go along."

"Good-bye," she said.

She saw him make his way through the mob. She backed away from the table, to a corner of the room that was less crowded. She saw Howard take some more food, and say something to Roland, who glanced distractedly from some other conversation. The doors were standing open to the summer brightness, and she saw Howard go out. Windows were open near her, giving some breeze, but she turned to open one wider. It stuck. She gave it up. When she looked about she saw Fred Winkler over by another corner. He had a lounging, almost supercilious stance. The blue eyes were fixed on her, at once languid and bright, and he was smiling the way he always had, one eyebrow rising. He nodded, and straightened somewhat. I ought to say hello to him, she thought.

They made their way to each other, along the wall. He was holding a little glass of something. His collar was wrinkled with the heat.

"Hello," she said.

"Hello."

"What are you doing here?" she asked.

"Well, I knew you'd be here. I phoned the Herzlingers."

"Oh. Are the Herzlingers here?"

"No. They couldn't make it."

"Oh," she said.

"It's too bad. They missed a splendid performance."

"Yes. He was good, wasn't he."

"Fantastic."

"When did you get back?"

"Yesterday."

"Yesterday?"

"Yesterday morning. In New York. By ship."

There was a silence between them. He did not seem to mind it but she did. "Did you climb the Matterhorn?" she asked. Her voice had begun quavering.

"A lesser peak." He named it, but it was unfamiliar to her.

"Oh. Was it beautiful?"

"Yes."

"How long were you away, altogether?"

He told her. She wondered what to ask next.

"I brought back a car," he said. "Come on out and see it. I drove up in it last night, from New York."

She was uncertain what to answer.

"Come on," he said. "It's warm here. It'll get us out of the crowd for a minute."

"Well, for a minute, if it's very nearby."

He gave a slight nod and began to find a path for her, squeezing as politely as possible between people's backs and around people, but it was slow, as there were many for her to smile at and exchange a few words with along the way. But as often as she did so he kept his distance, and she did not have to introduce him.

He had somehow gotten rid of his glass, and she followed him behind some people standing on the steps down into the sunlight. They crossed the grass in the speckled shade, and then went alongside the building and around the back of the parking lot, where spots of chromium gleamed blindingly. He led her to the sidewalk of Sumner Street. There were parked cars here too, in a line under shade trees. The houses were older here and closer together than on Muckanaug Street, and despite a certain seediness their side porches and gables gave them some stateliness. They walked up the sidewalk. There were many parked cars, but no people.

"And what did you do all summer?" he asked.

"Well, I still have my job, you know."

He stopped at a car so small she had not seen it behind the others. It had seats for only two, open to the air, and it was brilliant red, though its design seemed charmingly old-fashioned. The brown leathery seats, side by side with a gear-shift rising between them, seemed very low, scarcely above the street, and leaned back, as though invisible occupants had been jolted by a powerful sudden start. The low doors added to the openness, and the whole car looked to her like a low-cut shoe. The dash was full of meters.

"It's a darling little car," she said. "Does it really go?"

"Of course. Thirty-three miles to the gallon. It's noisy though. It sounds like an airplane."

"Where did you get it?"

"Switzerland. But the car's English."

"And did you drive it all around in Europe?"

"That's right."

She saw the strange foreign license plate, long and black with silver lettering.

"Why did you try to get me a job as a governess in Europe?" she asked.

"Why not?"

"But you hardly know me. I mean, what made you think of me?"

"Well, that's just it. I'd like to get to know you."

"Why?"

"I'll tell you when I know you."

"You wouldn't have gotten to know me anyway. You'd have been in Switzerland and I'd be traveling with that professor's family."

"I'd have run down to Venice. Paris, wherever you were."

"Then you wouldn't have climbed your alp."

"It would keep."

"I wouldn't have wanted to keep you from doing that. It's what you went for."

"No, I mean it. One thing I'd rather have done is spend time with you and get to know you. What little I know of you I like, so I want to know more. I've climbed before. And it can be a lonely thing. The more beautiful the lonelier."

She felt herself color a little at the ears. She thought of telling him he was mad, but it did not seem polite.

"You'd have met girls in the mountains," she said.

"Being with a woman can be lonesome too."

"It's nice talk, but you wouldn't have wanted to help me shepherd children around museums. Not with all Europe at your feet."

"Well, we'd have broken up if we didn't like it."

"You'd have gone off to the European fleshpots that young men are so fond of."

"I've been to the fleshpots already. And so what? There are other things involved."

Her fingers were touching the square windshield.

"My brother would have loved this car," she said. "The one that died, I mean."

"Get in."

"No, really, I couldn't."

"I mean it. It's a perfect day. We'll go down the Cape."

She made an annoyed little sigh and took her hand from the metal.

"Why not?" he said.

"Because it's ridiculous. It's impossible."

"Because it's too far? We'll be back when you say."

"Because I couldn't go today, for one thing. It's a special day, after all."

"Well, come with me, and it'll be even more special."

"You're a lunatic," she told him.

But she realized as she said it that it was tactically wrong. Her willingness to take the liberty of name-calling had in fact a sound of closeness.

"I couldn't anyway," she explained. "I've already turned down one invitation today. I told somebody I was spending the day with my family."

"You mean the one that was with you at the table? My competition?"

"I beg your pardon." She felt a wave of color at the ears again.

"Make it up to Artie another time."

"His name isn't Artie."

"What is it?"

"Howard."

"Well, you changed your mind. When you told him you were spending it with your family you thought you were."

"I don't do things like that."

"Well, I'm sorry. I didn't mean to be offensive. It was just a suggestion."

"It's ridiculous. We don't even know each other."

"I know. But I'd been intending to call you, and I thought, well, here we are."

She was looking at the car.

"All right, I'll phone you later," he said.

She glanced up at him. He was still looking at her. But his expression had sobered. He looked gentle, and serious. She fingered the deep curve of the door, to avoid looking at him.

"On the other hand, why wait till later," he said.

"I'm not going to the beach," she told him. "I can't walk in on my family to get a bathing suit and then walk right out again."

"We don't have to go to the beach. We could take a ride, and look around, and have dinner, and catch some summer theater, maybe."

She didn't answer.

"Or we don't even have to be out that long," he said. "We can just take a little spin. For an hour. Whatever you say."

She glanced back down the street, toward the corner. There was no one about.

"I don't even know you," she said.

"That can be remedied."

She sighed, with a little shake of her head, and fingered the car again. It had an old-fashioned fender.

"How fast can this thing go?" she asked him without turning.

"I'll stay within speed limit."

Her palm was resting on the red metal. The sun had warmed it.

"Okay," she said.